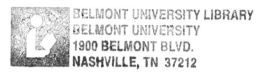

D1609641

Traumatic Brain Injury
Rehabilitation

Traumatic Brain Injury
Rehabilitation

Edited by

Mark J. Ashley
Centre for Neuro Skills
Bakersfield, California

David K. Krych
Centre for Neuro Skills
Irving, Texas

CRC Press
Boca Raton   London   New York   Washington, D.C.

Library of Congress Cataloging-in-Publication Data

Traumatic brain injury rehabilitation / edited by Mark J. Ashley and
   David K. Krych.
         p.   cm.
      Includes bibliographical references and index.
      ISBN 0-8493-9463-5 (alk. paper)
      1. Brain damage--Patients--Rehabilitation. I. Ashley, Mark J.
   II. Krych, David K.
      [DNLM: 1. Brain Injuries--rehabilitation. 2. Brain Injuries-
   -physiopathology. 3. Brain Injuries--complications. 4. Cognition
   Disorders--physiopathology. 5. Cognition Disorders--rehabilitation.
   WL 354 T7779 1995]
   RC387.5.T74 1995
   617.4'81044—dc20
   DNLM/DLC
   for Library of Congress   95-7284
                                                                              CIP

© 1995 by CRC Press LLC

No claim to original U.S. Government works
International Standard Book Number 0-8493-9463-5
Library of Congress Card Number 95-7284
Printed in the United States of America   3 4 5 6 7 8 9 0
Printed on acid-free paper

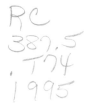

FOREWORD

The first question to be asked on seeing yet another book on traumatic brain injury is, "Why another book?" After all, there are now many books on TBI, and a newcomer has to offer something particularly enticing to make it worth reading. So, what is there in this book that makes it worth reading?

Happily, the book is a very well thought out combination of relevant neuroscience theory, medical practice, rehabilitation practice, and case management. In fact, any non-TBI specialist wanting a high quality introduction to current concerns and current rehabilitation practice will find it in this text.

The book begins with an outstanding chapter on assessment. Many chapters on assessment have been written already, but this one (by the two Editors of the book) addresses the issue of "Field Evaluation" in which an examiner has to make an appraisal of a potential client outside of the clinic or office and often in a hospital, rehabilitation facility, or the client's home. Many professionals have to do this, and many are anxious about their ability to do a thorough professional job. Clearly, this issue is becoming a major concern, with a major European research initiative devoted to the development of a generic TBI evaluation model, and the concerns dealt with in that initiative[1] are well illustrated in this chapter, which is a model of comprehensive clarity.

From field evaluation, the book progresses to more neurological and medical issues, including issues rarely dealt with comprehensively and rarely dealt with in the same volume. For example, problems of visual function (Ronald Morton, M.D.) and visual rehabilitation (Penelope Suter, O.D., F.C.O.V.D.), vestibular function (Peter Roland, M.D. and Erik Otto, R.P.T.), and epilepsy (Dean Naritoku, M.D. and Theresa Hernandez, Ph.D.) can all have very significant impacts on the TBI person's ability to function in daily life, as can heterotropic ossification, also dealt with in this section by Douglas Garland, M.D., yet such problems are often missed, misdiagnosed, or mismanaged. These five chapters, together with the chapter on the neurologic examination (David Gelber, M.D.), contain excellent summaries of current clinical practice and best practice in diagnosis, assessment, and treatment.

A recurring theme in the book is the link between laboratory findings, theory, and clinical rehabilitation practice. In fact, much rehabilitation is carried out in a theoretical vacuum, resulting in much inefficiency and reduced clinical effectiveness. Two chapters deal specifically with the link between theory and practice. The first is on neurotransmitters (Ronald Browning, Ph.D.), and the second is on the neurophysiology of learning (Robert Lehr, Ph.D.). It is obvious that the Editors had some concerns about introducing the topic of neurotransmitters, as there is an Editors' Note (really an apologia) at the beginning, and an Editors' Summarizing Note (a further apologia) at the end of the chapter. In fact, the chapter is excellent. It gives a clear and simple overview of neural transmission, deals with the main known and putative transmitters, and clearly puts the laboratory work into a clinical perspective. This chapter is a gem. The chapter on learning contains a clear exposition of the fundamentals of rehabilitation using low level functional skills as building blocks for higher level conceptual activity. This is written in the context of simple learning, but could serve as a general model of neurorehabilitation.

After dealing with basic assessment, medical, and neuroscience matters, the book moves to more clearly clinical chapters beginning with another gem — the chapter on applied behaviour analysis by Craig Persel, B.A. and Chris Persel. This topic is often superficially presented and ill digested. It can have an alluring air of simplicity making rehabilitation staff feel that they are all experts in applied behaviour analysis — a route to unprofessional, unethical, and ineffective clinical practice. The authors take a highly ethical approach to this topic, identifying a wide range of possible interventions, stating quite clearly the principal of minimal aversiveness, and stressing the need for meticulous operationalising of treatment components and meticulous recording of behaviour. Three further rehabilitation chapters follow — one on cognition, language, and communication (John Muma, Ph.D. and William Harn, Ph.D.), one on diagnosis and treatment of cognitive disorders (written by the Editors), and one on the management of residual physical deficits (Velda Bryan, P.T.). The first of these presents a model of communication, and in so doing, identifies and challenges other models. The authors are keen to deal with the issue of functional communication and to criticise naïve and simplistic approaches to assessment and treatment, particularly those that rely on a modular view of the organisation of cognition. All well and good until one remembers the invaluable insights gained from intensive neuropsychological studies of patients with specific agnosias, demonstrating very clearly a hierarchical and modular organisation of cognition. The Editors give a broad and practical model of cognitive processing, showing clearly how this can guide rehabilitation practice, and Bryan gives an excellent, thorough, and practical account of the presentation, diagnosis, assessment, and treatment of a wide range of physical problems post TBI.

The book finishes with two excellent chapters — the first on vocational rehabilitation (Joe Ninomiya, M.A., CRC, Mark Ashley, M.S., CCC-SLP, CCM, Michael Raney, B.A., CIRS, and David Krych, M.S., CCC-SLP, CCM), and the second on case management by Jan Wood, CRC, CIRS, CCM. The vocational rehabilitation chapter gives a good account of the different models of vocational rehabilitation, a sensible account of real life practical issues (should a client be blamed for not wishing to return to work, when the return may be financially disadvantageous?), and an excellent account of vocational rehabilitation planning. The case management chapter is worth its weight in gold, if only for the wonderful check list of issues to consider in assessing a facility prior to referring a patient. As a non-American practitioner, I was a little disappointed that this chapter dealt exclusively with American concerns, but that is a small point. I would also have liked a (brief) discussion of accreditation of facilities, although appreciate that this issue was implicit in the facility check list.

So, back to the question raised at the beginning. Why this book? The Editors tell us that its purpose is "...to provide the reader with a reference tool for use in developing and implementing treatment approaches in TBI rehabilitation...". This it does succinctly, informatively, and excellently. A pleasure to read.

References

¹   Truelle, J.-L., Brooks, D.N., Potagas, C., and Joseph, P.-A., A European chart for evaluation of patients with traumatic brain injury, in *Brain Injury and Neuropsychological Rehabilitation: International Perspectives;* Christensen, A.-L. and Uzzell, B.P. (Eds.), Lawrence Erlbaum, New Jersey, 1994, chap. 19.

Neil Brooks, Ph.D.
Director, Case Management Services
President, European Brain Injury Society
Edinburgh, Scotland

PREFACE

In the late 1970's, a specialty field emerged in rehabilitation focusing on survivors of traumatic brain injury (TBI). It was recognized, largely by private concerns who were financially liable for the considerable costs of care associated with survivors of traumatic brain injury, that rehabilitation strategies available in most rehabilitation centers were not adequate to address the long-term residual deficits observed following TBI. People who survived TBI were faced with debilitating physical, communicative, cognitive, social, and emotional impairments. Their medical condition was complicated by the fact that the brain, the organ of behavior, was so poorly understood and much of our knowledge about pharmacological intervention was derived from interventions with substantially different populations. Mechanisms of injury were not clearly understood, the neurophysiological substrates to learning and memory were ill-defined, and the overall physiology of the brain was, for the most part, vague.

Yet, despite significant shortcomings in our knowledge of such matters, families and professionals alike were faced with the real question of how best to help those persons who had sustained TBI. Professionals applied techniques developed for other neurologically compromised populations in an effort to deal with seemingly similar signs and symptoms but those interventions met with relatively poor success. The sequelae of traumatic brain injury proved to be far more complicated and resistant to treatment techniques of the day. The disabilities arising from TBI were far more extensive than any seen with more commonly observed strokes or other conditions and the persons affected were, on average, much younger and more numerous.

Pervasive disabilities translated to complicated long-term care requirements, often far more expensive to provide for than most people could afford. In fact, private insurers were instrumental in the push to develop more effective means for reduction of disability so as to reduce long-term cost of care.

As the effort to identify specific treatment approaches to the TBI population began, it was commonly held that neurological recovery was restricted to a relatively short period of time following injury of approximately six months. Slowly, this time period extended to twelve months, and eventually it became necessary to differentiate neurological recovery from "social" recovery. "Social" recovery would come to encompass recovery of physical, communicative, cognitive, and emotional functions after the natural course of neurological recovery had been completed.

Early treatment approaches were guided by historical perspectives of specific techniques used with other populations. As such, specific treatment approaches to TBI rehabilitation developed from observation of both the successes and limitations of adapted treatments. Demand increased for treatment facilities specializing in treating persons surviving TBI as persons needing rehabilitative services increased in number and research efforts focused almost exclusively on emergency and acute medical treatment techniques. Rehabilitation treatments were implemented essentially on an educated, trial-and-error basis.

Today, information is available from which to develop rationales upon which to base rehabilitation treatments and techniques. Not only do we have knowledge gained from experiences of the last 15 to 20 years, but science has also made tremendous gains in the study of neuroanatomy, neurophysiology, and neuropharmacology. Similar advances have occurred in medical technologies associated with acute medical treatment. We now need to review available resources to bring together this information in a useable format, together with information from other fields which will impact the rehabilitation of persons who have sustained TBI.

The purpose of this text is to provide the reader with a reference tool for use in developing and implementing treatment approaches in TBI rehabilitation. The subjects chosen were those subjects which have been neglected or have been dealt with sparingly in the literature to date.

The subjects represent areas of interest wherein diagnosis and treatment are frequently poorly guided by available training and can be gained largely by experiential means only. The hope is that this text will shorten the learning curve of its readers in many of the areas addressed.

This text is not intended to review the advances of emergency and acute medical management of the traumatically brain-injured patient as these subjects have been dealt with by other authors. Instead, the focus for this text is rehabilitation of relatively persistent sequelae associated with TBI. The text has been organized to provide the reader with relevant literature reviews which form a basis of support or "construct validity" for the diagnostic and/or treatment approaches presented. The text provides pragmatic treatment information as well as important information which can be used to define a philosophical orientation to rehabilitation in TBI and development of refined treatment approaches therein.

Chapter Descriptions

1. **"An Overview of Traumatic Brain Injury Rehabilitation: The Field Evaluation"** — The chapter on field evaluation is particularly novel. Patients are often evaluated for potential admission to a facility by staff who travel to the patient. Many times, training for this important work is minimal. This chapter strives to provide a framework from which the evaluator can attempt to collect information which will address most areas of deficit, providing valuable orienting information for a treatment staff who may become involved with the patient. Additionally, the chapter emphasizes the comprehensive overview of the patient's condition which should underscore not only diagnosis but treatment as well.

2. **"The Neurologic Examination of the Traumatically Brain-Injured Patient"** — This chapter provides valuable information pertaining to the neurological examination addressing the traumatically brain-injured patient. Since such patients rarely have small, discrete lesions, the examination must focus on numerous areas which are not often evaluated in a more abbreviated examination. The chapter alerts the practicing neurologist to the range of frequently observed deficits, discusses their identification and treatment, and discusses the role of allied health professionals in the management of these cases. This chapter serves another important role in that it describes the facets of the neurological examination for the non-neurologist. Since this field is made up of almost equally represented allied health, medical, and case management professionals, the portrayal of the neurologist's role is particularly valuable for the non-neurologist team member. Finally, the chapter serves the important role of cautioning all readers regarding the all too frequent assumption that all problems observed are a direct result of the original trauma rather than an ongoing, as yet undiagnosed complication such as posttraumatic epilepsy, hydrocephalus, degenerative neurological condition, or iatrogenic complication.

3. **"Posttraumatic Epilepsy and Neurorehabilitation"** — This chapter is a natural follow-up to the chapter on neurological examination. As with much in the field of traumatic brain injury, information has been gleaned from associated areas. We are in our infancy, however, in understanding the role and nature of posttraumatic epilepsy. Many conditions are inappropriately attributed to seizure conditions with still another group of seizure-related problems being treated psychiatrically or behaviorally without success. Pharmacological management of seizures is dependent upon a thorough understanding of the nature of the seizure condition itself. This chapter addresses epidemiology, description, diagnosis, and treatment of posttraumatic epileptic conditions. It offers insights into physiological, behavioral, and psychiatric manifestations of posttraumatic epilepsies. This information is crucial to

all treating professionals in that the diagnosis of posttraumatic epilepsy is often begun through clinical and behavioral observation. The case manager and allied health professional, together with the physiatrist, psychiatrist, psychologist, and neurologist must all be able to provide information as to what occurs during "apparent episodes" as well as what changes occur following initiation of a treatment protocol. Diagnostic and pharmacologic procedures are discussed in detail.

4. **"Neurotransmitters and Pharmacology"** — In keeping with the medically-oriented beginnings of the text, this chapter follows well. The chapter is complex and thorough in its treatment of the subject matter. It is intended to serve as a reference tool for the prescribing physiatrist, neurologist, neurosurgeon, and/or psychiatrist. The information offers insights for allied health professionals as to the neuropsychological consequences associated with pharmacological management of behavioral, attention, arousal, motor, or psychiatric conditions observed in the TBI population. The chapter is intended to provide the prescribing physician with an armamentarium of rationale for sound implementation of pharmacological management rather than the all too often utilized approach of intuitive prescription of medications based upon suggested usages derived from alternative populations.

5. **"Heterotopic Ossification in Traumatic Brain Injury"** — Early on in the development of this field, heterotopic ossification (HO) became known as a frustrating clinical entity. As HO formed, the logical solution was surgical resection; however, regrowth was more frequently observed than not. Dr. Garland has researched and published extensively in this area. The chapter is designed to educate the reader as to variables which impact incidence, review prevalence, and discuss diagnosis and treatment protocols. As managed care takes hold in the U.S., clinicians will need to recognize the appropriate management of this condition and the financial benefits to same. This chapter will be important to the physiatrist, orthopedist, physical therapist, occupational therapist, and case manager.

6. **"Vestibular Dysfunction After Traumatic Brain Injury: Evaluation and Management"** — Vestibular dysfunction following traumatic brain injury represents a frequently overlooked and under-diagnosed sequela. This clinical problem can be seen in a vast array of patients regardless of the severity of brain injury. The symptoms associated with vestibular dysfunction can mimic many other problems including those associated with psychiatric, emotional, visual, and perceptual disorders. The chapter begins with a review of literature and moves on to provide a review of the basic anatomical and physiological underpinnings of the vestibular system. A review of signs and symptoms associated with vestibular dysfunction is provided, together with extensive information about clinical evaluative and laboratory diagnostic procedures. Therapeutic and pharmacologic treatment procedures for vestibular rehabilitation are reviewed in detail, with relative application strengths and weaknesses discussed. This chapter provides valuable information for the physiatrist, otolaryngologist, neurologist, psychiatrist, neuropsychologist, physical therapist, occupational therapist, and case manager.

7. **"Visual Dysfunction Following Traumatic Brain Injury"** — This chapter begins with an extensive review of the anatomy of the eye and the neuroanatomical substrates to visual and visual motor dysfunction. Considerable emphasis is placed on lesion localization. Therapeutic intervention options such as lens design and manipulation, visual motor therapies, visual perceptual therapies, and surgery are discussed. Rehabilitation of the visual motor and visual perceptual system is emphasized.

8. **"Rehabilitation and Management of Visual Dysfunction Following Traumatic Brain Injury"** — This chapter provides for a thorough review of both the evaluative and treatment aspects of visual motor and visual perceptual disturbances to complete the text's address of visual system sequelae to TBI. The chapter provides a review of the physical substrates of vision together with the prevalence of visual dysfunction in the TBI population. A model is provided for organization of visual rehabilitation. Sensory input or reception, perception or integration, and motor output or behavior are discussed separately and as they relate to one another. Useful case studies are incorporated for the reader's consideration.

9. **"Neurophysiological Substrates of Learning"** — This chapter addresses the neurophysiological mechanisms which are active during learning. The chapter attempts to introduce the information to the non-neuroscientist for the purpose of developing an understanding of the interplay between therapy, learning, pharmacology, and neuronal anatomy and physiology. The chapter provides for a transition from the "hard sciences" of the early chapters to the "soft sciences" of the therapeutically-oriented chapters which follow. Correlations are drawn between issues of sensitization and habituation and behavioral schemas associated with learning. These are later approached in detail in the chapter on behavior modification. In its final pages, the chapter provides insights into the importance of neurodevelopmental issues as they relate to design and implementation of therapeutic plans. This chapter is excellent for physiatry, neurology, psychiatry, psychology, social work, physical therapy, occupational therapy, speech/language pathology, educational therapists, special educators, and case management professionals.

10. **"The Use of Applied Behavior Analysis in Traumatic Brain Injury Rehabilitation"** — This chapter is written to illustrate and simplify the concepts, techniques, and uses of applied behavior analysis with the TBI population. Disordered behavior is a common correlate to TBI and management options consist of pharmacology and behavior modification. As a process, behavior modification is not well understood by medical and allied health professionals. It is frequently observed to have been attempted, though with little to no success. This chapter provides information necessary to understand principles of behavior modification and to successfully implement behavioral programs. It provides information to allow integration of pharmacological and behavioral approaches. This chapter will serve as an invaluable reference tool for program directors, allied health professionals, physiatrists, neuropsychologists, and psychiatrists. Case managers will be able to critically evaluate the sophistication of behavioral programs as they consider their efficacy and the need for further intervention. Useful forms for program implementation are provided as well as a concise group of tables which allow for easy conceptualization of behavioral programming prior to and during program design.

11. **"Cognition, Language, Communication: Some Challenging Issues"** — This chapter addresses the relationships existing between language and cognition. It provides a review of literature hallmarking the existence of ties between language, cognition, and communication. The chapter is provided to encourage treaters to understand the incredible wealth of information available about the cognitive systems through use and review of language systems. Language can be used as a diagnostic and therapeutic modality for cognitive rehabilitation interventions. The chapter is of particular interest to neuropsychologists, speech/language pathologists, educational therapists, special educators, physiatrists, and neurologists. The chapter also serves as an introduction to the chapter on cognitive disorders which follows.

12. **"Cognitive Disorders: Diagnosis and Treatment in the TBI Patient"** — This chapter provides a review of neuroanatomical substrates to basic cognitive functions. The chapter focuses on frequently impaired cognitive skills and does not elaborate on diagnostically labeled deficits, but rather on functionally interrelated processes amenable to therapeutic intervention. It provides theoretical constructs for an approach to cognitive rehabilitation which is remediative in nature versus compensatory. The chapter provides information encouraging the view of cognition as a process rather than an entity and provides useful insight into the relationships between attention, perceptual feature identification, categorization, and cognitive distance skills. The chapter gives a detailed treatment approach for cognitive rehabilitative efforts. The chapter will be of interest to educational therapists, special educators, speech/language pathologists, cognitive rehabilitation therapists, and neuropsychologists. Case managers will find that the chapter provides insights into how cognitive rehabilitation can be viewed, measured, and monitored.

13. **"Management of Residual Physical Deficits"** — This chapter provides for an historical overview of the development of effective physical therapy interventions for the traumatically brain-injured patient. A focus is placed on developmental issues with a review of diagnostic categories often seen in TBI. The chapter emphasizes aggressive rehabilitative efforts designed to approach normalization of function as opposed to compensation for dysfunction. This chapter is of primary interest to physiatry, neurology, physical and occupational therapy, and exercise physiology. It provides useful information for the case manager as well.

14. **"Vocational Rehabilitation"** — This chapter deals with application of vocational rehabilitation practice to the brain-injured patient. The chapter reviews prevocational counseling and preparation. It deals extensively with identification of prerequisites to initiation of vocational rehabilitation services. Specifics of vocational testing, work evaluation, and vocational rehabilitation planning and execution are discussed. An appendix is provided reviewing tests utilized and recommended. This chapter will be of appeal to vocational rehabilitation counselors, case managers, physiatrists, neurologists, and psychologists.

15. **"Case Management of Brain Injury: An Overview"** — The field of case management is in its comparative infancy. This chapter is designed to provide information to the new as well as experienced case manager about program evaluation for TBI patients. The chapter reviews various payer types and their respective priorities. Information is imparted about funding sources, overview of the brain-injured patient's care from injury through recovery, and facility/program evaluation criteria. The role of the case manager is discussed as it pertains to the patient, family, funding source, and facility staff. This chapter will be of primary interest to case managers, physiatrists, program directors, and allied health professionals interested in understanding the role of case management in TBI.

Mark J. Ashley
David K. Krych

THE EDITORS

Mark J. Ashley, M.S., CCC-SLP, CCM, is Co-Founder and Executive Director of the Centre for Neuro Skills (CNS), which provides post-acute brain injury rehabilitation programs at their facilities in Bakersfield, California, and Irving, Texas. Mr. Ashley resides in Bakersfield, heading that program, while his Co-Executive Director, David Krych, supervises the daily operations in Irving. In addition to his responsibilities with CNS, Mr. Ashley serves on the Board of Directors of the Western Institute of Rehabilitation and serves as its Executive Director. He also serves on the Board of Directors for the Association for Community Integrated Neuro Rehabilitation.

Mr. Ashley received his Masters Degree in Speech Pathology from Southern Illinois University in Carbondale, Illinois. He is an Adjunct Professor for the University's Department of Communication Disorders and Sciences, specializing in brain injury and cognitive deficits. Mr. Ashley is a licensed Speech/Language Pathologist in California and Texas and is also a Certified Case Manager.

Mr. Ashley has specialized in head injury rehabilitation since 1978 and is recognized by his peers as an expert in the field. He has lectured at more than 100 national and international professional education activities to promote and refine therapeutic endeavors for the traumatically brain injured.

Mr. Ashley is a member of numerous professional associations including the American Speech, Language and Hearing Association; the American Academy of Clinical Neurophysiology; the American Congress of Rehabilitation Medicine; the California Speech and Hearing Association; the National Association for Independent Living; the National Association of Rehabilitation Professionals in the Private Sector; the National Head Injury Foundation; the National Rehabilitation Association; the National Rehabilitation Administration Association; and the Texas Speech and Hearing Association. Mr. Ashley is also co-recipient with Mr. Krych of the Southern Illinois University Distinguished Alumni Award for 1995.

This volume is Mr. Ashley's second book. The first was *Behavior Analysis: Applications for Traumatic Brain Injury Rehabilitation.* In addition to his books, Mr. Ashley has been published in numerous research publications in articles and case studies dealing with neurological rehabilitation, neuroembryological development, and rehabilitative outcomes. Mr. Ashley's current research interests include post-acute TBI (traumatic brain injury) efficacy and long-term outcomes.

Previous publications co-authored with Mr. Krych include Changes in Reimbursement Climate: Relationship Between Outcome, Cost, and Payor Type in the Post-Acute Rehabilitation Environment appearing in the *Journal of Head Trauma Rehabilitation;* Cost/Benefit Analysis for Post-Acute Rehabilitation of the Traumatically Brain Injured Patient appearing in the *Journal of Insurance Medicine;* and Considerations in the Purchase of Post-Acute Rehabilitative Services for the Head Injured also appearing in the *Journal of Insurance Medicine.*

David K. Krych, M.S., CCC-SLP, CCM, is Co-Founder and Executive Director of the Centre for Neuro Skills, residing in Irving, Texas.

He graduated from Southern Illinois University at Carbondale with a Masters Degree in Speech Pathology. He is currently an Adjunct Professor for the Department of Communication Disorders and Sciences at Southern Illinois University, specializing in brain injury and cognitive deficits. Mr. Krych is a licensed Speech/Language Pathologist in the states of Texas, California, and Florida. He is also a Certified Case Manager.

Mr. Krych is a member of the American Speech, Language and Hearing Association; the International Affairs Association; the American Congress of Rehabilitation Medicine (ACRM); the American Subacute Care Association; the California Speech and Hearing Association; the National Association for Independent Living; the National Association of Rehabilitation Professionals in the Private Sector; the National Head Injury Foundation; the National Rehabilitation Association; the Texas Speech and Hearing Association; the Florida Speech and Hearing Association; the California Speech and Hearing Association; the Texas Head Injury Association; and the Vestibular Disorders Association.

Awards and honors include National Distinguished Service Registry of Rehabilitation Professionals, 1988–1989; Blue Ribbon Faculty at the International Brain Injury Symposium: Advances in Clinical Practice, 1991; and 1994 recipient of the American Speech, Language and Hearing Association's Award for Continuing Education (ACE).

This is Mr. Krych's second book. The first was *Behavior Analysis: Application for Traumatic Brain Injury Rehabilitation*, co-authored with Mr. Ashley. In addition, Mr. Krych is the Editor of *Inside View,* a publication of the Centre for Neuro Skills. He is also the Treasurer for the Brain Injury Interdisciplinary Special Interest Group of the ACRM, and the Editor of its newsletter, *Moving Ahead.* He is also past chair of the Post-Acute Guidelines Committee of the Brain Injury Interdisciplinary Special Interest Group of the ACRM. Mr. Krych was recently named a member of the 1994 Southern Illinois University Foundation's President's Council. He is also co-recipient with Mr. Ashley of the Southern Illinois University Distinguished Alumni Award for 1995.

Mr. Krych's current research interests include verifying outcome data and functional outcome statistics.

CONTRIBUTORS

Mark J. Ashley, M.S., CCC-SLP, CCM
Centre for Neuro Skills
Bakersfield, California

Ronald A. Browning, Ph.D.
Departments of Physiology and Pharmacology
Southern Illinois University School of
  Medicine
Carbondale, Illinois

Velda L. Bryan, P.T.
Centre for Neuro Skills
Bakersfield, California

Douglas E. Garland, M.D.
Central Nervous System Division
Department of Surgery
Rancho Los Amigos Medical Center
Downey, California
and
Department of Orthopedics
University of Southern California
Los Angeles, California

David A. Gelber, M.D.
Department of Neurology
Southern Illinois University School of
  Medicine
Traumatic Brain Injury Rehabilitation
  Program
Memorial Medical Center
Springfield, Illinois

William E. Harn, Ph.D.
Speech and Hearing Sciences
Texas Tech University
Lubbock, Texas

Theresa D. Hernandez, Ph.D.
Department of Psychology
University of Colorado
Boulder, Colorado

David K. Krych, M.S., CCC-SLP, CCM
Centre for Neuro Skills
Irving, Texas

Robert P. Lehr, Jr., Ph.D.
Department of Anatomy
Southern Illinois University School of
  Medicine
Carbondale, Illinois

Ronald L. Morton, M.D.
Bakersfield, California

John R. Muma, Ph.D.
Speech Pathology and Audiology
University of Alberta
Edmonton, Alberta, Canada

Dean K. Naritoku, M.D.
Departments of Neurology and Pharmacology
Center for Epilepsy
Southern Illinois University School of
  Medicine
Springfield, Illinois

Joe Ninomiya, Jr., M.A., CRC
Centre for Neuro Skills
Bakersfield, California

Erik Otto, PT
Oldenzaal, Netherlands

Chris H. Persel
Centre for Neuro Skills
Bakersfield, California

Craig S. Persel, B.A.
Centre for Neuro Skills
Bakersfield, California

Michael L. Raney, B.A., CIRS
Centre for Neuro Skills
Bakersfield, California

Peter S. Roland, M.D.
Department of Otolaryngology
The University of Texas
Southwestern Medical Center
Dallas, Texas

Penelope S. Suter, O.D., F.C.O.V.D.
Vision Laboratory
Department of Psychology
California State University, Bakersfield
Bakersfield, California

Jan Wood, CRC, CIRS, CCM
State Compensation Insurance Fund
Monterey Park, California

ACKNOWLEDGMENT

The Editors would like to express their gratitude to Nancy Payne for her assistance in the preparation of this manuscript. Her attention to detail was of considerable assistance.

TABLE OF CONTENTS

1

An Overview of Traumatic Brain Injury Rehabilitation: The Field Evaluation

David K. Krych and Mark J. Ashley

CONTENTS

INTRODUCTION

Not only does this first chapter act as an overview of issues associated with traumatic brain injury (TBI) in general, it is also meant to be a structured look at the comprehensive data collection process needed prior to initiation of in-depth diagnostics and therapeutics. Collection of such information is crucial to development of an appropriately targeted diagnostic and therapeutic rehabilitation plan for minor and severe TBI. Yet, the clinical world whirls at a pace that often disallows such a deliberate consideration of numerous factors which, when pondered, can serve to sharpen the approach to be undertaken in planning diagnostics and therapeutics alike. Persistent and pervasive deficits such as those produced by TBI act independently of one another and interact with one another to produce a very complicated clinical picture.

Persons sustaining traumatic brain injury come to the injury with other significant life experience, most or all of which will need careful deliberation to determine the degree to which those life experiences will impact a rehabilitative process. This chapter provides an

1

overview of a system of data collection which has proven beneficial in design of clinical diagnostic and treatment programs with maximum efficiency and reasonable completeness. The information presented should be viewed as preliminary to the in-depth and more comprehensive and accountable diagnostic efforts to be undertaken by individual therapists following admission. The treatment team will obviously find it necessary to collect more complete diagnostic information prior to initiating a treatment program.

The field evaluation — the initial evaluation of the TBI individual — should be reflective of the range of therapeutic possibilities available for rehabilitation. Assessment of the individual for his/her individual strengths and weaknesses in the professional domains of physical therapy, occupational therapy, speech pathology, cognition, counseling, vocational rehabilitation, and, of course, medical condition, is essential for successful rehabilitation. A thorough field evaluation will point to the most productive areas of rehabilitation.

The advent of numerous facilities and differing program concepts for the treatment of individuals with brain injuries, together with ever-increasing emphasis on community reintegration, has increased the need for effective field evaluations. Whether a patient's program is accomplished as part of an "inpatient" scenario in a traditional transitional living facility, or is focused on the home environment, a definitive understanding of the clinical and medical needs of the individual to be served is of paramount importance. The field evaluation must go beyond a mere determination of whether the individual falls within the spectrum of given admission criteria. Rather, the evaluation process should be objective, as well as descriptive and prescriptive, in nature.

The field evaluation must take into consideration the environmental circumstance of the person being evaluated as well as the nature of the referral questions. This includes such questions as, "Why is the evaluation being done?" "Who has requested the evaluation?" "What is the expected outcome of the evaluation process?" and "What are the environmental influences which impact the patient on a regular basis and/or can be expected to influence the patient following any rehabilitation effort?" For example, an evaluation being requested by a workers' compensation carrier for the purpose of enrolling a patient in a vocational rehabilitation program would answer questions of a fairly narrow scope. An evaluation performed at the request of a family member for the purpose of determining whether the person in question could be managed at home — for example, under family supervision with an outpatient treatment component — would be much broader in nature. The evaluator, therefore, must have a very clear picture of the nature of the evaluation questions, and the system used to gather information must be flexible, yet comprehensive enough to address all questions posed.

Information regarding medical, therapeutic, family, social, academic, and vocational history is not likely to be complete in the medical record. To that end, the evaluator will need to conduct a professional interview of the patient, family, friends, employer, fellow workers, and treaters. The most effective interview will be conducted by the evaluator who has extensive knowledge in any of the areas in question. This is a vital component of the entire evaluation process and should not be underestimated.[1] The would-be field evaluator, then, would be well-advised to review professional interview techniques and develop good skills in this venue.

The most important thing for the field evaluator to keep in mind throughout the entire review process is that he/she may be the first person to closely review the medical record in its entirety. The medical history and current medical circumstance have important relationships to the ongoing process of rehabilitation and the future options for care/treatment. The responsibility, therefore, is not simply to represent the best interests of a facility but to represent the best interests of the patient in an advocacy fashion and to recognize a role in quality control. The field evaluator must be a mixture of facility representative, patient advocate, and payer auditor.

This is a tall order to fill. Individuals with experience in nursing and allied health professions are in a good position to fit all three roles. Individuals of a business background with an emphasis in marketing are ill-prepared to take on the significant responsibility of objective reporting and making recommendations that will potentially affect an individual's future. The role of the field evaluator is broad in its scope, technical in its focus, and not to be underestimated in its complexity.

PRE-EVALUATION PREPARATION

It is always useful, regardless of the evaluation question, to have access to current information and previous medical history. Basic information, such as name, birthdate, date of injury, age, and insurance or case management contact person are necessary bits of information. Likewise, less obvious information, such as social security number, appropriate claim numbers referring to respective insurance carriers or other agencies, maiden name, and determination of whether legal counsel is involved, as well as the legal status of the person, are equally basic matters, though they are sometimes difficult to ascertain. The pre-evaluation time frame can, therefore, be utilized to ferret out this less obvious information.

Analysis of records prior to the actual field evaluation provides ample time to define potential conflicts in the records and clarify these issues. Frequently, discrepancy between age and actual birth date can be found in records as well as more critical issues such as coma duration, length of posttraumatic amnesia, and important information concerning the injury itself and the circumstances leading up to it. Conflict in the medical records, however, may not always be apparent in the absence of careful review.

It is not uncommon for potentially serious implications concerning mechanism of injury to be hidden by a medical diagnosis given in the absence of a description of accident circumstances. An individual being considered for admission to a pain program, diagnosed as suffering from "whiplash" and also suffering from vague complaints of nausea and blurred vision, yields one image for the evaluator. Knowing that the individual's car was hit in the rear by an 18-wheel truck going 35 miles an hour, while the individual's Volkswagen stood still at a stoplight, yields a much different understanding of the nature of the injury. Therefore, information concerning the nature of the incident leading to injury and the condition of the individual at the scene and at the time of emergency room intervention could be quite meaningful.

Similarly, serious errors can be avoided by conducting a thorough review of medical records. Laboratory and radiologic records, together with surgical and consultative reports, should be reviewed in their entirety rather than by reviewing only diagnostic impressions or recommendations. A great deal of relevant information can be found in such reports, sometimes uncovering subtle inaccuracies in historical information reporting as well as revealing the basis for a particular specialist's opinions and conclusions. The necessity for review of medical records prior to seeing a patient cannot be overstated. It should be understood, however, that a lack of complete medical records cannot necessarily delay the evaluation in the real-world setting. Every attempt should be made to collect complete medical records for review, preferably either before or during the evaluation or, if necessary, immediately following the evaluation.

A history of multiple hospital admissions may be important and should be reported thoroughly. Reporting all hospital and facility stays in chronological order, with admission and discharge status as well as discussion of medical events occurring during the stay at each facility, lends valuable depth to understanding an individual's current needs. A good understanding of available therapeutic treatment techniques and their relative effectiveness is crucial to developing a meaningful rationale and justification for future care and treatment. Prognostication of outcome and expected treatment duration can be derived more readily with a thorough understanding of treatment interventions which have preceded the field evaluation.

Discharge dates should be reported along with a thorough description of medication trials and secondary medical issues that might have an impact on rehabilitation potential or that might become problematic in the future. For example, the development of diabetes insipidus or the existence of a prediagnosed hydrocephalus could cause difficulties in later stages of rehabilitation. Likewise, a patient with a history of phlebitis or cardiac problems may need a significantly altered approach to be taken in postacute rehabilitation, particularly from a physical restoration standpoint.

Unfortunately, there is a tendency for field evaluators to underestimate the need to review medical issues and describe the full scenario of previous medical and rehabilitation treatments. There is the perspective that, once the patient is ready for transfer from one treatment setting to another, review of basic-level medical concerns relating to earlier stages of recovery is no longer important. Indeed, in some situations, the field evaluation has become nothing more than a quick glance at a patient and a marketing effort with the family and professional staff who are involved in making decisions about the patient's discharge. This is unfortunate because it allows important issues to slip by and not be taken into consideration in the continuing rehabilitation effort. When a field evaluation is nothing more than another marketing call, the best interests of the family and patient cannot be served, nor can the best interests of the field of rehabilitation, as a whole, be served. If the evaluation process becomes an opportunity for the marketing representative to make promises on behalf of his facility in order to secure another patient, a gross breech of ethics has occurred.[2]

There is really no substitute for a complete and accurate review of the individual's medical and rehabilitative history. This is not to suggest that current medical status is any less important. This is simply to state that current medical status is better understood in perspective with prior medical history.

CURRENT MEDICAL STATUS

Current medical status includes issues such as bowel and bladder concerns, dietary and nutritional needs and habits as well as data concerning height, weight, and allergies. It is also appropriate to review behavioral health matters such as current or premorbid substance abuse as well as whether the individual is now, or was previously, a smoker. Sleep-wake cycles, frequency of naps, and quality of sleep are important to document as well as any familial medical history of significance.

Dental status is a frequently overlooked area of medical review. Individuals who have suffered trauma to the head often have associated broken or malaligned teeth. Furthermore, medication, such as Dilantin, can cause hyperplasia of the gums[3] and subsequent oral hygiene difficulties. If oral hygiene is problematic, special attention will need to be paid to activities of daily living associated with tooth brushing and dietary concerns. An individual who exhibits tactile defensiveness to oral stimulation may be reacting to gums or teeth which are painful.

A full review of current medications and a summary of nursing notes is, in the least, required. It is sometimes difficult to define, chronologically, the distinction between medical "history" and current medical issues. The important differentiation for the field evaluator is the basic delineation of medical issues which have been resolved (history) and the medical issues which may continue to require attention in future rehabilitation efforts (current medical status).

AUDIOMETRY/VISION

Audiometry and vision are two medically associated areas requiring attention in the evaluative process. First of all, being aware of whether hearing and vision have been formally tested, and by whom, is important. From a diagnostic standpoint, one should determine whether evoked-potential studies have been performed. Some indication of the severity of the blow to the head may be suggested if blood was viewed either behind the tympanic membrane or in the external auditory meatus. A blow of significant force to the temporal region may also alert the reviewer to the possibility of vestibular dysfunction, tympanic membrane rupture, or ossicular chain disarticulation and subsequent deficits in hearing and/or balance.[4,5] This knowledge should lead the examiner to evaluate lacrimation and salivation and to determine any differentiated damage to distributions of cranial nerve VII.[6,7] The seventh cranial nerve is particularly susceptible to damage in traumatic head injury due to the manner in which the nerve exits the skull.[7] If vestibular testing or tympanometry has not been performed, the alert evaluator may be in a position to recommend these informative tests, either prior to admission to the postacute environment or soon after. Further discussion of potential vestibular dysfunction is found in later sections of this chapter and in Chapter 6 of this volume.

Audiometry

Audiometric evaluation is rarely performed in the acute stage of hospitalization. If the patient has not been specifically evaluated by audiometry, observation can lead to important preliminary conclusions. Observe the patient's reaction to conversational speech and whether the individual localizes to environmental sound appropriately. Determine whether the person exhibits an abnormal auditory startle reaction to lend insight into the status of hearing. Orienting by turning the head left, regardless of where the source of sound is, may indicate that there is a hearing loss of some type on the right. Likewise, observation of an auditory startle reaction in an adult, adolescent, or an older child may suggest the individual is unable to effectively filter auditory information or might be hypersensitive to sound.

There are several behaviors that would suggest a deficit in an individual's hearing status. An individual who constantly turns his head to one side with a given ear toward the speaker, intently watches the lips of the speaker, continually asks for repetitions, or looks from one speaker to another as if trying to determine who is speaking is obviously having some difficulty. Failure to appreciate "finger rub" can signal hearing loss and assist in localization of side of loss.

Two issues that too often go undescribed are a history of hearing loss and identification of an individual who has worked in a noisy environment all his life, such as construction workers, auto mechanics, individuals with a long history of military service (being near gunfire or explosive concussions), factory workers, sport shooters, etc. Such individuals are likely to have sustained noise-induced sensorineural hearing loss as a result.[4,5] The evaluator should review prescription and nonprescription drug history for potential ototoxicity as well.[5]

Tinnitus can be described by patients as whistling, buzzing, or just as "noises in my head". A carefully taken history can lead to investigation of vestibular end-organ states, temporal bone integrity, and behavioral habits, such as caffeine intake or noise exposure, all of which can impact tinnitus. The evaluator should determine how severe the tinnitus is and whether it is constant or variable. If tinnitus is described as variable, the patient's appraisal of the variability may be helpful in further diagnostic undertakings.

Vision

There are several fairly obvious issues which are necessary to delineate with regard to vision as a whole. First of all, it is important to determine whether prescriptive lenses were worn prior to or after injury as well as whether the person being evaluated has any visual complaints. Comparing the patient's complaints of any visual problems with formal ophthalmological examination findings can sometimes be very revealing. Often, although the ophthalmologic evaluation determines no gross abnormalities and may even yield a determination that the patient has 20/20 vision, the individual may still complain of "acuity" problems. Careful observation and further questioning can sometimes reveal that the visual problem is actually a manifestation of vestibular, oculomotor, or ocular alignment deficits. These may result in difficulties with depth perception, visual figure-ground difficulties, diplopia, and problems with reading, visual scanning, and visual tracking.[8,9] Determining the precise nature of the visual deficit is typically beyond the purview of the field evaluation. Important information can be brought back to the team concerning these potential issues, however.

There are several easy field activities which can yield important diagnostic information concerning visual integrity. Evaluating visual fields to confrontation is easy and requires no invasive process. If the patient is able to follow some simple directions, instruct the individual to focus on the evaluator's nose. Move a pencil from the patient's ear forward, first on one side and then the other, and ask the patient to indicate when the pencil appears (without moving the eyes from the fixed focal point and maintaining the head position in neutral) to obtain gross determination of temporal visual fields. Next, while the patient covers one eye, bring the pencil into view from behind the patient's ear on the same side as the covered eye to obtain a gross understanding of nasal field integrity for the uncovered eye. Performing the same activity superiorly from the forehead out and from the chin out can give information about the upper and lower quadrants of vision. Obviously, this technique does not replace the diagnostic value of visual field testing that might be performed in the ophthalmologist's office; however, it can at least give a gross measure and point the way for the possible need for more in-depth testing.

Observing the individual in activity can yield information concerning visual field integrity, e.g., seeing the person eating only half of a portion of food that is presented can indicate that part of the visual field is not seen. Also, an individual consistently bumping into the left door jamb when passing from one room to another can indicate that he is not seeing the door jamb due to a visual field defect or a visual field neglect.

Observing how the individual tracks people in the environment or how the person tracks a pencil going through a visual field are two ways of gaining information about ocular motility. The evaluator is looking for the eyes to follow in "smooth pursuit" without obvious jumps or jerks. If it is observed that the object has stopped moving and the individual's eyes have continued to track, this "overshooting" phenomenon may be indicative of vestibular dysfunction.[10,11] Both eyes should track at the same rate and with continued focus. Deviation of one eye from the focal plane can cause blurred vision as well as a distinct double image. If divergence, as opposed to convergence, is noted in ocular alignment, either during tracking or at rest, the person may complain of blurred vision or of double vision. If not, the visual image from one eye may be suppressed cortically or there may be reduced or absent vision in the diverged eye. Information regarding such phenomena can sometimes be gleaned from further review of medical records (preferably a neuro-ophthalmology examination). If no information is discovered concerning this observation, this certainly raises a major area for further diagnostic investigation.

From a perceptual standpoint, it is appropriate to determine how well an individual can render a three-dimensional observation into a two-dimensional representation. Have the individual draw a floor plan of the room that he is in, including windows, walls, doors, and placement of furniture. Also, have the person draw a floor plan of someplace other than the room he is currently in to reveal information about visual praxis,[12] visual imagery skills, and cognitive distance.[13] Carrying a visual perceptual measurement tool, such as the Hooper Adult Visual Organization Test*,[14] is quite feasible and is easily performed.

COGNITION

There is no better technique to determine orientation to person, place, time, and date than to simply ask the person. It is strongly recommended, however, that orientation to person not be determined by the patient being asked to remember the evaluator's name. It is more valid to give the name of someone with whom he/she is familiar.

---

* *The Hooper Adult Visual Organization Test* determines a person's ability to form concepts from pieces presented in a random field.

Determining whether attentional deficits are present is a simple process of observation. If the individual does not maintain attention to ongoing conversation or to tasks, the evaluator must consider competitive stimuli in the environment. Determining whether the individual is more susceptible to competing visual or auditory stimuli is helpful. Observation of whether the person is able to perform concentration or persistence tasks more effectively is diagnostically informative. "Concentration" refers to activities of a mental nature, while "persistence" refers to the individual's ability to continue in physical activities. People perform in different ways depending on whether tasks are physical or nonphysical in nature, essentially due to differences in cognitive distance.[15] There is an expected difference between concentration and persistence abilities, with concentration being more difficult.

Just as important as determining whether the individual can persist or concentrate is determining whether the individual can desist with an activity and change to a new task. Being able to perform one task and shift to a new task without a loss of accuracy, even for a very short period of time, is more important diagnostically than is a person's ability to attend to a single, ongoing task for a longer period of time. "Attention span", therefore, is less the issue than a description of the environment in which attention is being maintained, whether the activity is physical or mental in nature, and whether the individual is able to change efficiently from one activity to another without loss of information or accuracy.

Further observations regarding the cognitive status of the patient must be driven by the philosophy of the treating facility which, obviously, should be the same as the evaluator's. Contrary to popular belief, there is no single, universal cognitive approach. The idea of "traditional cognitive testing" is a fallacy. Depending on the training of the individual, cognition takes on different meanings. The philosophy of the authors is well described in the chapter in this volume on cognition (Chapter 12), as well as the information contained in the chapter pertaining to language and cognition (Chapter 11). With this bias in mind, the following description is indicative of the evaluative process for a program with a commensurate philosophical orientation.

The first arena to be considered is the patient's ability to readily identify features across three objects. The person is asked to deliver an assay across three objects with an example performed by the examiner, i.e., a pair of scissors may be silver in color, approximately four inches in length, weigh approximately two ounces, have an overall oblong shape, be functional at cutting paper, have rounded ends on the points, and be constructed of some kind of metal. The overall time to describe these seven features for someone without neurological damage is easily under 30 seconds. A new object is then presented to the patient (a lead pencil, a plastic tumbler, a comb, etc.). Determining whether the individual can perform this task after demonstration is important. Also, determining whether the individual requires cues for certain features and not others is revealing. Does the person orient to color, but always miss shape? The evaluator would look for a decrease in time necessary to provide the features, as well as an increase in the number of features that are given spontaneously, across the three trials. It is important to note repetitions. Does the person always come back to the object's function as opposed to giving information concerning other features?[16,17]

Have the person name three other items not currently in the room that share a single feature with Object 1, 2, or 3. This provides a good indication of the individual's cognitive functioning and provides insight into cognitive distance. Often the individual will be able to give an appropriate description of the object at hand but not be able to name other items which share common features and are not in view.

Ask the individual how given objects can be used in alternative fashions to gain some understanding of the person's ability to expand categories and deal with more cognitively distant information. Ask the individual if a chair can be used as a ladder or whether a pen can be used as a weapon, etc. If the person knows that the function can be changed even though he/she may not be able to describe the features necessary to make the change possible, the reviewer knows that there is some emergent understanding of category overlap. Look for an ability to alter the usual function of an object using one or more of its perceptual features to derive a novel use.

Create categories of several objects (up to four) and ask the individual what the items have in common. A coin, a key, and a paper clip are obviously similar in that all are made of some kind of metal. Very often, individuals will look at the group, begin to spread them out, and talk about them individually as opposed to describing them as a group. Keeping track of the individual's responses will provide insight into categorizational skills. Patients will sometimes become fixed on minute details but miss the most obvious common feature. Next, present three new objects with a fourth that does not fit to allow evaluation of categorical negation. Negation is a two-step cognitive process and is, therefore, more cognitively challenging. Observing the person's ability to shift between feature inclusion and feature exclusion, i.e., what do all the objects have in common or which object does not belong, gives considerable insight into the individual's cognitive flexibility.

It is also important to determine the individual's ability to deal with more cognitively distant concepts. An easy and fast evaluative tool is the use of proverbs such as "That's the way the cookie crumbles," "Don't cry over spilled milk," "You have the cart before the horse," "People who live in glass houses shouldn't throw stones," etc. The person's rendering of the concrete interpretation vs. the proverbial meaning of these sayings is very revealing and worth the time for presentation. Likewise, having the individual go through a multistep process to describe a given activity, such as the steps involved in changing a tire or the steps involved in baking a cake, gives the evaluator a fairly clear understanding of the ability to sequence. Iconic store mechanisms can be grossly evaluated using several 3 × 5 cards with three rows of three letters.[18] Present the card for a brief period (two to five seconds), noting the length of presentation. Following the presentation and removal of the card from sight, name a row and have the person list the letters contained in that row. Of course, the row chosen should be randomized. Keep track of the percentage of correct responses for the letters on the named line. The percentages should be in the neighborhood of 75% accuracy for a three- to five-second presentation. Likewise, a random presentation of a series of numbers can be presented auditorially. Have the person repeat the numbers in appropriate forward order and, in a separate testing, backward. Percentage of accuracy can be kept and should run in a range of six to seven numbers forward and four to five numbers backward.[19]

A very important prognostic indicator, from the standpoint of determining the likelihood of a person's ability to show improvement in cognitive areas, is whether the person is rule-governed or nonrule-governed in their learning.[17] It is very easy to get some basic insight into this area with a deck of cards. Deal the playing cards slowly into two piles in the patient's visual field and ask the person to determine the rule you are using to put a card into one pile as opposed to another. First deal the cards into red and black piles. If the person is initially unable to determine that the rule is black vs. red, some coaching or cueing may be necessary. How well or how poorly the person does with this step will determine whether it is necessary to go to the next step. Obviously, if the person is very quickly able to describe the reason for the cards being separated, then a shift is necessary. If the person does not understand the activity or has difficulty maintaining attention, there is no need to continue the activity. In the first shift, simply change red to the opposite pile and black to the previously red pile. This is called a "reversal shift".[15] Again, some coaxing and cueing may be necessary. Depending on the difficulty this shift creates for the patient, further activity may be unnecessary. Should the person be able to describe this reversal shift, evaluation of "nonreversal shift"[15] is the next step. Changing from color to number concept is suggested, i.e., odd numbers vs. even numbers or face cards vs. nonface cards. This tends to be a very difficult shift because the individual is frequently overly-focused on color.[15] This activity is a very good clinical measure of the individual's rule or nonrule governed status. Some indication of cognitive tempo (i.e., whether the person is a reflective or impulsive thinker) can also be gleaned.

Following the above activity with a more cognitively distant task gives a good indication of how well the person can shift from one activity to another. Ask the individual what he would do if he came home and found a family member lying on the floor unconscious and bleeding from a deep cut on the arm. Complications can be added as the person describes his problem-solving scenario, e.g., cannot awaken the person, the phone does not work, neighbors are not home, etc. Not only does this give good measure of problem-solving ability, it also describes some ability to establish priorities as well as provide insight into frustration tolerance.

Obviously, not every patient who is evaluated can go through the above described tasks. Determining the individual's cognitive ceiling and/or behavioral boiling point, as the case may be, is up to the evaluator. Many aspects of cognitive tempo, speed of processing, rule- vs. nonrule-governed learning, or the ability to include and exclude categories can be observed while the individual is participating in ongoing therapeutic activity or from review of therapy records. That behavior is a manifestation of cognition is not a new concept.[20] Interviews with appropriate therapists can lend insight into these arenas as well; however, there is no real substitute for spending as much time as possible with the patient. Performing some of the described activities can be invaluable to the treating staff who will be expected to pick up with this individual at the time of admission and perform additional diagnostic activities. The more the evaluator can bring the therapeutic staff into the "ballpark", the more likely it is that well-tuned and efficient evaluative procedures can follow the admission.

EDUCATION

To some (educators, in particular), cognitive skills are measured in terms of traditional academic skills. However, for the purpose of the field evaluation, it is recommended that the area of cognition be separated from academic issues. One area that is notoriously lacking in most evaluative processes is a description of the individual's academic history. Unfortunately, this information is sometimes difficult to unearth, and family members are not always the best historians with regard to describing the patient's academic history. Collecting enough information to be able to eventually obtain high school/college records is helpful. In fact, it is important, in some cases, to review elementary and junior high school records to identify premorbid behavioral and learning disorders in younger patients and their potential contribution to difficulties in the rehabilitation process.

From a life skills standpoint, several issues require attention. First of all, does the person currently, or did he before the injury, manage his own finances, including check writing, depositing, and bill paying? Determine if there has been a change in the situation or whether the person is still able to fulfill the same responsibilities as he or she did premorbidly.

On a much more basic level are issues of coin identification and making change. Determine whether the person can count a random number of objects, add and subtract concrete objects, write number symbols upon request, and count by twos, fives, and tens. If time permits, information about adding and subtracting with larger numbers and with carrying can be meaningful as well as knowing whether the individual can multiply, divide, and distinguish decimal values and whole number fractions. It may be helpful to carry a few pages of math and reading exercises of various grade level equivalents for this segment of the evaluation. Certainly, depending on the individual's premorbid vocational history, there may be greater or lesser expectation in these regards. Depending on vocational expectations after treatment, more or less emphasis may be required in this particular area from a treatment standpoint and, therefore, from the field evaluation.

Determine whether the individual can recognize random letters of the alphabet, read simple sight words, or simple sentences. Reading and writing require the same commonsense approach as described above. Is the person able to read materials such as labels, newspapers, or signs? Again, depending on the individual's premorbid history and current vocational expectations, reading comprehension tasks should be evaluated and weighed appropriately.

OCCUPATIONAL/PHYSICAL/RECREATIONAL THERAPY

The field evaluator should have some grasp of the occupational and physical therapy histories, both of an acute and postacute nature. Comparison of past history with current observation should include as much of the following information as possible. Comments regarding range of motion in all extremities, trunk rotations, and head and neck rotations are important and can often lead to the discovery of not only undiagnosed difficulties in joint mobility but, also, the possibility of vestibular dysfunction. For example, although heterotopic ossification and other joint-limiting circumstances should be investigated, it cannot be assumed that a pathology in limb mobility is the sole cause of observed range of motion restrictions. If passive and active ranges of motion throughout the body are full, but in dynamic circumstances such as climbing stairs or community ambulation the individual walks with reduced hip rotation, lack of trunk flexibility, fixed shoulder and neck, and overall lack of fluidity, consideration should be given to the possibility of vestibular hypersensitivity.[21]

Strengths in all extremities, as well as overall muscle endurance, require investigation. Strength and endurance can have direct impact on the kind of care and/or treatment a given patient can tolerate. Sensation should be tested throughout the extremities together with the degree of proprioceptive loss that the individual may be experiencing. The evaluator can glean much information from careful observation of the patient while he goes through his daily rehabilitation or living routine. Noticing that the individual must concentrate when grasping an object, that the individual is overly cautious with regard to foot placement when walking, or the existence of a wide-based gait in the absence of apparent cerebellar or motor dysfunction, may raise the suspicion of proprioceptive and/or sensory loss. Likewise, the inability to recognize common objects when presented to the hands of an individual with eyes closed (stereognosis) may indicate proprioceptive and/or sensory loss.[19] Stereognostic impairments can lead to the suggestion of impaired callosal fiber tracts.[22] These signs, together with other diagnosed apraxia, may significantly alter prognostic potentials for a given patient.

One frequently overlooked arena of impairment is the olfactory sense. It has been noted that lack of olfactory sense is a frequent sequela of even minor head injury.[23] Obviously, difficulties with the olfactory sense can cause changes in appetite and gustatory response. The olfactory sense is easily tested in the field with eyes closed and presentation of a small vial containing cloves or coffee. A history which includes a loss of appetite, difficulty in amount of meal consumption, or weight loss may increase the index of suspicion for changes in olfaction and gustatory sensation, overall.

Observations of fine vs. gross motor skills should be made. Considerable information can be gained with regard to the person's ability to manipulate objects, from a dexterity standpoint, simply by watching the person in his daily routine. It is not necessary to do peg tests or bring other standardized tests with you into the field. Likewise, gross motor activities are easily observed in an environmentally valid fashion simply by being with the patient for a period of time. If there is ongoing physical or occupational therapy activity that requires movement, observation can yield information regarding the quality of movement and many other areas. Likewise, determination of how an individual transfers from wheelchair to car, from car to wheelchair, or from bed to wheelchair does not require the evaluator to perform these activities in the field. Observation over time can provide a great deal of information for documentation.

Balance, although usually described in terms of "good" or "poor" in relation to how much assistance an individual might need in walking, is actually a multilevel task that requires careful observation and evaluation. First of all, general observations regarding posture in standing and sitting should be made. The person's ability to shift weight in standing and sitting should also be observed. If the individual is restricted to a wheelchair, sitting balance with and without support should be observed. Differentiation between trunk strength/endurance and balance should be made. Unchallenged standing balance is also easily observed. When challenging standing balance, heel-to-toe walking can be quite helpful. It is not absolutely necessary to observe one-foot standing balance; however, if the opportunity arises and this activity can be performed, be sure the individual is protected from falling and is away from sharp corners in the environment. The ability to go from standing to tall-kneeling and, eventually, to a four-point position (on hands and knees) provides a good diagnostic review of overall balance and coordination. With the individual in four-point stance, ipsilateral and reciprocal balance can be evaluated easily. Have the individual balance on left knee/left hand and then right knee/right hand for ipsilateral balance. Next, alternate right hand/left knee and left hand/right knee for reciprocal balance observation. The evaluator will need to consider any orthopedic restrictions or obvious neuromuscular impairments which may preclude a pure assessment of balance and coordination skills alone. If observations are occurring in the physical or occupational therapy gym, this task can be evaluated by simply asking the treating therapist to help you.

Comment should be made with regard to the individual's quality of gait, both at a normal and an increased pace and on smooth and uneven surfaces. If the person is observed outside the confines of the physical therapy gym, observe the differences in gait between indoor and outdoor ambulation.

Complaints of headache, nausea, dizziness, and blurred vision after activity and/or plane change can indicate vestibular dysfunction.[21] To provide further information relative to vestibular function (the evaluator should have already determined balance with eyes closed while guarding the patient against falling before performing this activity), an easy and safe activity is allowing the individual to march in place with and without vision. If the individual is able to maintain position with vision but, without vision, tends to rotate to the left or right, there is, very likely, vestibular involvement. If there is room for the individual to take five or six steps forward and backward in all directions, the activity of having the individual march in a line, with and without vision, is also informative. Any light or sound sources which could assist in maintaining spatial orientation should be neutralized prior to this test. If the individual is able to maintain straight line forward and straight line backward with eyes open but, with eyes closed, inscribes a star-shaped pattern, a vestibular dysfunction is almost a certainty.[24] Again, the evaluator should be able to consider the potential influences of orthopedic issues in this testing which might contribute to a less-than-accurate test finding. The reader is referred to Chapter 6 of this volume for a more in-depth discussion of vestibular system diagnostics.

A somewhat more difficult evaluative technique is the measure of nystagmus. This is a very good indicator of vestibular dysfunction, though, in some situations, it may be dangerous to have the person stand in place, with eyes closed, and rotate in a semirapid fashion. The idea is to then watch for a nystagmus (rapid pulsating of the eyes to left or right). If nystagmus continues for more than 30 seconds or if the individual complains of significant dizziness, headache, nausea, or blurred vision, this raises the suspicion that the vestibular system is overly sensitive to stimulation. Determining whether the nystagmus beat is quicker to left or right is not necessary, at this point, and can be better evaluated at a later date via a diagnostic tool called an electronystagmography or ENG.[24] It is more important in the field evaluation to simply determine whether the nystagmus continues for an unexpectedly long or short period of time. Remember that visual fixation can suppress nystagmus, so this procedure should not serve as a sole measure of vestibular impairment. One needs to consider that oculomotor innervation may also be impaired, making nystagmus difficult to observe. It is possible for nystagmus to be caused by a number of drugs and/or alcohol in the system, as well.

A note of caution — if evaluating an individual who is prone to seizure activity, it is recommended that vestibular testing of the nature described above not be performed in the field due to the possibility that photic stimulation could stimulate seizure activity.[25] Probably the best way to evaluate vestibular function in the field is to have the therapist, who is familiar with the patient, perform at least some of the above described activities as part of the ongoing therapeutic process. Unfortunately, the field evaluator is often faced with professional staff who do not know the importance of vestibular testing and evaluation. The evaluator, therefore, is left to his own devices in determining the degree to which vestibular dysfunction may be affecting the patient's status. Considerable caution in this regard is recommended.

As always, historical information can be quite helpful in determining any problems with the vestibular system. A history which includes falling at night, disorientation at night, use of night-lights or leaving lights on since the injury, loss of balance in the shower, fear of stairs or heights, discomfort following car rides, motion sickness, irritability following activities requiring plane changes (e.g., dressing, toileting, car riding), and so on, may be suggestive of an intolerance for normal vestibular stimulation. These complaints alone are enough to warrant documentation to allow for later in-depth investigation via a neuro-otologic evaluation.

RESIDENTIAL SKILLS/ACTIVITIES OF DAILY LIVING (ADL's)

Activities of daily living include the areas of hygiene, toileting, dressing, grooming, feeding, meal planning, meal preparation, shopping, laundry, taking of medications, telephone usage, kitchen clean-up, household security and safety, household cleaning, mail, leisure pursuits, time management, and travel planning and arrangement. An important consideration for differentiation in ADL arenas is the difference between the person's ability to perform the activity and opportunity. Also of importance is the separation of the person's ability to perform the activity from behavior that may interfere with that person's willingness to perform those activities. An individual who has severe frontal lobe injury may not be able to perform some activities of daily living which require one routine to follow another because of difficulties with persistence and initiation.[26] Furthermore, some individuals who exhibit verbal and physical aggression may not be particularly functional in their performance of activities of daily living, not because they are unable to perform the task per se, but because the behavior they are exhibiting precludes measurement of ADL skills. Determining the difference between competence and performance is the field evaluator's task.

It is, of course, important to fully characterize the individual's abilities for performance of ADL's. The evaluator should include in this description the source from which information was obtained. Information regarding the amount and the type of assistance required and the nature of any initiation observed is helpful.

Likewise, evaluation of community skills, e.g., driving, community transportation, leisure pursuits, and current social interactions, will require discussion of the environment in which the person resides as well as a description of the person's ability to establish performance in a given activity. In other words, if an individual is restricted in his comings and goings, there is no opportunity for the development of social activities and, thus, no real way to determine the person's true social capabilities. Finally, not to be left out is the arena of special needs and equipment. Making comments concerning the current or anticipated use of prosthetic and adaptive devices for accomplishment of ADL's is important.

PSYCHOSOCIAL

The psychosocial portion of the field evaluation is not only an opportunity to review neuropsychological testing and psychological status but, also, a chance to review the individual's life as a whole. Where he/she was born and raised and comments conveying the general tone of the person's life are appropriate. Military service history and religious affiliation are important. Any social history concerning involvement with the legal system should be reported.

The field evaluator cannot be expected to bring along a full array of neuropsychological testing equipment. Neuropsychological evaluations can take several days, in and of themselves, and are not the essence of the field evaluation. Too much emphasis on neuropsychological evaluation during a field examination can be detrimental to evaluating the patient as a whole. There is importance to the establishment of rapport between the evaluator and the individual being evaluated, in any given circumstance. The field evaluator is trying to glean as much information in as many areas and from as many sources as is possible and is not necessarily concerned about pinpointing specific areas of psychological concern.

Of great value is determining (in a nonthreatening manner) if the client can describe his deficits and his limitations. Determine if the individual can give examples of how the disabilities affect his personal lifestyle. Many times, the ability to self-analyze is hampered by cognitive processing problems, denial, rationalization, or level of acceptance of disability at the time of the evaluation. It is important to be nonjudgmental and to focus on general perceptions of self-concept in terms of how the person sees himself and what he is "about". It can be quite helpful to gain an understanding of the person's emotional reaction to the current disability and to the changes in lifestyle which have occurred. Does the person have any current accomplishments of which he/she is particularly proud? There may be areas of accomplishment within the therapeutic realm or within the living environment that lends to the individual's positive self-image. Is there indication that there is realignment of premorbid level of self-concept with current level of circumstance? The evaluator should attempt to gain insight into the goals the person may have for the immediate and foreseeable future. The information above will bear substantially upon not only the duration of a rehabilitation program but, also, the likelihood of success of such a program and avenues which will require further exploration and treatment to achieve a successful outcome.

Family Relations and Sexuality

An area closely aligned with self-esteem and self-concept is perception of self from a sexuality standpoint. This perception goes far beyond mere questions of performance, although these issues are certainly important to mention. Sexuality should not be confused with what the treater might describe as sexually inappropriate behavior. Unfortunately, as some individuals go through the recovery process, social confusion can lead to behaviors that are not time and place appropriate. Although it is appropriate to make comment concerning these behaviors, in no way should judgmental bias arising from social, religious, or personal convictions cloud the reviewer's perspective. It is much more important for the field evaluation process to focus on sexuality from the standpoint of specific behaviors, relationships, and intimacy. Does the individual have close relationships that are still functional and how does the person's premorbid personality match his current perception of himself? This is difficult to evaluate and it is important that the evaluator not blunder into this arena without preparation. In many cases, these matters will require further, in-depth review in later stages of treatment. Just as it is important to avoid confusion of sexually aberrant behavior with sexuality, it is important to realize that the presence of such behavior should not preclude a patient from further treatment.

Family/Social

Marital status and the names and ages of children should be recorded as well as the individual's family of origin information, i.e., his parents' names and their current relationship with the patient and siblings' names, ages, and relationship to the patient. Changes in relationships should be discussed if they are pertinent to the current circumstance.

The family's education and awareness of the problems, their roles, goals, and concerns for the patient should be reviewed. Determination of whether any family members are involved in counseling or involved directly in the therapeutic process should be made.

Family issues weigh heavily on discharge options. If this information is available, some description of how the family would like to be involved and their perceptions of the discharge process should be discussed. For example, does the family want the client returned to the home? If yes, what roles do they see themselves playing and, if not, why? Determining the role of the family at discharge during the field evaluation can aid in evaluating the appropriateness of a given individual for a particular type of rehabilitation. Understanding from the outset that the family is not going to be involved in discharge options might change the perception of appropriate settings for discharge from acute care. In this scenario, it is possible that a more long-term environment than that of a transitional living program should be sought. Determination of how the client sees the family, that is, does he see them as being supportive or obstructive to the rehabilitation process, can lend insight into potential problem areas of the family or potentially positive aspects of family involvement that may not have been considered.

Another problem that is often overlooked is conservatorship or guardianship concerns. If conservatorship or guardianship has been established, the individual's freedom to make his own choices with regard to discharge and financial matters may be significantly impacted. Furthermore, at some point in the rehabilitation process, it may become necessary to review the continued necessity for the conservatorship or guardianship that is in place over the individual. In this type of situation, the facility finds itself in an awkward position. The need to respect the conservator or guardian's wishes with regard to discharge options may be in direct conflict with the need to take an advocacy position for the patient. Going into the process aware of these dynamics can help prepare a smoother treatment process and sometimes avoid confrontations and difficult conflicts between conservator/guardian and patient, patient and facility, or conservator/guardian and facility.

Friendships should be documented. Quality and quantity of visitations or interactions can point to potential problems such as social isolation, opportunistic relationships, or to potentially beneficial discharge scenarios, i.e., placement with, or supervision by, a close family friend. If the patient has been able to maintain high quality, premorbid friendships through the ordeal of the injury and recovery, it speaks highly of the preserved and potential social skills of the individual and the quality of friendships. Friendships which are able to prevail in the face of such adversity may hold additional promise when discussions are held pertaining to discharge living or vocational scenarios. Networking with family and friends for such issues can increase the number of options available and impact the nature of the rehabilitation goals and process.

How the individual reacts in group or social settings, as well as noting overall socially appropriate behavior, is an important psychosocial issue. If there is opportunity for the client to have social interaction, how successful is this process? Did he prior to the accident, or does he continue to, belong to church or social organizations? Also, are there hobbies, clubs, or defined goals which the individual was pursuing prior to the injury and to which he continues to aspire? All too often, these social issues fall by the wayside. However, the survival of these interests and goals can point to a very positive psychosocial outcome.

Behavior

The problems that patients have with impulsive anger of a verbal or physical nature should be carefully and fully described. Discussion should include the individual's social and family behavior prior to the injury. Determine, if possible, whether the individual used or abused alcohol or other substances prior to the injury and whether he continues to do so.

Some understanding of the patient's coping mechanisms, premorbidly and currently, sets the stage for the future counseling process. If the individual shows frustration or anger, anxiety or nervousness, or guilt complexes concerning the injury, these emotional responses can complicate an already difficult treatment scenario. If the individual is experiencing depression, level of functioning is subject to misinterpretation. If the individual is very frustrated about his circumstance, the ensuing withdrawal or aggressive behavior may also be misinterpreted. Obtaining some indication of whether the individual is motivated, or able to be motivated, to improve is very important to any ongoing rehabilitation process. What needs to be kept in mind, however, is that individuals with frontal lobe or right hemisphere damage frequently appear to be "unmotivated" and "difficult" to actively engage in the rehabilitation process.[26] Reference to the Medical History section is recommended in this regard and the evaluator is warned to be cognizant of right hemisphere lesions which may impair the individual's ability to measure himself socially against a norm.[19] Likewise, frontal lobe injury can cause difficulty with an individual's apparent lack of motivation or initiation. It is very important that this be taken into consideration and that no judgmental perspective be taken with regard to the patient's motivational status. Indeed, such subjective terms (motivated, unmotivated, etc.) should be avoided in the field evaluation. Subjective labels can only hurt the ongoing evaluation/rehabilitation process.

SPEECH/LANGUAGE PATHOLOGY

Although the speech pathologist may share some responsibilities in the areas of cognition and education with others from their allied health professional team, there are several other traditional areas for consideration in the role of the speech/language pathologist. First is the area of oral motor apraxia and dysarthria. There is no substitute for a thorough oral peripheral examination. The oral peripheral examination may not be fully performed while in the field; however, familiarity with the process is of considerable importance. Again, as in previous sections of this chapter, it is suggested that considerable insight can be gained into this arena through observation and discussion with current treating therapists. If the individual is not in an ongoing therapeutic endeavor, a greater degree of familiarity with speech/language issues may be necessary. Careful observation, however, can reveal much in the passage of a few hours' time.

An example of an oral peripheral examination is available in Figure 1.1. The purpose of the oral peripheral examination is to review the structures and functions of the speech mechanism and is limited mainly to the production of speech — that is, intelligibility (how easily is speech understood?) and articulation of speech (how well are individual speech sounds made?).

The evaluator must determine if impairments of voice are present. This includes a review of volume, breath support, and clarity of voice. The evaluator should be familiar with hypernasal voice in order to be able to make comment regarding velopharyngeal integrity.[27] Evaluate whether intonation changes are utilized in speech production. Such intonational or prosodic changes can substantially alter communicative intent and, as such, are critical to the success of social commerce (interaction with other human beings).[28]

The fluency of speech is another area for observation. It is important not to confuse fluency with intelligibility. An individual may actually use neologisms (words that are either phonetically or linguistically incorrect) but the production of speech may continue to be fluent.[29] The question to ask is, "Does speech move smoothly from one utterance to another or is it broken, halting, or full of stops and starts and/or broken words?" It is important to remember that the field evaluator is not trying to determine the etiology of the problem. He/she is simply making an observation of how fluent or dysfluent the person is.

From the standpoint of language, there are several rather helpful observations that the field evaluator can make. First of all, establish some sense of how the patient uses language. Is it used mainly for aggressive or threatening statements or is it used to fulfill personal needs? Is it used effectively? If the person cannot communicate effectively using oral means, is he/she able to communicate through some combination of graphic skills or gestures? Also, observing whether the individual initiates communicative acts with familiar people and unfamiliar people alike is important. It should be kept in mind that, while the person may have difficulty with anomia (word finding difficulties), paraphasias (words that are incorrectly used or words that have speech sounds substituted such as "chair" for "table" or "sable" for "table") or neologisms (words that have no particular meaning),[30] the attempt to communicate is important

ORAL PERIPHERAL EXAMINATION

Facial Symmetry

Rest:	Normal_____	Rt. Droop_____	Lt. Droop_____
Smile:	Normal_____	Rt. Weak_____	Lt. Weak_____
Labial Strength:	Normal_____	Weak_____	
Pucker:	Normal_____	Weak_____	

Facial Sensation: 1 (V)_____   2 (V)_____   3 (V)_____

Mandible

Rest Position:	Normal_____	Low_____	
Jaw Extension:	Normal_____	Right_____	Left_____
Jaw Lateralization:	Normal_____	Rt. Absent_____	Lt. Absent_____
Resistive Closure:	Normal_____	Weak R_____	Weak L_____

Tongue

Rest:	Normal_____	Rt. Atrophy_____	Lt. Atrophy_____
Tremor:	Absent_____	Present_____	
Protrusion:	Normal_____	Rt. Dev._____	Lt. Dev._____
Fasciculations:	Absent_____	Present_____	
Protrusion Strength:	Normal_____	Weak_____	
Elevation:	Normal_____	Weak_____	
Lateralization:(in cheek)	Normal_____	Rt. Weak_____	Lt. Weak_____

Diadochokinetics:	Normal_____	Depressed_____
Oral Mucosa:	Normal_____	
Lesion(s)	Describe:_____	
Mass	Describe:_____	

Velopharyngeal Mechanism

Rest:	Normal_____	Rt. Droop_____	Lt. Droop_____
Clefts:	Absent_____	Present_____	
Ah:	Normal_____	Rt. Droop_____	Lt. Droop_____
Hypernasality:	Yes_____	No_____	
Gag:	Absent_____	Present_____	
Swallowing:	Normal_____	Impaired_____	Absent_____

Has there been fluoroscopy?_____
Results:_____
_____

FIGURE 1.1   Oral peripheral examination.

in and of itself. Furthermore, the effectiveness of communication is not always dependent upon the quality of speech or language. The determination of the existence of aphasia or other language problems is really not a question that must be answered by field evaluation. It is better to get a global view of the individual's ability to involve himself in social commerce than to determine if there is a component of Broca's or Wernicke's aphasia per se.

VOCATION

The vocational history section of the field evaluation is, depending upon the referral question, either more or less important to the overall evaluation. Obviously, if the field evaluation is being done to determine the vocational potential of an individual, the importance of this section cannot be overstated. On the other hand, if evaluating an individual coming from a hospital environment in the early stages of rehabilitation and before a clear pattern of recovery has been defined, the importance of the vocational section takes on more of a psychosocial tone than one of potential return to work.

If appropriate, some chronological history of vocational endeavors since high school is suggested. Also, a listing of the states that the individual has worked in, some idea of wages earned, and a description of job positions, as well as a listing of companies and company locations, is suggested. It is recommended that some indication be obtained of positive and negative aspects, from the patient's perspective, concerning the jobs that he/she has held. Identifying what job(s) the individual enjoyed most and the reasons can be helpful. This is true not only from a purely vocational standpoint but also from a psychosocial perspective. It is appropriate to determine, in a general way, what the client sees himself doing vocationally in the future. How does this observation or perception weigh against future hopes and goals or against practical realities imposed by physical or cognitive disabilities? A subjective measurement on the reviewer's part with regard to the degree to which the patient's future hopes are based in reality is appropriate. The evaluator should consider the potential for psychological, emotional, financial, and/or legal incentives and disincentives for return to work which may impact the rehabilitative effort.

In all likelihood, a field evaluation will not be complete enough to make definitive comment about return-to-work scenarios. Indeed, all too often, the field evaluator appears to be under some pressure from payer sources to make comment about return-to-work potential. It is strongly recommended that such comments not be made in lieu of a more complete vocational evaluation, which is beyond the purview of the field evaluation.

IMPRESSIONS AND RECOMMENDATIONS

In this day and age of rapid communication, fax machines, and conference calls, all too often the body of the evaluation is left to molder in a file while the Impressions and Recommendations section of the report is read. While the Impressions and Recommendations section of the report is based upon the knowledge and information contained in the body of the field evaluation, the reader may be left without a full appreciation of the patient's circumstance when only the Impressions and Recommendations section of the report is considered. However, field evaluators must live with the realities of the environment in which they work and, therefore, must recognize that, in all likelihood, the Impressions and Recommendations section will need to stand on its own. The Impressions and Recommendations section must pull all the components of the evaluation together in a cohesive fashion and bring the reader to a set of reasonable conclusions.

The Impressions and Recommendations section must also connect the observations of the field evaluator with a broader rehabilitation perspective. It is, therefore, suggested that some form of broadly accepted rating system be used in association with the findings in the Impressions and Recommendations section. Such a scale may be the Disability Rating Scale,[31] as shown in Figure 1.2, or some other scale familiar to the field evaluator. In this way, a more broadly defined "level of disability" can be associated with the more descriptive findings reported in the field evaluation. This practice provides a common reference point for multiple treaters from a disability measurement perspective.

Appropriate attention must be paid in the initial portion of the Impressions and Recommendations section to ensure that the referral question is clearly answered. If the referral question had to do with the appropriateness of the candidate for postacute rehabilitation, reference to this question is mandatory. If the individual is found to be an appropriate candidate, a general statement of how this conclusion was derived is appropriate. If not, any appropriate alternatives should be provided with a rationale about why they may be more appropriate. Also, in association with the referral question, what is the potential treatment scenario, and its anticipated outcome, that is being recommended by the evaluator? It is not enough for the evaluator to answer the referral question, "Is this individual an appropriate candidate for postacute rehabilitation?", without describing how that determination was made and how the proposed treatment process will positively influence the outcome of the case.

DISABILITY RATING (DR) SCALE•

Name _____ Sex _____ Birthdate _____ Brain Injury Date _____

Cause of Injury: _____ MVA/MCA*   _____ Head Trauma**   _____ Infection   _____ Stroke   _____ Anoxia

_____ Developmental (Congenital)   _____ Degenerative   _____ Metabolic   _____ Drowning

_____ Other (Specify) _____

*MVA = Motor Vehicle Accident; MCA = Motorcycle Accident. *Circle one.*

**Gun shot, blunt instrument, blow to head, fall, etc.

DATE OF RATING

CATEGORY	ITEM▲							
Arousability	Eye Opening[1]							
Awareness and	Communication Ability[2]†							
Responsivity••	Motor Response[3]							
Cognitive Ability for	Feeding[4]							
Self Care	Toileting[4]							
Activities	Grooming[4]							
Dependence on Others•••	Level of Functioning[5]							
Psychosocial Adaptability	"Employability"[6]							

COMMENTS: **Total**

[1]Eye Opening

0	Spontaneous
1	To Speech
2	To Pain
3	None

[2]Communication Ability†
Either Verbal; Writing or Letter Board;
or Sign (viz. eye blink, head nod, etc.)

0	Oriented
1	Confused
2	Inappropriate
3	Incomprehensible
4	None

[3]Best Motor Resp.

0	Obeying
1	Localizing
2	Withdrawing
3	Flexing
4	Extending
5	None

[4]Cognitive Ability for Feeding,
Toileting, Grooming (Does patient
know how and when? Ignore motor disability.)

0	Complete
1	Partial
2	Minimal
3	None

†In presence of tracheostomy (place T next to score); for voice or speech dysfunction (place D next to score if there is dysarthria, dysphonia, voice paralysis, aphasia, apraxia, etc.)

[5]Level of Functioning
(Consider both physical &
cognitive disability)

0	Completely independent	
1	Independent in special environment	
2	Mildly dependent	- (a)
3	Moderately dependent	- (b)
4	Markedly dependent	- (c)
5	Totally dependent	- (d)

[6]"Employability"
(As a full time worker,
homemaker or student)

0	Not restricted
1	Selected jobs, competitive
2	Sheltered workshop, non-competitive
3	Not employable

Disability Categories

Total DR Score	Level of Disability
0	None
1	Mild
2-3	Partial
4-6	Moderate
7-11	Moderately severe
12-16	Severe
17-21	Extremely severe
22-24	Vegetative state
25-29	Extreme vegetative state
30	Death

a needs limited assistance (non-resident helper)
b needs moderate assistance (person in home)
c needs assistance with all major activities
**   at all times**
d 24-hour nursing care required

▲ See over for item definitions
Revised 8/87

•Rappaport et al. Disability Rating Scale for Severe Head Trauma Patients: Coma To Community. Arch Phys Med Rehab. 63:118-123, 1982
••Modified from Teasdale, Jennett, Lancet 2:81-83, 1974
•••Modified from Scranton et al. Arch Phys Med Rehab. 51:1-21, 1970

FIGURE 1.2 Disability rating scale. (Reprinted with permission from Rappaport, M., Hall, K., Hopkins, K., Belleza, T., and Cope, D. (1982). Disability rating scale for severe head trauma: Coma to community. *Arch. Phys. Med. Rehabil.*, 63, 118–123.)

The field evaluator must show support for his/her determination, in this regard, by describing potentially positive factors which might influence outcome (uncomplicated medication regimen, lack of seizure disorder, the patient's positive attitude toward his circumstance, a positive family situation, realistic vocational/educational expectations, etc.). There may also be deficits or issues influencing outcome that will make the goals of rehabilitation difficult to achieve. These must also be delineated in succinct form (premorbid personality issues, i.e., substance abuse, poor medical status, unsuccessful vocational ventures, etc.).

Specific recommendations for care/treatment programming must be addressed to clearly define deficits and influencing factors that will become germane as the postevaluation period unfolds. Following are several examples of recommendations addressing a variety of hypothetical concerns and their potential management in the postacute arena:

1. Currently, this individual is taking 2 mg of Haldol BID, plus 2 mg of Haldol, HS, PO. Review of this medication regimen in conjunction with any potential behavioral management approach will be important.
2. As is mentioned in the Audiology section of this report, there is some indication of hearing loss, both of a historical nature and also associated with the current temporal skull fracture. Audiological evaluation is recommended after this individual has established and maintained behavioral control to the point where he can participate appropriately in the evaluative process.
3. There have been vague complaints of visual acuity problems. As is the case with hearing status concern, visual evaluation is recommended when participation in evaluative procedures is tolerated.
4. Behavior management strategies will be imposed with attention to environmental validity, rhythm of living, and overall structure on a day-to-day basis. Furthermore, initiation of routine activities of daily living expectations will be a part of the ongoing behavioral management process. Withdrawal of attention to verbal aggression will be initiated.
5. Cognitive work with this individual is required regarding his difficulty with cognitive distance. Furthermore, important areas of concern are issues of categorization, both inclusion and exclusion as it relates to iconic features, as well as emergently rule-governed behavior.
6. As improvements have been noted in visual acuity, reading and simple math activities are felt to be appropriate, at this time, from a survival skills standpoint, i.e. reading signs, making change, reading warning labels, etc.
7. Occupational therapy will focus mainly on activity of daily living issues. In a less restricted environment, more information can be gleaned regarding this individual's ability to care for himself and to manage his personal environment. Work in the area of visual praxis is recommended.
8. Physical therapy issues include balance and gait concerns as well as overall endurance and strength issues. A neurodevelopmental program to address gross motor planning may assist in developing muscle balance and coordination.
9. As part of the ongoing postacute process, it is recommended that more opportunity for social interaction be accomplished. It is understood that this individual was an active Rotarian prior to his injury as well as an active member of the Lutheran Church. Establishing liaisons with these two groups is felt to be of primary importance.
10. It will be important, from a psychosocial standpoint, to develop a counseling approach with this individual that will help him deal with adjustment to disability, self-concept, and personal pride issues. Adjustment to disability is particularly important, considering the right frontal temporal lesions, as well as the bifrontal lesions which will likely make it very difficult for him to identify his own deficits and perceive his own difficulties in relationship to the social circumstance that he finds himself in. A concrete approach to orientation will be required.
11. Speech pathology activities will focus mainly on cognitive deficits reported above (see Recommendation 5), but will also address mild-moderate dysarthria. Strengthening of oral structure, tongue and lips in particular, should increase intelligibility of speech significantly.
12. It is also suggested that a vocational component be added to the ongoing therapeutic perspective due to the fact that this individual has so much of his self-worth tied up in his past vocational prowess. Although vocational and prevocational issues are felt to be very important at this point in time, it is difficult, if not impossible, to make projections regarding the ultimate vocational outcome at this time. Evaluation of vocational potential would be an ongoing process, hopefully, leading to a full vocational evaluation and appropriate vocational recommendations.

Indeed, each section of the field evaluation should be separately reviewed, its essence translated into recommendations for programming, and listed clearly in order that the reader (reviewing the report only from the Impressions and Recommendation section) is, figuratively, brought up to speed by the evaluator's conclusions.

Appropriate discussion of projection of time frame for the recommended treatment process is important. Payers, as well as the patient and his/her family, need to have predictable time frames. Vague recommendations with regard to program time frames can lead to unnecessarily long rehabilitation stays in transitional facilities and also increase the length of interventions from outpatient and community and home scenarios. Obviously, the field evaluator is not able to make exact length-of-stay determinations solely on the basis of the initial evaluation; however, some indication of time frame, with recommendations for appropriate review after admission, is imperative.

Finally, closing remarks should serve to bring together any remaining loose ends. Reiteration of communication links between evaluator and referral source are appropriately made at this time. Future communication processes between payer and potential treaters should also be set out at this time. A reminder concerning the role of the field evaluator may also be appropriate as well as a recapping of particularly difficult or special areas of concern regarding the patient, the evaluative process, or the essence of the recommendations being made.

REFERENCES

1. Emerick, L. L. and Hatten, J. T., *Diagnosis and Evaluation in Speech Pathology*, Prentice-Hall, Inc., Englewood Cliffs, NJ, 1974.
2. McMahon, B. T. and Shaw, L. R., *Work Worth Doing: Advances in Brain Injury Rehabilitation*, PMD Press, Orlando, FL, 1991.
3. *Physicians' Desk Reference*, Medical Economics Data, Montvale, NJ, 1993, 1762.
4. Martin, F. N., *Introduction to Audiology*, Prentice-Hall, Inc., Englewood Cliffs, NJ, 1975, 286.
5. Goodhill, V. and Guggenheim, P., Pathology, diagnosis, and therapy of deafness, in *Handbook of Speech Pathology and Audiology*, Travis, L. E., Ed., Prentice-Hall, Inc., Englewood Cliffs, NJ, 1971, 279.
6. Willis, W. D., Jr., and Grossman, R. G., *Medical Neurobiology*, 2nd edition, C. V. Mosby Company, St. Louis, MO, 1977.
7. Smith, C. H. and Beck, R. W., Facial nerve, in *Biomedical Foundations of Ophthalmology*, Volume 1, Tasman, W. and Jaeger, E. A., Eds., J. B. Lippincott Company, Philadelphia, 1992.
8. Bouska, M. J., Kauffman, N. A. and Marcus, S. E., Disorders of the visual perceptual system, in *Neurological Rehabilitation*, 2nd edition, Umphred, D. A., Ed., C. V. Mosby Company, St. Louis, MO, 1990.
9. Lepore, F. E., The neuro-ophthalmologic case history: Elucidating the symptoms, in *Duane's Clinical Ophthalmology*, Volume 2, Tasman, W. and Jaeger, E. A., Eds., J. B. Lippincott Company, Philadelphia, 1992.
10. Farber, S. and Zoltan, B., Visual-vestibular systems interaction: Therapeutic implications, *J. Head Trauma Rehabil.*, 4, 9, 1989.
11. Goodwin, J. A., Eye signs in neurologic diagnosis, in Weiner, W. J. and Goetz, C. G., Eds., *Neurology for the Non-Neurologist*, 2nd edition, J. B. Lippincott Company, Philadelphia, 1989.
12. Fisher, A., Murray, E. and Bundy, A., *Sensory Integration: Theory and Practice*, F. A. Davis Company, Philadelphia, 1991.
13. Muma, J. R., *Language Acquisition: A Functionalistic Perspective*, Pro-Ed, Austin, TX, 1986.
14. Hooper, H. E., *Hooper Visual Organization Test (VOT) Manual*, Western Neuropsychological Services, Los Angeles, 1958, revised 1983.
15. Muma, J. R., *Language Handbook: Concepts, Assessment, Intervention*, Prentice-Hall, Inc., Englewood Cliffs, NJ, 1978.
16. McCarthy, J. and Kirk, S., *Illinois Test of Psycholinguistic Abilities — Examiner's Manual*, Revised edition, University of Illinois Press, Urbana, IL, 1968.
17. Muma, J. R. and Muma, D., *Muma Assessment Program — MAP*, Natural Child Publishing Company, Lubbock, TX, 1979.
18. Anderson, J. R., *Cognitive Psychology and Its Implications*, W. H. Freeman & Company, San Francisco, 1980.
19. Lezak, M. D., *Neuropsychological Assessment*, Oxford University Press, New York, 1976.

20. Mann, L. and Sabatino, D. A., *Foundations of Cognitive Process in Remedial and Special Education*, Aspen Publishers, Rockville, MD, 1985.
21. Pender, D. J., *Practical Otology*, J. B. Lippincott Company, Philadelphia, 1992.
22. Guyton, A. C., *Basic Neuroscience*, 2nd edition, W. B. Saunders Company, Philadelphia, 1991.
23. Jennett, B. and Teasdale, G., *Management of Head Injuries*, F. A. Davis Company, Philadelphia, 1981, 273.
24. Mumenthaler, M., *Neurology*, Thieme Medical Publishers, Inc., New York, 1990.
25. Vogt, G., Miller, M. and Esluer, M., *Mosby's Manual of Neurological Care*, C. V. Mosby Company, St. Louis, MO, 1985.
26. Levin, H. S., Grafman, J. and Eisenberg, H., *Neurobehavioral Recovery from Head Injury*, Oxford University Press, New York, 1987.
27. Boone, D. R., *The Voice and Voice Therapy*, 2nd edition, Prentice-Hall, Inc., Englewood Cliffs, NJ, 1977.
28. Moncur, J. P. and Brackett, I. P., *Modifying Vocal Behavior*, Harper & Row, New York, 1974.
29. Clark, H. and Clark, E., *Psychology and Language*, Harcourt, Brace, Jovanovich, Inc., New York, 1977.
30. Goodglass, H. and Kaplan, E., *The Assessment of Aphasia and Related Disorders*, Lea & Febiger, Philadelphia, 1972.
31. Rappaport, M., Hall, K., Hopkins, K., Belleza, T. and Cope, D., Disability rating scale for severe head trauma: Coma to community, *Arch. Phys. Med. Rehabil.*, 63, 118,1982.

2

The Neurologic Examination of the Traumatically Brain-Injured Patient

David A. Gelber

CONTENTS

0-8493-9463-5/95/$0.00+$.50
© 1995 by CRC Press Inc.

INTRODUCTION

The neurologist often has a key role in the evaluation and management of patients with traumatic brain injury, especially in the emergent and acute phases of care delivery. As rehabilitation commences, the neurologist may be involved as a consultant or may play a more active role overseeing the rehabilitation process, depending upon the nature of his or her practice and the degree to which physiatric services are available. The role of the neurologist in the rehabilitation of the traumatically brain-injured (TBI) patient often includes defining the extent of neurologic damage, reviewing pharmacological issues as they impact central nervous system function, identifying and managing posttraumatic epilepsies and other neurological complications, and presenting information in a manner which is of maximal use to allied health professionals, family members, and the patient. This chapter allows the allied health professional insight into aspects of the neurologic examination, which will provide enhanced opportunity for interaction between the neurologist and other rehabilitation professionals.

The brain and supporting structures are extremely vulnerable to traumatic injury. Patients with severe brain injury are often left with significant physical and neuropsychological sequelae requiring prolonged hospitalization and the need for postacute rehabilitation programs. In the postacute setting, it is the physician's role to perform an adequate patient evaluation, including detailed history, physical and neurologic examinations, and, in conjunction with the rest of the rehabilitation team, to develop a comprehensive rehabilitation program to address each particular patient's needs.

The extent of brain injury and residual deficits varies from patient to patient, depending on the nature of the insult and localization of brain injury. Penetrating, or open, head wounds (e.g., skull fracture or gunshot wound) most often cause focal brain injury at the site of impact due to contusion, laceration, hemorrhage, or necrosis of underlying brain tissue.[1] Closed head acceleration/deceleration injuries typically cause coup or contrecoup insults to the brain, resulting in polar injuries to the frontal, temporal, and, occasionally, the occipital lobes. Diffuse axonal injury may also occur, as a result of shearing of axons within myelin sheaths, leading to injury to the subcortical white matter.[2] Brain structures most vulnerable to this type of injury include the corpus callosum, superior cerebellar peduncles, basal ganglia, and periventricular white matter.[3] In addition to the direct traumatic injury, the brain may also be damaged as a result of complications of the head injury, including edema, hypoxia, posttraumatic infarction, and hydrocephalus.[4]

The severity of brain injury also varies amongst patients. Poorer functional outcomes are associated with increased patient age, presence of intracranial hemorrhage, abnormal motor responses, impaired eye movements or pupillary responses, hypotension, hypoxemia, hypercarbia, and increased intracranial pressure.[5] With the most severe injuries, patients may have prolonged coma, severe cognitive and behavioral sequelae, and marked motor and sensory deficits leading to profound functional impairments. At the other end of the spectrum, mild head injuries may result in the "postconcussion syndrome" with slight memory and behavioral manifestations, headache, and vertigo, but with little in the way of motor deficits or functional impairments.[6]

The neurologic examination is a key element in the evaluation of the traumatically brain-injured patient. The focus of the examination, however, differs depending on the stage of patient recovery. In the acutely brain-injured patient, the neurologic examination serves to localize the site and extent of brain injury allowing the physician to develop a plan of acute medical and surgical management. In addition, serial neurologic examinations performed in the first few weeks following injury provide useful information regarding prognosis for recovery.

The purpose of the neurologic examination in the postacute rehabilitation setting is different from that performed in the acute stages following traumatic brain injury. The most important aspect of the examination in the postacute setting is to identify the specific physical, neurologic, cognitive, and behavioral deficits that will potentially limit the patient from a functional standpoint. Hemiparesis, for example, may affect a patient's ability to perform independent transfers, ambulate safely, or dress himself without help. Spasticity may impede nursing care, limit bed mobility, and cause difficulty with wheelchair seating and ambulation. Identifying these deficits and related functional impairments allows the rehabilitation team to set appropriate rehabilitation goals and to develop a comprehensive rehabilitation program to address the patient's needs. It is also important for the rehabilitation team to be able to identify specific deficits and potential limitations to the patient's family members and caregivers to allow them to adjust to these changes and make adequate plans for the patient's return to home and reentry into the community.

In the postacute setting, the physician must also be able to distinguish deficits that are a direct consequence of the traumatic brain injury from those that are due to medical complications. These potential complications include heterotopic ossification, posttraumatic hydrocephalus, posttraumatic epilepsy, intracranial and systemic infections, and medication side effects. Failure to identify medical complications will delay appropriate treatment and could place the patient at risk of permanent impairments.

This chapter will detail the neurologic examination of the traumatically brain-injured patient in the postacute recovery period. Emphasis will be placed on identifying neurologic deficits that are common in the head-injured patient. Functional impairments, particularly as they relate to rehabilitation, will be reviewed. Finally, medical complications that are commonly encountered in the traumatically brain-injured patient will be briefly discussed.

EVALUATION OF THE TRAUMATICALLY BRAIN-INJURED PATIENT IN THE POSTACUTE SETTING

The initial evaluation of the traumatically brain-injured patient should include a detailed history. Since most of these patients have some cognitive impairment, the history may need to be obtained from medical records and from family members. Important details of the injury include the nature of the head injury (open or closed), whether the brain injury was focal or diffuse, duration of posttraumatic amnesia, whether there were complicating factors (hemorrhage, hypoxia, hypertension, posttraumatic seizures) or associated systemic injuries (including spinal cord or peripheral nerve injury).

One of the most important factors in assessing patients with traumatic brain injury is the patient's premorbid cognitive and behavioral status. Assessment should include a history of drug or alcohol abuse or psychiatric illness. Level of education and employment status should also be obtained. Younger patients may have school records, including results of previous formal cognitive testing, which can provide some objective picture of premorbid cognitive skills. Additional information should be sought from family members or employers.

A general physical examination should be performed on all patients. General observation should include assessment of the patient's level of consciousness; posture in bed, sitting, or standing; and the presence of any external catheters or tubes (tracheostomy, gastrostomy tube, Foley catheter). The skin should be carefully examined for signs of breakdown (decubitus ulcers) or rash. Since concomitant skeletal injuries are common, a thorough musculoskeletal examination should be performed with careful attention to any abnormal posturing of limbs, skeletal deformities, or limited range of motion at joints. Careful examination of the lungs,

**TABLE 2.1 Components of the Neurologic Examination
in the Traumatically Brain-Injured Patient**

Mental status
    Level of consciousness
    Orientation
    Attention and concentration
    Memory
    Calculations
    Speech and language
    Spatial orientation/perception
    Affect and behavior
Cranial nerves
Motor
    Muscle bulk
    Muscle tone
    Muscle strength
    Abnormal movements
Sensation
    Primary sensory modalities
    Cortical sensory function
Coordination
Reflexes
Posture and gait

heart, and abdomen should also be performed to rule out infection or other pathological processes.

Finally, a detailed neurologic examination should be performed. This should include a detailed assessment of mental status, cranial nerves, motor system, sensory system, reflexes, coordination, and posture and gait (Table 2.1).

THE NEUROLOGIC EXAMINATION

Examination of Mental Status

Cognition and behavior are often affected in the traumatically brain-injured patient. Manifestations include disorders of intellect, learning and memory, language, perception, and executive functions (planning and goal setting). Although a formal, detailed cognitive assessment is usually performed by the neuropsychologist and speech pathologist, useful information may be obtained from simple testing. Areas that should be assessed include level of consciousness, orientation, attention and concentration, memory, calculations, speech and language, spatial orientation and perceptual skills, and affect and behavior.

Level of Consciousness

An altered level of consciousness may occur in the acute stage following traumatic brain injury as a result of diffuse injury to the cerebral hemispheres or damage to the brainstem reticular formation. Other contributing factors include hypoxia, cerebral edema with increased intracranial pressure, and infection. Altered consciousness is often accompanied by confusion, disorientation, and retrograde amnesia, particularly if the limbic structures are affected.

Impairment in the level of consciousness may also be evident in the postacute rehabilitation setting, either because of residual brain injury or secondary factors such as metabolic abnormalities (hypernatremia, hypoglycemia, uremia, etc.), posttraumatic seizures, posttraumatic hydrocephalus, or medication side effects. A deterioration in level of consciousness should always alert the physician to the possibility of one of these complications. From a functional standpoint, an altered or deteriorating level of consciousness will obviously interfere with a patient's ability to actively participate in rehabilitation therapies and will shift the focus of therapy to more passive activities such as muscle stretching and range of motion exercises.

Level of consciousness is easily assessed by observation and is best described by noting the patient's response to various levels of stimulation. Terms often used to describe altered levels of consciousness include lethargy (arousal to voice), stupor (arousal to vigorous physical stimulation), or coma (unresponsiveness to pain or other external stimuli).[7]

Orientation

Confusion and disorientation are common sequelae of traumatic brain injury and are often associated with an altered level of consciousness. Disorientation most often results from diffuse cerebral injury, particularly that involving limbic structures, but can also be caused by factors such as metabolic abnormalities (discussed above).

Orientation is assessed by asking the patient his name, the date (day of week, month, year), and location (name of hospital, floor number, room number, etc.).

Attention and Concentration

Attention and concentration are often impaired in patients with diffuse head injuries, particularly with insults to the frontal lobes.[3,8] Slowing of cognitive functioning and distractibility are also common findings.[9] These impairments can significantly affect a patient's progress in therapies because of inattention, slowness in performing cognitive tasks, and diminished ability to carry over information from day to day.

Attention and concentration may be informally evaluated during the course of the patient examination. Patients may have difficulty attending to the interview and may be easily distracted by external stimuli such as hallway activity or roommates. Speed of cognitive processing may also be grossly assessed by noting the patient's response time to questions or commands.

Memory

Both long- and short-term memory may be affected in the head-injured patient due to injury to the mesial temporal lobes and thalamus.[3] Old (retrograde) memory as well as new learning (anterograde memory) may be involved. Verbal memory skills are affected in patients with left hemispheric injury, while spatial/perceptual memory skills are affected in patients with right hemispheric lesions. Other cognitive impairments, such as poor concentration and apathy, may also interfere with encoding of new memories.

The duration of anterograde memory impairment, i.e., posttraumatic amnesia, is an important early prognostic factor with regard to recovery. Patients with prolonged posttraumatic amnesia tend to have more residual cognitive impairment and overall poorer functional outcome.[10] Memory impairment may impact patients' progress in the rehabilitation program, especially if the ability to learn new information is affected and the carryover of information learned in therapies is limited.

Immediate memory is primarily a function of information registration and is most dependent on attention and concentration. It is usually spared following traumatic brain injury,[8] except in the early recovery period or when other factors, such as medication side effects or metabolic encephalopathy, affect patients' ability to attend to task. Immediate memory can be assessed by asking the patient to immediately repeat three objects named. Alternatively, one can use digit span testing. The examiner gives a series of digits at a rate of one per second and asks the patient to repeat these both forward and backward. A normal individual can repeat seven digits forward and six in reverse order. In testing recent memory, the patient can be asked to recall three objects in three or five minutes. Recent memory can also be assessed by asking the patient simple historical questions such as, "What did you have for breakfast this morning?". Remote memory may be assessed by asking the patient about events in the past, his/her address or phone number, names of children, anniversary dates, etc.

Calculations

Focal injury to the dominant parietal lobe may result in impairment of mathematical skills. Deficits may limit the patient functionally in terms of his ability to manage finances or participate in basic community activities such as shopping.

Calculation skills can easily be assessed by having patients perform serial subtraction of sevens from one hundred. Other tasks, such as counting change or more complex multiplication or division problems, can be administered. One must take premorbid educational history into account when interpreting the results of these tests.

Speech and Language

Language skills are commonly impaired in traumatic brain injuries that involve the dominant hemisphere. Difficulty with spoken and written language or problems with language processing result. Language deficits are usually accompanied by other cognitive impairments.[11] The most common feature of traumatic aphasia is anomia (characterized by difficulty naming, word-finding deficits, and paraphasic errors).[12,13] Wernicke's (fluent or receptive) aphasia occurs less commonly following traumatic brain injury. It is caused by focal injury to the dominant temporal lobe and is characterized by fluent paraphasic speech with impaired comprehension and repetition.[14] Broca's (nonfluent or expressive) aphasia, is more common in penetrating-type head injuries due to a lesion of the dominant frontal lobe. Broca's aphasia is characterized by nonfluent speech, with disturbed prosody, and perseveration. Other language disorders associated with traumatic brain injury include mutism (usually seen following head injury in children and in recovery from coma), stuttering, echolalia (repetition of others), and palilalia (repetition of self).[4] Higher level language skills may also be affected, often becoming apparent as the aphasia resolves. Problems include difficulty with complex auditory processing, spelling, sentence construction, synonyms, antonyms, and with abstract language skills such as picture description.[12]

Dysarthria, or impairment in articulation, is also a common sequela of traumatic brain injury and is caused by weakness and incoordination of the tongue and pharyngeal muscles. Deficits range from mild inarticulation to unintelligible speech, with the pattern depending on the location of brain injury.[14] Lesions of the hypoglossal nerve cause unilateral tongue weakness and difficulty articulating lingual consonants *(t,d,l,r,n)*. Weakness of the soft palate results in nasal speech characterized by an abnormal resonance to sounds.[15] Patients with pronounced facial weakness often have difficulty with labial and dentilabial consonants *(p,b,m,w,f,v)*. Bilateral involvement of corticobulbar pathways results in "pseudobulbar" speech, characterized by slow, labored speech, with imprecise articulation, and a harsh, "strained" quality. Cerebellar lesions are associated with dysrhythmic speech with irregularity of pitch and loudness. Injury to the basal ganglia may result in jerky, dysrhythmic speech with associated choreoathetosis, or slowed, slurred speech lacking inflection and modulation, associated with parkinsonian features.

Speech and language deficits clearly cause functional impairments, limiting a patient's ability to communicate effectively and to interact verbally with those around them. This not only affects the rehabilitation program but has serious implications in terms of a patient's interaction with others and in eventually being able to live independently in the community. Although a comprehensive evaluation is typically performed by the speech pathologist, basic aspects of speech and language can be assessed during the neurologic examination. The physician should observe the patient's spontaneous speech for fluency and syntax. Receptive language skills can be evaluated by having the patient follow one-, two-, and three-step verbal and written commands. Patients should be asked to name various common objects. Repetition can be assessed by asking the patient to repeat "no ifs, ands, or buts". Patients can be asked to read the newspaper or daily menu aloud and to write from dictation. Articulation can be grossly assessed by listening to the patient's speech during the interview and by having the patient repeat certain test phrases such as "Methodist Episcopal".

Spatial Orientation/Perception

Patients with focal injuries to the nondominant parietal lobe will often have difficulty with spatial orientation and perceptual tasks. This may be manifest as constructional apraxia, characterized by difficulty drawing or copying geometric designs. Disorders of body image may also be evident and manifest by a dressing apraxia, or neglect of the contralateral side of the body. The most serious form of neglect is anosognosia or the inability of one to recognize his own deficits.

Perceptual impairments and neglect are a serious hindrance to progress in the rehabilitation program. Patients with poor spatial orientation often wander or get lost. Patients with neglect are a safety risk because they often do not appreciate or pay attention to their deficits. Inattention to the affected side may cause a patient to accidentally roll over on a paretic arm or dangle it in the spokes of a wheelchair. Patients may be unable to safely negotiate their wheelchairs down a hallway or turn into an open doorway without striking a wall.

Constructional praxis may be assessed by having the patient draw simple geometric figures, such as a square or triangle, or more complex forms such as two intersecting pentagons. Patients should be able to bisect a line at the midline and draw an accurate clock face. Neglect can often be identified by observation. The patient may not attend to his affected side or may ignore his motor or sensory deficits.

Affect and Behavior

Psychiatric disorders are most common in the early recovery period following traumatic brain injury, especially upon recovery from coma,[3,16] but may be seen even years after injury.[17] Patients may experience delirium with disorientation and confusion, distractibility, restlessness, irritability, hallucinations, and delusions. These manifestations are most common in patients who have evidence of frontal or temporal lobe damage.[18] Delirium may also be caused by medication side effects, metabolic abnormalities, or infection.

Later in the recovery period, a change in personality, affect, and mood may be evident as a result of damage to the frontal lobes and limbic structures. Patients may be irritable and aggressive, demonstrate childish behavior, and show exaggeration of their premorbid personality. Other common features of frontal lobe injury include emotional disinhibition, emotional blunting, diminished drive and initiative, egocentricity, perseveration, mental rigidity, affective lability, loss of temper control, and impatience.[3,8] Patients with lesions of the basio-medial frontal cortices demonstrate impairment in social judgment and in sexual control.[3] Patients with injury to the dorsolateral frontal cortices also demonstrate difficulty with "executive skills", or the ability to plan and execute a complex task.[8]

Patients who demonstrate abnormal behavior may be difficult to manage. Those that are apathetic and lack initiative often do not put forth the maximum effort in therapies. Patients who demonstrate lack of impulse control, aggressiveness, and sexual inappropriateness are often disruptive, not only to staff but to other patients participating in the program. Furthermore, family members may have difficulty adjusting to a change in their behavior. It is important for the physician and rehabilitation team to identify these behavioral abnormalities, to develop an optimal behavioral modification program to minimize disruptive behavior, and to design the most effective overall rehabilitation strategies to address these problems.

Although not usually assessed formally in the neurologic examination, behavior and affect can be observed during the patient interview. Further information regarding patient behavior can be obtained from nursing staff and from more detailed testing performed by the neuropsychologist. Premorbid behavioral status should be ascertained from family members.

Cranial Nerve Examination

Cranial Nerve I

Olfactory dysfunction occurs in approximately 7% of patients with traumatic brain injury. This figure approaches 20% in head-injured patients who have suffered loss of consciousness.[19,20] Furthermore, the olfactory nerve is the most commonly affected cranial nerve in mild head injury. Impairment in detection of smell (anosmia) is usually caused by frontal or occipital blows causing direct injury to the olfactory pathways, which extend from the olfactory epithelium to the entorhinal cortex.[21] Impaired olfactory recognition or distortion of the normal sense of smell (parosmia) results from injury to the orbitofrontal and temporal lobes.[22,23] Olfactory dysfunction can lead to functional impairment including diminished pleasure, interference with certain occupations, and potential safety problems due to inability to detect dangerous smells such as gas.[20]

Smell may be assessed by having the patient identify various common odors such as tobacco or cloves. Noxious stimuli, such as ammonia, should be avoided since these stimulate the trigeminal nerve rather than the olfactory nerve.

Cranial Nerve II

The optic nerve and anterior visual pathways are affected in approximately 5% of TBI patients[24] with 3% experiencing persistent visual field defects, impaired visual acuity, or blindness.[25] Loss of vision occurs most commonly following frontal injuries, particularly if there are fractures of the orbital bones. The optic nerve and pathways may be injured due to shearing forces, mechanical stretching, contusion, or vascular insufficiency.[26,27] Deficits include monocular blindness, due to optic nerve injury; bitemporal hemianopia, due to ischemia of the optic chiasm; homonymous hemianopia, due to injury to the optic radiations; and cortical blindness, due to lesions of the calcarine cortex. The latter is particularly common after head injury in children and is usually transient.[20]

Functionally, visual impairment results in diminished personal pleasure and may limit the patient's mobility due to impaired visual acuity and altered depth perception. In the rehabilitation setting, visual impairments may lead to difficulty with wheelchair propulsion and ambulation and may cause safety concerns. Patients may have difficulty performing daily care activities, ultimately leading to a loss of independence. Community reentry skills, such as returning to work or resumption of driving, may also be affected.

Optic nerve function is assessed by pupillary response, fundoscopic examination, visual field testing, and measurement of visual acuity. In comatose patients, optic nerve function is best assessed by the pupillary response. In the case of unilateral optic nerve injury, neither the ipsilateral nor the contralateral pupil constrict when light is shone in the affected eye. Both pupils constrict, however, when light is shone in the unaffected eye. An afferent pupillary defect may also be demonstrated by the swinging flashlight test. When the light is swung back and forth from eye to eye, the pupil on the affected side will dilate as the light is swung to that eye (Marcus-Gunn phenomenon). In longstanding optic nerve atrophy, the optic disc may appear pale on fundoscopic examination. The presence of papilledema suggests the possibility of posttraumatic hydrocephalus or increased intracranial pressure of other causes and warrants further investigation.

Visual acuity may be impaired as a result of traumatic injury to the orbit and optic nerve or due to diffuse injuries to the occipital lobe. Acuity may be assessed by having the patient read a hand-held Snellen acuity chart or Rosenbaum near-vision card[26] or by reading materials such as a newspaper or menu. Visual fields are assessed by confrontation testing. Each eye should be tested separately with comparison of the patient's visual fields to the examiner's.

Cranial Nerves III, IV, and VI

Injury to the oculomotor, trochlear, or abducens nerves occurs in 2 to 8% of patients following head injury. These nerves may be injured in the orbit as the result of orbital wall fractures or in the cavernous sinus due to basilar skull fractures.[28,29] The cranial nerve nuclei, or intranuclear pathways, may be injured as a result of brainstem injury.[30] Injury may result in eye deviation, dysconjugate gaze, or abnormal head postures with subjective complaints of diplopia. Supranuclear, or conjugate gaze paresis, may result from injury to the gaze centers in the frontal or parietal lobes, horizontal gaze center in the pons, or vertical gaze center in the midbrain. Diplopia, or gaze paresis, may cause functional impairment by interfering with the patient's visuomotor tasks.

Eye movements are evaluated by having the patient track an object in the six cardinal positions of gaze. The inability to move the eye upward, inward, or downward, with preserved lateral movement, suggests injury to the oculomotor nerve. This is often accompanied by ptosis and pupillary dilatation. Injury to the trochlear nerve is manifest by the inability to intort the eye or move it downwards, often accompanied by head tilt to the nonaffected side.[31,32] The inability to move the eye laterally, with preservation of other ocular movements, suggests injury to the abducens nerve. In the comatose individual, eye movements can be assessed by oculocephalic or oculovestibular testing (see below).

Cranial Nerve V

A trigeminal nerve lesion occurs in 3.6% of head-injured patients.[33] The injury is most commonly extracranial due to facial fracture and can involve any or all of the branches of the trigeminal nerve. Rarely, the trigeminal nerve may be injured as a result of trauma to the brainstem or due to basilar skull fracture involving the petrous bone.[34] In the latter instance, associated hearing loss and ipsilateral facial weakness are common.

Injury to the sensory branches of the trigeminal nerve results in hemianesthesia of the face. Involvement of the ophthalmic branch leads to corneal anesthesia and potential corneal abrasion. Motor branch involvement results in weakness of the muscles of mastication and impairment of chewing. Loss of sensation in the mouth may cause pocketing of food and increases the risk of aspiration.

In the comatose patient, trigeminal nerve sensory function can be assessed by testing the corneal reflex (sensory limb). In alert, attentive patients, facial sensation can be evaluated with pinprick or cotton swab in the three nerve divisions. Trigeminal motor function can be tested by assessing masseter and pterygoid muscle strength. With trigeminal nerve injury, the jaw will deviate toward the affected side.

Cranial Nerve VII

The facial nerve is injured in approximately 3% of head-injured patients, most commonly due to temporal bone fractures. Associated hearing loss is common. Brainstem trauma may also result in injury to the facial nerve nucleus. Facial nerve injury results in ipsilateral weakness of muscles of the upper and lower face. Injury to the corticobulbar pathways due to lesion of the frontal lobe, internal capsule, or upper brainstem also results in facial weakness, but spares the upper facial musculature.

Facial nerve injury can cause significant functional impairments. The inability to close the eye fully can lead to corneal dryness, abrasion, and pain. Facial weakness may impair swallowing or cause a flaccid dysarthria.

Facial nerve function can be assessed in the comatose patient by the corneal reflex (motor limb). In the attentive patient, facial muscle strength can be assessed by asking the patient to smile, purse his/her lips, whistle, raise the eyebrows or forehead, and close the eyes.

Cranial Nerve VIII

Both the cochlear and vestibular nerves may be injured as a result of head trauma. Hearing loss occurs in 18 to 56% of head-injured patients[35] as a result of injury to the inner ear and related structures. Longitudinal fractures of the temporal bone, most commonly caused by a blow to the temporoparietal area, result in conductive hearing loss due to dislocation and disruption of the ossicles.[36] Transverse fractures of the temporal bone, caused by occipital or frontal blows, cause sensorineural hearing loss, vertigo, and disequilibrium due to direct injury to the acoustic nerve or trauma to the cochlea or labyrinth.[37] Lesions of the auditory or vestibular nuclei can occur as a consequence of brainstem contusions. There is, generally, not much functional impairment seen due to hearing loss since the deficit, when it occurs, is usually unilateral. Vestibular insults are usually more problematic, leading to dizziness and difficulties with balance and coordination.

Hearing may be evaluated by whisper or finger rub. Air and bone conduction are assessed by the Rinne and Weber tests. Patients with suspected hearing loss should be referred for more detailed audiometric evaluation.

The presence of direction-fixed horizontal nystagmus usually suggests unilateral vestibular injury. Vertical nystagmus usually results from direct brainstem injury. Nystagmus may also occur as a consequence of medications, particularly anticonvulsants. In the comatose individual, vestibular function may be assessed by testing the oculocephalic reflexes (doll's eyes) and oculovestibular reflexes (ice water calorics). In testing the oculocephalic reflex, rapid turning of the head results in conjugate eye deviation to the opposite side. Injury to the vestibular apparatus or vestibular pathways results in absence of eye deviation. Dysconjugate eye movements suggest injury to the internuclear pathways in the brainstem. In performing oculovestibular testing, the patient's head is tilted to 30 degrees and the external auditory canal is irrigated with ice water. A normal response is characterized by tonic conjugate deviation of the eyes toward the side of irrigation. In an awake individual, there may be nystagmus, with the fast component directed away from the site of irrigation. Injury to the vestibular pathways results in failure of eye deviation, while injury to the internuclear brainstem pathways results in dysconjugate eye movements. Patients with suspected injury to the vestibular pathways may be more formally assessed with electronystagmography.

Cranial Nerves IX and X

The glossopharyngeal and vagus nerves are only rarely affected in traumatic brain injury, usually as a result of basilar skull fracture with extension into the foramen magnum.[33] These nerves are responsible for laryngeal and pharyngeal sensory and motor function, respectively, with injury resulting in impaired phonation and swallowing.

Glossopharyngeal and vagus nerve function are assessed by the gag reflex. The reflex is diminished or absent on the side of nerve injury. In addition, the palate and uvula may be deviated to the opposite side. The gag reflex may be pathologically brisk when there are lesions of the corticobulbar pathways bilaterally, usually a consequence of extensive injury to the frontal lobes or deep white matter. There is usually an associated "pseudobulbar affect," characterized by emotional lability and spastic tetraparesis.

Cranial Nerve XI

The spinal accessory nerve supplies motor function to the ipsilateral sternocleidomastoid and trapezius muscles. This nerve is affected only rarely in head injury, with an effect occasionally seen following basilar skull fractures.

Spinal accessory nerve function is assessed by testing sternocleidomastoid muscle (lateral neck rotation to the opposite side) and trapezius muscle (ipsilateral shoulder shrug) strength. Impairment results in weakness of these muscles.

Cranial Nerve XII

The hypoglossal nerve provides motor function to the ipsilateral tongue. This nerve is also only rarely affected in head-injury patients, as a result of basilar skull fractures or injury to the atlanto-occipital region.[38] Injury results in swallowing difficulties due to inability to manipulate the food bolus in the mouth.

The hypoglossal nerve is tested by having the patient stick out the tongue. Injury results in deviation of the tongue to the ipsilateral side.

Motor Examination

Muscle Bulk

In the traumatically brain-injured patient, generalized muscle atrophy may occur as a result of disuse following prolonged coma or immobility. Focal muscle atrophy always suggests lower motor neuron injury and should alert the physician to possible peripheral nerve, plexus, or nerve root injury. A peroneal neuropathy, for example, may arise secondary to a dislocated knee or as a consequence of an excessively tight lower extremity cast, resulting in footdrop and atrophy of the anterior compartment of the lower leg. The median, ulnar, radial, and sciatic nerves may also be injured as a result of skeletal injury or impingement by heterotopic bone. Brachial plexus or cervical root injuries are common in motorcycle accidents, particularly when the patient lands on his neck and shoulder.

Muscle bulk is generally assessed by observation. Focal atrophy can be discerned by comparing the circumference of the limb in question to the opposite side.

Muscle Tone

Various abnormalities of muscle tone may develop in the head-injured patient. Spasticity is the most common type of tone abnormality seen in brain-injured patients. "Spasticity" is defined as a velocity-dependent increase in resistance to passive movement, predominantly affecting the flexor groups in the upper extremities and extensor groups in the lower extremities. Tone may also be increased in the truncal muscles. Spasticity results from injury to the corticospinal tracts and is usually associated with muscle weakness, hyperreflexia, and an extensor plantar reflex response (Babinski sign). "Rigidity" is defined as an increase in resistance to passive movement, independent of velocity, and is most prominent in the flexor muscle groups of the upper and lower limbs. Cogwheel rigidity may result from direct injury to the basal ganglia; however, this is more common as a consequence of anoxia or a side effect of neuroleptic medications. Paratonia, or the inability of a patient to voluntarily relax his muscles during passive movement, is seen as a consequence of bilateral frontal lobe injury. Hypotonia, or diminished muscle tone, is occasionally seen as a consequence of cerebellar injury.

Increased tone may cause pain in the affected limb and may impede rehabilitation by limiting mobility and transfer skills, performance of nursing care, and activities of daily living. Spasticity in the upper extremity may hamper fine dexterity and limit the ability to perform daily care activities. Neck and head control may be impaired leading to difficulties with grooming and feeding skills. Spasticity of the pharyngeal and laryngeal muscles may impair articulation, phonation, swallowing, and breathing. Increased tone in the trunk musculature leads to problems in positioning in bed, wheelchair seating, standing, and ambulation.

If a routine program of passive stretching is not performed, fixed joint contractures may develop. These occur most commonly at the wrist, elbow, knee, and ankle. Patients with ankle plantar flexion contractures may not have an adequate base of support in order to transfer safely. Contractures of the hip and knee may limit a patient's ability to stand and ambulate. Contractures of the hip adductors may limit access to the perineal area causing problems with catheter care and skin breakdown. Patients may have difficulty turning in bed or positioning themselves properly in the wheelchair, ultimately leading to pressure ulcerations on contact points (greater trochanters, sacrum, and heels).

Muscle tone is evaluated by passively moving the upper and lower extremities with the patient fully relaxed. Movements that are commonly tested include flexion/extension of the wrist, pronation/supination of the forearm, flexion/extension of the elbow, and flexion/extension of the knee or hip.

Range of motion of all joints should also be carefully assessed. Limited range of motion is suggestive either of contracture of that joint or heterotopic ossification, particularly if there is evidence of bony overgrowth in the joint region.[39] Heterotopic ossification is discussed in more detail in Chapter 5 of this volume.

Muscle Strength

The two most common patterns of muscle weakness following traumatic brain injury are hemiparesis and tetraparesis due to injury to the corticospinal tracts in the cerebral hemispheres or brainstem. Weakness is usually accompanied by spasticity and hyperreflexia. Focal muscle weakness should raise the suspicion of a superimposed nerve root, plexus, or peripheral nerve injury.[25]

Muscle weakness causes obvious functional limitations, depending on its distribution and severity. Patients with severe tetraparesis often are unable even to roll in bed without assistance and may need help with simple daily care activities such as feeding and grooming. Although patients with hemiparesis usually require less physical assistance, they are often unable to transfer or ambulate independently and usually require help with daily care activities.

Primary movers of the fingers, wrists, elbows, shoulders, neck, ankles, knees, and hips should be assessed. It is important to position the patient properly while conducting muscle strength testing in order to assure that the muscle being tested is appropriately isolated from other muscles with similar function. Strength is most commonly graded on the following scale:[15] 0 = no muscle contraction noted; 1 = flicker of movement (0 to 10% of normal movement); 2 = movement through partial range of motion with gravity eliminated (11 to 25% of normal movement); 3 = movement through full range of motion against gravity (26 to 50% of normal movement); 4 = movement through full range of motion against gravity, together with minimal resistance from the examiner (51 to 75% of normal movement); 5 = normal muscle power (76 to 100% of normal movement).

Abnormal Movements

Abnormal postures or motor movements may result directly from traumatic brain injury or as a consequence of medication side effects (Table 2.2). "Dystonia", defined as inappropriate prolonged contraction of muscles resulting in distortion of the limb,[40] can occur secondary to injury to the basal ganglia or as a side effect of neuroleptic medications.[40,41] Similarly, dyskinesias (characterized by insuppressible, stereotyped, automatic movements of the limbs or orofacial musculature) may also result from basal ganglia injury or from medication side effects. Choreoathetosis (slow, writhing, spasmodic, involuntary movements of the limbs or facial musculature) is most commonly seen as a side effect of anticonvulsants, dopaminergic medications, adrenergic medications, oral contraceptives, or antipsychotic medications but may also result from traumatic injury to the basal ganglia.[42] Ballismus (characterized by violent flinging of the proximal upper extremity) may occur from direct injury or hemorrhage in the subthalamic region. Tremor has also been reported as a consequence of head injury.

TABLE 2.2 Movement Disorders Associated with Traumatic Brain Injury

Dystonia
Dyskinesia
Choreoathetosis
Ballismus
Tremor
Myoclonus
Asterixis
Parkinsonism

Most frequent is a postural or kinetic tremor which may involve the head, upper extremities, or lower extremities.[43]

"Myoclonus" is defined as sudden, brief, shock-like, involuntary muscle contractions. These can be focal, segmental, or generalized and may be stimulus induced.[44] Myoclonus has also been reported as a direct consequence of head injury, often associated with cerebellar, basal ganglia, or pyramidal signs.[45-47] Myoclonus may also result from complications, including metabolic abnormalities (renal or hepatic failure, hyponatremia, or hypoglycemia), medication side effects (L-Dopa), or hypoxic brain injury.[44] "Asterixis" is defined as an involuntary lapse of posture occurring at a joint during tonic muscle contraction.[48] This is usually detected as a wrist flap while holding the arms outstretched with the wrists extended. Asterixis has been reported as a consequence of injury to the thalamus, internal capsule, midbrain, or parietal cortex but is more commonly associated with toxic/metabolic encephalopathy (hepatic or renal failure) or use of anticonvulsant medications.[48] Posttraumatic parkinsonism has also been described as a result of blunt head injury.[49]

Abnormal movements interfere with both gross and fine motor function by inhibiting normal coordinated movements. These hamper the ability to perform activities of daily living such as feeding or grooming and interfere with fine motor activities such as buttoning buttons or pulling zippers. Abnormal postures may interfere with wheelchair positioning, sitting balance, standing, and ambulation.

Sensory Examination

Sensory perception is often affected in patients with traumatic brain injuries, although the sensory deficits are usually overshadowed by the motor and cognitive impairments. Injury to the thalamus results in impairment of all sensory modalities on the contralateral face and body. With parietal lobe injuries, there is preservation of pain and temperature sensation, although patients are unable to localize the site of sensory stimulation. In addition, joint position sense, stereognosis (the ability to identify shapes and objects by touch), and graphesthesia (the ability to recognize figures written on the skin) are also impaired. Sensory neglect is often apparent, particularly if the nondominant parietal lobe is involved.

Sensory deficits may lead to serious functional impairments. A patient's inability to detect or localize pain may result in body injury as the result of the patient's lack of awareness and inability to protect the affected extremity. This is even a greater problem in patients who demonstrate neglect. Impaired upper extremity joint position sense may significantly affect a patient's ability to perform daily care activities such as feeding or grooming because of the inability to accurately detect and control limb position in space. Lack of feeling in the hands may also impair fine motor movements, making buttoning or fastening snaps difficult. Lower extremity sensory deficits may lead to difficulties with transfers and ambulation because of difficulties with accurate foot placement and balance. Patients with impaired sensation are at increased risk of developing pressure ulcerations, particularly if there is associated spasticity and impaired mobility.[50]

Patients' responses to sensory testing are highly subjective and dependent on factors such as level of consciousness, attention, and concentration. In a patient with a depressed level of consciousness, only gross sensory testing can be performed. In this case, sensory testing involves evaluation of the patient's grimace or motor response (e.g., withdrawal of limb) to a painful stimulus.

In an alert, cooperative patient, sensory testing should include assessment of the primary sensory modalities, which include pain, light touch, vibration, and joint position sense. Responses should be compared from side to side and between upper and lower extremities. If the primary sensory modalities are intact, higher cortical sensory functions can be assessed. Graphesthesia can be evaluated by asking the patient to identify a letter or number traced in the palm of the hand. Stereognosis is tested by having the patient identify an object or shape placed, unseen, in the hand. Localization of a sensory stimulus can be evaluated by touching a body part, with either a pin or cotton swab, and asking the patient to specifically identify the area of stimulation. Sensory neglect can be assessed by double simultaneous stimulation. Patients with neglect will be able to detect a stimulus on either limb when tested individually but will neglect the affected side when the limbs are stimulated at the same time.

Coordination

Coordination is modulated by various central and peripheral nervous system structures, including the corticospinal tracts, basal ganglia, cerebellum, and sensory pathways. Most severe traumatic brain injuries cause diffuse structural injury and can affect any of these systems. Injury to the corticospinal tracts results in muscle weakness and slowing of gross and fine motor tasks. Basal ganglia lesions cause slowed initiation of movement and bradykinesia. Cerebellar injury may result in limb and truncal ataxia, dysmetria (inability to gauge distance, speed, and power of movement, resulting in an overshoot or undershoot of the target), dysdiadochokinesia (impairment in performance of rapid alternating movements), dyssynergia (decomposition of movement, resulting in lack of speed and skill in performing complex motor movements), and intention tremor.[15] Sensory pathway insults, particularly those involving the posterior columns, cause ataxia due to impaired proprioception.

Incoordination can affect a patient's ability to perform either gross or fine hand movements necessary to perform daily care activities. Patients may have difficulty bringing food to their mouths and may need assistance with dressing, particularly with buttons, snaps, and shoelaces. Writing may be illegible. Truncal ataxia may impair sitting and standing balance causing problems with wheelchair seating, standing, and ambulation.

Upper extremity coordination can be assessed by various tests. On finger-to-nose testing, the patient alternates between touching his nose and touching the examiner's finger held at arm's length from the patient. The smoothness and accuracy of the movement are noted, looking for evidence of dysmetria, dyssynergia, or intention tremor. Rapid alternating movements can be evaluated in several ways. Patients can be asked to rapidly flex and extend the fingers, rapidly oppose the tips of the index finger and thumb, alternate hand patting between the palmar and dorsal surface (pronation/supination), or alternate touching the tip of the thumb to the tips of each finger in succession. The speed of movement, rhythm, smoothness of movement, and accuracy should be assessed.

Lower extremity coordination can be evaluated by the heel-to-knee-to-toe test. The patient is asked to touch his heel to his knee and slide his heel up and down his lower leg. Again, the smoothness and accuracy of movement are assessed. Alternatively, the patient can be asked to draw a figure eight or circle in the air with his great toe. Rapid alternating movements can be evaluated by asking the patient to tap his foot rapidly or repeat a pattern of tapping.

Reflexes

Evaluation of muscle stretch reflexes helps localize the sites of brain injury. Hyperactive reflexes suggest injury to the corticospinal tracts and are associated with muscle weakness, spasticity, and an extensor plantar response (Babinski sign). Hypoactive reflexes occur most commonly with diseases or injuries of the lower motor neuron. Focal hyporeflexia, particularly if involving one reflex or reflexes in a single limb, should always raise the suspicion of a spinal root, plexus, or peripheral nerve injury. Diffuse hyporeflexia is most often associated with peripheral neuropathy, e.g., secondary to diabetes, chronic alcohol abuse, or renal disease, but also occurs with cerebellar injury.

The presence or exaggeration of other reflexes also helps localize brain injury. A hyperactive jaw jerk (masseter reflex) suggests bilateral corticospinal tract injury above the level of the mid pons. The presence of primitive reflexes, also called *frontal release signs,* i.e., sucking, grasp, and snout reflexes, suggests bifrontal or diffuse cerebral injury.

The biceps, triceps, brachioradialis, patellar, and Achilles muscle stretch reflexes are most commonly tested. Responses are graded on a 0 to 4 scale: 0 = absent reflex; 1 = diminished reflex; 2 = normal reflex; 3 = hyperactive reflex, although not necessarily pathologic; 4 = pathologically hyperactive reflex, with clonus or spread to other muscles in the ipsi- or contralateral limb.[15] The plantar response can be elicited in a number of ways. The most common maneuvers are the Babinski technique, performed by stimulating the sole of the foot with a blunt object, and the Chaddock maneuver, by stimulating the lateral aspect of the foot. A normal response is plantar flexion of the toes, whereas an abnormal response is characterized by dorsiflexion of the great toe with fanning of the other toes.

Posture and Gait

Traumatic brain injury, because of injury to the motor and sensory systems, commonly results in abnormalities in posture and stance and difficulty walking. Patients with spastic hemiparesis may have difficulty standing because of trunk instability and may be unable to adequately weight shift in order to ambulate safely. If ambulation is possible, there may be significant gait deviation. Weak hip flexors and ankle dorsiflexors result in impaired swing-through of the limb and inadequate toe clearance during the swing phase of gait. Spasticity and contractures may limit range of motion at the hip, knee, and ankle. Decreased arm swing and circumduction of the lower extremity may be noted. Assistive devices (walker, cane) and lower extremity orthoses may be necessary. Patients with basal ganglia injury often demonstrate stooped posture and shuffling gait. Patients with marked proprioceptive deficits may have difficulty with foot placement and balance.

The patient should be observed in a sitting and, if possible, a standing position for assessment of posture and static balance. Patients can be asked to stand with their feet together and arms outstretched or to stand on one leg to maintain their balance. Dynamic balance reactions can be tested by pushing the patient off balance, noting whether he is able to maintain his position and whether he demonstrates protective reflex reactions. If the patient is able to ambulate, gait should be assessed. Attention should be given to position of the patient's head and trunk and whether arm swing is normal and symmetrical. The movement of the patient's pelvis and hip, knee, ankle, and foot should also be observed. Balance and coordination can be further assessed by having the patient attempt to walk heel-to-toe in a straight line (tandem gait).

CHANGE IN STATUS

One of the difficulties in patient assessment is distinguishing deficits that are due directly to the traumatic brain injury from those that are secondary to systemic disease or complications of the head injury. At any point during the patient's recovery, deterioration in a neurologic status should always alert the physician to the possibility of such a complication. These include development of posttraumatic epilepsy, hydrocephalus, central nervous system or systemic infections, and toxic/metabolic encephalopathies.

Posttraumatic Epilepsy

Epileptic seizures occur in 2.5 to 5% of patients with traumatic brain injury. These are most commonly secondarily generalized tonic-clonic seizures, although approximately 20% are of complex partial type, manifested by staring, interruption of speech, and automatisms.[51] Early epilepsy, i.e., seizures occurring within the first week following injury, are most common in children under age five and in adults with depressed skull fracture or intracranial hemorrhage. Late epilepsy begins months to years following injury and is thought to be secondary to an epileptogenic scar.

Any alteration in level of consciousness, particularly if intermittent and associated with abnormal motor movements, should raise the suspicion of an epileptic seizure. An EEG is necessary to document seizure activity electrically and to localize the seizure focus. Urgent neuro-imaging (CT or MRI) is warranted to rule out the possibility of an acute structural brain lesion such as hemorrhage or abscess. The possibility of metabolic abnormalities, such as hypoglycemia, hyponatremia, or hypomagnesemia, or underlying infection (systemic or central nervous system), can lower seizure threshold and should also be considered.

Hydrocephalus

Ventricular dilatation is seen in 29 to 72% of patients following traumatic brain injury.[52] This is most often a consequence of diffuse brain injury with compensatory ventricular enlargement (hydrocephalus ex vacuo). Hydrocephalus may also develop as a result of impairment in the flow or absorption of cerebrospinal fluid.[53] The true incidence of posttraumatic extraventricular obstructive hydrocephalus, characterized by ventricular enlargement without concomitant enlargement of the sulci, is probably approximately 8%,[54] with the incidence of symptomatic hydrocephalus less than 1%.[55]

Symptoms of hydrocephalus range from loss or alteration of consciousness to the classic triad of normal-pressure hydrocephalus, which includes urinary incontinence, gait apraxia, and memory deficits. Any patient with a deteriorating level of consciousness or the clinical features of normal-pressure hydrocephalus should be evaluated with a head CT or MRI scan. Additional studies (lumbar puncture, radionuclide cisternography) may also be necessary for diagnosis.

Infection

Intracranial infections, including meningitis, brain abscess, or encephalitis, can occur in patients following traumatic brain injury. Most susceptible are patients with a basilar skull fracture with extension into the paranasal sinuses or middle ear or those who have had intracranial surgery.[56] Signs and symptoms of intracranial infection include fever, nuchal rigidity, depressed level of consciousness, and focal neurologic signs, including seizures. Workup should include a head CT or MRI. If there is no evidence of a mass lesion, a lumbar puncture should be performed.

Systemic infections, e.g., urinary tract infection or pneumonia, can also cause fever and depressed level of consciousness, especially in patients with underlying brain injury. Seizure threshold is also lowered in these individuals. Any change in patient behavior, deterioration in level of consciousness, or development of breakthrough seizures should raise the possibility of infection. Workup should be guided toward locating the source of infection in order to institute appropriate treatment as quickly as possible.

Toxic/Metabolic Encephalopathy

Toxic encephalopathy, due to medication side effects, is common in the head-injured population. Any change in a patient's behavior, depressed level of consciousness, or sudden appearance of a movement disorder should raise the suspicion of a medication side effect. The most common offenders include sedative/hypnotics, neuroleptics, and anticonvulsants. Fortunately, these side effects are usually reversible upon cessation of the medication. Other causes for encephalopathy, such as infection or metabolic abnormalities (hyponatremia, hypernatremia, hypocalcemia, hypoglycemia, hyperglycemia, etc.), should be ruled out.

SUMMARY

The neurologist has a key role to play in the medical and therapeutic management of the TBI patient in the postacute rehabilitation environment. The role extends beyond cursory neurological examination, encompassing occasionally complex neurological diagnosis and management. The neurologist should be comfortable in interfacing with physiatry, otolaryngology, psychiatry, and all allied health professionals to form an optimum approach to comprehensive postacute rehabilitation of the TBI patient.

REFERENCES

1. Adams, J. H., Graham, D., Scott, G., Parker, L. S., and Doyle, D., Brain damage in fatal non-missile head injury, *J. Clin. Pathol.*, 33, 1132, 1980.
2. Adams, J. H., Mitchell, D. E., Graham, D. I., and Doyle, D., Diffuse brain damage of immediate impact type: Its relationship to "primary brain-stem damage" in head injury, *Brain*, 100, 489, 1977.
3. McAllister, T. W., Neuropsychiatric sequelae of head injuries, *Psychiatr. Clin. North Am.*, 15, 395, 1992.
4. Levin, H. S., Aphasia after head injury, in *Acquired Aphasia*, Sarno, M. T., Ed., Academic Press, Inc., San Diego, 1991, 455.
5. Miller, J. D., Butterworth, J. F., Gudeman, S. K., Faulkner, J. E., Choi, S. C., Selhorst, J. B., Harbison, J. W., Lutz, H. A., Young, H. F., and Becker, D. P., Further experience in the management of severe head injury, *J. Neurosurg.*, 54, 289, 1981.
6. Auerbach, S. H., The post-concussive syndrome: Formulating the problem, *Hosp. Pract.*, 9, 1987, October 30.
7. Plum, F. and Posner, J. B., *The Diagnosis of Stupor and Coma*, F. A. Davis Company, Philadelphia, 1980.
8. Brooks, N., Behavioral abnormalities in head injured patients, *Scand. J. Rehabil. Med. Suppl.*, 17, 41, 1988.
9. Bennett-Levy, J. M., Long-term effects of severe closed head injury on memory: Evidence from a consecutive series of young adults, *Acta Neurol. Scand.*, 70, 285, 1984.
10. Chadwick, O., Rutter, M., Brown, G., Shaffer, D., and Traub, M., A prospective study of children with head injuries. II: Cognitive sequelae, *Psychol. Med.*, 11, 49, 1981.
11. Groher, M. E., Communication disorders in adults, in *Rehabilitation of the Adult and Child with Traumatic Brain Injury*, Rosenthal, M., Griffith, E. R., Bond, M. R., and Miller, J. D., Eds., F. A. Davis Company, Philadelphia, 1990, 148.
12. Thomsen, I. V., The patient with severe head injury and his family, *Scand. J. Rehabil. Med.*, 6, 180, 1974.
13. Levin, H. S., Grossman, R. G., and Kelly, P. J., Aphasic disorder in patients with closed head injury, *J. Neurol. Neurosurg. Psychiatry*, 39, 1062, 1976.
14. Sarno, M. T., Buonaguro, A., and Levita, E., Characteristics of verbal impairment in closed head injured patients, *Arch. Phys. Med. Rehabil.*, 67, 400, 1986.
15. Haerer, A. F., *DeJong's The Neurologic Examination*, 5th edition, J. B. Lippincott Company, Philadelphia, 1992.
16. Lishman, W. A., Brain damage in relation to psychiatric disability after head injury, *Br. J. Psychiatry*, 114, 373, 1968.
17. Lezak, M. D., Relationships between personality disorders, social disturbances, and physical disability following traumatic brain injury, *J. Head Trauma Rehabil.*, 2, 57, 1987.
18. Thomsen, I. V., Late outcome of very severe blunt head trauma: A 10–15 year second follow-up, *J. Neurol. Neurosurg. Psychiatry*, 47, 260, 1984.
19. Sumner, D., Disturbances of the senses of smell and taste after head injuries, in *Handbook of Clinical Neurology*, Volume 24, Vinken, P. J. and Bruyn, C. W., Eds., North-Holland Publishing, Amsterdam, 1976, 1.
20. Jennett, B. and Teasdale, G., *Management of Head Injuries*, F. A. Davis Company, Philadelphia, 1981.

21. Hendricks, A. P. J., Olfactory dysfunction, *Rhinology*, 26, 229, 1988.
22. Sarangi, P. and Aziz, T. Z., Post-traumatic parosmia treated by olfactory nerve section (letter), *Br. J. Neurosurg.*, 4, 358, 1990.
23. Levin, H. S., High, W. M., and Eisenberg, H. M., Impairment of olfactory recognition after closed head injury, *Brain*, 108, 579, 1985.
24. Gjerris, F., Traumatic lesions of the visual pathways, in *Handbook of Clinical Neurology,* Volume 24, Vinken, P. J. and Bruyn, C. W., Eds., North-Holland Publishing, Amsterdam, 1976, 27.
25. Roberts, A. H., *Severe Accidental Head Injury: An Assessment of Long-Term Prognosis*, The Macmillan Press, Ltd., London, 1979.
26. Kline, L. B., Morawetz, R. B., and Swaid, S. N., Indirect injury of the optic nerve, *Neurosurgery*, 14, 756, 1984.
27. Crompton, M. R., Visual lesions in closed head injury; *Brain*, 93, 785, 1970.
28. Baker, R. S. and Epstein, A. D., Ocular motor abnormalities from head trauma, *Surv. Ophthalmol.*, 35, 245, 1991.
29. Shokunbi, T. and Agbeja, A., Ocular complications of head injury in children, *Child's Nerv. Syst.*, 7, 147, 1991.
30. Hardman, J. M., The pathology of traumatic brain injuries, in *Advances in Neurology: Complications of Nervous System Trauma*, Volume 22, Thompson, R. A. and Green, J. R., Eds., Raven Press, New York, 1979, 15.
31. Kushner, B. J., Ocular causes of abnormal head postures, *Ophthalmology*, 86, 2115, 1979.
32. Sydnor, C. F., Seaber, J. H., and Buckley, E. G., Traumatic superior oblique palsies, *Ophthalmology*, 89, 134, 1982.
33. Yadav, Y. R. and Khosla, V. K., Isolated 5th to 10th cranial nerve palsy in closed head trauma, *Clin. Neurol. Neurosurg.*, 93, 61, 1991.
34. Schecter, A. D. and Anziska, B., Isolated complete post-traumatic trigeminal neuropathy, *Neurology*, 40, 1634, 1990.
35. Kochhar, L. K., Deka, R. C., Kacker, S. K., and Raman, E. V., Hearing loss after head injury, *Ear, Nose Throat J.*, 69, 537, 1990.
36. Sakai, C. S. and Mateer, C. A., Otological and audiological sequelae of closed head trauma, *Semin. Hear.*, 5, 157, 1984.
37. Nelson, J. R., Neuro-otologic aspects of head injury, in *Advances in Neurology: Complications of Nervous System Trauma,* Volume 22, Thompson, R. A. and Green, J. R., Eds., Raven Press, New York, 1979, 107.
38. Delamont, R. S. and Boyle, R. S., Traumatic hypoglossal nerve palsy, *Clin. Exp. Neurol.*, 26, 239, 1989.
39. Garland, D. E. and Rhoades, M. E., Orthopedic management of brain-injured adults: Part II, *Clin. Orthopaed. Relat. Res.*, 131, 111, 1978.
40. Marsden, C. D., Obeso, J. A., Zarranz, J. J., and Lang, A. E., The anatomical basis of symptomatic hemidystonia, *Brain*, 108, 463, 1985.
41. Pettigrew, L. C. and Jankovic, J., Hemidystonia: A report of 22 patients and a review of the literature, *J. Neurol. Neurosurg. Psychiatry,* 48, 650, 1985.
42. Robin, J. J., Paroxysmal choreoathetosis following head injury, *Ann. Neurol.*, 2, 447, 1977.
43. Biary, N., Cleeves, L., Findley, L., and Koller, W., Post-traumatic tremor, *Neurology*, 39, 103, 1989.
44. Fahn, S., Marsden, C. D., and Van Woert, M. H., Definition and classification of myoclonus, in *Advances in Neurology: Myoclonus*, Volume 43, Fahn, S., Marsden, C. D., and Van Woert, M. H., Eds., Raven Press, New York, 1986, 1.
45. Lance, J. W., Action myoclonus, Ramsay Hunt syndrome, and other cerebellar myoclonic syndromes, in *Advances in Neurology: Myoclonus*, Volume 43, Fahn, S., Marsden, C. D., and Van Woert, M. H., Eds., Raven Press, New York, 1986, 33.
46. Hallett, M., Chadwick, D., and Marsden, C.D., Cortical reflex myoclonus, *Neurology*, 29, 1107, 1979.
47. Starosta-Rubenstein, S., Bjork, R. J., Snyder, B. D., and Tulloch, J. W., Posttraumatic intention myoclonus, *Surg. Neurol.*, 20, 131, 1983.
48. Young, R. R. and Shahani, B. T., Asterixis: One type of negative myoclonus, in *Advances in Neurology: Myoclonus*, Volume 43, Fahn, S., Marsden, C.D., and Van Woert, M. H., Eds., Raven Press, New York, 1986, 137.
49. Nayernouri, T., Posttraumatic parkinsonism, *Surg. Neurol.*, 24, 263, 1985.
50. Donovan, W. H., Garber, S. L., Hamilton, S. M., Krouskop, T. A., Rodriguez, G. P., and Stal, S., Pressure ulcers, in *Rehabilitation Medicine*, DeLisa, J. A., Ed., J. B. Lippincott Company, Philadelphia, 1988, 476.
51. Jennett, B., Post-traumatic epilepsy, in *Rehabilitation of the Adult and Child with Traumatic Brain Injury*, Rosenthal, M., Griffith, E. R., Bond, M. R., and Miller, J. D., Eds., F. A. Davis Company, Philadelphia, 1990, 89.
52. Beyeri, B. and Black, P. McL., Posttraumatic hydrocephalus, *Neurosurgery*, 15, 257, 1984.
53. Kishore, P. R. S., Lipper, M. H., Girevendulis, A. K., Becker, D. P., and Vines, F. S., Post-traumatic hydrocephalus in patients with severe head injury, *Neuroradiology*, 16, 261, 1978.

54. Gudeman, S. K., Kishore, P. R. S., Becker, D. P., Lipper, M. H., Girevendulis, A. K., Jeffries, B. F., and Butterworth, J. F., Computed tomography in the evaluation of incidence and significance of post-traumatic hydrocephalus, *Neuroradiology*, 141, 397, 1981.

55. Narayan, R. K., Gokaslan, Z. L., Bontke, C. F., and Berrol, S., Neurologic sequelae of head injury, in *Rehabilitation of the Adult and Child with Traumatic Brain Injury*, Rosenthal, M., Griffith, E. R., Bond, M. R., and Miller, J. D., Eds., F. A. Davis Company, Philadelphia, 1990, 94.

56. Miller, J. D., Pentland, B., and Berrol, S., Early evaluation and management, in *Rehabilitation of the Adult and Child with Traumatic Brain Injury*, Rosenthal, M., Griffith, E. R., Bond, M. R., and Miller, J. D., Eds., F. A. Davis Company, Philadelphia, 1990, 21.

3

Posttraumatic Epilepsy and Neurorehabilitation

Dean K. Naritoku and Theresa D. Hernandez

CONTENTS

Although epilepsy has been long recognized as a common sequela to head injury, progress in understanding its pathophysiology and treatment has been slow. As a result, clinicians have focused little attention on improving outcome and therapy of posttraumatic epilepsy, and in most institutions, therapy of posttraumatic epilepsy has remained irrational and arbitrary. The decision to initiate or withhold antiepileptic drug therapy has far-reaching implications for rehabilitation of the traumatically brain-injured (TBI) patient. Inappropriate use of anticonvulsants may cause unnecessary cognitive impairment in persons not requiring medication. On the other hand, experimental data suggest that uncontrolled seizures retard functional improvement during recovery from brain injury. Thus, it is crucial to positively discriminate patients that will require and benefit from antiepileptic drug therapy from those who will not.

EVALUATION OF EPISODIC BEHAVIORAL CHANGES

Episodes of abnormal behavior occur commonly after severe head injuries and present a diagnostic challenge for the treating physician. There are many potential etiologies for these episodes; therefore, it is crucial to determine the correct diagnosis in order to select the most appropriate and efficacious therapies and avoid iatrogenic complications. Several disease entities result in fluctuations of mental status in the posttraumatic brain-injured state. These include posttraumatic encephalopathy, seizures, postictal state, and numerous encephalopathies of toxic and metabolic etiologies. The encephalopathy caused by the posttraumatic state is discussed in detail in other chapters in this book. Mentation tends to fluctuate in the TBI patient and may be mistaken for seizures, especially when there is a superimposed encephalopathy of another etiology. Metabolic encephalopathies are characterized by fluctuating mentation and may also be mistaken for seizures. Inappropriate use of antiepileptic drugs in these situations will not only be ineffective but may result in worsening of confusion or agitation.

There are many common etiologies for acute encephalopathies. Medication-induced encephalopathies rank among the most common and easily remedied causes of confusional states. As a result of the brain injury, TBI patients possess a lower tolerance to the central nervous system side effects of psychotropic drugs and other medications. Medications with anticholinergic properties are tolerated especially poorly and should be avoided because of their tendency to cause confusion, hallucinations, and memory loss, especially in older patients.[1,2] Antihistamines and many over-the-counter preparations fall into this category and are often overlooked as causes of transient or prolonged confusion. Several centrally acting sedatives, especially benzodiazepines and barbiturates, have extremely long half-lives. From a pharmacokinetic standpoint, long half-lives result in a greater interval before steady state is achieved; thus, adverse effects on the central nervous system may not be apparent until several days after the start of medications and cause-and-effect may not be apparent. As a general rule, sedative agents (including benzodiazepines, opioids, and barbiturates) exacerbate encephalopathies; therefore, they frequently aggravate confusion or agitation in TBI patients and should be avoided. Other drugs commonly used in the TBI patient may have profound effects on the central nervous system. The medication list should always be reviewed for histamine antagonists (i.e., cimetidine) and narcotics, for the possibility that they are inducing the confusional state.

Several systemic derangements are commonly associated with the posttraumatic state. Head injury may cause the syndrome of inappropriate antidiuretic hormone (SIADH) and result in hyponatremia, which in turn may cause confusion. Systemic infections are common in the TBI patient because of reduced mobility and presence of indwelling catheters. Any infection may manifest as an abrupt decline in mental status or agitation. An acute decline or fluctuation in mental status may herald a pulmonary, urinary tract, or wound infection. In patients with open head injuries and skull fractures, the possibility of a central nervous system infection should always be considered when there is an abrupt decline in mental status. When in doubt, a lumbar puncture must be performed, after careful assessment of intracranial pressure. Hypoxia may also cause agitation and confusion and is commonly caused by pulmonary emboli from deep venous thrombosis or fat emboli. Stroke is usually not a cause of global cognitive dysfunction except in cases of multifocal, brainstem, or diencephalic strokes.

Panic disorder may closely mimic epilepsy and is frequently seen in patients after trauma. The resulting panic episodes may be mistaken for complex partial seizures because of the loss of consciousness that may occur as a result of associated vasovagal attacks. Panic episodes are often misdiagnosed as medically intractable seizures, and this diagnosis should be considered in patients who are not responsive to antiepileptic medications. A careful history will help sort out this differential diagnosis. Typically, in the case of a panic attack, the patient complains of feeling dissociated, smothered, and in need of fresh air. The patient may have perioral numbness, tingling of digits, and a feeling of impending doom. Generally, full awareness of surroundings is retained and the patient is able to maintain conversation. When syncope occurs, it is usually brief and vasovagal in nature. As the patient loses consciousness, there is dimming of vision and the patient appears pale and clammy. The patient generally falls limply

TABLE 3.1 International Classification of Seizures[a]

Current terminology	Old terminology
I. Partial onset seizures	
A. Simple partial seizures (consciousness not impaired) Include:	
Motor symptoms	Focal motor, jacksonian
Sensory symptoms	Focal sensory
Autonomic or psychic symptoms	"Auras"
B. Complex partial seizures (consciousness impaired)	Temporal lobe, psychomotor seizures
C. Secondarily generalized seizures	Grand mal
II. Primarily generalized seizures Include:	
Typical absence	Petit mal
Atypical absence	
Myoclonic	
Tonic-clonic (primary generalized)	Grand mal
Clonic	
Clonic-tonic-clonic	
Atonic	Akinetic

[a] Adapted from Commission on Classification and Terminology of the International League Against Epilepsy (1981).

to the ground or slumps over, if sitting. Occasionally, a brief clonic or tonic-clonic seizure occurs, adding to the confusion of whether the episode resulted from a true seizure disorder. In contrast to true epileptic seizures, the patient with a syncopal episode generally regains consciousness and orientation rather quickly. A key difference between complex partial seizures and panic attacks is that, in the latter instance, the patient generally retains full awareness and can maintain a conversation until the loss of consciousness. Antiepileptic drugs are ineffective for panic disorder, whereas alprazolam and imipramine are very effective.[3]

CLINICAL EVALUATION OF SEIZURES

Seizures should be considered when episodes of discrete and stereotypic behavioral changes occur with altered or lost consciousness. Because there are no specific tests for epilepsy, the diagnosis must be made on clinical grounds. However, seizures are transient episodes and result in loss of consciousness. Thus, the patient can provide only a vague or incomplete history and much of the diagnosis lies in a careful history taken from observers. When taking a history, a key point to remember is that seizures are distinct episodes, with a definite start and end. With the exception of status epilepticus, the usual seizure lasts only a few minutes and, afterwards, there is generally clearing of mentation over the duration of minutes with return to baseline. Prolonged confusion of an hour to days' duration is only rarely caused by seizures and should alert the clinician to the possibility of other causes outlined above.

Under the International Classification of Seizures,[4] seizures are classified by whether they appear to start from a localized cortical region (partial onset seizures) or over the entire brain at once (primarily generalized seizures). The classification scheme is outlined in Table 3.1. Partial seizures are caused by localized cortical abnormalities and tend to be acquired in nature, whereas primarily generalized seizures appear to be caused by genetic factors. The partial onset seizure category encompasses seizure types that previously went under several terminologies, including Jacksonian, psychomotor, and temporal lobe seizures. Tonic-clonic (grand mal) seizures that result from spread of the ictus from a focal onset are included in the partial onset seizure category as secondarily generalized tonic-clonic seizures. Partial seizures are further divided by whether they impair consciousness (complex partial seizures) or not (simple partial seizures).

The distinction in seizure onset has important implications for the pathophysiology and therapy of the seizure. Antiepileptic drugs tend to be selective for the seizure type and are analogous to cardiac antiarrhythmic drugs, which are fairly selective for arrhythmia type. Because posttraumatic seizures occur as a result of localized injury to the cerebral cortex, the resulting seizures are of partial onset, with or without secondary generalization. The behavioral manifestations of posttraumatic seizures relate to area of onset, usually in the penumbra of injury. Thus, injuries to the convexity of the brain often result in sensory or primary motor manifestations at seizure onset, such as a migrating paresthesias or twitching and jerking of an extremity. Seizures of the temporal lobe may result in psychic phenomena such as a sensation of fear or *déjà vu*, followed by automatisms, whereas frontal seizure foci often result in aversive motor or more complex behaviors.

During typical complex partial seizures, the patient will often stare and become nonresponsive or poorly responsive to commands. Automatisms frequently occur and take the form of lip smacking, chewing, and fidgeting with objects. Although the patient may spontaneously speak or seem to respond to commands, the language is inappropriate to the situation. The patient may affirm or disagree when questioned but, generally, gives little more than simple responses and does not follow complex commands. Generally, combativeness occurs only when the person is restrained. Thus, when directed aggression occurs, such as seeking out and striking a staff member, the episode most likely is a conscious act and not the result of a seizure. After a complex partial seizure, there is often a several-minute period of confusion and disorientation which represents the postictal state. The patient will often feel tired or exhausted and will frequently go to sleep. When present, a history of postepisode confusion and lethargy often helps to identify episodes as seizures, as it generally does not occur or is brief with spells of other etiologies.

In TBI patients, tonic-clonic (grand mal) seizures result from secondary generalization, i.e., spread of the seizure from the seizure focus at the site of trauma to other parts of the brain, especially the brainstem, which appears to moderate the initial tonic phase of the convulsion.[5] Thus, the tonic-clonic seizure episode often begins as a brief simple or complex partial seizure. The warning, or "aura", that patients often describe is actually the beginning of a seizure that is perceived while the person is conscious and is actually a simple partial seizure.

Tonic-clonic seizures consist of two behavioral phases — the tonic phase and the clonic phase. These phases are easily identified with a careful history. During the tonic phase, there is a sudden stiffening of all extremities. The epileptic cry may occur during this phase as a result of sudden diaphragmatic contraction. After a brief period, the extremities become tremulous. As the tremor slows in frequency, it evolves into a coarse jerking motion resulting in the clonic phase. At the end of the seizure, the jerking slows and ceases. After a tonic-clonic seizure, the person is invariably groggy and disoriented for several minutes. Absence of the tonic phase or postepisode confusion in a person with convulsive behavior should raise the question of nonepileptic episodes, including psychogenic seizures, in patients with a history of convulsive spells. However, the postictal state may be fleeting or indiscernible after brief complex partial seizures. Thus, a minimal postictal state does not exclude seizures when convulsive activity does not occur.

Acute medical management is similar for both partial or tonic-clonic seizures. During the convulsion, the patient should be rolled to one side to avoid aspiration if vomiting occurs. If semiconscious, the patient should be gently directed away from harm. Contrary to common belief, the tongue cannot be swallowed or bitten off and objects should never be forced into the patient's mouth. Insertion of hard objects, such as spoons or "bite sticks", may break teeth and cause serious complications of fragment aspiration and pneumonia. A soft oral airway may be used if it is easily inserted.

Primarily generalized seizures, including absence (petit mal), myoclonic seizures, and tonic-clonic seizures without localized cerebral cortical onset, commonly begin in childhood or adolescence and appear to be idiopathic or genetic in etiology. These epilepsies are diagnosed by their distinctive patterns on the electroencephalogram (EEG), which consist of bilateral synchronous spike-wave patterns. Their onset in patients following traumatic brain injury is highly unusual and should be considered coincidental. It is important to identify these seizure types since absence and myoclonic seizures do not respond to, or may be worsened by, medications used for partial onset seizures, such as phenytoin and carbamazepine.[6,7]

ETIOLOGIC CONSIDERATIONS

Risk factors for posttraumatic epilepsy have been examined in several population studies. However, it is difficult to resolve the relative risk of specific characteristics of injury, such as presence of bleeding and depth of injury, because these markers tend not to be independent variables. For example, although concussion (loss of consciousness) has been considered a risk factor for posttraumatic epilepsy, patients with mild concussive injury alone have only a 0.6% risk of seizures within five years, which is not significantly increased over the incidence of new seizures in the general population.[8]

Data from World War II, the Korean War, and the Vietnam War have provided several data points on risk factors for posttraumatic epilepsy. Overall, the risk for nonmissile head injury was 24% in World War II[9] and 12% during the Korean War.[10] Interestingly, the risk of epilepsy following penetrating missile injury was about 35% for both World War II and the Korean War but was much higher (53%) in the Vietnam War.[11] The differences between studies on Vietnam War veterans and previous war veterans may relate to both improved care of head injury and differences in the nature of injuries. In particular, high-velocity rifles were used in combat and, when combined with improved surgical care, may have resulted in a greater percentage of survivors with epileptogenic lesions.

Risk factors have also been studied in nonmilitary injuries. As outlined above, mild head injuries do not present an increased risk of posttraumatic epilepsy. The incidence of posttraumatic epilepsy after moderate head injuries is 1.6%, and 11.6% after severe injuries.[8] In review of military and nonmilitary injuries, similar risk factors appear. Early seizures (onset less than one week) also appear to be a risk factor for subsequent seizures in several series,[12] but the increased risk appears to be dependent on the severity of head injury.[8] In civilian head injuries, early seizures are not predictive of seizure recurrence when the head injury is mild but do appear to increase risk in moderate to severe injuries.[8] The time of seizure onset also appears to be predictive of seizure recurrence. In wartime injuries, early seizures are associated with seizure recurrence, but the risk of seizure recurrence increases if the onset is greater than one week.[13]

The risk of posttraumatic epilepsy in the presence of an intracerebral hematoma was estimated at 21% in nonmilitary injuries.[8] However, Guidice and Berchou[14] found intracerebral hematomas not to be predictive of posttraumatic epilepsy. This may be due to the fact that CT scans were used routinely in all head-injured patients at their center. Earlier studies, which did not utilize CT scanning, would not have detected intracerebral hemorrhage in milder cases that did not require surgery or were not evident on cerebral angiogram. Alternatively, recent studies have argued that the most predictive factor for posttraumatic seizures is focal CT abnormalities.[12,15] In one small series, the development of posttraumatic epilepsy was correlated with the presence of bone fragments on CT scan studies;[16] however, the scope of this study could not establish whether the risk of bone fragments was independent of injury severity. The type of skull fracture also tends to predict the likelihood of posttraumatic epilepsy. Greater risk occurs in patients with depressed skull fractures[8,12] with intermediate risk for linear convexity or basilar fractures.

The duration of coma appears to be a high risk factor in several studies.[8,14] Genetic susceptibility to epilepsy has been proposed as an important risk factor for posttraumatic epilepsy.[17,18] Although a recent Veterans' Administration (VA) cooperative study indicated a significant familial predisposition in patients with partial onset seizures as a group, there did not appear to be an increased prevalence of epilepsy in families of patients with posttraumatic epilepsy.[19]

When the epidemiologic studies are viewed as a group, it appears that the severity of brain injury best predicts whether posttraumatic epilepsy will occur. While there is debate on the relative risk of any single factor, it is likely that most identified risk factors are indicators of a high degree of brain injury, rather than being specific etiologies. Furthermore, posttraumatic epileptogenesis is probably dependent on several pathophysiologic mechanisms (see below) which may partially explain the large number of identified risk factors.

LABORATORY INVESTIGATIONS FOR POSTTRAUMATIC SEIZURES

When faced with the new onset of seizures, laboratory studies should screen for conditions that may have lowered seizure threshold. Serum chemistries should be drawn to exclude electrolyte imbalances and, minimally, should include sodium, glucose, and calcium levels. A complete blood count may detect a subclinical infection and an arterial blood gas will exclude hypoxia. Imaging studies, consisting of either computerized tomography (CT) or magnetic resonance imaging (MRI) may help identify new lesions contributing to epileptogenesis. Prior to initiation of antiepileptic drug therapy, a complete blood count and liver function studies should be measured to exclude the possibility of an underlying blood dyscrasia or liver disease.

The electroencephalogram (EEG) is a useful tool for evaluating patients with episodic behavioral changes. Interictal abnormalities, such as epileptiform spikes or sharp waves, are often present in patients with epilepsy. A difficulty arises in that interictal abnormalities are transient, much like the seizures they attempt to detect. Thus, a normal EEG does not exclude the possibility of epilepsy. Conversely, an abnormal EEG alone does not diagnose epilepsy. As outlined in later sections, there are important consequences of antiepileptic drug therapy; thus, it is crucial that the TBI patient not be treated solely on the basis of EEG findings. The EEG does provide supportive evidence of a seizure disorder when it is clinically suspected, and its greatest utility lies in its ability to help identify whether the seizure onset is partial or generalized. Despite its limitations, the EEG is one of the most important tests in evaluating epilepsy as it provides electrophysiologic information that cannot be obtained from any other laboratory investigation. Its predictive value in patients with traumatic brain injury is still debated.

A retrospective study of EEG findings in patients with head injury revealed no predictive value of focal or generalized EEG abnormalities.[20] However, this study included all abnormalities and did not specifically assess the risk of epileptiform patterns; thus, the predictive value of EEG in asymptomatic patients remains to be determined. The EEG is valuable as a prognostic factor in persons who have already experienced a seizure. The interictal hallmark of epilepsy is the epileptiform spike or sharp wave. When well-formed and definite, focal spikes are predictive of seizure recurrence in both brain-injured patients[21] and in patients with seizures of unidentified causes.[22]

The EEG study technique should follow the guidelines of the American EEG Society.[23] To briefly summarize, all studies should utilize at least 16 channels of EEG recording to allow for adequate spatial resolution and localization of EEG abnormalities. Gold disk electrodes should be used and attached to the scalp with either collodion or electrode paste to assure low electrical impedance. Needle electrodes should not be used because of their high impedance and the potential risk of blood-borne pathogens. Standard EEG montages should be used, per recommendations of the American EEG Society.[23] Drowsiness and sleep-enhanced expression of epileptiform abnormalities and recording during these stages of consciousness must be performed. The patient should be sleep deprived for the entire night prior to the EEG study as this will increase the probability of recording epileptiform abnormalities and avoid the need for sedation.

There has been much debate over the advantages of special EEG electrodes used to improve the detection of interictal abnormalities. Nasopharyngeal electrodes have been popular for their reported increased sensitivity over standard scalp electrodes. The nasopharyngeal electrode consists of an angled shaft with a small ball-tipped end. They are inserted into each nostril and rotated so that they appose the mesial temporal regions. Insertion of nasopharyngeal electrodes is extremely uncomfortable and may prevent the patient from falling asleep. Nasopharyngeal recordings are highly susceptible to respiration and movement artifact.

Critics of nasopharyngeal electrodes point out that their apparent increased sensitivity results from the montages typically used, rather than their location. Nasopharyngeal montages typically utilize high interelectrode distances, whereas conventional montages utilize closely spaced scalp electrodes. Because differential amplifiers subtract common signals, a weak spike signal may be canceled by conventional bipolar montages which utilize small interelectrode distances. Accordingly, standard scalp electrodes with high-distance electrode montages are probably as effective as nasopharyngeal electrodes at detecting epileptiform abnormalities and are considerably more comfortable.[24,25]

An example of the greater sensitivity of high-distance referential montages over the commonly used bipolar chain montages is shown in Figure 3.1. Other surface electrodes that have been demonstrated to increase sensitivity to temporal spikes include the true anterior temporal (T1 and T2) scalp electrodes[26] and anterior cheek electrodes.[27] Sphenoidal electrodes are fine wires passed through a skin puncture under each zygomatic arch and placed over the foramen ovale. They provide excellent, low-noise recordings but are invasive and uncomfortable. In most cases, sphenoidal electrodes are not routinely utilized in EEG laboratories. At our center, we routinely use standard scalp electrodes with high-distance montages and record referentially from the temporal leads and ear electrodes to the vertex (Cz) in cases of suspected temporal lobe epilepsy.

Prolonged EEG recording may be extremely useful in cases where the cause of altered mental status episodes cannot be ascertained by conventional means and the spells occur with enough frequency to be detected within the designated recording period. Twenty-four-hour ambulatory EEG monitoring is usually available at larger medical centers. These devices continuously record EEG and EKG activity for one day and may be performed on an outpatient basis. There are several limitations to ambulatory recording. In most cases, a total of only eight channels of data may be recorded (usually seven EEG channels and one EKG channel) which limits the ability to localize interictal abnormalities or seizure onset. Thus, an ambulatory EEG recording should not replace a routine 16-channel EEG study for initial workup, just as a cardiac Holter monitor should not replace a standard EKG. The paucity of channels also means that loss of a single recording channel or electrode during the recording session may cause irreplaceable loss of data and render the study inconclusive. As EEG technicians or other health care staff are not present to observe the recording, it may be difficult to later sort artifact from true abnormalities during playback. Moreover, if a diary is not carefully maintained during the recording period or the patient is unable to trigger the alarm on the recording unit reliably, it may not be possible to correlate the episodes in question with the EEG or EKG, or the episode may even be missed entirely. This limitation of ambulatory EEG recording may pose a problem for diagnosis, especially if the patient is unaware of the episodes or they are nonepileptic in etiology. Recent technologic developments now allow 16 channels of ambulatory recording, which provides better spatial resolution of EEG abnormalities; however, the limitations associated with a lack of trained observers remain.

Intensive neuromonitoring involves continuous 16- to 64-channel recording of electroencephalographic, electrocardiographic, and other electrophysiologic data with simultaneous video recording of behavior. It is available at most epilepsy centers and many tertiary

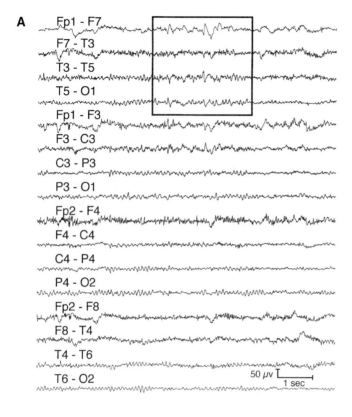

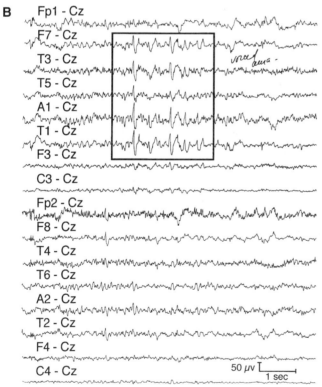

FIGURE 3.1 Effects of EEG montage on detection of epileptic discharges. Two EEG tracings are from the same seizure event (aura) in a patient with intractable complex partial seizures and have been reformatted by computer to standard bipolar and high-distance referential recordings. (A) The EEG has been reformatted to the commonly used bipolar chain montage. The left temporal epileptiform discharge is outlined in the box. Note the minimal change in the tracing during the aura; this is the result of cancellation of epileptiform signals due to the small interelectrode distances. These abnormalities could potentially be ignored or dismissed as insignificant. (B) The same recording has been reformatted with high-distance referential montages so that the temporal leads are referenced to the vertex (Cz). The left temporal epileptiform discharges are again outlined with a box. Note that the EEG changes are now much more obvious and are seen maximally in the left ear (A1) and true anterior temporal (T1) leads. High-distance referential montages are recommended in patients with suspected temporal lobe seizure onset.

care facilities. These studies allow precise correlation of behavioral changes with electrophysiologic data to determine the exact etiologies of the behavioral episodes. In addition, most units allow computer-assisted reformatting of EEG signals to help delineate epileptiform abnormalities. The main drawback of intensive neuromonitoring is the relatively high cost and need for a hospital facility, but in many cases it provides the only means to obtain definitive and conclusive information. It should be reserved for situations where the diagnosis cannot be determined by usual means or when nonepileptic spells are suspected. Intensive neuromonitoring is essential for localization of epileptic foci when epilepsy surgery is contemplated.

POTENTIAL EPILEPTOGENESIS OF PSYCHOTROPIC MEDICATIONS

Behavioral and affective disorders are common after traumatic brain injury, and it is often necessary to treat the brain-injured patient with psychotropic medications. Of concern is whether these agents lower seizure threshold. In overdose, tricyclic antidepressants induce seizures and status epilepticus, but it is less clear to what extent they are proconvulsant at clinically effective doses. Many reports of tricyclic-induced seizures are retrospective and do not take into account the normal incidence of new onset seizures. When drug monitoring has been instituted to avoid high levels, the risk has been estimated at only 0.4%.[28] Although a 0.2% risk of seizures has been estimated for fluoxetine therapy on the basis of preclinical trials, fluoxetine is anticonvulsant in experiments using epileptic rodents with convulsive seizures.[29] In a retrospective study of persons with depression and established epilepsy, antidepressant therapy actually improved seizure frequency in the majority (56%) of patients.[30] This raises the question of whether this positive effect on seizure control occurs indirectly, i.e., through improvement of depression or, instead, by directly raising seizure threshold. Interestingly, a double-blind placebo study has demonstrated imipramine to be effective adjunctive antiepileptic therapy in intractable atonic, myoclonic, and absence epilepsy in subjects without affective problems.[31,32] Thus, at nontoxic levels, tricyclic antidepressants may possess anticonvulsant properties for certain seizure types, despite being proconvulsant at toxic levels. This bimodal response is frequently seen in other drugs with anticonvulsant properties, most notably phenytoin, carbamazepine, and lidocaine.

The ability of tricyclic antidepressants to increase seizure frequency may be selective for seizure type. For example, a selective increase of tonic-clonic seizures may occur with use of imipramine or maprotiline in patients with mixed seizure types.[32] Neuroleptics are frequently utilized in the posttraumatic state for agitated behavior and there are several reports of their proconvulsant effect. Unfortunately, little data exist on the actual risks of antidepressants and neuroleptics in the setting of traumatic brain injury. However, from existing information on these agents, it appears that the actual clinical risk of seizure exacerbation by psychotropic medications is small and is usually far outweighed by the need to effectively manage a severe affective or disruptive state in the TBI patient. Thus, these medications should be used when necessary for psychiatric and behavioral problems.

THERAPY OF POSTTRAUMATIC SEIZURES

Initiation of antiepileptic drug therapy should begin only after careful evaluation of the patient and seizures have been clearly identified. Almost all clinicians will begin therapy once two seizures have occurred, but there is debate on whether therapy should be initiated after the first seizure. Many clinicians will not treat a single seizure without recurrence; others will treat, depending on the situation. As outlined in later sections, there are clearly no firm data to justify antiepileptic drug therapy in TBI patients who have not experienced a seizure.

TABLE 3.2 Antiepileptic Drugs Useful in the Treatment of Posttraumatic Epilepsy

Drug	Efficacy	Toxicity	Pros	Cons
Phenytoin	+++	++	Inexpensive Long half-life	Nonlinear kinetics Cosmetic, gait problems
Carbamazepine	+++	++	Linear kinetics	Hyponatremia common Dizziness Short half-life
Valproic acid	+++	++	Linear kinetics	Tremor Nausea Divided doses Short half-life
Felbamate	+++	++	Linear kinetics Long half-life	Nausea, anorexia Weight loss Insomnia Headaches Aplastic anemia
Gabapentin	++	+	Linear kinetics Not metabolized by liver Very low toxicity No antiepileptic drug interactions	Short half-life Currently approved for add-on therapy only
Primidone	+++	+++[a]	Linear kinetics Possibly less sedating than phenobarbital	Short half-life; metabolized to phenobarbital Sedation, psychosis Severe cognitive impairment
Phenobarbital	+++	+++[a]	Linear kinetics Inexpensive Long half-life	Sedation Severe cognitive impairment

[a] Phenobarbital and primidone are not recommended for therapy of posttraumatic epilepsy because of their high neurotoxicity.

Selection of antiepileptic drug therapy must be based on several factors, including efficacy for seizure type and side effects. A specific antiepileptic drug may be quite selective for seizure type, thus necessitating seizure classification. Posttraumatic epilepsy is caused by focal or multifocal injury and consists of partial onset seizures and secondarily generalized tonic-clonic seizures. Accordingly, appropriate antiepileptic drugs for posttraumatic epilepsy are those used for partial onset seizures. The most commonly used antiepileptic drugs are listed in Table 3.2.

A multicenter, double-blind, randomized study compared the efficacy of phenytoin, carbamazepine, primidone, and phenobarbital against partial onset seizures. All of the drugs were equally efficacious in terms of seizure control.[33] However, barbiturates were tolerated poorly, resulting in a high dropout rate in these treatment groups. It is likely that there are also individual differences in response to any given antiepileptic drug. Thus, a nonresponder to one medication should be systematically tried on each of the other major antiepileptic drugs.

Similar results were obtained in a British study involving patients with newly diagnosed partial onset epilepsy which compared the efficacy of carbamazepine, phenytoin, and valproic acid.[34] Valproic acid exhibited the same efficacy as phenytoin and carbamazepine against partial onset seizures and convulsion, suggesting its usefulness for these seizure types.

However, a recent VA cooperative study compared the efficacy of carbamazepine to valproic acid for partial onset seizures and indicated a modest but significantly lower efficacy of valproic acid against complex partial seizures.[35] Valproic acid appeared to be equally effective to carbamazepine against secondarily generalized tonic-clonic seizures. Nonetheless, valproic acid is generally well tolerated; thus, it should be considered for patients who are unresponsive or intolerant to phenytoin and carbamazepine.

All antiepileptic drugs may cause significant problems with neurotoxicity and pose problems for the TBI patient. Indeed, all antiepileptic drugs commonly cause ataxia at high levels and may also exacerbate gait abnormalities at lower levels, in some patients. This may present a problem to the patient who is returning to ambulation. There is a significant incidence of hyponatremia in carbamazepine-treated patients over the age of 25.[36] A common side effect of valproic acid that may pose a problem to the TBI patient is postural tremor. In general, the tremor does not cause problems with daily activities but can be troublesome in patients who are prone to postural tremor. The tremor is reversible, dose dependent, and responds to a dose reduction or other medications that block essential tremor (propranolol, primidone). Because the barbiturates, including phenobarbital and primidone, are poorly tolerated and result in a high incidence of cognitive impairment, they should be used only as a last resort in TBI patients, when they are unable to take other medications or are completely refractory to other antiepileptic medications.

Three anticonvulsants (felbamate, gabapentin, lamotrigine) have been recently approved for use in partial onset seizures. They appear to have high therapeutic indices, i.e., a wide window between efficacy and toxicity, and have been demonstrated to be effective in double-blind controlled studies.[37-39] However, use of felbamate has been restricted by the FDA for use in severe intractable epilepsy only, because of an increased risk of aplastic anemia. This risk is estimated by the FDA to be 1:2000. The addition of these new drugs will provide alternatives for patients who do not tolerate or respond to current antiepileptic drugs and will, it is hoped, eliminate the need for the highly toxic barbiturates. Undoubtedly, they will be tested in posttraumatic epilepsy and may provide a better armamentarium for this problem.

In general, antiepileptic drugs should be introduced slowly to avoid problems with neurotoxicity. If introduced too quickly, carbamazepine may cause severe dizziness and valproic acid may cause nausea. When multiple seizures or status epilepticus occurs, phenytoin is easiest to rapidly introduce. After initiation, the dose should be upwardly titrated until seizures are controlled or clinical neurotoxicity is reached. The latter should be assessed clinically by periodic examination of gait, intentional tremor, and presence of drowsiness, cognitive impairment, or nystagmus. Drug plasma levels may be utilized to provide a rough guideline for therapy but should not be used as the sole indicator of therapy or toxicity.[40]

Phenytoin is unique among the commonly used antiepileptic drugs in that it saturates its metabolic enzymes at therapeutic levels which results in zero-order kinetic elimination. As a result, the effective half-life is variable and becomes longer with higher levels of phenytoin. As a result of nonlinear kinetics, there is a proportionate increase of serum level at low doses of phenytoin, but at therapeutic levels small increments result in marked elevations of levels.[41] This phenomenon is responsible for what is mistakenly identified as wild fluctuations in phenytoin levels. The long half-life resulting from higher levels means that steady state may not be achieved for weeks. This often causes the patient to become toxic despite the fact that "therapeutic levels" were obtained one week after the dose change. Pediatric tablets (50 mg) and 30 mg capsules are often very useful for these situations.

In all cases, the therapeutic plan should strive for a single antiepileptic drug regimen. Monotherapy has been shown to be more efficacious than polytherapy and minimizes toxicity, drug interactions, and cost.[42,43]

NEURAL MECHANISMS OF POSTTRAUMATIC EPILEPSY

Brain damage resulting from traumatic head injury can significantly impair physical, cognitive, and social function. Recovery from deficits caused by the brain damage can be variable, and permanent neurological disability occurs in as many as 90,000 survivors of head injury in the United States.[44] These disabilities are further compounded by posttraumatic epilepsy, which results not only in spontaneous and unpredictable seizure recurrence but also in toxicities associated with antiepileptic drug therapies. Given the high incidence of head injury and the degree to which posttraumatic epilepsy can impact on quality of life, a better understanding of mechanisms underlying posttraumatic epileptogenesis is warranted. An improved understanding could lead to therapies that decrease the likelihood of posttraumatic epilepsy without compromising recovery from brain injury.

Studies on posttraumatic epileptogenesis implicate several pathologic etiologies that may induce a seizure focus. These etiologies may be broadly separated into those related to the acute insult (i.e., penetration of parenchyma, shearing forces, and disruption of blood-brain barrier) and those caused by late sequelae (i.e., vascular disruption, cicatricial pulling, and synaptic reorganization). Given the wide variations of brain injury and complications, it is unlikely that any single mechanism is responsible for posttraumatic epileptogenesis. Thus, posttraumatic epileptogenesis probably utilizes combinations of several mechanisms, especially those that are supported by scientific studies and concur with clinical aspects of posttraumatic epilepsy.

In 1930, Foerster and Penfield induced seizure activity by electrical stimulation of areas surrounding a gunshot lesion of cerebral cortex. These findings suggested the presence of an epileptic zone or penumbra surrounding the site of brain injury. Furthermore, retraction of dura that had become adherent to the damaged cortex also triggered seizures. They concluded that posttraumatic seizures are most likely to occur after dural penetration, which induces formation of scar tissue between brain and dura, and subsequent pulling of the ipsilateral and, sometimes, contralateral hemispheres toward the lesion, as a result of contraction brought about by normal maturation of the scar (cicatricial contraction).[45] This hypothesis is supported by clinical findings that head injuries associated with dural penetration are associated with the highest incidence of posttraumatic epilepsy (27 to 43%).[18]

Additional putative mechanisms include glial cell proliferation and damage to blood vessels, axon collaterals, and blood-brain barrier, each of which is known to precipitate brain injury.[46] Jasper hypothesized that the toxicity of extravasated blood increases neuronal activity abnormally in some brain regions and disrupts blood flow in others. These pathophysiologic changes could result in the alternating periods of seizure activity and functional neuronal depression that characterize acute status epilepticus induced by brain contusion.[46] Alternatively, damage to inhibitory axon collaterals by shearing forces may result in reduction of inhibitory tone and excessive depolarization that ultimately produce seizure discharges.[46] However, overt penetration of dura and disruption of brain parenchyma may not be absolute requisites for posttraumatic epilepsy.

Lowenstein and colleagues recently reported that extradural fluid percussion induces profound decreases in hippocampal hilar neurons and hyperexcitability of dentate granule cells in rodents.[47] Thus, even nonpenetrating brain injury can cause pathologic changes in brain structures with aberrant excitability that induces posttraumatic seizures. These findings could help explain the emergence of posttraumatic epilepsy in persons with milder, low velocity head injuries who do not appear to have frank penetration of dura or intracerebral bleeding.

Perhaps one of the more intriguing hypotheses of posttraumatic epilepsy has been the implication of blood breakdown products, particularly hemosiderin, in the cellular events that lead to epileptogenesis. An important role for iron deposition has been supported by experimental studies in animals. Subpial iontophoresis of ferrous or ferric chloride into sensorimotor cortex of cat or rat induces a chronic epileptic focus with many striking similarities to lesions in human posttraumatic epilepsy.[48,49] Electrocorticographic seizure activity is observed within 48 hours after injection and behavioral convulsions occur between 48 hours and five days. These abnormalities recur spontaneously and persist for more than twelve weeks after injection.[49] Examination of the iron-induced focus reveals many histopathologic changes found in posttraumatic epileptic foci from humans:[48] a meningocerebral cicatrix, consisting of fibroblasts and iron-laden macrophages, surrounds the iron injection cavity with neuronal loss and gliosis occurring next to the injection site. Hypertrophied astrocytes encompass the entire iron focus. It has been hypothesized that a cascade of events is initiated by the iron focus and results in the genesis of a posttraumatic epileptic focus. Breakdown of blood from brain injury-induced extravasation creates iron deposits that may induce free-radical oxidant formation and subsequent lipid peroxidation.[50] In support of this hypothesis is the finding that antioxidant administration reduces the incidence of iron-induced seizure activity,[51] although it remains unclear exactly how lipid peroxidation induces posttraumatic epileptogenesis.

The mechanisms discussed so far largely address seizure activity that occurs acutely following brain injury. However, the onset of posttraumatic seizures is bimodal — the highest peak in incidence occurs during the first week (early onset seizures) and a secondary peak occurs at about six months.[52] This latency suggests there is a maturation process resulting in the genesis of an epileptic focus. Thus, the notion that posttraumatic epilepsy may be prevented remains attractive and has been the subject of many studies (see below).

Not all persons who have exhibited posttraumatic seizures in the acutely injured state develop epilepsy (i.e., spontaneous recurrent seizures), and it is quite probable that additional neuronal mechanisms are involved in the transition from a single symptomatic seizure episode to an epileptic state where seizures recur spontaneously. That is, events linked specifically to the brain injury may initiate posttraumatic seizures which subsequently induce a sequence of events that facilitate further recurrences.

An attractive explanation is based upon the long-standing belief that "seizures beget seizures." This notion is supported by a prospective study of unselected patients with new onset of seizures which demonstrated that the probability of seizure control was inversely related to the number of seizures experienced prior to initiation of antiepileptic drug therapy.[53,54] Furthermore, the time interval between seizures appears to decrease with subsequent episodes in untreated patients.[55] This concept has been explored in the animal model of "kindling".

Kindling refers to a phenomenon in which a brain region may be rendered permanently epileptic when subjected to brief, repeated electrical stimulations that, alone, would not induce behavioral seizures.[56] This paradigm, in which the brain "learns" to seize, has been used to study epileptogenesis and neuronal plasticity. Typically, electrical stimulation is administered by an implanted depth electrode and, initially, results only in a brief localized epileptiform discharge on EEG, without a behavioral response. With continued daily stimulation, there are progressive increases in duration of both EEG epileptiform discharges and motor seizure activity.

The resulting convulsive behavior evolves through stages that are highly reproducible from animal to animal and may be graded by levels of behavioral severity.[57] Stage 0 is no behavioral response; Stage 1 consists of chewing motion; and Stage 2 consists of head nodding. At Stage 3, the animal displays clonus (jerking) of forelimbs, and at Stage 4, there is forelimb clonus with rearing onto hind limbs. The fifth and most severe stage consists of forelimb clonus with rearing and falling.

Thus, kindling of seizure activity induces neuronal changes within the brain that result in more severe generalized seizures from a stimulus that initially produced only focal seizure activity. Similar mechanisms may be utilized in the genesis of posttraumatic epilepsy. If this is the case, then an understanding of the kindling phenomenon in experimental animals could shed light on the causes of posttraumatic epileptogenesis.

Numerous transient and long-term changes occur in several neurotransmitter systems during electrical kindling.[58] The most dramatic and enduring changes are seen within the excitatory and inhibitory amino acid transmitter systems. Indeed, kindled seizures are dependent upon, and further produce, overactivation of excitatory amino acid transmission and reduction of inhibitory amino acid transmission. Because sequelae of brain injury bring about aberrations in the excitatory and inhibitory systems, this discussion will focus on how these abnormalities may underlie posttraumatic epileptogenesis.

The *N*-methyl-D-aspartate (NMDA) receptor is a glutamate receptor subtype. It is activated under conditions of high neuronal synaptic activity, including seizures. When activated, the NMDA receptor opens a channel that permits calcium entry into the neuron. This calcium influx may then signal further biochemical changes within the neuron that mediate neuronal plasticity, including long-lasting enhancement of excitatory amino acid transmission (long-term potentiation), neurite outgrowth, and neuronal migration.[59,60] An NMDA receptor mediated increase of excitatory neurotransmission also appears to play a crucial role in the hippocampal slice model of epileptogenesis *in vitro*[61] and during kindling *in vivo*.[62,63]

Gamma-aminobutyric acid (GABA) is the major inhibitory neurotransmitter within the brain. It exerts its inhibitory effect, directly, by opening a chloride channel or, indirectly, by a potassium channel. Kindling significantly reduces neuronal sensitivity to GABA; the changes are long lasting and may be seen at four and twelve weeks after the last fully kindled (Stage 5) seizure.[64-67] Loss of sensitivity to GABA evolves during the course of kindling and correlates with seizure severity.[64] These changes are believed to result from a compensatory desensitization of the receptor in response to increased GABA release during the electrical kindling process.[68,69] Thus, the very mechanisms utilized by the brain to suppress kindling may be counterproductive and ultimately facilitate the kindling process.

How might traumatic brain injury bring about the imbalances between neuronal excitation and inhibition that lead to posttraumatic epileptogenesis? One possibility is that shearing forces during the head injury damage inhibitory axon collaterals and result in loss of neuronal inhibition. The decreased inhibitory control would increase network excitability which, in the short term, would result in seizure activity and, in the long term, could lead to a chronic epileptic state. Alternatively, posttraumatic epileptogenesis may not be dependent on axonal loss but, rather, aberrant neurite sprouting and regeneration. Structural reorganization of synapses occurs during kindling. Specifically, kindling causes sprouting of mossy fibers in the hippocampus.[70,71]

Another plausible explanation for posttraumatic epileptogenesis is alterations in blood flow that occur following brain injury. Brain injury disrupts vascularization at the site of damage as well as in areas "downstream" from the insult. Disruption in blood flow could bring about both ischemic and hypoxic conditions which produce significant increases in synaptic glutamate release and decreased inactivation of glutamate. Overactivation of glutamate receptors, including NMDA receptor activation, results in excessive Ca^{2+} influx[72] which promotes phosphorylation of the $GABA_A$ receptor to its nonfunctional, desensitized state.[73] Taken together, trauma-induced disruption of normal brain function could result in a state that both primes the brain for acute seizures and provides the foundation for long-term changes that render the brain chronically epileptic.

PROPHYLAXIS OF SEIZURES: PROS AND CONS

There is much controversy concerning the practice of antiepileptic drug prophylaxis after head injury. Although clinicians commonly institute antiepileptic drugs after head injury, there is little evidence that they are effective in preventing posttraumatic epilepsy. Several early studies suggested a beneficial effect of prophylactic anticonvulsant therapy,[74,75] but later controlled studies failed to support these findings. Recently, the effects of phenytoin on the incidence of posttraumatic seizures were studied in a double-blind, randomized fashion.[76] Unlike previous studies, phenytoin levels were maintained in the high therapeutic range to reduce the possibility that the reported lack of efficacy was caused by inadequate dosaging. This study demonstrated that, although phenytoin prophylaxis reduces the incidence of early seizures (i.e., those occurring within the first week after injury), there was no difference in long-term outcome over the placebo group.

The lack of effectiveness of antiepileptic drugs in preventing posttraumatic epilepsy is also paralleled in experimental kindling studies. Although many antiepileptic drugs may block fully kindled convulsions in animals, they do not prevent the kindling process and do not prevent the increases in seizure severity. Accordingly, phenytoin and carbamazepine may block seizures but do not consistently prevent epileptogenesis from occurring.[77,78] In contrast, phenobarbital and benzodiazepines do appear to be antiepileptogenic in that they are effective in slowing the progression of amygdala-kindled seizures.[79-81] Valproic acid has also been found to retard the rate of amygdala kindling but only when used at high doses with significant toxicities.[82,83] Currently, there are no data from controlled studies regarding the use of barbiturates or benzodiazepines in humans for seizure prophylaxis. However, the high toxicity of these medications would make their long-term use impractical in the TBI population. Clinical trials for valproic acid have been proposed but results from such a trial will not be available for several years.

Perhaps the largest obstacle in the quest for effective pharmacologic prophylaxis is the high probability that neural mechanisms that underlie the development of the epileptic state are not the same as those utilized during acute seizure initiation. It should be noted that seizures may occur in normal persons under extreme conditions such as hypoxia or hypoglycemia; it is the condition of spontaneous seizure recurrence that defines the epileptic condition. Thus, the key to achieving prophylaxis for posttraumatic epilepsy may lie in studying mechanisms that regulate seizure propensity, i.e., those mechanisms that chronically raise or lower seizure threshold in brain regions. It is likely that posttraumatic epilepsy is the result of altered regulation of critical neuronal networks, which then permits spontaneous seizure initiation under normal conditions. At present, drug development paradigms screen for drugs that block chemically induced seizures or electroshock in normal animals. Potential drugs are initially selected only for their ability to antagonize seizures of acute symptomatic causes rather than prevent maturation of a chronic epileptic network. This is clearly a limitation of current drug screening programs.

Furthermore, clinical testing of new drugs generally involves persons with established epilepsy and, again, does not discern if medications can prevent the development of the epileptic state. In contrast, use of paradigms that involve inhibition of epileptogenesis as an endpoint could result in drugs with antiepileptogenic properties, i.e., the ability to prevent epilepsy. At present, there are only a few algorithms that could screen drugs for antiepileptogenic properties. In animals, this would mean using inhibition of kindling as an endpoint or the ability to reverse predisposition to seizure in genetically epilepsy-prone animal models. Clinical testing would prove more difficult since it would require prospective testing in persons at risk for epilepsy who have not had seizure recurrences.

The notion that antiepileptogenic agents may be identified is supported by the electrical kindling paradigm. As outlined above, the NMDA receptor appears to play a key role in events that underlie long-term neuronal changes. Antagonists that directly compete for this receptor inhibit the progression of electrically kindled seizures but have relatively less effect on seizures once kindling has been achieved.[84] This suggests a potential antiepileptogenic role of NMDA receptor antagonists that is independent of its ability to block acute seizures. Similarly, administration of the alpha$_1$ adrenergic receptor agonist, clonidine, can significantly retard the rate of evolution of kindled seizure stage but, by itself, does not block the fully established kindled seizure.[85,86] A key role of noradrenergic neurotransmission in the regulation of epileptogenesis has been proposed.[87,88] In contrast, currently used antiepileptic drugs may not affect the pathophysiologic processes resulting in spontaneous seizure recurrence. Thus, the need for more satisfactory antiepileptogenic therapy will necessitate a change in current experimental drug development paradigms so that potential prophylactic drugs may be screened. Use of models of epilepsy, rather than acute seizures, holds great promise for future development of antiepileptogenic drugs. These models include the electrical kindling paradigm and studies in genetically seizure-prone animals. Ultimately, the effectiveness of a drug as an antiepileptogenic agent will require prospective, placebo-controlled trials in the TBI and other high-risk patients.

POSTTRAUMATIC EPILEPSY: IMPLICATIONS FOR NEUROLOGIC RECOVERY

The appearance of posttraumatic epilepsy poses significant problems for rehabilitation of the TBI patient. The uncertainty caused by randomly occurring loss of consciousness places yet an additional barrier to independence. At worst, uncontrolled epilepsy may necessitate placement in specialized care facilities and, at the least, may prohibit driving privileges. Some data suggest the impact of posttraumatic epilepsy on neurorehabilitation may extend beyond these social aspects and could actually impede brain recovery. World War II veterans with head injury who developed posttraumatic epilepsy had a lower survival rate than veterans without epilepsy.[89] The incidence and severity of cognitive deficit in hemiplegic children is highly correlated with the presence of seizure activity, independent of the amount of cerebral damage.[90] A recent retrospective study on head-injured patients demonstrated that functional measures were lower in patients that developed posttraumatic epilepsy upon entry into rehabilitation than those who did not. Although both groups improved significantly, functional outcome remained lower in the epileptic group.[91]

However, this study could not address the question of whether seizures directly affect brain recovery or whether posttraumatic epilepsy only reflects the severity of brain injury. Because posttraumatic epileptogenesis is most likely to occur after the most severe head injuries, it is difficult to isolate the effect of posttraumatic epilepsy on brain recovery from the many other variables, including potential negative effects of antiepileptic drug therapy. This is a major limitation for most studies that attempt to understand the effects of seizures on cognitive or behavioral deficits in humans. Several experimental animal studies have addressed this question and provide evidence that certain types of seizures adversely affect brain recovery while other types do not.

Although brief seizures do not cause brain damage, prolonged seizures cause neuronal death by excitotoxic mechanisms.[92] It is possible that neurons previously compromised by trauma are rendered susceptible to seizure activity that would otherwise be tolerated. Learning is impaired in young rodents undergoing repetitive and frequent audiogenic seizures.[93] In contrast, repetitive kindled seizures do not appear to affect learning and memory.[94] Clinical studies have shown that simple abnormal EEG activity is associated with impaired cognition[95] and that response time is impaired even during single focal interictal spikes in humans.[96] These results suggest that, at least in some situations, seizures may inhibit learning.

Interestingly, posttraumatic seizures may be the result of adaptive mechanisms initiated by the injured brain in its attempt to restore normal neuronal activity. Experimental data in animal studies suggest that mild, infrequent seizures are beneficial to a recovering brain.[97-99] As can be seen in Figure 3.2, animals that experienced "mild" (Stage 0) amygdala-kindled seizures in the first six days after frontal cortex damage recovered from deficits slightly faster than nonkindled/lesioned controls.[99] In contrast, animals that experienced a more severe seizure type (Stage 1) within the first six days after lesion failed to recover from somatosensory deficits in the first three months.[99] Similarly, the effects of amygdala kindling on spatial memory (working and reference) have been investigated in animals.[100] Kindled seizures, of any severity, have no effect on spatial working memory or established reference memory but do impair acquisition of spatial reference memory when the transition from partial to generalized kindled seizure activity occurs.

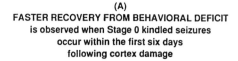

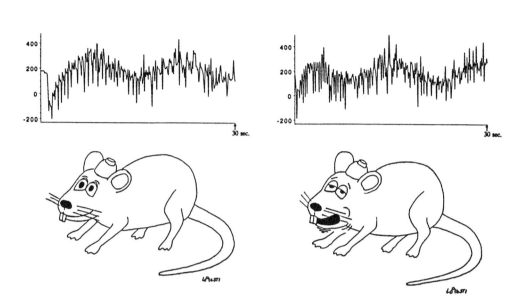

FIGURE 3.2   Effect of seizure severity on outcome of experimental brain injury. The tracings display representative amygdala-kindled EEG seizure activity (AD = after discharge) and ictal behavior observed in rats during the first six days after lesion. (A) Typical EEG activity (total AD=38 sec) is displayed during a Stage 0 kindled seizure. The rat is immobile and exhibits no convulsive behavior. When Stage 0 kindled seizure activity occurs during the first six days after brain damage, recovery from behavioral deficits occurs at a slightly faster rate than nonkindled/lesioned controls, and significantly faster than rats that experienced Stage 1 kindled seizures. (B) EEG activity (total AD=50 sec) is displayed during a Stage 1 kindled seizure. During these seizures, the rat exhibits pronounced chewing. When Stage 1 kindled seizure activity occurs during the first six days after brain damage, recovery from behavioral deficits is significantly delayed when compared to nonkindled/lesioned control rats or rats that experienced Stage 0 kindled seizures.

In summary, experimental data suggest the effect of seizures on functional recovery of the injured brain may be bimodal. While recurrent and/or severe seizures may have a negative impact on recovery, mild, infrequent seizures can facilitate behavioral recovery. Thus, it is only when the seizures are severe enough to cause further brain damage, or frequent enough to develop into intractable epilepsy, that they are detrimental to the behavioral recovery and quality of life.

ANTIEPILEPTIC DRUG-INDUCED COGNITIVE IMPAIRMENT AND NEUROREHABILITATION

Because traumatic brain injury may theoretically lead to kindling of epilepsy and seizure-induced inhibition of functional recovery, it would seem justified to place all severely head-injured patients on antiepileptic prophylaxis. However, antiepileptic drug therapy is not without neuropsychologic costs to the TBI patient. It has been argued that, since brain injury carries only an approximate 5% risk for posttraumatic epilepsy, the remaining 95% needlessly receive anticonvulsant medication.[101] This group of patients is exposed to the toxicities of anticonvulsant administration without any potential benefit. It has been fairly well established that, even in normal volunteers, antiepileptic drugs cause significant cognitive impairment, albeit minor in many cases.[102] Barbiturates commonly cause problems with cognitive impairment. Although an earlier study suggested that carbamazepine induced less cognitive impairment than phenytoin,[103] this may have been due to toxic levels of phenytoin in this series. When the data was reexamined so that patients with toxic phenytoin levels were removed from the previous study, no significant differences in cognitive impairment could be found between each treated group.[104] A later study, which maintained levels in therapeutic ranges, verified these findings.[105] In addition, phenobarbital was shown to induce marked cognitive impairment, even at low levels. Although valproic acid is thought to cause minimal problems with cognition, withdrawal of this medication improved psychometric scores.[106] In TBI patients, antiepileptic drug-induced impairment could cause further compromise of cognitive function. In experiences at our center, several TBI patients have had improvement of concentration and cognitive complaints following withdrawal of antiepileptic drugs.

A potential mechanism by which anticonvulsants may adversely affect the recovering brain could be their ability to suppress repetitive firing, which is important for long-term potentiation, a phenomenon associated with learning (see Chapter 9 of this volume). Suppression of repetitive firing could be counterproductive following brain injury, especially since neuronal depression already occurs as a consequence of brain injury. This condition of postinjury neuronal depression has been referred to as *diaschisis,*[107] which is the temporary disruption of neuronal activity in undamaged areas functionally related to injured areas.

Evidence that diaschisis occurs after brain injury has been well established with measures of blood flow, metabolism, electrical activity, and neurotransmitter levels.[108-111] Moreover, this depression of neuronal activity after brain injury has been correlated with behavioral deficits, and restoration of normal neuronal activity correlates with behavioral recovery.[112,113] In support of this notion, Dikmen and colleagues[114] demonstrated that phenytoin prophylaxis impairs recovery from cognitive deficits in both moderately and severely head-injured patients. When combined with the lack of efficacy in preventing seizures beyond the first week, it is extremely difficult to justify the practice of phenytoin prophylaxis.

Barbiturates and benzodiazepines directly modulate the $GABA_A$ receptor and increase neuronal inhibition. This receptor appears to be important in modulating memory processes within the brain.[115] Drugs affecting this receptor inhibit learning in normal animals, whereas antagonists of this site improve memory tasks.[116,117] The amnestic effect of benzodiazepines is also seen readily in humans who have received intravenous benzodiazepines for brief surgical procedures, and even single doses cause memory impairment and attention deficits in normal persons.[118]

Data from animal studies provide further evidence that barbiturates and benzodiazepines inhibit recovery from brain injury. If diazepam is administered during the first three weeks after unilateral anteromedial cortex damage, recovery from somatosensory deficits is delayed indefinitely.[119] Even if diazepam is administered only for the first seven days after brain damage, recovery is significantly delayed.[120,121] Phenobarbital also appears to interfere with somatosensory and motor recovery following brain damage in rats and nonhuman primates.[122,123]

Several anticonvulsants currently under investigation for human epilepsy also appear to augment GABA mechanisms and could conceivably cause problems for recovery in TBI patients. These drugs include GABA reuptake inhibitors, GABA-transaminase inhibitors, and GABA agonists. Less experimental data are available on the effects of other antiepileptic drugs on functional recovery after brain injury. However, since most antiepileptic drugs either inhibit repetitive firing or increase GABA mediated inhibition, they should be used judiciously and not given for prophylaxis until studies identify effective antiepileptogenic therapies.

CONCLUSIONS

The accurate diagnosis of episodic behaviors is crucial to providing the most appropriate therapy for TBI patients. Although posttraumatic epilepsy is a common entity, it may be difficult to recognize. Posttraumatic epilepsy must be carefully distinguished from other types of behavioral spells because either unnecessary antiepileptic drug therapy or uncontrolled seizures may potentially impair neurologic recovery. At present, there is little evidence to support prophylactic use of anticonvulsants in TBI patients as they do not prevent epileptogenesis clinically and much data implicates a negative effect on cognition and recovery of brain function. Thus, antiepileptic drug therapy should be withheld until there is a *bona fide* diagnosis of epilepsy, i.e., at least two separate seizure events that are not due to transient metabolic derangements. Once the diagnosis of epilepsy is secure, effective therapy should be initiated promptly to prevent the deleterious effects of uncontrolled seizures on brain recovery. Future research will need to address whether control of posttraumatic epilepsy improves functional outcome and if these gains outweigh the adverse effects of antiepileptic drug therapy. In addition, the mechanisms of posttraumatic seizures will need to be better understood so that therapies that prevent epileptogenesis may be achieved.

ACKNOWLEDGMENT

The authors thank David LoPresti for his help in preparing the illustrations for this chapter.

REFERENCES

1. McEvoy, J. P., McCue, M., Spring, B., Mohs, R. C., Lavori, P. W., and Farr, R. M., Effects of amantadine and trihexyphenidyl on memory in elderly normal volunteers, *Am. J. Psychiatry,* 144, 573, 1987.
2. Potamianos, G. and Kellett, J. M., Anti-cholinergic drugs and memory: The effects of benzhexol on memory in a group of geriatric patients, *Br. J. Psychiatry,* 140, 470, 1982.
3. Cross-National Collaborative Panic Study, Second Phase Investigators, Drug treatment of panic disorder. Comparative efficacy of alprazolam, imipramine, and placebo, *Br. J. Psychiatry,* 160, 191, 1992.
4. Commission on Classification and Terminology of the International League Against Epilepsy, Proposal for revised clinical and electroencephalographic classification of epileptic seizures, *Epilepsia,* 22, 268, 1981.
5. Browning, R. A. and Nelson D. K., Modification of electroshock and pentylenetetrazol seizure patterns in rats after precollicular transections, *Exp. Neurol.,* 93, 546, 1986.
6. Levy, L. L. and Fenichel, G. M., Diphenylhydantoin activated seizures, *Neurology,* 15, 716, 1965.
7. Snead, O. C., III, and Hosey, L. C., Exacerbation of seizures in children by carbamazepine, *N. Engl. J. Med.,* 313, 916, 1985.
8. Annegers, J. F., Grabow, J. D., Groover, R. V., Laws, E. R., Elveback, L. R., and Kurland, L. T., Seizures after head trauma: A population study, *Neurology,* 30, 683, 1980.
9. Walker, A. E. and Jablon, S., A follow-up study of head wounds in World War II. *Veterans' Administration Monograph,* Veterans Administration, Washington, DC, 1961.
10. Caveness, W. F., Walker, A. E., and Ascroft, P. B., Incidence of post-traumatic epilepsy in Korean veterans as compared with those from World War I and World War II, *J. Neurosurg.,* 19, 122, 1962.
11. Salazar, A. M., Jabbari, B., Vance, S. C., Grafman, J., Amin, D., and Dillon, J. D., Epilepsy after penetrating head injury. I. Clinical correlates: A report of the Vietnam Head Injury Study, *Neurology,* 35, 1406, 1985.
12. Pagni, C. A., Posttraumatic epilepsy. Incidence and prophylaxis, *Acta Neurochir.,* S50, 38, 1990.
13. Weiss, G. H. and Caveness, W. F., Prognostic factors in the persistence of posttraumatic epilepsy, *J. Neurosurg.,* 37, 164, 1972.
14. Guidice, M. A. and Berchou, R. C., Post-traumatic epilepsy following head injury, *Brain Injury,* 1, 61, 1987.
15. D'Alessandro, R., Tinuper, P., Ferrara, R., Cortelli, P., Pazzaglia, P., Sabattini, L., Frank, G., and Lugaresi, E., CT scan prediction of late post-traumatic epilepsy, *J. Neurol. Neurosurg. Psychiatry,* 45, 1153, 1982.
16. Askenasy, J. J. M., Association of intracerebral bone fragments and epilepsy in missile head injuries, *Acta Neurol. Scand.,* 79, 47, 1989.
17. Hughes, J. R., Post-traumatic epilepsy in the military, *Mil. Med.,* 151, 416, 1986.
18. Caveness, W. F., Meirowsky, A. M., Rish, B. L., Mohr, J. P., Kistler, J. P., Dillon, J. D., and Weis, G. H., The nature of posttraumatic epilepsy, *J. Neurosurg.,* 50, 545, 1979.
19. Treiman, D. M., Genetics of the partial epilepsies, in *Genetics of the Epilepsies*, Beck-Mannagetta, G., Anderson, V., Doose, H., and Janz, D., Eds., Springer-Verlag, Berlin, 1989, 74.
20. Jennett, B. and van de Sande, J., EEG Prediction of post-traumatic epilepsy, *Epilepsia,* 16, 251, 1975.
21. Courjon, J., A longitudinal electro-clinical study of 80 cases of post-traumatic epilepsy observed from the time of the original trauma, *Epilepsia,* 11, 29, 1970.

22. van Donselaar, C. A., Schimsheimer, R.-J., Geerts, A. T., and Declerck, A. C., Value of the electroencephalogram in adult patients with untreated idiopathic first seizures, *Arch. Neurol.,* 49, 231, 1992.

23. American EEG Society Guidelines in EEG, 1–7, *J. Clin. Neurophysiol.,* 3, 131, 1986.

24. Starkey, R. R., Sharbrough, F. W., and Drury, I., A comparison of nasopharyngeal with ear and scalp electrodes using referential and bipolar technique, *Electroencephalogr. Clin. Neurophysiol.,* 58, 117, 1984.

25. Sperling, M. R. and Engel, J., Jr., Electroencephalographic recording from the temporal lobes: A comparison of ear, anterior temporal, and nasopharyngeal electrodes, *Ann. Neurol.,* 17, 510, 1985.

26. Sharbrough, F. W., Commentary: Extracranial EEG evaluation, in *Surgical Treatment of the Epilepsies,* in Engel, J., Jr., Ed., Raven Press, New York, 1987, 167.

27. Krauss, G. L., Lesser, R. P., Fisher, R. S., and Arroyo, S., Anterior "cheek" electrodes are comparable to sphenoidal electrodes for the identification of ictal activity, *Electroencephalogr. Clin. Neurophysiol.,* 83, 333, 1992.

28. Preskorn, S. H. and Fast, G. A., Tricyclic antidepressant induced seizures and plasma drug concentration, *J. Clin. Psychiatry,* 53, 160, 1992.

29. Dailey, J. W., Yan, Q. S., Mishra, P. K., Burger, R. L., and Jobe, P. C., Effects of fluoxetine on convulsions and on brain serotonin as detected by microdialysis in genetically epilepsy-prone rats, *J. Pharmacol. Exp. Ther.,* 260, 533, 1992.

30. Ojemann, L. M., Baugh-Bookman, C., and Dudley, D. L., (1987). Effect of psychotropic medications on seizure control in patients with epilepsy, *Neurology,* 37, 1525–1527.

31. Fromm, G. H., Amores, C. Y., and Thies, W., Imipramine in epilepsy, *Arch. Neurol.,* 27, 198, 1972.

32. Fromm, G. H., Wessel, H. B., Glass, J. D., Alvin, J. D., and Van Horn, G., Imipramine in absence and myoclonic-astatic seizures, *Neurology,* 28, 953, 1978.

33. Mattson, R. H., Cramer, J. A., Collins, J. F., Smith, D. B., Delgado-Escueta, A. V., Browne, T. R., Williamson, P. D., Treiman, D. M., McNamara, J. O., McCutchen, C. B., Homan, R. W., Crill, W. E., Lubozynski, M. F., Rosenthal, N. P., and Mayersdorf, A., Comparison of carbamazepine, phenobarbital, phenytoin and primidone in partial and secondarily generalized tonic-clonic seizures, *N. Engl. J. Med.,* 313, 145, 1985.

34. Callahan, N., Kenney, R. A., O'Neill, B., Crowley, M., and Goggin, T., A prospective study between carbamazepine, phenytoin and sodium valproate as monotherapy in previously untreated and recently diagnosed patients with epilepsy, *J. Neurol. Neurosurg. Psychiatry,* 48, 639, 1985.

35. Mattson, R. H., Cramer, J. A., and Collins, J. F., A comparison of valproate with carbamazepine for the treatment of complex partial seizures and secondarily generalized tonic-clonic seizures in adults. The Department of Veterans' Affairs Epilepsy Cooperative Study No. 264 Group, *N. Engl. J. Med.,* 327, 765, 1992.

36. Kalff, R., Houtkooper, M. A., Meyer, J. W. A., Goedhart, D. M., Augusteijn, R., and Meinardi, H., Carbamazepine and serum sodium levels, *Epilepsia,* 25, 390, 1984.

37. UK Gabapentin Study Group, Gabapentin in partial epilepsy, *Lancet,* 335, 1114, 1990.

38. Leppik, I. E., Dreifuss, F. E., Pledger, G. W., Graves, N. M., Santilli, N., Drury, I., Tsay, J. Y., Jacobs, M. P., Bertram, E., Cereghino, J. J., Cooper, G., Sahlroot, J. T., Sheridan, P., Ashworth, M., Lee, S. I., and Sierzant, T. L., Felbamate for partial seizures: Results of a controlled clinical trial, *Neurology,* 41, 1785, 1991.

39. Loiseau, P., Yuen, A. W. C., Duche, B., Ménager, T., and Arné-Bès, M. C., A randomized double-blind placebo-controlled crossover add-on trial of lamotrigine in patients with treatment-resistant partial seizures, *Epilepsy Res.,* 7, 136, 1990.

40. Pellock, J. M. and Willmore, L. J., A rational guide to routine blood monitoring in patients receiving antiepileptic drugs, *Neurology,* 41, 961, 1991.

41. Browne, T. R. and Chang, T., Phenytoin biotransformation, in *Antiepileptic Drugs,* 3rd Edition, Levy, R., Mattson, R., Meldrum, B., Penry, J. K., and Dreifuss, F. E., Eds., Raven Press, New York, 1989, 197.

42. Schmidt, D., Reduction of two-drug therapy in intractable epilepsy, *Epilepsia,* 24, 369, 1983.

43. Mirza, W., Credeur, J., and Penry, J. K., Results of antiepileptic drug reduction in institutionalized epileptic patients with multiple handicaps, *Epilepsia,* 305, 663, 1989.

44. Goldstein, M., Traumatic brain injury: A silent epidemic, *Ann. Neurol.,* 27, 327, 1990.

45. Foerster, O. and Penfield, W., The structural basis of traumatic epilepsy and results of radical operation, *Brain,* 53, 99, 1930.

46. Jasper, H. H., Pathophysiological mechanisms of post-traumatic epilepsy, *Epilepsia,* 11, 73, 1970.

47. Lowenstein, D. H., Thomas, M. J., Smith, D. H., and McIntosh, T. K., Selective vulnerability of dentate hilar neurons following traumatic brain injury: A potential mechanistic link between head trauma and disorders of the hippocampus, *J. Neurosci.,* 12, 4846, 1992.

48. Willmore, L. J., Sypert, G. W., and Munson, J. B., Recurrent seizures induced by cortical iron injection: A model of posttraumatic epilepsy, *Ann. Neurol.,* 4, 329, 1978.

49. Willmore, L. J., Sypert, G. W., Munson, J. B., and Hurd, R. W., Chronic focal epileptiform discharges induced by injection of iron into rat and cat cortex, *Science,* 200, 1501, 1978.

50. Willmore, L. J., Post-traumatic epilepsy: Cellular mechanisms and implications for treatment, *Epilepsia*, 31, S67, 1990.

51. Rubin, J. J. and Willmore, L. J., Prevention of iron-induced epileptiform discharges in rats by treatment of antiperoxidants, *Exp. Neurol.*, 67, 472, 1980.

52. Paillas, J. E., Paillas, N., and Bureau, M., Post-traumatic epilepsy: Introduction and clinical observations, *Epilepsia*, 11, 5, 1970.

53. Reynolds, E. H., Early treatment and prognosis of epilepsy, *Epilepsia*, 28, 97, 1987.

54. First Seizure Trial Group, Randomized clinical trial on the efficacy of antiepileptic drugs in reducing the risk of relapse after a first unprovoked tonic-clonic seizure, *Neurology*, 43, 478, 1993.

55. Elwes, R. D., Johnson, A. L., and Reynolds, E. H., The course of untreated epilepsy, *BMJ*, 297, 948, 1988.

56. Goddard, G. V., McIntyre, D. C., and Leech, C. K., A permanent change in brain function resulting from daily electrical stimulation, *Exp. Neurol.*, 25, 295, 1969.

57. Racine, R. J., Modification of seizure activity by electrical stimulation: II. Motor seizure, *Electroencephalogr. Clin. Neurophysiol.*, 32, 281, 1972.

58. McNamara, J. O., Bonhaus, D. W., Shin, C., Crain, B. J., Gellman, R. L., and Giacchino, J. L., The kindling model of epilepsy: A critical review, *CRC Crit. Rev. Clin. Neurobiol.*, 1, 341, 1985.

59. Lipton, S. A. and Kater, S. B., Neurotransmitter regulation of neuronal outgrowth, plasticity and survival, *Trends Neurosci.*, 12, 265, 1989.

60. Komuro, H. and Rakic, P., Modulation of neuronal migration by NMDA receptors, *Science*, 260, 95, 1993.

61. Stasheff, S. F., Anderson, W. W., Clark, S., and Wilson, W. A., NMDA antagonists differentiate epileptogenesis from seizure expression in an in vitro model, *Science*, 245, 648, 1989.

62. Martin, D., McNamara, J. O., and Nadler, J. V., Kindling enhances sensitivity of CA3 hippocampal pyramidal cells to NMDA, *J. Neurosci.*, 12, 1928, 1992.

63. McNamara, J. O., Bonhaus, D. W., and Nadler, J. V., Novel approach to studying N-methyl-D-aspartate receptor function in the kindling model of epilepsy, *Drug Dev. Res.*, 17, 321, 1989.

64. Hernandez, T. D. and Gallager, D. W., Development of long-term subsensitivity to GABA in dorsal raphe neurons of amygdala-kindled rats, *Brain Res.*, 582, 221, 1992.

65. Hernandez, T. D., Rosen, J. B., and Gallager, D. W., Long-term changes in sensitivity to GABA in dorsal raphe neurons following amygdala kindling, *Brain Res.*, 517, 294, 1990.

66. Kamphuis, W., Gorter, J. A., and Lopes da Silva, F. H., A long-lasting decrease in the inhibitory effect of GABA on glutamate responses of hippocampal pyramidal neurons induced by kindling epileptogenesis, *Neuroscience*, 41, 425, 1991.

67. Kapur, J., Michelson, H. B., Buterbaugh, G. G., and Lothman, E. W., Evidence for chronic loss of inhibition in the hippocampus after kindling: Electrophysiological studies, *Epilepsy Res.*, 4, 90, 1989.

68. During, M. J., Craig, J. S., Hernandez, T. D., Anderson, G. M., and Gallager, D. W., Effect of amygdala kindling on the in vivo release of GABA and 5-HT in the dorsal raphe nucleus of freely moving rats, *Brain Res.*, 584, 36, 1992.

69. Kamphuis, W., Huisman, H., Dreijer, A. M. C., Ghijsen, W. E. J. M., Verhage, M., and Lopes da Silva, F. H., Kindling increases the K+-evoked Ca2+-dependent release of endogenous GABA in area CA1 of rat hippocampus, *Brain Res.*, 511, 63, 1990.

70. Sutula, T., Xiao-Xian, H., Cavazos, J., and Scott, G., Synaptic reorganization in the hippocampus induced by abnormal functional activity, *Science*, 239, 1147, 1988.

71. Represa, A. and Ben-Ari, Y., Kindling is associated with the formation of novel mossy fibre synapses in the CA3 region, *Exp. Brain Res.*, 92, 69, 1992.

72. Choi, D. W., Calcium-mediated neurotoxicity: Relationship to specific channel types and role in ischemic damage, *Trends Neurosci.*, 11, 465, 1988.

73. Chen, Q. X., Stelzer, A., Kay, A. R., and Wong, R. K. S., GABA-A receptor function is regulated by phosphorylation in acutely dissociated guinea-pig hippocampal neurones, *J. Physiol.*, 420, 207, 1990.

74. Wohns, R. N. W. and Wyler, A. R., Prophylactic phenytoin in severe head injuries, *J. Neurosurg.*, 51, 507, 1979.

75. Servit, Z. and Musil, F., Prophylactic treatment of posttraumatic epilepsy: Results of a long-term follow-up in Czechoslovakia, *Epilepsia*, 22, 315, 1981.

76. Temkin, N. R., Dikmen, S. S., Wilensky, A. J., Keihm, J., Chabal, S., and Winn, H. R., A randomized, double blind study of phenytoin for the prevention of post-traumatic seizures, *N. Engl. J. Med.*, 323, 497, 1990.

77. McNamara, J. O., Rigsbee, L. C., Butler, L. S., and Shin, C., Intravenous phenytoin is an effective anticonvulsant in the kindling model, *Ann. Neurol.*, 26, 675, 1989.

78. Weiss, S. R. B. and Post, R. M., Carbamazepine and carbamazepine-10,11-epoxide inhibit amygdala-kindled seizures in the rat but do not block their development, *Clin. Neuropharmacol.*, 10, 272, 1987.

79. Schmutz, M., Klebs, K., and Baltzer, V., Inhibition or enhancement of kindling evolution by antiepileptics, *J. Neural Transm.*, 72, 245, 1988.

80. Löscher, W. and Hönack, D., Comparison of the anticonvulsant efficacy of primidone and phenobarbital during chronic treatment of amygdala-kindled rats, *Eur. J. Pharmacol.*, 162, 309, 1989.

81. Silver, J. M., Shin, C., and McNamara, J. O., Antiepileptogenic effects of conventional anticonvulsants in the kindling model of epilepsy, *Ann. Neurol.*, 29, 356, 1991.

82. Löscher, W., Fisher, J. E., Nau, H., and Honack, D., Valproic acid in amygdala-kindled rats: Alterations in anticonvulsant efficacy, adverse effects and drug and metabolite levels in various brain regions during chronic treatment, *J. Pharmacol. Exp. Therap.*, 250, 1067, 1989.

83. Young, N. A., Lewis, S. J., Harris, Q. L. G., Jarrot, H. B., and Vajda, F. J. E., The development of tolerance to the anticonvulsant effects of clonazepam, but not sodium valproate, in the amygdaloid kindled rat, *Neuropharmacology*, 26, 1611, 1987.

84. Holmes, K. H., Bilkey, D. K., Laverty, R., and Goddard, G. V., The N-methyl-D-aspartate antagonists amionphosphonovaerate and carboxypiperazephosphonate retard the development and expression of kindled seizures, *Brain Res.*, 506, 227, 1990.

85. Gellman, R. L., Kallianos, J. A., and McNamara, J. O., Alpha-2 receptors mediate an endogenous noradrenergic suppression of kindling development, *J. Pharmacol. Exp. Ther.*, 241, 891, 1987.

86. Pelletier, M. R. and Corcoran, M. E., Intra-amygdaloid infusions of clonidine retard kindling, *Brain Res.*, 598, 51, 1992.

87. Burchfiel, J. and Applegate, C. D., Stepwise progression of kindling: Perspectives from the kindling antagonism model, *Neurosci. Behav. Rev.*, 13, 289, 1989.

88. Dailey, J. W., Mishra, P. K., Ko, K. H., Penny, J. E., and Jobe, P. C., Noradrenergic abnormalities in the central nervous system of seizure-naive genetically epilepsy-prone rats, *Epilepsia*, 32, 168, 1991.

89. Walker, A. E. and Blumer, D., The fate of World War II veterans with posttraumatic seizures, *Arch. Neurol.*, 46, 23, 1989.

90. Vargha-Khadem, F., Issacs, E., van der Werf, S., Robb, S., and Wilson, J., Development of intelligence and memory in children with hemiplegic cerebral palsy, *Brain*, 115, 315, 1992.

91. Armstrong, K. K., Sahgal, V., Bloch, R., Armstrong, K. J., and Heinemann, A., Rehabilitation outcomes in patients with posttraumatic epilepsy, *Arch. Phys. Med. Rehabil.*, 71, 156, 1990.

92. Ben-Ari, Y. E., Limbic seizure and brain damage produced by kainic acid: Mechanisms and relevance to human temporal lobe epilepsy, *Neuroscience*, 14, 375, 1985.

93. Holmes, G. L., Thompson, J. L., Marchi, T. A., Gabriel, P. S., Hogan, M. A., Carl, F. G., and Feldman, D. S., Effects of seizures on learning, memory, and behavior in the genetically epilepsy-prone rat, *Ann. Neurol.*, 27, 24, 1990.

94. Holmes, G. L., Chronopoulos, A., Stafstrom, C. E., Mikati, M., Thurber, S., and Hyde, P., Long-term effects of kindling in the developing brain on memory, learning, behavior, and seizure susceptibility, *Epilepsia*, 33, S42, 1992.

95. Binnie, C. D., Channon, S., and Marston, D., Learning disabilities in epilepsy: Neurophysiological aspects, *Epilepsia*, 31, S2, 1990.

96. Shewmon, D. A. and Erwin, R. J., The effect of focal interictal spikes on perception and reaction time. I. General considerations, *Electroencephalogr. Clin. Neurophysiol.*, 69, 319, 1988.

97. Feeney, D. M., Bailey, B. Y., Boyeson, M. G., Hovda, D. A., and Sutton, R. L., The effects of seizures on recovery of function following cortical contusion in the rat, *Brain Injury*, 1, 27, 1987.

98. Hernandez, T. D. and Schallert, T., Seizures and recovery from experimental brain damage, *Exp. Neurol.*, 102, 318, 1988.

99. Hernandez, T. D. and Warner, L. A., Kindled seizures and the recovering brain: Delineation of a critical period, *Soc. Neurosci. Abstr.*, 19, 393, 1993.

100. Beldhuis, H. J. A., Everts, G. J., Van der Zee, E. A., Luiten, P. G. M., and Bohus, B., Amygdala kindling-induced seizures selectively impair spatial memory. 1. Behavioral characteristics and effects on hippocampal neuronal protein kinase C isoforms, *Hippocampus*, 2, 397, 1992.

101. Pellock, J. M., Who should receive prophylactic antiepileptic drug following head injury? *Brain Injury*, 3, 107, 1989.

102. Meador, K. J., Loring, D. W., Allen, M. E., Zamrini, M. D., Moore, B. A., Abney, O. L., and King, D. W., Comparative cognitive effects of carbamazepine and phenytoin in healthy adults, *Neurology*, 41, 1537, 1991.

103. Dodrill, C. B. and Troupin, A. S., Psychotropic effects of carbamazepine in epilepsy: A double-blind comparison with phenytoin, *Neurology*, 27, 1023, 1977.

104. Dodrill, C. B. and Troupin, A. S., Neuropsychological effects of carbamazepine and phenytoin: A reanalysis, *Neurology*, 41, 141, 1991.

105. Meador, K. J., Loring, D. W., Huh, K., Gallagher, B. B., and King, D. W., Comparative cognitive effects of anticonvulsants, *Neurology*, 40, 391, 1990.

106. Gallassi, R., Morreale, A., Lorusso, S., Procaccianti, G., Lugaresi, E., and Baruzzi, A., Cognitive effects of valproate, *Epilepsy Res.*, 5, 160, 1990.

107. von Monakow, C., *Die Lokalisation im Grosshim und der Abbau der funktiondurch kortikale Herde*. J. F. Bergman, Wiesbaden, 1914. Translated and excerpted by Harris, G., in *Mood States and Mind*, Priebam, K. H., Ed., Penguin, London, 1949, 27.

108. Boyeson, M. B. and Feeney, D. M., Striatal dopamine after cortical injury, *Exp. Neurol.*, 89, 479, 1985.

109. Hovda, D. A., Sutton, R. L., and Feeney, D. M., Recovery of tactile placing after visual cortex ablation in cat: A behavioral and metabolic study of diaschisis, *Exp. Neurol.*, 97, 391, 1987.

110. Kempinsky, W. H., Experimental study of distal effects of acute focal injury, *Arch. Neurol. Psychiatry*, 79, 376, 1958.

111. Meyer, J. S., Shinohara, M., Kanda, T., Fukuuchi, Y., Ericson, A. D., and Kok, N. H., Diaschisis resulting from acute unilateral cerebral infarction, *Arch. Neurol.*, 23, 241, 1970.

112. Deuel, R. K. and Collins, R. C., The functional anatomy of frontal lobe neglect in the monkey: Behavioral and quantitative 2-deoxyglucose studies, *Ann. Neurol.*, 15, 521, 1984.

113. Glassman, R. B. and Malamut, D. L., Recovery from electroencephalographic slowing and reduced evoked potentials after somatosensory cortical damage in cats, *Behav. Biol.*, 17, 333, 1976.

114. Dikmen, S. S., Temkin, N. R., Miller, B. M., Machamer, J., and Winn, R., Neurobehavioral effects of phenytoin prophylaxis of posttraumatic seizures, *J. Am. Med. Assoc.*, 265, 1271, 1991.

115. Izquierdo, I. and Medina, J., GABA$_A$ receptor modulation of memory: The role of endogenous benzodiazepines, *Trends Neurosci.*, 12, 260, 1991.

116. Castellano, C. and McGaugh, J. L., Retention enhancement with post-training picrotoxin: Lack of state dependency, *Behav. Neural Biol.*, 51, 165, 1989.

117. Castellano, C. and McGaugh, J. L., Effects of post-training bicuculline and muscimol on retention: Lack of state dependency, *Behav. Neural Biol.*, 54, 156, 1990.

118. Satzger, W., Engel, R. R., Ferguson, E., Kapfhammer, H., Eich, F. X., and Hippius, H., Effects of single doses of alpidem, lorazepam and placebo on memory and attention in healthy young and elderly volunteers, *Pharmacopsychiatry*, 23(S3), 114, 1990.

119. Schallert, T., Hernandez, T. D., and Barth, T. M., Recovery of function after brain damage: Severe and chronic disruption by diazepam, *Brain Res.*, 379, 104, 1986.

120. Hernandez, T. D., Jones, G. H., and Schallert, T., Co-administration of the benzodiazepine antagonist R$_o$ 15-1788 prevents diazepam-induced retardation of recovery, *Brain Res.*, 487, 89, 1989.

121. Hernandez, T. D., Kiefel, J., Barth, T. M., Grant, M. L., and Schallert, T., Disruption and facilitation of recovery of function: Implication of the gamma-aminobutyric acid/benzodiazepine receptor complex, in *Cerebro-vascular Diseases*, Ginsbergand, M. and Dietrich, W. D., Eds., Raven Press, New York, 1989, 327.

122. Hernandez, T. D. and Holling, L. C., Disruption of behavioral recovery by the anti-convulsant phenobarbital, *Brain Res.*, 635, 300, 1994.

123. Watson, C. W. and Kennard, M. A., The effect of anticonvulsant drugs on recovery of function following cerebral cortical lesions, *J. Neurophysiol.*, 8, 221, 1945.

4

Neurotransmitters and Pharmacology

Ronald A. Browning

CONTENTS

EDITORS' NOTE

The following chapter was solicited for inclusion in this volume for some very specific reasons. The field of neurorehabilitation is a young one, developing at a time when neuroscience is likewise growing exponentially. Early efforts at neurorehabilitation were directed by limited knowledge of medical and therapeutic techniques which had been applied to neurologically impaired populations other than the traumatically brain-injured. These techniques were often of some use in initiation of treatment; however, their efficacy was soon challenged and techniques specific to traumatic brain injury were developed.

Likewise, pharmacological management of the traumatically brain-injured population began by drawing upon clinical observations of drug effects in other neurologically impaired populations. Pharmaceuticals were often applied in an experimental fashion, directed by symptomatology rather than pharmacological principles underlying specific drug action within the CNS.

The information which follows is intended to provide the reader with highly detailed information pertaining to specific drug action within the CNS relative to neurotransmitter synthesis, storage, release, and inactivation. It is hoped that this information will provide the clinician with the necessary theoretical and neuroanatomical constructs to develop and apply sound pharmacological approaches in augmentation of medical and rehabilitative efforts for the traumatically brain-injured population.

INTRODUCTION

Most drugs that are used for an action on the central nervous system (CNS), such as those employed in neurology and psychiatry, exert their action at the site where neurons communicate with one another, namely, the synapse (Figure 4.1). These drugs, therefore, exert their effect by modifying the process of neurotransmission. The exceptions to this rule are those classes of neuroactive agents known as 1) *local anesthetics,* which prevent nerve conduction by blocking sodium channels, thereby alleviating pain, 2) *general anesthetics,* which produce a reversible loss of consciousness by an unknown mechanism, and 3) some *antiepileptic agents,* which prevent seizures by an, as yet, unidentified mechanism.

Drug classes whose mechanism of action involves a modification of synaptic neurotransmission include analgesics (used to alleviate pain), antipsychotic agents (used to treat schizophrenia), antidepressants, antianxiety agents (e.g., **diazepam** or Valium®*), some antiepileptic drugs, antispasmodics, and muscle relaxants. In addition, due to the ubiquitous role of the peripheral autonomic nervous system in the regulation of organ-system function such as cardiovascular, respiratory, gastrointestinal, nasal congestion, and the like, it is not surprising to find that drugs altering peripheral neurotransmission are used to treat a wide variety of disorders such as hypertension, heart disease, gastrointestinal disorders, hiccups, asthma, hay fever, etc.

The question of whether a substance functions as a neurotransmitter is not an easy one to answer and requires extensive experimental testing by neuroscientists. Neurobiologists have set specific criteria that must be fulfilled before a substance is accepted as a neurotransmitter. These criteria were established in the mid-1960's by Werman,[1] and while they have been extremely useful for the last 26 years, they may not be entirely adequate since nitric oxide, a gas, has recently been suggested to function as a neurotransmitter, but does not fulfill the previously established criteria.[2]

Nevertheless, there are about seven chemicals that have been well-established as neurotransmitters and another 20 to 30 substances that are highly suspected to be neurotransmitters

*Registered Trademark of Roche Products, Inc., Manati, Puerto Rico.

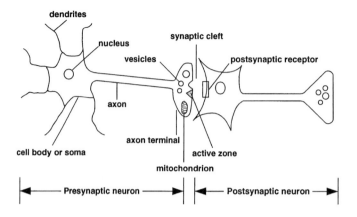

FIGURE 4.1   Diagram of a typical synapse between two neurons. The neuron synapsing on another neuron is referred to as the *presynaptic neuron*, while the neuron receiving the input is called the *postsynaptic neuron*. In the diagram, the synapse is axosomatic. Various subcellular structures associated with the synapse are labeled. The active zone is believed to be the site at which vesicles attach to the presynaptic membrane just prior to release.

or neuromodulators in the nervous system. The seven well-established or classical neurotransmitters include:

1. acetylcholine
2. norepinephrine
3. dopamine
4. 5-hydroxytryptamine (5-HT, serotonin)
5. gamma aminobutyric acid (GABA)
6. glycine
7. glutamate/aspartate

All of these have been associated with the action of drugs that exert an effect on the nervous system. In addition, there are several prominent peptides which serve as neurotransmitters or neuromodulators (i.e., modify the action of the classical neurotransmitters) that have been associated with the action of drugs and these will be discussed.

In order to appreciate the physiological and/or biochemical mechanisms by which drugs alter neurotransmission, one must have considerable knowledge of the events involved in synaptic neurotransmission. Thus, we will begin with a description of the physiology of chemical neurotransmission and then proceed to discuss each individual neurotransmitter and the drugs that mediate their effects through each neurotransmitter. It should be kept in mind that synaptic transmission is not only important for understanding the action of drugs, it is vital for all functions of the nervous system, and the synapse appears to be the site at which learning and memory take place in the CNS (see Chapter 9 of this volume).

CHEMICAL NEUROTRANSMISSION

In the mammalian nervous system (both central and peripheral), the predominant form of communication between two nerves and between nerve and muscle (or nerves and glands) is chemical. The site at which this chemical transmission occurs is called the *synapse*. From Figure 4.1, it can be seen that the synapse consists of several cellular and subcellular structures. Although synapses can occur at several locations on a neuron which is receiving information from another neuron, the more typical arrangement is that described in Figure 4.1. Thus, the axon terminal of one neuron generally synapses on the cell body (soma, or perikaryon, called *axosomatic synapses*) or dendrites of another neuron (called *axodendritic synapses*). Axons may also synapse on other axons, especially at the nerve terminals (called *axo-axonic synapses*), and under unusual circumstances, dendrites may synapse with other dendrites (*dendrodendritic synapses*) or cell bodies may synapse with one another (*soma-somatic synapses*). At the prototypical synapse, the neurotransmitter, which is usually a small water-soluble organic amine, is synthesized from precursors within the axon terminal, taken up into and stored in a small round or ovoid vesicle, and released from the nerve terminal in a calcium-dependent process when an action potential or nerve impulse reaches the nerve terminal.

Indeed, the steps associated with neurotransmission at a chemical synapse are as follows:

Step 1: The first step is the release of the neurotransmitter from its storage site in a vesicle due to the arrival of an action potential which, in turn, opens voltage-dependent calcium channels and allows the influx of calcium from the extracellular fluid. The calcium then triggers a release process called *exocytosis*. Exocytosis involves fusion of the vesicle membrane with the nerve membrane and the opening of the vesicle into the synaptic cleft (Figure 4.1). Thus, the vesicle extrudes its contents into the synaptic cleft. The release process can be regulated by receptors found on the nerve terminal (called *presynaptic receptors* or *autoreceptors*).

Step 2: The next step in neurotransmission involves binding of the neurotransmitter to *receptors* in the postsynaptic membrane and the initiation of postsynaptic events, i.e., a depolarization or a hyperpolarization. Receptors give both neurotransmitters and drugs their selectivity and specificity. The receptors, which are typically membrane proteins or glycoproteins, only recognize and bind chemicals of the "correct" chemical structure. Thus, just as only one key opens a lock, only one chemical structure can initiate postsynaptic events via the receptors. The receptors come in two varieties: 1) those that actually form an ion channel in the membrane (such as the nicotinic cholinergic receptor) and mediate rapid events when the transmitter binds and are called *ligand-gated ion channels* or 2) those that are connected to ion channels indirectly via "second messenger" molecules that become activated inside the cell when the transmitter binds to the receptor. In the latter case, the receptor is linked to a guanine nucleotide binding protein (called a *G-protein*) which functions as the link between the receptor protein and the enzyme(s) that synthesize the second messenger. This class of receptors is referred to as *G-protein linked receptors* or *metabotropic receptors*.

Potentials that develop in the postsynaptic cell either move the membrane potential further from the threshold for triggering an action potential (hyperpolarization) or move it closer to the threshold (depolarization). Hyperpolarization (inhibitory postsynaptic potentials or IPSP's) results from the opening of chloride or potassium channels in the membrane, allowing chloride to flow in or potassium to flow out. Hyperpolarization, then, inhibits postsynaptic firing. Depolarization (excitatory postsynaptic potentials or EPSP's) results from the opening of channels that allow both sodium and potassium to flow down their concentration gradients through the same channel. This is different from the sodium-selective channel that is involved in the propagation of the action potential down the axon. If the depolarization is great enough, the threshold for an action potential is reached and an action potential (regenerative, sodium current) is propagated down the axon to initiate more synaptic transmission.

In the central nervous system, a neuron can only respond in one of two ways: 1) it either reaches threshold and fires an action potential, which, in turn, propagates information to the next neuron via synaptic transmission or 2) it is inhibited and does not fire an action potential.

Step 3: The third step of the neurotransmission process consists of the postsynaptic response. The postsynaptic response can consist of an action potential in the neuron, the contraction of muscle, or the secretion of a gland.

Step 4: This step consists of inactivation of the neurotransmitter in the synaptic cleft. The transmitter must be removed from the synaptic cleft in order for the postsynaptic cell to repolarize, which is necessary for the synapse to regain responsiveness to incoming information. The two most important mechanisms for removing the neurotransmitter from the cleft are: 1) reuptake into the neuron from which it was released and 2) enzymatic degradation. In addition, other mechanisms include diffusion away from the cleft and uptake (transport) into other cells (e.g., glial cells, muscle cells in the periphery, or other neurons).

SITES WHERE DRUGS ACT

Drugs may either facilitate or inhibit neurotransmission. Some of the mechanisms by which drugs can facilitate neurotransmission include:

1. Stimulation of the release of the neurotransmitter into the cleft.
2. Increased synthesis of the neurotransmitter in the presynaptic terminal.
3. Prevention of inactivation of the neurotransmitter following release, e.g., blocking reuptake or blocking enzymes of degradation.
4. Stimulation of the postsynaptic receptors directly to produce a response. A drug that does this is called an *agonist*.

Some of the mechanisms by which drugs inhibit neurotransmission include:

1. Inhibition of the synthesis of the neurotransmitter.
2. Prevention of transmitter release.
3. Interference with neurotransmitter storage in the vesicle.
4. Blocking of the neurotransmitter receptor.

A drug which binds to a receptor, blocking neurotransmitter action but producing no effect, is called an *antagonist*.

In the sections that follow, we will review each individual neurotransmitter and the drugs that produce clinical effects by altering chemical neurotransmission.

ACETYLCHOLINE

Acetylcholine (ACh) is phylogenetically one of the oldest and most widely studied neurotransmitters. It was, in fact, the neurotransmitter for which chemical neurotransmission was originally demonstrated, when it was found to be released from nerves innervating the frog heart by Loewi in 1921.[3] It has been most thoroughly studied in the peripheral nervous system where it functions as a neurotransmitter of the motoneurons innervating skeletal muscle (those muscles involved in the voluntary control of movement). ACh is also the neurotransmitter of the preganglionic sympathetic and parasympathetic fibers as well as the postganglionic parasympathetic fibers.[3] The response to stimulating parasympathetic nerves innervating various organs in the body is shown in Table 4.1. As you can see, these nerves affect every organ of the body. Drugs which alter neurotransmission at these synapses can have very profound effects.

ACh is also a neurotransmitter in the central nervous system where specific pathways have recently been identified in the rat brain. Basically, there are two groups of ACh pathways: 1) those innervating the forebrain (cell bodies in the basal forebrain around the medial septum and nucleus basalis of Meynert) as well as the interneurons in the striatum (basal ganglia) and 2) those innervating the brainstem and diencephalon (cell bodies in the laterodorsal tegmental nucleus and the pedunculopontine tegmental nucleus). Some of the proposed functions of ACh in these CNS pathways are listed in Table 4.2, but it is clear that we have much to learn about the intricate details of how ACh regulates such things as learning and memory, sleep, seizures, and emotional states.

TABLE 4.1 Organ Response To Parasympathetic Nerve Stimulation[a]

Organ receiving innervation	Response to stimulation	Receptor type
Eye		
Iris, sphincter	Pupillary constriction (miosis)	Muscarinic
Ciliary muscle	Contraction-near vision	Muscarinic
Heart		
SA node	Decrease in heart rate	Muscarinic
Atrium	Shortens refractory period	Muscarinic
AV node	Slows conduction	Muscarinic
Ventricles	No response-poor innervation	Muscarinic
Vasculature	No parasympathetic innervation (has muscarinic receptors which can respond with vasodilation)	Muscarinic
Trachea and bronchioles	Constriction	Muscarinic
Stomach and intestine	Increase in motility, tone and secretions; relaxation of sphincters	Muscarinic
Urinary bladder		
Detrusor muscle	Contraction, bladder emptying	Muscarinic
Trigone and sphincter	Relaxation	Muscarinic
Sex organs, male	Erection	Muscarinic
Sweat glands	Secretion	Muscarinic
Lacrimal glands	Secretion	Muscarinic
Nasopharyngeal glands	Secretion	Muscarinic

[a] See Lefkowitz et al.[3] for more detail.

TABLE 4.2 Some Proposed Functions of ACh in the CNS

Learning and memory (cholinergic neurons
  lost in Alzheimer's disease)
Sleep and arousal states
Body temperature
Susceptibility to seizures
Affective states (mood)
Cardiovascular function via hypothalamus
Motor disorders (Parkinson's disease)

Synthesis, Storage, Release, and Inactivation of ACh

Neurons that utilize ACh as a neurotransmitter are referred to as *cholinergic* neurons, and a schematic diagram of such a neuron is shown in Figure 4.2. Acetylcholine is synthesized within cholinergic neurons from the precursor, *choline*, which comes from the diet and/or the breakdown of phospholipids, primarily in the liver.[4] Some of the choline that is taken up into cholinergic neurons for synthesis of ACh comes from the enzymatic degradation of released ACh. In fact, about 50% of the choline released as ACh is recaptured by the neuron after enzymatic degradation for the synthesis of more ACh.[5]

Choline is transported into the nerve by a transporter or "carrier" protein in the membrane. This transporter or carrier has a high affinity for choline, which means that it avidly picks up choline from the surrounding area. It has, however, a limited number of transport sites, meaning that it can get filled up or saturated. Increasing the concentration of choline to the point at which the sites become filled results in a proportional increase in the rate of choline transport. However, once all transporters are occupied, the rate of transport becomes constant.

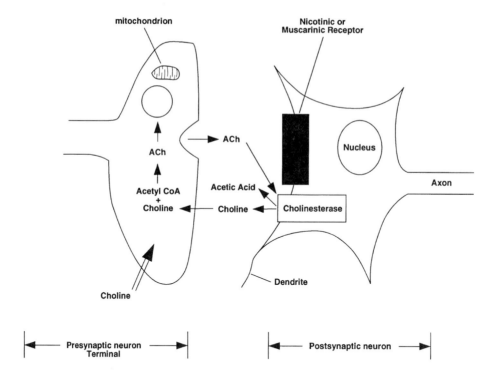

FIGURE 4.2   Diagram of a cholinergic synapse, showing fate of ACh after release into the synaptic cleft. Note that the neuron utilizes choline from two sources: (1) the blood and (2) the breakdown of released ACh. Cholinesterase found in the postsynaptic membrane terminates the action of released ACh.

Theoretically, one should be able to increase the synthesis of ACh by increasing the availability of choline, especially since the enzyme that converts choline to ACh during enzymatic synthesis, choline acetyltransferase, is not saturated with substrate (choline).

A co-substrate to choline is utilized in the synthesis of ACh. This co-substrate is called *acetylcoenzyme A* (acetylCoA). AcetylCoA derives from pyruvate via the breakdown of glucose and, as such, is in plentiful supply in the neuron.

Experimental studies have established that the rate-limiting factor in the overall ACh synthesis is the uptake of choline by the neuron.[5,6] Since ACh neurons are lost in Alzheimer's disease, it has been of interest to attempt to increase ACh synthesis in brains of Alzheimer's patients. Although some studies have suggested that this is possible, choline has not been found terribly useful for improving memory in this or other populations.[7] The reason for this may be that the choline uptake transporter saturates and that the intracellular or cytoplasmic choline concentration can only be increased to a limited extent. There are no drugs known to increase the uptake of choline, though there are experimental drugs which inhibit the uptake of choline and interfere with the synthesis of ACh, such as hemicholinium and triethylcholine, both of which are competitive inhibitors of choline uptake.

Choline can also get into neurons by another mechanism, called *"low-affinity" uptake*, which may account for the increase in synthesis of ACh that is seen in some peripheral organs following the administration of high doses of choline. Much higher concentrations of choline are required to saturate the transport proteins involved in low-affinity transport.

It has recently been hypothesized that the selective vulnerability of cholinergic neurons in Alzheimer's disease may be due to the dual role of choline in forming both membrane phospholipids and ACh in these neurons and the selective breakdown of cell membrane to shunt choline into the neurotransmitter leading to cell membrane damage.[8] If the latter is true, treatment with choline may be beneficial. There is new evidence that giving choline to rats can

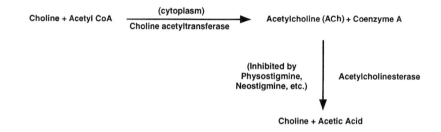

FIGURE 4.3 Synthesis and enzymatic degradation of acetylcholine (ACh). Shows the enzymes involved.

increase the release of ACh in the striatum[9] and this effect can apparently be enhanced by caffeine.[10]

The enzyme that catalyzes the synthesis of ACh is choline acetyltransferase (ChAT), which is a soluble enzyme (nonmembrane bound) found in the cytoplasm of cholinergic neurons. The gene responsible for forming ChAT is expressed only in cholinergic neurons, and this enzyme therefore serves as a phenotypic marker for cholinergic neurons. The overall synthetic scheme is given in Figure 4.3.

Once ACh is synthesized, it is stored in small spherical vesicles along with several other constituents, including adenosine triphosphate (ATP) and a protein called *vesiculin.* The sequestration of the ACh within these tiny vesicles serves to protect it from destruction by the enzyme acetylcholinesterase. Although there appears to be some ACh in the cytoplasm of the neuron, the vast majority is found within the vesicles from which it is released directly into the synaptic cleft. This is accomplished by the complex process called *exocytosis.*

Exocytosis requires that the vesicle membrane fuse with the neuron membrane and "dump" its contents into the cleft in an all-or-none process. Some of the ACh that is free within the cytoplasm of the neuron may have just been synthesized en route to being taken up by the vesicle membrane transporters for storage within the vesicle. The ACh is believed to be transported into the vesicle by an ATPase that pumps protons (hydrogen ions) into the vesicle so the inside does not become charged and also maintains an isotonic state, in spite of the high concentration of ACh in the vesicle.[11] The only drug currently known to interfere with the storage of ACh is **vesamicol,** which blocks the uptake of ACh into the vesicle and prevents the release of newly synthesized ACh.[12]

The latter findings greatly strengthened the hypothesis that ACh is released from the neuron by exocytosis. Exocytosis is a calcium-dependent process and calcium is necessary for fusion to occur between the vesicle membrane and the cell membrane. The voltage change that occurs in the nerve terminal with the arrival of the action potential opens calcium ion channels allowing calcium to enter the nerve terminal and initiate the exocytotic process. Electrophysiological and morphological evidence also indicates that ACh is released from neurons by exocytosis.[5,11]

Once ACh has been released from the neuron, it can diffuse to the postsynaptic receptor to mediate a response in the postsynaptic neuron. However, it must then be inactivated if the synapse is to remain functional. In the case of ACh, inactivation occurs by enzymatic degradation of the neurotransmitter. Almost all other neurotransmitters (except for the peptides) are inactivated by reuptake into a neuron. Thus, ACh is unique among neurotransmitters in terms of the mechanism of inactivation following release into the synaptic cleft.

The enzyme that degrades ACh is called *acetylcholinesterase.* However, several cholinesterases have been found in the body. One of them circulates in plasma and is known as *pseudocholinesterase* or *butyrylcholinesterase,* which hydrolyzes butyrylcholine faster than ACh.[5] Acetylcholinesterase is associated with the synaptic cleft and is attached both to the presynaptic and postsynaptic membranes. This enzyme has been shown to exist in several molecular forms that differ in their lipid solubility and in the way they attach to membranes.

Several inhibitors of acetylcholinesterase are available and these produce a dramatic increase in the concentration of ACh in the body. Such drugs are widely used in medicine and are discussed below.

Acetylcholine Receptors

Like other neurotransmitters, ACh produces its effects and obtains its selectivity by binding to specific receptors in the postsynaptic cell membrane. These receptors chemically recognize ACh and allow it to interact with specific functional groups in the receptor. Based on the studies of Dale,[13] it has long been known that there are two major types of ACh receptors, which were first identified in the peripheral nervous system: 1) ACh receptors at which nicotine can mimic the action of ACh that were termed *nicotinic* by Dale and 2) ACh receptors that respond to the alkaloid muscarine (from mushrooms) and were called *muscarinic* receptors. The nicotinic receptors were found to be localized at the neuromuscular junction (voluntary nerves to skeletal muscle), the autonomic ganglia, and the adrenal medulla, while muscarinic receptors were found at the effector organs innervated by the postganglionic parasympathetic fibers. Both types of ACh receptors have been found in the brain.

Nicotinic Receptors

Nicotinic receptors have been widely studied, and most of our knowledge about nicotinic receptors comes from work on electric fish such as the Torpedo which uses its electric organ to kill prey. It turns out that the high voltage in these fish is generated by ACh receptors, which are highly concentrated in the electric organ. Thus, the electric fish has served as a rich source of nicotinic receptor protein for biochemists to study.

The nicotinic receptor was found to be a ligand-gated ion channel composed of four subunits (termed *alpha, beta, gamma,* and *delta*). However, it takes five subunits to form the ion channel, so the channel is formed by two alphas, one beta, one gamma, and one delta subunit.[14] ACh binds to the alpha subunit of the receptor, and since there are two alpha subunits, it takes two molecules of ACh to open the channel. Modern techniques of molecular biology (genetic engineering) have contributed greatly to our knowledge of the nicotinic receptor as well as to our knowledge of the molecular structure of other receptors. These studies have led to a widely accepted model of the nicotinic receptor at the electric organ of fish and at the neuromuscular junction of mammals.

However, the nicotinic receptor on neurons (e.g., the autonomic ganglia and in the brain) appears to be different. For example, it has long been known that they are not blocked by the classical neuromuscular nicotinic antagonist, d-tubocurarine, but are blocked by hexamethonium, another nicotinic antagonist. Research on neuronal nicotinic receptors is very active, indeed, and has important bearing on nicotine addiction and even Alzheimer's disease, since nicotine has been shown to increase the release of ACh in the cerebral cortex.[15,16] A greater understanding of the different subtypes of neuronal nicotinic receptors, which is now unfolding, is certain to have a big impact on the future treatment of CNS disorders. There is now some evidence that nicotinic receptor agonists may be beneficial in restoring memory that has been impaired due to Alzheimer's disease.

Muscarinic Receptors

Muscarinic receptors are thought to make up the majority of the ACh receptors (95%) in the mammalian brain. Unlike nicotinic receptors, the muscarinic receptors are linked to G-proteins and second messengers that carry the signal to ultimately produce a response or change in the cell. Based on recent molecular cloning technology, five subtypes of muscarinic receptor have been identified. The basic chemical structure (i.e., the amino acid sequence) of these muscarinic receptors has been determined.[17] The best described of the muscarinic receptors are the so-called M1, M2, and M3 which correspond to the m1, m2, and m3 cloned receptors.[14] Inasmuch as the muscarinic receptors are G-protein linked, they mediate their effects through second messengers. Muscarinic receptors may be involved in mediating either excitation or inhibition in the brain, which is usually produced by the opening (inhibition) or closing (excitation) of K^+ channels (i.e., potassium channels).

All G-protein coupled receptors consist of a polypeptide chain (protein) with seven hydrophobic regions (i.e., areas containing amino acids that are more lipid than water soluble). It has been found that these hydrophobic regions of the molecule correspond to positions where the protein loops (crosses) through the cell membrane. So, these receptors loop back and forth through the membrane seven times and are said to contain *seven membrane-spanning regions*. Other G-protein linked receptors with seven membrane-spanning regions include the adrenergic, dopaminergic, and serotonergic receptors (see below).

The M2 receptor found in the heart is most often the one involved in inhibition. The M1, M3, and cloned m5 subtypes increase intracellular cyclic adenosine monophosphate (AMP), a second messenger, via a G-protein. However, in some neurons, these same receptors seem to activate phospholipase C through another G-protein, which results in the hydrolysis of phosphatidyl inositol and the formation of diacylglycerol (DAG) or inositol triphosphate (IP3), which, in turn, function as second messengers. M2 and M4 receptors result in the inhibition of adenylate cyclase by acting through a G-protein and, in addition, may activate (open) K^+ channels directly. These effects lead to a slowing of the heart and a decrease in the force of myocardial contraction.[3]

Atropine is a nonselective antagonist for all muscarinic receptors, while **pirenzepine** is selective for the M1 receptor. **AFDX 116** and **methoctramine** are antagonists for the M2 receptor. The release of ACh and other neurotransmitters may be partially regulated by the activation of M2 receptors located on presynaptic nerve terminals.[18]

Clinically Useful Drugs That Act by Altering Cholinergic Neurotransmission

Facilitators of Cholinergic Neurotransmission

Cholinergic Agonists

There are a number of cholinergic agonists (drugs which bind to the receptor and produce a response or mimic the action of ACh), but only the muscarinic agonists find significant clinical usefulness. These drugs are primarily used in ophthalmology to treat glaucoma or to treat bowel and bladder retention postoperatively.

Muscarinic agonists include **acetylcholine**, which is not used because it is rapidly destroyed by acetylcholinesterase or butyrylcholinesterase; **methacholine**, which is only partially sensitive to the action of acetylcholinesterase and is available as a diagnostic tool; **bethanechol** (Urecholine®*), which is used for bowel and bladder retention; **carbachol**, which is used to treat glaucoma and has some nicotinic agonist activity as well; and **pilocarpine**, a naturally occurring alkaloid found in plants, which is a potent muscarinic agonist used to treat glaucoma. Pilocarpine is generally given in eye drops applied topically to the eye.

All of these drugs are used for their effect on the peripheral autonomic nervous system rather than the CNS. Presumably, some of these agonists have some difficulty crossing the blood-brain barrier. However, when given in high doses, pilocarpine gets into the brain and causes seizures in experimental animals.[19] Another muscarinic agonist, **oxotremorine**, seems to produce marked effects on the brain at low doses in that it produces many of the symptoms of Parkinson's disease. Based on the apparent role of the ascending cholinergic neurons in the brain in regulating states of consciousness, it seems possible that cholinergic agonists that

---

* Registered Trademark of Merck & Company, Inc., West Point, Pennsylvania.

enter the brain produce arousal and insomnia. Indeed, even small doses of pilocarpine given intravenously in cats have been shown to produce arousal.[20]

There are no therapeutically useful nicotinic agonists except nicotine itself, which is used in patches or gum to treat smokers' dependence. However, clinical trials are being conducted to test the efficacy of nicotine in the treatment of Alzheimer's disease. Given the fact that the neuronal nicotinic receptor is different from the muscle receptor and that there are several subtypes of neuronal nicotinic receptors, it is likely that we will soon see some new nicotinic drugs that are useful in various neurological disorders.

Cholinesterase Inhibitors

Other than agonists, the only drugs used clinically to facilitate cholinergic neurotransmission are the inhibitors of acetylcholinesterase. These include the reversible cholinesterase inhibitors such as **physostigmine** (Antilirium®*), **neostigmine** (Prostigmin®**), **pyridostigmine** (Mestinon®***), and **edrophonium** (Tensilon®****) that are used to treat myasthenia gravis. Physostigmine crosses the blood-brain barrier while others do not, due to the fact that they are highly charged molecules. **Tacrine** (Cognex®*****) is a lipid-soluble reversible cholinesterase inhibitor that easily reaches the brain. It was recently introduced for the treatment of Alzheimer's disease. Tacrine also appears to act as a partial agonist at muscarinic cholinergic receptors. It has a short half-life (two to four hours) and is metabolized in the liver, where it can interfere with the metabolism of other drugs. There are also several irreversible inhibitors of cholinesterase such as the **organophosphates** (e.g., diisopropylfluorophosphate or DFP), which irreversibly phosphorylate the enzyme and are used primarily as insecticides. However, some of these are present in eye drops for the treatment of glaucoma. Obviously, the irreversible cholinesterase inhibitors are extremely toxic and are of interest because of their toxicological effects. They are too dangerous for systemic use.

Inhibitors of Cholinergic Neurotransmission

Muscarinic Antagonists

Alkaloids present in the belladonna plant have long been used as muscarinic antagonists. These include atropine and **scopolamine** (hyoscine) both of which are nonselective muscarinic antagonists. These drugs readily enter the brain after systemic administration, and some antimuscarinic agents, like **benztropine** (Cogentin®******), are used exclusively for their effect on the brain. The latter compound has been used to prevent the Parkinsonian-like side effects associated with antipsychotic drugs like Haldol®*******. In the days before H_2 histamine receptor antagonists (e.g., **cimetidine**), which are among the most commonly used ulcer drugs), atropine and other belladonna alkaloids were used to treat gastric ulcers and other conditions associated with increased gastrointestinal (GI) activity. However, **pirenzepine**, the M1 selective antagonist, has been found to be better at reducing gastric secretion. A new muscarinic antagonist, **ipratropium** (Atrovent®********), is delivered in an aerosol in the treatment of bronchial asthma. Anticholinergic drugs reduce bronchial secretions and cause bronchodilation, while decreasing GI activity and dilating the pupils. Hence, they are also used by ophthalmologists to dilate the pupils for examination

---

* Registered Trademark of Forest Pharmaceuticals, Inc., St. Louis, Missouri.
** Registered Trademark of ICN Pharmaceuticals, Inc., Costa Mesa, California.
*** Registered Trademark of ICN Pharmaceuticals, Inc., Costa Mesa, California.
**** Registered Trademark of ICN Pharmaceuticals, Inc., Costa Mesa, California.
***** Registered Trademark of Parke–Davis, Morris Plains, New Jersey.
****** Registered Trademark of Merck & Company, Inc., West Point, Pennsylvania.
******* Registered Trademark of McNeil Consumer Products Company, Fort Washington, Pennsylvania.
******** Registered Trademark of Boehringer Ingelheim Pharmaceuticals, Inc., Ridgefield, Connecticut

of the retina. When there is hypersecretion of saliva or bronchiolar secretions, as there is during general anesthesia, atropine or other antimuscarinic drugs are also used to reduce secretions and to dilate bronchiolar passages.

Nicotinic Antagonists

Nicotinic antagonists, at the present time, may be divided into two general categories: 1) those that are muscle nicotinic receptor antagonists, so-called *neuromuscular blockers,* such as **d-tubocurarine** (curare, the South American arrow poison) and 2) the neuronal nicotinic antagonists or so-called *ganglionic blockers* such as **hexamethonium** or **mecamylamine**. The neuromuscular blockers and the ganglionic blockers interfere with neurotransmission by acting on the postsynaptic nicotinic receptor (ion channel) and binding to it in a competitive or noncompetitive manner to prevent the binding of ACh to the receptor. The drugs that act at the neuromuscular junction to produce muscle paralysis bind directly to the nicotinic receptor, preventing access of ACh. This is also how some of the ganglionic blocking agents work (e.g., mecamylamine, **trimethaphan**). However, some of the ganglionic blockers (e.g., hexamethonium) enter the ion channel and form a plug, which also effectively interferes with neurotransmission by preventing influx of sodium ions.[21]

The neuromuscular blocking agents are also classified into two types: 1) depolarizing blockers and 2) nondepolarizing blockers. **Succinylcholine** (Anectine®*) is the most commonly used and best-known depolarizing blocker. It binds to the nicotinic receptor at the neuromuscular junction and produces a depolarization of the membrane, which remains in persistent depolarization for a long time, rendering the synapse nonfunctional. After a period of time, the neuromuscular block actually converts to a competitive-type block which is called *Phase II*. Giving a cholinesterase inhibitor will not antagonize the action of a depolarizing blocker and, in fact, may make the block worse. d-Tubocurarine, **gallamine**, **vecuronium**, and **pancuronium** are, on the other hand, competitive neuromuscular blockers which compete with ACh at the receptor. Thus, administering a cholinesterase inhibitor (e.g., physostigmine or neostigmine) can reverse the block produced by competitive antagonists such as d-tubocurarine. All neuromuscular blockers and most ganglionic blockers have a charged nitrogen atom and therefore do not get into the brain when injected systemically. In fact, if they are injected into the cerebrospinal fluid, they typically cause seizures. Mecamylamine, on the other hand, is a secondary amine which can enter the brain. Ganglionic blockers are used to lower blood pressure during removal of tumors of the adrenal gland, and neuromuscular blockers are used to relax muscles during endoscopic examinations, surgery, and electroconvulsive shock therapy.

NOREPINEPHRINE

Norepinephrine (NE) is one of three endogenous chemicals known as *catecholamines* that function as neurotransmitters in the mammalian nervous system. The other two are epinephrine, which is a neurotransmitter in the brain but a hormone in the periphery, and dopamine, which is a neurotransmitter in the brain (see below). NE is the neurotransmitter of the sympathetic postganglionic fibers of the autonomic nervous system, where it is involved in such things as increasing heart rate, constricting blood vessels or raising blood pressure, reducing gastrointestinal motility, and dilating pupils (see Table 4.3 for the response of various organs to sympathetic nerve stimulation). There are some exceptions to the rule that all postganglionic sympathetic nerves are "adrenergic" (i.e., use NE as a transmitter), namely, those postganglionic fibers going to sweat glands and the ones going to certain blood vessels in lower mammals. These both use ACh as a transmitter.

---

* Registered Trademark of The Brown Pharmaceutical Co., Inc., Research Triangle Park, North Carolina.

TABLE 4.3 Organ Response to Sympathetic Nerve Stimulation[a]

Organ receiving innervation	Response to stimulation	Receptor type
Eye		
Iris, radial muscle	Dilation (mydriasis)	Alpha$_1$
Iris, ciliary muscle	Relaxation for far vision	Beta$_2$
Heart		
Sa node	Increase in heart rate	Beta$_1$
Atrium	Increase in contractility	Beta$_1$
Av node	Increased conduction velocity	Beta$_1$
Ventricle	Increased contractility	Beta$_1$
Vasculature		
Skin and mucosa	Constriction	Alpha$_1$
Skeletal muscle	Constriction, dilation	Alpha$_1$; beta$_2$
Cerebral	Constriction	Alpha$_1$
Abdominal viscera	Mostly constriction, some dilation	Alpha$_1$; beta$_2$ for dilation
Trachea and bronchioles	Relaxation	Beta$_2$
Stomach and intestine	Decrease in motility and tone and secretion; contraction of sphincters	Alpha$_1$, alpha$_2$, Beta$_2$
Urinary bladder		
Detrusor muscle	Relaxation	Beta$_2$
Trigone and sphincter	Contraction	Alpha$_1$
Sex organ, male	Ejaculation	Alpha$_1$
Sweat glands	Localized secretion (palms of hands)	Alpha$_1$
Lacrimal glands	Slight secretion	Alpha$_1$
Nasopharyngeal glands	No direct innervation	—

[a] See Lefkowitz et al.[3] for detail.

The finding that catecholamines form fluorescent compounds in tissue exposed to formaldehyde gas greatly facilitated the mapping of such neurons in the brain. The technique, known as *fluorescence histochemistry,* was developed by Falck and Hillarp in Sweden in the early 1960's.[22]

The noradrenergic neurons in the brain are found in one of two systems: 1) the locus ceruleus system and 2) the lateral tegmental system. A description of these two systems is beyond the scope of this chapter, but can be found in an excellent review by Moore and Bloom.[23] Histochemical studies showed that the noradrenergic axons have a very widespread distribution reaching essentially all levels of the neuraxis. For example, neurons in the nucleus locus ceruleus of the pons innervate everything from the cerebral cortex to the spinal cord. The diffuse nature of the noradrenergic innervation allows this system to have global influences on brain function. The NE system in the brain has been implicated in a wide variety of functions, including anxiety, affective states (mood), arousal, REM sleep, aggression, pain perception, pleasure experience, seizures, and endocrine function.

Synthesis, Storage, Release, and Inactivation of NE

Neurons which synthesize and use NE as a neurotransmitter are referred to as *adrenergic* neurons or *noradrenergic* neurons. NE is synthesized in postganglionic sympathetic neurons and in neurons of the brain from tyrosine, an amino acid which is formed from phenylalanine in the liver. Phenylalanine is referred to as an essential amino acid because it must be supplied in the diet. Tyrosine is transported into adrenergic neurons by a high-affinity uptake transporter.[24] Once inside the neuron, tyrosine is converted to NE by the reactions shown in Figures 4.4 and 4.5.

The rate-limiting enzyme in the overall synthesis of catecholamines (both NE and dopamine) is tyrosine hydroxylase, which is found in the cytoplasm of the neuron. This enzyme utilizes molecular oxygen and tyrosine as substrates and requires iron and tetrahydrobiopterin as cofactors. Under most conditions, the concentration of tyrosine in the neuron saturates the enzyme. Thus, increasing the tyrosine concentration will not enhance the rate of NE synthe-

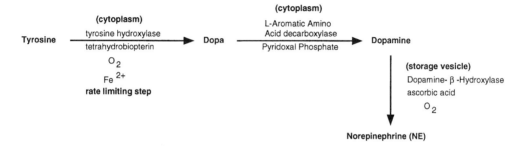

FIGURE 4.4 Synthesis of norepinephrine (NE) in the adrenergic nerve terminal. Shows the enzymes involved, the co-factors needed and their location within the neuron.

sis.[24] However, under conditions of increased utilization (e.g., stress), it may be possible to increase the rate of NE synthesis by administering tyrosine.[24]

The second step in the pathway, the conversion of DOPA (dihydroxyphenylalanine) to dopamine requires aromatic-L-amino acid decarboxylase, which uses pyridoxal phosphate (vitamin B_6) as a cofactor (Figure 4.5).

The third step in the pathway utilizes dopamine-β-hydroxylase (DBH) to convert dopamine to NE. DBH is a copper-containing enzyme which uses ascorbic acid as a cofactor and is located in the membrane of the storage vesicle. Thus, as dopamine is actively transported into the vesicle, it gets converted to NE.[5] Apparently, there is some soluble DBH inside the vesicle which is co-released with NE. Inhibition of DBH should reduce the levels of NE without affecting the levels of dopamine. In the adrenal medulla and in some neurons of the brain, NE is converted to epinephrine by the enzyme phenylethanolamine-N-methyltransferase (PNMT), which is found in the cytoplasm of cells.[3] Synthesis of NE within a neuron is regulated by a wide variety of factors, including the intracellular concentration of NE and the firing rate of the neuron.

Once synthesized, the catecholamines (NE, dopamine, and epinephrine in the brain) are stored in either small (200–300 Å) or large (500–1200 Å) membrane-bound vesicles. Inside the vesicle, NE is stored in a complex with ATP (adenosine triphosphate), as shown in Figure 4.4. NE is actively transported into the vesicle from the surrounding cytoplasm by an ATP-Mg^{++}-dependent process.[25] Uptake of NE into the vesicle, as well as storage inside the vesicle, is inhibited by the drug **reserpine**, which ultimately leads to the depletion of the tissue content of NE.

The release of NE from nerve terminals occurs when the terminal is depolarized by an incoming action potential. This results in the opening of voltage-dependent Ca^{2+} channels that trigger the process of exocytosis, similar to the release of ACh described above.

Many drugs can facilitate the release of NE from nerve endings to increase the concentration in the synaptic cleft and at the postsynaptic receptors. These include the **amphetamines** and **methylphenidate** (Ritalin®*), which stimulate the release of NE and dopamine (see below) by a Ca^{2+}-independent mechanism that does not involve exocytosis.

Following release of NE into the synaptic cleft and interaction with the postsynaptic receptors, the neurotransmitter action is terminated primarily by reuptake into the presynaptic terminal from which it was released.[5,24] The reuptake process for NE involves a sodium-dependent process which is inhibited by **antidepressants** and **cocaine**, but not by drugs like reserpine which inhibit the vesicular uptake. Recently, the molecular characteristics of the uptake transporter protein have been studied in great detail, and the chemical structure of this protein has been determined from cloning experiments.[26] Although reuptake has been shown to be the major process responsible for terminating the action of NE, enzymatic degradation also takes place via the enzymes monoamine oxidase (MAO) and catechol-O-methyltransferase (COMT).

----

* Registered Trademark of Ciba Pharmaceutical Company, Summit, New Jersey.

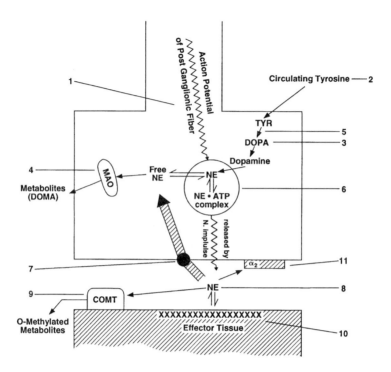

FIGURE 4.5 Schematic diagram of an adrenergic (sympathetic) neuron terminal synapsing on an effector organ in the peripheral autonomic nervous system. This also serves as a model for adrenergic synapses in the central nervous system (CNS). However, most of our knowledge about adrenergic synapses has come from studies on the peripheral sympathetic nervous system. The numbers shown indicate the sites where drugs are known to act to modify neurotransmission. These are as follows: (1) Some drugs (e.g., guanethidine and bretylium) inhibit the release of NE by blocking the propagation of the action potential (essential for release) into the nerve terminal; (2) under conditions of stress, it may be possible to increase NE synthesis by increasing the concentration of circulating tyrosine (i.e., by administering tyrosine); (3) a more effective way to increase dopamine and NE synthesis is to administer L-dopa because it bypasses the rate-limiting step involving tyrosine hydroxylase; (4) inhibitors of monoamine oxidase (MAO; e.g., tranylcypromine) act at Site 4 to prevent the degradation of NE; (5) inhibitors of tyrosine hydroxylase (e.g., alpha methyltyrosine) act here to block synthesis of NE; (6) drugs which interfere with the storage of NE (e.g., reserpine) act on the vesicle and eventually deplete the neuron of NE; (7) drugs which block reuptake of NE (e.g., cocaine and tricyclic antidepressants) act to increase the concentration of NE in the synapse; (8) NE in the synaptic cleft can act as an agonist on the postsynaptic receptors as can other agonists for alpha or beta receptors; (9) inhibitors of COMT can increase the availability of NE for agonist action; (10) NE, as well as other directly acting agonists, initiates a response; however, antagonists can also act here to block the response; (11) presynaptic alpha-2 receptors decrease the release of NE when these receptors are activated by NE or drugs such as clonidine.

MAO, which is present in the outer membrane of the mitochondrion, is involved in the intraneuronal degradation of free NE that is present in the cytoplasm of neurons. The MAO found in human and rat brain is present in two forms that are referred to as *Type A* and *Type B,* based on the fact that they have different substrate specificity and different sensitivity to specific inhibitors. For further discussion of the different types of MAO, the reader is referred to Cooper et al.[5] COMT is present in most cells of the body and takes care of the extraneuronal metabolism of catecholamines (NE and dopamine) before they reach the urine.[5,24]

Drugs which act as inhibitors of MAO cause elevations in the intraneuronal content of catecholamines (NE and dopamine) and eventually enhance the concentration of neurotransmitters reaching the receptors. MAO inhibitors are employed as antidepressant drugs.

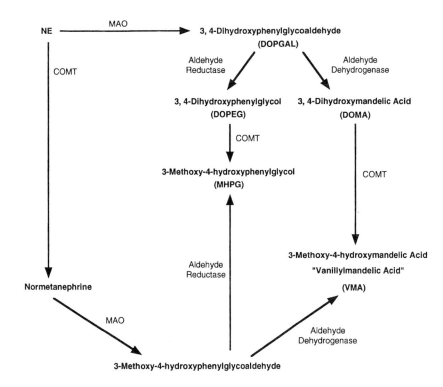

FIGURE 4.6 Enzymatic degradation of NE by monoamine oxidase (MAO) and catecholamine-*O*-methyltransferase (COMT).

The metabolic products resulting from the action of COMT and MAO on NE and dopamine are shown in Figure 4.6. These products represent clinically important metabolites that can be measured in cerebrospinal fluid (CSF) or urine to provide an index of how the catecholamine systems have been altered by disease or drug treatment. Weiner and Molinoff[24] can be reviewed for more details.

Norepinephrine Receptors

Norepinephrine receptors (adrenoceptors) mediate the effects of NE. Adrenoceptor subtypes that respond to NE include alpha$_1$, alpha$_2$, and beta$_1$. Beta$_2$ receptors have a lower affinity for NE, but have a high affinity for epinephrine and are involved in mediating some of the effects of the latter neurotransmitter or hormone. Specific agonists and antagonists exist for each receptor and some of these are described below.

In recent years, a great deal of information has been gained about the molecular nature of the adrenoceptors, both in terms of their coupling to second messenger systems (so-called *signal transduction mechanisms*) and their chemical structure. Each receptor is known to be an integral membrane glycoprotein with seven membrane-spanning regions and a molecular weight of 64,000 to 80,000 daltons.[27]

Unlike the nicotinic cholinergic receptor, which forms an ion channel and produces ultra-rapid effects, the adrenoceptors mediate their effects through second messenger systems and guanine nucleotide regulatory proteins or G-proteins.[3,24]

Both beta$_1$ and beta$_2$ adrenoceptors are linked to adenylate cyclase in the membrane by a G$_s$ (stimulatory G) protein which is activated by a combination between the receptor protein and an adrenergic agonist. The alpha subunit of the G$_s$ protein with guanosine triphosphate (GTP) bound to it can then interact with adenylate cyclase and activate it, leading to the conversion of

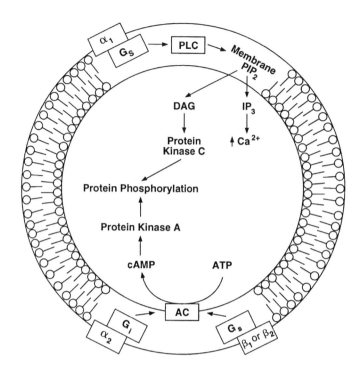

FIGURE 4.7   Schematic diagram of second messenger (signal transduction) systems linked to alpha and beta adrenergic receptors in a cell (neuron or effector cell) containing such receptors. The α_1 receptor is linked by a G-protein to phospholipase C (PLC) which, when activated (by agonist binding to α_1 receptor), leads to the breakdown of phosphatidylinositol 4,5-biphosphate (PIP_2) to form two second messengers (diacylglycerol or DAG and inositol triphosphate or IP3). The DAG activates protein kinase C which can, in turn, phosphorylate proteins including those in ion channels, while the IP3 causes an increase in intracellular calcium by releasing it from various stores. The calcium can activate calcium/calmodulin-dependent protein kinase which can phosphorylate other proteins. $Beta_1$ and $beta_2$ receptors act through a G_s protein to stimulate adenylyl cyclase (AC) leading to an increase in the formation of cyclic adenosine monophosphate (cAMP) which can activate protein kinase A to increase the phosphorylation of various proteins. Note that the α_2 receptor acts through a G_i protein (inhibitory G-protein) which leads to inhibition of adenylyl cyclase and a decrease in the intracellular concentration of cAMP. As can be seen here, protein phosphorylation is the major mechanism by which receptors act through signal transduction systems to alter cell function.

ATP to cyclic AMP. The latter can, in turn, activate various protein kinases which are involved in the phosphorylation (i.e., the addition of a phosphate group or PO_4^-) of various proteins that regulate membrane ion transport to alter membrane potentials (Figure 4.7).

The $alpha_2$ adrenoceptors, which are usually located presynaptically, also mediate their effect on membrane potential through a G-protein and adenylate cyclase activity, but unlike the beta receptors, the $alpha_2$ receptor is linked to a G_i (inhibitory G) protein which causes an inhibition of adenylate cyclase and a reduction in the amount of cyclic AMP (and presumably a reduction in protein phosphorylation) in the neuron.

The $alpha_1$ adrenergic receptor mediates its action through another second messenger system which is also linked to the receptor by a G_s protein. The second messengers produced when an agonist binds to the $alpha_1$ receptor are actually metabolites of phosphoinositide breakdown mediated by phospholipase C and include inositoltriphosphate (IP3) and diacylglycerol (DAG), as was the case for certain muscarinic receptors described above. IP3 causes the release of Ca^{2+} from intracellular storage sites, and the Ca^{2+} can then activate protein kinases to produce phosphorylation of membrane proteins (Figure 4.6). The DAG activates protein kinase C which, in turn, phosphorylates various proteins to mediate various cellular responses of alpha$_1$ agonists.[5,28]

There are now subtypes of alpha$_1$ receptors (e.g., α_{1a}, α_{1b}, α_{1c}) and it is likely that we will soon see subtypes of alpha$_2$ as well as the beta$_1$ and beta$_2$ receptors. Selective agonists and antagonists are available for alpha$_1$, alpha$_2$, beta$_1$, and beta$_2$ receptors, and these drugs are primarily used for their effects on the peripheral autonomic nervous system, especially in the area of cardiovascular disease.

Clinically Useful Drugs Which Alter Noradrenergic Neurotransmission

Facilitators of Noradrenergic Neurotransmission

Adrenergic Agonists

These are also referred to as *direct-acting sympathomimetic amines* and they are classified as either alpha or beta agonists. There are both alpha$_1$ and alpha$_2$ agonists available but many are nonselective. **Norepinephrine** (Levophed®*) itself is available and is an agonist for alpha$_1$, alpha$_2$, and beta$_1$ receptors, while epinephrine is an agonist for all adrenergic receptors. **Phenylephrine** is an alpha$_1$ agonist that is used in nose drops (Neo-Synephrine®**) as a nasal decongestant, where it acts to vasoconstrict the mucosal blood vessels and reduce congestion. Other alpha agonists that are predominantly alpha$_1$ selective include **methoxamine** and **metaraminol**. **Clonidine** (Catapres®***) is an alpha$_2$ agonist used as an antihypertensive agent because of its action on the brain, where stimulation of alpha$_2$ receptors presumably decreases the activity of the peripheral sympathetic nervous system. Other alpha$_2$ agonists include **guanfacine** and **guanabenz**.

Isoproterenol (Isuprel®****) is a beta agonist that stimulates both beta$_1$ and beta$_2$ receptors and has been used as a bronchodilator because of the beta$_2$ receptors in the bronchioles that mediate bronchiolar relaxation (Table 4.3). Indeed, most of the beta agonists are used for the treatment of diseases such as asthma that are associated with bronchoconstriction. Selective beta$_2$ agonists are also available and have the advantage of not causing cardiac stimulation when used in asthma. These include **metaproterenol** (Metaprel®*****), **terbutaline** (Brethine®******), and **albuterol** (Proventil®*******).

Drugs Which Block NE Reuptake

Inasmuch as reuptake is the major mechanism for inactivating released NE, drugs which block this process have a marked ability to facilitate noradrenergic neurotransmission. The classical example of a drug that does this is **cocaine**. Cocaine, however, also blocks dopamine and serotonin reuptake. Many of the antidepressant drugs (so-called *tricyclic antidepressants*) are potent and selective inhibitors of NE uptake and presumably mediate some of their beneficial effects in depression via this mechanism.[29] Selective NE uptake inhibitors include **desipramine** (Norpramin®********), **protriptyline** (Vivactil®*********), **nortriptyline** (Aventyl®**********), and **maprotiline** (Ludiomil®***********). All of these are used to treat depression. Side

---

* Registered Trademark of Sanofi Winthrop Pharmaceuticals, New York, New York.
** Registered Trademark of Sanofi Winthrop Pharmaceuticals, New York, New York.
*** Registered Trademark of Boehringer Ingelheim Pharmaceuticals, Inc., Ridgefield, Connecticut.
**** Registered Trademark of Sanofi Winthrop Pharmaceuticals, New York, New York.
***** Registered Trademark of Sandoz Pharmaceuticals, East Hanover, New Jersey.
****** Registered Trademark of Geigy Pharmaceuticals, Ardsley, New York.
******* Registered Trademark of Schering Corporation, Kenilworth, New Jersey.
******** Registered Trademark of Marion Merrell Dow, Inc., Kansas City, Missouri.
********* Registered Trademark of Merck & Company, Inc., West Point, Pennsylvania.
********** Registered Trademark of Eli Lilly & Company, Indianapolis, Indiana.
*********** Registered Trademark of Ciba Pharmaceuticals Company, Summit, New Jersey.

effects of these drugs include their ability to increase heart rate and blood pressure due to peripheral effects on the cardiovascular system. At plasma concentrations that exceed the recommended level, these drugs can also lower seizure threshold or precipitate seizures.

Drugs Which Increase NE Release

Several drugs are available to increase the release of NE (as well as dopamine in the CNS) from nerve endings. The mechanism by which this is accomplished is not entirely clear. However, it appears to involve the release of NE from a nonvesicular pool which does not require calcium and does not involve exocytosis. The current hypothesis is that these drugs are taken up by the uptake transporter for NE, bringing the carrier to the inside of the neuron where NE can bind to it for exchange transport. They also interfere with the uptake of NE by vesicles, increasing the cytoplasmic concentration of NE and making more available for reverse transport.[3] Drugs that facilitate the release of NE include **amphetamine**, **dextroamphetamine** (Dexedrine®*), **methamphetamine** (Desoxyn®**) and **methylphenidate** (Ritalin®). These drugs also increase the release of dopamine from nerve terminals, which is believed to be responsible for many of their effects and will be discussed below.

Amphetamine is the racemic mixture of D- and L-amphetamine. Dextroamphetamine is three to four times more potent in stimulating the CNS than is L-amphetamine. All amphetamine analogues have powerful cardiovascular stimulating effects leading to an increase in blood pressure and the work of the heart. The CNS stimulating effects of amphetamine on arousal and locomotor activity are dependent on newly synthesized NE or dopamine since these effects are blocked by alpha methyltyrosine, a tyrosine hydroxylase inhibitor used to block NE synthesis.[21]

The amphetamines, as a group, are used to suppress appetite in the treatment of obesity and to treat narcolepsy and attention deficit hyperactivity disorder (ADHD). These drugs are regulated as controlled substances because of their abuse potential. High doses can produce a psychosis that is indistinguishable from an acute paranoid schizophrenic syndrome. Moreover, it has been shown, in both rats and nonhuman primates, that repeated injections of methamphetamine can produce neurotoxicity leading to the loss of both dopamine- and serotonin-containing neurons in the brain.[30-33] The mechanism responsible for this neurotoxicity remains unknown, although several hypotheses have been proposed.

Drugs That Decrease the Enzymatic Degradation of NE

NE is degraded intraneuronally by the enzyme monoamine oxidase (MAO), as indicated above. Inhibiting this enzyme should eventually increase the concentration of NE in the synaptic cleft. Several MAO inhibitors are used clinically as antidepressants. These include **tranylcypromine** (Parnate®***), **phenelzine** (Nardil®****), and **isocarboxazid** (Marplan®*****). Some MAO inhibitors are being used experimentally to prevent further deterioration of Parkinson's disease. One drug in the latter category is **selegiline** (deprenyl), which is selective for MAO-B. Patients on MAO inhibitors cannot eat foods containing tyramine (a potent NE releaser). Normally, tyramine is metabolized by MAO in the intestine but this enzyme is inactive in patients on an MAO inhibitor. The tyramine reaching the circulation causes a hypertensive crisis with very dangerous consequences. Thus, individuals taking MAO inhibitors must avoid foods containing tyramine, such as wine, beer, cheese, and other fermented products.

---

* Registered Trademark of SmithKline Beecham Pharmaceuticals, Pittsburgh, Pennsylvania.
** Registered Trademark of Abbott Laboratories, North Chicago, Illinois.
*** Registered Trademark of SmithKline Beecham Pharmaceuticals, Pittsburgh, Pennsylvania.
**** Registered Trademark of Parke-Davis, Morris Plains, New Jersey.
***** Registered Trademark of Roche Laboratories, Nutley, New Jersey.

Inhibitors of Noradrenergic Neurotransmission

Adrenoceptor Antagonists

There have long been available drugs that are selective antagonists of either alpha or beta adrenergic receptors. Now, we have drugs that are even selective for a specific subtype of alpha or beta receptor. The main advantage of a subtype-selective antagonist is that it will have fewer side effects. Nonselective alpha antagonists include **phenoxybenzamine** and **phentolamine**, while nonselective beta antagonists include **propranolol** (Inderal®*), **sotalol**, and **pindolol**. Of interest for the treatment of hypertension are the alpha$_1$ selective antagonists, **prazosin** (Minipress®**) and **terazosin** (Hytrin®***). Beta$_1$ selective antagonists are useful because they can be used to reduce blood pressure, stop cardiac arrhythmias, or prevent subsequent heart attacks with minimal effects on bronchiolar smooth muscle. **Metoprolol** (Lopressor®****), **atenolol** (Tenormin®*****), **acebutolol** (Sectral®******), and **esmolol** (Brevibloc®*******) are all currently marketed beta$_1$ selective antagonists used to treat cardiovascular disorders.

Inhibitors of NE Release

Some drugs are selectively taken up into noradrenergic nerve terminals and then prevent the release of NE apparently by blocking the invasion of the action potential into the terminal (i.e., a local anesthetic-like effect). Drugs in this category are referred to as *adrenergic neuronal blocking agents* and include **guanethidine** (Ismelin®********), **guanadrel** (Hylorel®*********), and **bretylium**. Initially, these drugs cause a transient release of NE prior to the inhibition of release. When used chronically, guanethidine also has a reserpine-like effect (see below) by interfering with NE storage and depleting the neurons of NE. Such drugs are primarily used as antihypertensive agents.

Inhibitors of Storage

Reserpine is the classical drug for inhibiting the storage of catecholamines (NE, epinephrine, and dopamine) and serotonin (see below). Reserpine interferes with the uptake of monoamines into the vesicle and also blocks storage inside the vesicle. When NE is not stored, it leaks out of the vesicle into the cytoplasm and is degraded by MAO. Thus, reserpine leads to a depletion of the NE from the nerve terminals (see Figure 4.5). It is primarily used in combination with other drugs as an antihypertensive agent.[21]

Inhibitors of NE Synthesis

There are two sites within the NE synthetic pathway where drugs can be used to block synthesis: 1) the tyrosine hydroxylase step (which is the rate-limiting enzyme) and 2) the dopamine-β-hydroxylase step. The latter is more selective and can be accomplished with the drug **disulfiram** (Antabuse®**********) or its active metabolite, diethyldithiocarbamate (DDTC). Unfortunately, these drugs inhibit a lot of other enzymes and have many side effects.

---

* Registered Trademark of Wyeth–Ayerst Laboratories, Philadelphia, Pennsylvania.
** Registered Trademark of Pfizer Consumer Health Care, Parsippany, New Jersey.
*** Registered Trademark of Abbott Laboratories, North Chicago, Illinois.
**** Registered Trademark of Geigy Pharmaceuticals, Ardsley, New York.
***** Registered Trademark of Zeneca Pharmaceuticals, Wilmington, Delaware.
****** Registered Trademark of Wyeth–Ayerst Laboratories, Philadelphia, Pennsylvania.
******* Registered Trademark of Anaquest, Inc., Liberty Corner, New Jersey.
******** Registered Trademark of Ciba Pharmaceutical Company, Summit, New Jersey.
********* Registered Trademark of Fisons Corporation, Rochester, New York.
********** Registered Trademark of Wyeth–Ayerst Laboratories, Philadelphia, Pennsylvania.

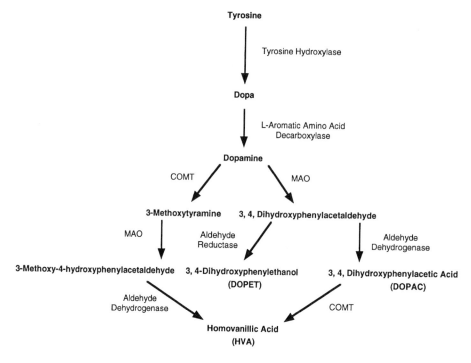

FIGURE 4.8 Synthesis and degradation of dopamine. Note that HVA is the major metabolite. COMT, catechola-mine-*O*-methyltransferase; DOPA, dihydroxyphenylalanine; MAO, monoamine oxidase.

The most common way to interfere with synthesis of NE is to inhibit tyrosine hydroxylase with **α-methyltyrosine** (Metyrosine®*). However, this drug also blocks the synthesis of epinephrine and dopamine and is, therefore, not very selective.

DOPAMINE

Although dopamine can be found in the peripheral nervous system in such places as the carotid body and sympathetic ganglia, it is of interest primarily for its neurotransmitter role in the CNS, where it is involved in a wide variety of functions from regulating motor function (basal ganglia) to inhibiting the release of prolactin from the pituitary gland. Most of the dopamine neurons in the brain have their cell bodies either in the midbrain (e.g., substantia nigra), where they are involved in the regulation of emotional states or motor activity (e.g., substantia nigra dopamine is lost in Parkinson's disease), or the hypothalamus, where they are involved in regulating endocrine function.[5] Thus, there are three major dopaminergic pathways in the CNS: 1) the nigrostriatal pathway (which projects from the substantia nigra to the striatum and is important in Parkinson's disease), 2) the mesocortical and mesolimbic system (which projects from the ventromedial aspect of the midbrain to the limbic system and the cerebral cortex, playing a key role in psychiatric disorders), and 3) the tuberoinfundibular pathway (which projects from the arcuate nucleus of the hypothalamus to the median eminence of the pituitary stalk, which regulates endocrine function).

Synthesis, Storage, Release, and Inactivation of Dopamine

Dopamine is an intermediate compound in the synthesis of NE and is, in fact, the immediate precursor of NE (see Figure 4.8). Thus, the synthesis is identical to that of NE up through the formation of dopamine, but does not proceed to NE because dopaminergic neurons lack the

* Registered Trademark of Merck & Company, Inc., West Point, Pennsylvania.

enzyme dopamine-β-hydroxylase. As was the case with NE synthesis, tyrosine hydroxylase is the rate-limiting enzyme in the synthetic pathway and, if one wants to block synthesis, this is the enzyme to block.

Dopamine synthesis is regulated somewhat differently than is NE synthesis. This is largely because dopaminergic neurons have autoreceptors on the dopamine nerve terminal that regulate both synthesis and release, whereas NE neurons have autoreceptors (which are α_2) that regulate release only.[5] However, like NE, the intracellular concentration of dopamine can regulate synthesis through end-product inhibition. Again, tyrosine hydroxylase is normally saturated with tyrosine, so administering tyrosine is not an effective way to enhance the synthesis of dopamine. However, DOPA decarboxylase is not saturated with substrate, and synthesis of dopamine can be increased by the administration of DOPA, given as levodopa, which is now the drug of choice in the treatment of Parkinson's disease. In Parkinson's disease, the nigrostriatal dopaminergic pathway degenerates and the administration of levodopa helps replace the dopamine in the striatum.

Dopamine is stored in vesicles in a manner similar to that of NE in a complex with ATP. Several soluble proteins, called *chromogranins*, are also present in the dopamine storage vesicle. The release of dopamine from nerve terminals, like that of NE, is triggered by the arrival of an action potential. Release occurs by a process of exocytosis and, therefore, is calcium dependent. The release of dopamine is apparently reduced by a negative feedback mechanism when excess dopamine in the synaptic cleft interacts with presynaptic receptors (autoreceptors). Activation of autoreceptors on the cell body reduces the firing rates of dopaminergic neurons.[5] All dopaminergic autoreceptors are believed to be of the D-2 or D-3 subtype (see below).

Dopamine is inactivated following release by a high-affinity uptake transporter (reuptake), which transports it back into the neuron from which it was released. This is an energy-requiring process that is dependent on sodium and is similar to the NE reuptake. As is the case with NE and most other neurotransmitters, the dopamine transporter has been cloned and found to be a member of a large family of transporter proteins that have twelve membrane-spanning regions. Indeed, much is known about the molecular characteristics of the dopamine transporter.[34]

Although reuptake into the neuron from which it was released is the primary mechanism for terminating the physiological effects of released dopamine, it may also undergo enzymatic metabolism similar to NE. Thus, both MAO and COMT can convert dopamine to inactive compounds according to the schema shown in Figure 4.8. Moreover, the resulting metabolites DOPAC and HVA (see Figure 4.8) are often used as indices of the rate of dopamine turnover in the CNS. Antipsychotic drugs (neuroleptics) which block dopamine receptors increase the concentration of dopamine metabolites in cerebrospinal fluid and in the brain (see below and Cooper, Bloom, and Roth[5] for more detail).

Dopamine Receptors

Two major types of dopamine receptors (D-1 and D-2) were identified and described in great detail using receptor binding techniques.[35] However, in the last four years, five additional dopamine receptors have been identified using molecular cloning techniques and all the dopamine receptors, including the new ones (D-3, D-4, and D-5), are now classified as either D-1-like or D-2-like receptors.[36-39] The D-1-like include the D-1 and D-5 receptors, while the D-2-like include D-2, D-3, and D-4 receptors. The D-1-like receptors appear to mediate their effects through a G_s protein which activates adenylate cyclase and increases cyclic AMP, while the D-2-like receptors appear to be negatively coupled to adenylate cyclase, producing an inhibition of the latter through a G_i protein. All of the dopamine receptors (D-1, D-2, D-3, D-4, and D-5) have seven hydrophobic regions corresponding to the predicted seven membrane-spanning regions of the other G-protein linked receptors in this family.

There is considerable sequence homology (similar sequence of amino acids in the protein) between the various dopamine receptors as well as between these receptors and other members of this family such as the beta$_1$ and muscarinic receptors.[36] The D-3 receptor appears to represent both an autoreceptor and postsynaptic receptor and is found in limbic areas of the brain.[36] The D-4 receptor is of great interest because it has been implicated in the effects of clozapine (an atypical antipsychotic agent) and may account for the unique effects of **clozapine** (Clozaril®*). For most antipsychotic drugs, there is a high correlation between their clinical potency and their D-2 receptor blocking action. However, clozapine is much more potent at blocking D-4 receptors and has fewer motor side effects than the other antipsychotic drugs. Moreover, clozapine is effective at alleviating the symptoms of schizophrenia in some patients that are refractory to other antipsychotic drugs. The D-4 receptor is largely found in the limbic system and there is some evidence that the D-4 receptor is markedly increased in the brains of schizophrenic patients.[39] There appear to be as many as seven different forms of the D-4 receptor in the human brain with each form having a different number of amino acids.[39] In general, the function of most subtypes of dopamine receptor are unknown. D-1 receptors have only been found postsynaptically, but D-2 receptors occur either pre- or postsynaptically and autoreceptors are usually of the D-2 subtype. The use of D-1 and D-2 agonists has shown that activation of both receptors may be necessary for expression of certain dopamine functions.

The dopamine neurons have been implicated in the abuse of stimulants such as cocaine and amphetamine. Mesolimbic dopaminergic neurons have also been implicated in the addiction to alcohol and nicotine. It has recently been proposed that variations in the gene for the D-2 receptor may contribute to inter-individual differences in vulnerability to alcoholism and polysubstance abuse.[40]

Clinically Useful Drugs Which Alter Dopaminergic Neurotransmission

Facilitators of Dopaminergic Neurotransmission

Dopamine Agonists

Dopamine itself does not cross the blood-brain barrier and therefore cannot be used for effects on the CNS. However, dopamine is used intravenously for its effects on the cardiovascular system, where it acts on beta$_1$ receptors in the heart to increase contractility and on dopamine receptors in the renal vasculature to cause vasodilation. Because of these two actions, dopamine is used to treat various forms of shock. **Apomorphine** is a nonselective dopamine agonist that does get into the brain and has been used to treat such things as Parkinson's disease. However, it is poorly absorbed from the gut and must be administered parenterally. Apomorphine achieves high concentrations in the chemoreceptor trigger zone (CTZ) in the area postrema of the medulla oblongata, which regulates vomiting. Because of its effects here, apomorphine produces nausea and vomiting, limiting its usefulness in the treatment of dopamine deficiency syndromes. Other nonselective dopamine agonists include **bromocriptine** (Parlodel®**) which has long been used to treat endocrine disorders such as hyperprolactinemia, where it acts in the anterior pituitary gland to inhibit the release of prolactin. Bromocriptine is also now recommended for the treatment of Parkinson's disease. **Lisuride** and **pergolide** (Permax®***) are two other dopamine agonists that, along with bromocriptine, have been used in Parkinson's disease.

Several new selective D-1 and D-2 agonists are now being examined experimentally. For example, **SKF 38393** is a D-1 agonist, while **LY 17155** is a D-2 agonist. These are being used as tools to learn more about the function of D-1 and D-2 receptors, but they could become clinically useful in the future. Drugs selective for the D-3, D-4, or D-5 receptor have not yet been developed.

---

* Registered Trademark of Sandoz Pharmaceuticals Corp., East Hanover, New Jersey.
** Registered Trademark of Sandoz Pharmaceuticals Corp., East Hanover, New Jersey.
*** Registered Trademark of Athena Neurosciences, Inc., So. San Francisco, California.

Drugs That Increase the Synaptic Concentration of Dopamine by Acting Indirectly

These include the indirectly-acting agents such as **amphetamine** and **methylphenidate** (Ritalin®), which increase the release of dopamine into the synaptic cleft, the dopamine reuptake inhibitors (**GBR 12909**, amphetamine, **nomifensine, benztropine, amantadine**), and the drugs which increase dopamine synthesis (**levodopa**, amantadine). The reader will note that some of these drugs have more than one action. For example, amphetamine and amantadine increase the release of dopamine from nerve endings as well as prevent the inactivation by reuptake.

Several reports, in recent years, suggest that enhancing dopaminergic neurotransmission may be beneficial to patients with traumatic brain injury (TBI). Improving dopaminergic function appears to be useful for two types of deficits in these patients. First, some TBI patients display parkinsonian-like symptoms and, second, dopaminergic agents may improve arousal and the ability to focus attention on the task at hand, including rehabilitation therapy. Just as L-DOPA (levodopa) is effective in Parkinson's disease, it may help similar symptoms in patients with TBI. However, the combination of L-DOPA with a peripheral decarboxylase inhibitor will reduce the metabolism of L-DOPA in the periphery and increase the amount that actually reaches the brain. Thus, the combination of levodopa and carbidopa (a decarboxylase inhibitor) is often used. Sinemet®* (a mixture of L-DOPA and **carbidopa**) has, in fact, been used successfully in some patients with TBI.[41,42]

Drugs That Block Enzymatic Degradation of Dopamine

Like other catecholamines, dopamine is degraded by MAO and COMT (see above). Therefore, MAO inhibitors can increase the synaptic concentration of dopamine. Selegiline (Eldepryl®**) (described above) is now being used to treat Parkinson's disease because it may prevent the formation of neurotoxins that destroy dopaminergic neurons and arrest the progression of the disease. All of the MAO inhibitors described above under NE will also prevent the enzymatic degradation of dopamine. There are currently no COMT inhibitors available for clinical use. However, several new COMT inhibitors are being examined experimentally in animal studies.[43]

Inhibitors of Dopaminergic Neurotransmission

Drugs That Interfere with Dopaminergic Neurotransmission

In this category, we have just two groups of drugs: 1) the receptor antagonists or blockers and 2) the drugs which interfere with storage (e.g., reserpine). As would be expected, the only ones that provide selective effects on dopaminergic neurotransmission are the receptor blockers, since reserpine-like drugs interfere with the storage of all monoamines. We will, therefore, consider only the dopamine antagonists here.

Antagonists of dopamine receptors are primarily used as antipsychotic drugs (also called *neuroleptics*) to treat schizophrenia. The fact that all of the drugs effective in schizophrenia are dopaminergic antagonists has led to the hypothesis that schizophrenia is caused by too much dopamine at certain synapses, a hypothesis that has been difficult to prove. Essentially all of the dopamine antagonists block D-2 receptors, but D-1 and D-4 receptors may be affected by selected drugs. A list of the dopamine antagonists is given in Table 4.4.

Dopamine antagonists have many side effects because they block dopamine receptors not only in the limbic system, which regulates emotion, but, also, in the basal ganglia, where loss of dopamine function causes parkinsonian-like symptoms, and in the pituitary where they cause endocrine-related side effects. **Metoclopramide** (Reglan®***) is a dopamine antagonist

---

* Registered Trademark of DuPont Pharmaceuticals, Wilmington, Delaware.
** Registered Trademark of Somerset Pharmaceuticals, Inc., Tampa, Florida.
*** Registered Trademark of A. H. Robins Company, Richmond, Virginia.

TABLE 4.4 Dopamine Receptor Antagonists (Blockers)[a]

Chemical class	Examples of drugs	Receptor type
Phenothiazines	Chlorpromazine Thioridazine Perphenazine	D-1 and D-2
Thioxanthenes	Chlorprothixene Thiothixene	D-2
Butyrophenones	Haloperidol (Haldol®)	Some selectivity for D-2
Dihydroindoles	Molindone	D-2
Dibenzodiazepines	Clozapine (Clozaril®)	D-4(?)
Substituted benzamides	Metoclopramide (Reglan®) Sch 23390	D-2 Selective for D-1

[a] See Baldessarini et al.[29] for more detail.

used for its peripheral effects and its effects on the chemoreceptor trigger zone (which is outside the blood-brain barrier) to prevent nausea and vomiting. Although it penetrates the brain poorly, some does reach the basal ganglia which can cause some parkinsonian-like side effects. All of the D-2 dopamine receptor antagonists have antiemetic properties, but only some (e.g., metoclopramide and **prochlorperazine**) are approved for such use.

5-HYDROXYTRYPTAMINE (SEROTONIN)

5-Hydroxytryptamine or serotonin (5-HT) is an indolamine that is found both in the periphery and in the CNS. About 90% of the 5-HT in the body is found in the gastrointestinal tract (in enterochromaffin cells and neurons of the myenteric plexus), while 8% of the 5-HT of the body is found in platelets, and only 2% is found in the brain.[5] It is, however, the 2% in the brain that receives most of the attention and this is the fraction we will focus on.

Within the brain, 5-HT is localized in neurons that express the gene for tryptophan hydroxylase (Trp-OH). Extensive mapping of serotonergic neurons in the CNS of the rat has been performed using fluorescence histochemistry and immunocytochemistry. In general, the cell bodies of the serotonergic neurons are located along the midline of the brainstem in what are called *raphe nuclei*. Originally, nine separate groups of 5-HT cell bodies were described by Dahlstrom and Fuxe,[44] but more recently other cell groups have been detected in the area postrema (vomiting area) and in the caudal locus ceruleus as well as in the interpeduncular nucleus.[5] Like the noradrenergic neurons, the serotonergic neurons have a widespread distribution innervating most areas of the brain from the cerebral cortex to the spinal cord. The more caudal cell groups (B-1 to B-3) primarily innervate the spinal cord, while the rostral cell groups (B-6 to B-9) innervate the forebrain. A detailed description of the neuroanatomy of serotonergic neurons has been provided by Molliver.[45]

Synthesis, Storage, Release, and Inactivation of Serotonin

The amino acid precursor for 5-HT synthesis is tryptophan, which is an essential amino acid supplied in the diet. Tryptophan, like tyrosine, is a neutral amino acid that also gains entry into the brain by the large neutral amino acid transporter. Thus, plasma tryptophan will compete with other neutral amino acids such as tyrosine and phenylalanine for transport into the brain, which means that the concentration of brain tryptophan will be determined not only by the concentration of tryptophan in plasma but also by the plasma concentration of other neutral amino acids.[5,46] Once in the extracellular fluid of the brain, tryptophan is transported into the serotonergic neurons by a high-affinity and a low-affinity transport system where it can then be converted to 5-HT by a two-step reaction (Figure 4.9) with each step being catalyzed by a different enzyme.[47]

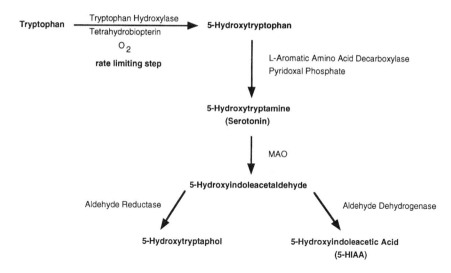

FIGURE 4.9 Synthesis and degradation of 5-hydroxytryptamine (serotonin) in the CNS. Note that 5-HIAA is the major metabolite. MAO, monoamine oxidase.

The rate-limiting step in the overall conversion of tryptophan to serotonin is the first step, which is catalyzed by tryptophan hydroxylase (Figure 4.9) and results in the conversion of tryptophan to 5-hydroxytryptophan (5-HTP). Like tyrosine hydroxylase, tryptophan hydroxylase is a cytoplasmic mixed-function oxidase, which requires molecular oxygen and a reduced pteridine as cofactors. It should also be noted that a membrane-associated form of tryptophan hydroxylase has been found, indicating that some of the enzyme may be membrane bound. Various inhibitors of tryptophan hydroxylase have been identified, the best known of which is **parachlorophenylalanine** (PCPA), which has been used experimentally to study the function of 5-HT.

Inasmuch as the Km of tryptophan hydroxylase (50–120 μM) is higher than the concentration of brain tryptophan (30 μM), the enzyme is not saturated with tryptophan, which means that increasing the concentration of brain tryptophan can increase the synthesis of 5-HT and lead to higher brain levels of serotonin.[47,48] Thus, it has been found that dietary manipulations of tryptophan can change the brain concentration of serotonin. The 5-HTP formed by the action of tryptophan hydroxylase on tryptophan is immediately converted to 5-HT (serotonin) by the action of aromatic-L-amino acid decarboxylase, the same enzyme that converts DOPA to dopamine in catecholaminergic neurons. The decarboxylation of 5-HTP, like that of DOPA, requires pyridoxal phosphate as a cofactor. Inasmuch as the decarboxylation takes place in the cytoplasm, the resulting 5-HT must then be transported into vesicles for storage (see below).

The rate of 5-HT synthesis appears to be regulated by the rate of neuronal firing. The latter control over 5-HT synthesis appears to be exerted on tryptophan hydroxylase by a Ca^{2+}-dependent phosphorylation of the rate-limiting enzyme.[48]

The available evidence suggests that serotonin, like the catecholamines, is stored in membrane-bound synaptic vesicles inside nerve terminals.[49] A substantial portion of the serotonin in the brain is found in isolated vesicles and these vesicles have been shown to take up serotonin.[50,51] Release of 5-HT, like that of other neurotransmitters, appears to occur by exocytosis in a calcium-dependent manner.[49] However, certain drugs, such as **p-chloroamphetamine**, are believed to release serotonin from the cytoplasmic pool rather than the vesicular pool,[52] and there is some evidence that the depolarization mediated release by neurons can involve either vesicular or cytoplasmic pools.[53] The available evidence suggests that 5-HT is stored in the vesicles in a complex with ATP and perhaps a serotonin-binding protein.[49]

The release of 5-HT from nerve endings is also believed to be regulated via a negative feedback mechanism through serotonin autoreceptors located on the presynaptic (serotonergic) nerve terminals. The evidence indicates that these 5-HT autoreceptors are of the 5-HT$_{1B}$ subtype (see below and Green).[48] Most of the postsynaptic effects of 5-HT are believed to be inhibitory, although it has been shown to facilitate excitatory neurotransmitters at some sites in the brain.[48]

Mechanisms similar to those of catecholamine inactivation (see above) have been shown to occur for serotonin inactivation. Thus, both reuptake into the neuron from which it was released and monoamine oxidase may be involved in the inactivation of 5-HT following its action in the synaptic cleft. A high-affinity, sodium-dependent, energy-dependent (requires ATP) uptake of 5-HT has been demonstrated in experimental studies,[46] and reuptake into serotonergic terminals appears to function as the primary inactivation mechanism for removing released serotonin from the synaptic cleft. This concept is supported by studies showing that inhibitors of serotonin uptake, such as **fluoxetine** (Prozac®*) or **clomipramine** (Anafranil®**), enhance the action of serotonin. However, others[54] believe that the primary fate of released 5-HT is uptake by nonserotonergic cells followed by degradation by monoamine oxidase to form 5-hydroxyindoleacetic acid (5-HIAA). The latter investigators have suggested that brain or CSF levels of 5-HIAA can be used as an index of serotonin turnover and utilization.[54] From Figure 4.8, it can be seen that 5-hydroxytryptophol can also be formed by the action of monoamine oxidase on serotonin in the brain, although the major metabolite is 5-HIAA.[48]

Serotonin Receptors

In the last four to five years, there has been an explosion of information about the 5-HT receptor. Three separate families of serotonin receptors have been identified.[55] These include the 5-HT$_1$ family (including 5-HT$_{1A}$, 5-HT$_{1B}$, 5-HT$_{1D}$, 5-HT$_{1E}$, etc.), the 5-HT$_2$ family, and the 5-HT$_3$ family.

The 5-HT$_1$ family is negatively coupled to adenylate cyclase through a G$_i$ protein and has seven membrane-spanning regions similar to other G-protein linked receptors. The 5-HT$_2$, and what was formerly called the 5-HT$_{1C}$ receptors, make up another family because of their molecular and biochemical similarities. Both of the latter receptors are linked to phospholipase C and the phosphoinoside second messenger system through G-proteins similar to the alpha$_1$ adrenergic receptor.

The 5-HT$_3$ family was originally identified in the periphery.[56] These receptors appear to be ligand-gated ion channels that mediate primarily excitatory effects of serotonin. At the present time, 5-HT$_3$ receptors are identified primarily by their affinity for specific agonists and antagonists.[55,56] The 5-HT$_3$ receptors appear to be present in the area postrema where they play a role in regulating vomiting. Indeed, the 5-HT$_3$ antagonist **ondansetron** (Zofran®***) is now used to treat the nausea and vomiting associated with cancer chemotherapy.

Clinically Useful Drugs Which Alter Serotonergic Neurotransmission

Facilitators of Serotonergic Neurotransmission

Drugs That Increase the Synthesis and/or Release of 5-HT

Since the rate-limiting enzyme Trp-OH is not saturated with tryptophan, it is possible to increase the synthesis of 5-HT by administering tryptophan. However, a number of factors

---

* Registered Trademark of Dista Products Company, Indianapolis, Indiana.
** Registered Trademark of Basel Pharmaceuticals, Summit, New Jersey.
*** Registered Trademark of Cerenex Pharmaceuticals, Research Triangle Park, North Carolina.

affect the amount of tryptophan that actually gets into the brain, such as the ratio of tryptophan to other neutral amino acids in the plasma that compete with tryptophan for transport into the brain and the concentration of free fatty acids in the plasma which compete with tryptophan for binding to plasma proteins.

Tryptophan administration has apparently been used in the treatment of depression, but its effectiveness has been questioned. It is also possible to increase the release of 5-HT from nerve terminals with **fenfluramine** (Pondimin®*), a drug that has been marketed as an appetite suppressant (anorexiant) to treat obesity. It is interesting that fenfluramine remains on the market despite the fact that it was shown to damage serotonergic neurons in rats.

Drugs That are 5-HT Agonists

The availability of agonists selective for specific subtypes of 5-HT receptors is low. Serotonin itself does not cross the blood-brain barrier and many of the other agonists are hallucinogenic. However, there are two partial agonists for 5-HT$_{1a}$ receptors (**ipsapirone** and **buspirone**) that are being used. Of these, buspirone (BuSpar®**) is the only one approved for use in the United States, where it is used as an antianxiety agent. **Sumatriptan** (Imitrex®***), an agonist for the 5-HT$_{1D}$ receptor, is now marketed for the treatment of migraine headache. The latter is believed to act by increasing cerebral vascular constriction during the vasodilatory phase of a migraine headache.[57,58]

Drugs That Block the Reuptake or Prevent Enzymatic Degradation of 5-HT

It is clear that the most common way to increase serotonergic neurotransmission, clinically, is to use a reuptake blocker. The ones approved for clinical use include **fluoxetine** (Prozac®) and **clomipramine** (Anafranil®), both of which are used as antidepressants. These drugs are also used to treat obsessive-compulsive disorder and could be used to suppress appetite, although they are not approved for the latter. Monoamine oxidase inhibitors, described above under norepinephrine, can also be used to enhance serotonergic neurotransmission, since they will prevent the degradation of this amine as well.[5] However, the MAO inhibitors are not selective and should result in an increase in the synaptic content of NE, dopamine, and 5-HT.

Inhibitors of Serotonergic Neurotransmission

There are few drugs clinically available for interfering with serotonergic neurotransmission and these fall into one of two categories: 1) drugs that interfere with storage of 5-HT and 2) drugs that block 5-HT receptors. The drugs that interfere with the storage of 5-HT are the same drugs that do this to NE and dopamine, namely, **reserpine** or **tetrabenazine**. The only one used clinically is reserpine, which is used to treat hypertension. A side effect of reserpine is depression with suicidal tendency, which apparently results from the depletion of brain NE and 5-HT.

There are a whole host of experimental drugs that block 5-HT receptors, but only two are available for clinical use at the present time. These include **methysergide** (Sansert®****), a nonselective (broad spectrum) 5-HT antagonist, which is used to prevent the onset of migraine headaches, and **ondansetron** (Zofran®), a 5-HT$_3$ antagonist which is used to treat nausea and vomiting (described above). Given the plethora of 5-HT receptors and the rate at which new ones are being discovered, it is clear that the drug companies have a difficult road ahead; however, it is also clear that a wide variety of new and, it is hoped, selective 5-HT antagonists will be available in the future.

---

* Registered Trademark of A. H. Robins Company, Richmond, Virginia.
** Registered Trademark of Mead Johnson Pharmaceuticals, Princeton, New Jersey.
*** Registered Trademark of Cerenex Pharmaceuticals, Research Triangle Park, North Carolina.
**** Registered Trademark of Sandoz Pharmaceuticals Corp., East Hanover, New Jersey.

Serotonin has been implicated in a wide variety of functions, including anxiety, sleep states, pain perception, affective states (depression), food intake, thermoregulation, seizures, vomiting, neuroendocrine functions, and blood pressure. New drugs to treat disorders of these functions may well come from selective agents for modifying serotonergic neurotransmission.

GAMMA AMINOBUTYRIC ACID

Gamma aminobutyric acid (GABA) is one of two amino acids (the other being glycine) that function as major inhibitory neurotransmitters in the mammalian brain. GABA is present in essentially all areas of the brain and has been implicated in the mechanism of action of several antiepileptic drugs as well as in the action of hypnotics (sleeping aids) and antianxiety drugs. The concentration of GABA in the brain is much higher than that of the monoamine neurotransmitters. Studying the neurotransmitter role of GABA and other amino acids has not been easy for researchers because these amino acids also play a metabolic role and are structural components of proteins. Thus, within the neuron, there is both a metabolic and a neurotransmitter pool of GABA. Determining whether one is dealing with the metabolic pool or the neurotransmitter pool of GABA is crucial, but not always easy.

GABAergic neurons are widely distributed throughout the brain and spinal cord. In most areas of the brain, GABAergic neurons are short interneurons (inhibitory interneurons) rather than long projection cells. However, some GABAergic pathways have been mapped, and these include the pathway from the striatum (caudate) to the substantia nigra and another from the globus pallidus to the substantia nigra. The purkinje cells of the cerebellum are also GABAergic and some of these project to the lateral vestibular nucleus in the medulla oblongata.[59]

Synthesis, Storage, Release, and Inactivation of GABA

GABA is synthesized from glutamic acid by the enzyme glutamic acid decarboxylase (L-glutamate decarboxylase, GAD), which serves as a biochemical marker for GABAergic neurons.[60] The glutamate is formed from glucose via the glycolytic pathway and the Krebs cycle.[60,61] Pyruvate, formed from glucose, enters the Krebs cycle as acetylCoA and is converted to alpha ketoglutarate, the first component of the "GABA Shunt", which leads to the synthesis of GABA (Figure 4.9).[61]

The GABA shunt represents an alternative pathway between two intermediates of the Krebs cycle. In this shunt, alpha ketoglutarate is converted to glutamic acid in a transamination reaction involving GABA-alpha ketoglutarate transaminase. Some authorities have suggested the transamination of alpha ketoglutarate to glutamate may involve the enzyme aspartate amino transferase which is coupled to the conversion of aspartic acid to oxaloacetic acid.[62,63] The glutamate is then converted to GABA by glutamate decarboxylase (GAD).

GABA is degraded by GABA-transaminase (GABA-T) which converts it to succinic semialdehyde. In this process, a molecule of GABA can be broken down only if a molecule of precursor is formed (Figure 4.10).[60] The succinic semialdehyde is then converted to succinic acid by the enzyme succinic semialdehyde dehydrogenase (SSADH), returning the shunt to the Krebs cycle (Figure 4.10).

Released GABA may also enter the glutamine loop. In the latter case, the GABA is taken up by glial cells where it is converted back to glutamate by a reverse transamination involving GABA-T. The glia cannot convert glutamate to GABA because they lack GAD, but they convert the glutamate to glutamine with glutamine synthetase. The newly formed glutamine can diffuse out of the glial cells and into the GABAergic nerve endings where it can be converted back to glutamate by glutaminase. This provides another mechanism by which neurons can conserve GABA.[60]

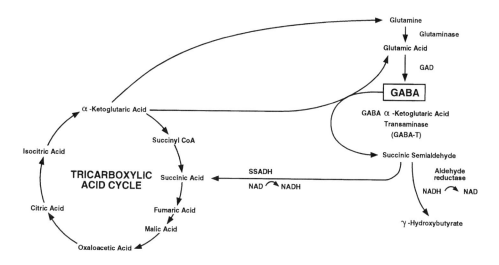

FIGURE 4.10 Synthesis and degradation of GABA via the GABA "shunt" off the tricarboxylic acid (Krebs) cycle.

GAD and GABA-T can be manipulated pharmacologically. Both enzymes require pyridoxal phosphate (vitamin B_6) as a cofactor, but the subcellular location of the enzymes differs for the two. GAD is a soluble enzyme found in cytoplasm and GABA-T is a mitochondrial enzyme.

Based on recent findings, it appears that there are two types of GAD, each of which is formed from a different gene. The two types of GAD are referred to as GAD_{65} and GAD_{67}.[64] These forms differ in molecular weight, amino acid sequence, interaction with pyridoxal phosphate, and expression in different parts of the brain. GAD_{65} appears to be localized to nerve terminals to a greater extent than GAD_{67}.

There is some controversy over whether GAD is saturated with glutamate. Some authorities[60] suggest that it is, while others[64] suggest that it is not. However, all investigators agree that there is no evidence that GABA synthesis is controlled by the availability of glutamate, which should be the case if GAD is unsaturated with substrate. Of interest is the finding that GAD is the target of antibodies present in people who later develop insulin-dependent diabetes mellitus (Type 1 diabetes). In these patients, the antibody which destroys the beta islet cells of the pancreas is directed at GAD.[65,66]

GABA-T is also a pyridoxal phosphate-dependent enzyme which has been purified to homogeneity and was shown to have a molecular weight of about 109,000. The availability of alpha ketoglutarate may regulate the tissue levels of GABA. Variations in the concentration of alpha ketoglutarate could be responsible for the postmortem changes in GABA levels that are known to occur. For example, when respiration stops, the dependence of the Krebs cycle on respiration results in a marked decline in the availability of alpha ketoglutarate and the consequent reduction in GABA-T activity, which depends on alpha ketoglutarate for transamination. However, GABA synthesis can still occur from glutamate via GAD, which is an anaerobic enzyme.[60]

Whether GABA and other amino acid neurotransmitters are stored in and released from synaptic vesicles remains somewhat controversial. Both a vesicular and a cytoplasmic pool of GABA exist within the neuron, and release occurs in both a Ca^{2+}-dependent and Ca^{2+}-independent manner.[67] However, synaptic vesicles isolated from the pig cortex contain a high concentration of GABA.[68] Based on differences in the rate of equilibration of ^{3}H-GABA between cytoplasmic and vesicular fractions, it has been concluded that the calcium-dependent release is from the vesicular fraction rather than the cytoplasmic fraction.[69]

As has been demonstrated for the uptake of NE and 5-HT into synaptic vesicles, GABA may be taken up into synaptic vesicles by an Na^+-independent mechanism that is driven by a proton gradient maintained by a Mg^{++}-ATPase.[70] Evidence also suggests that GABA is released from a cytoplasmic fraction,[71] both in a Ca^{2+}-dependent and Ca^{2+}-independent manner. The cytoplasmic release may involve an exchange transporter between cytoplasmic and extracellular compartments. The latter exchange system seems to be coupled to a Na^+ transporter.[67]

It has recently been suggested that the amino acidergic exchange transporter is responsible for the Ca^{2+}-independent release of GABA that is known to coexist with the Ca^{2+}-dependent release.[72] Thus, the available evidence suggests that the release of GABA (and other amino acid neurotransmitters) can occur by either of two Ca^{2+}-dependent mechanisms, vesicular or cytoplasmic, and also by a Ca^{2+}-independent mechanism. How these three systems interact with each other and which system, if any, predominates is yet to be determined (see detailed review by Nicholls[67]).

Following release from nerve endings, high-affinity uptake by neurons and glial cells is believed to be responsible for terminating the neurotransmitter action of GABA since no rapid enzymatic destruction system similar to that for ACh has been identified. Uptake of GABA is dependent on the Na^+/K^+ pump and the electrochemical Na^+ gradient.[73,74] The high-affinity uptake of GABA is capable of moving GABA against a concentration gradient and generally concentrates the amino acid three to four orders of magnitude higher in the intracellular compartment than in the extracellular compartment. The transporter involved utilizes energy, but does not require the splitting of ATP. The driving force for GABA (and other amino acid) transport is believed to be the simultaneous downhill movement of Na^+ ions which are maintained at a quasi steady state far from equilibrium.[73]

High-affinity uptake of GABA and excitant amino acids into glial cells has also been demonstrated by several laboratories.[75] The operation of the glial transporter is similar to the neuronal transporter and is in the direction of net uptake. In contrast to the neuronal transporter, no exchange of internal for external amino acid has been demonstrated for the glial transporter. The glial transporter is also less sensitive to changes in external K^+ or Na^+ concentration[76] and may be more sensitive to inhibition by β-alanine.[72,77] Despite these differences, both transporters are believed to produce inactivation of released amino acid neurotransmitter. In 1990, a cDNA clone encoding the GABA transporter was isolated from rat brain and its properties were examined in Xenopus oocytes.[78] The cloned transporter (called GAT-1) has all the properties of the neuronal GABA transporter including Na^+ and chloride dependence. The transporter is a 67-kDa protein with 11 to 13 transmembrane regions similar to other neurotransmitter transporters.

GABA Receptors

Two subtypes of GABA receptor have been described and are referred to as *GABA_A* and *GABA_B receptors*. The $GABA_A$ receptor has been more thoroughly investigated and is said to be one of a superfamily of ligand-gated ion channels that evolved from a common ancestral receptor.[76,79] This family also includes the nicotinic acetylcholine receptor and the glycine receptor. $GABA_A$ receptors are stimulated by GABA, **muscimol**, and **isoguvacine** and are inhibited by the convulsants **bicuculline** (competitively) and **picrotoxin** (noncompetitively). The $GABA_A$ receptor appears to exist in a macromolecular complex which consists of the GABA recognition site, the chloride channel, and the benzodiazepine binding site. Activation of the $GABA_A$ receptor causes an opening of the chloride channel, which usually results in hyperpolarization unless the membrane potential is already greater than the chloride equilibrium potential, in which case, GABA produces depolarization.

Molecular cloning has indicated that there are five major types of polypeptide subunits which range in weight from 50 to 60 kDa (alpha, beta, gamma, delta, and rho). Like the nicotinic ACh receptor, each subunit has four membrane-spanning regions, one of which is believed to contribute to the walls of the ion channel. Molecular cloning studies have provided evidence for the existence of six alpha, four beta, three gamma, one delta, and three rho subunits. Expression of the mRNAs for these subunits in Xenopus oocytes or cultured cells in various combinations has been carried out to see what subunits are required for full receptor function. It appears that, while GABA regulated chloride conductance (which is inhibited by bicuculline and picrotoxin) can be obtained with the expression of alpha and beta subunits only, full benzodiazepine sensitivity is obtained only if cultured cells contain the mRNAs for alpha, beta, and the gamma$_2$ subunits.[80] Thus, recombinant receptors containing α, β, and γ_2 subunits most closely resemble GABA$_A$ receptors found in the brain, and the subtype of α and β subunits expressed determines the various affinities for benzodiazepines found in different parts of the brain.[80] As was the case with the ACh receptor, it is believed that five subunits (e.g., two alphas, two betas, and a gamma$_2$) form the ion channel.

The GABA$_B$ receptor is insensitive to bicuculline, 3-aminopropanesulfonic acid, and isoguvacine, but has a weak sensitivity to muscimol and a stereospecific sensitivity to **(–)baclofen**. The GABA$_B$ receptor, unlike the GABA$_A$ receptor, is not a ligand-gated ion channel, but is, instead, linked through G-proteins to a second messenger system like the muscarinic cholinergic and the adrenergic receptors. Most of the early studies suggested that GABA$_B$ receptors were primarily presynaptic receptors involved in inhibiting the release of neurotransmitters; however, it is now clear that they may mediate postsynaptic inhibition as well.[81,82] Basically, two membrane effects have been attributed to the GABA$_B$ receptors: 1) a decrease in Ca^{2+} conductance (usually a presynaptic effect leading to decreased neurotransmitter release) and 2) an increase in K$^+$ conductance (usually leading to postsynaptic hyperpolarization) as occurs in hippocampal pyramidal cells following the application of baclofen. It has been suggested that the reason for the different effects may be related to the fact that the GABA$_B$ receptors are linked to different channels in different locations. Thus, they are probably linked via second messengers to Ca^{2+} channels on presynaptic terminals and to K$^+$ channels at postsynaptic sites.[82] The second messengers to which GABA$_B$ receptors have been suggested to be linked are cAMP (decreased) and phosphatidyl inositols.

The classical agonist for GABA$_B$ receptors is (–)baclofen. A number of studies have been carried out with baclofen to assess the function of GABA$_B$ receptors. However, one difficulty with the use of baclofen is that it crosses the blood-brain barrier rather poorly.[82]

Clinically Useful Drugs Which Alter GABAergic Neurotransmission

Facilitators of GABAergic Neurotransmission

GABA Agonists

Several experimental drugs are used as agonists for the GABA$_A$ receptor, including **muscimol**, **THIP**, and **isoguvacine**. In fact, there are no clinically approved drugs that act as GABA$_A$ agonists per se. However, the **benzodiazepines** are allosteric modulators of the GABA$_A$ receptor and, when bound to their high-affinity site on the GABA$_A$ receptor, enhance the binding of GABA to its binding site and increase the frequency of chloride channel opening. The benzodiazepines are by far the most popular clinically used drugs whose mechanism of action involves the GABA$_A$ receptor complex. The latter compounds have a wide variety of uses, including the treatment of anxiety, seizures, insomnia, and muscle spasms. The benzodiazepines bind with high affinity to a site on the chloride channel and enhance the inhibitory action of GABA.

Benzodiazepines used to treat anxiety include **diazepam** (Valium®), **oxazepam** (Serax®*), **alprazolam** (Xanax®**), and **lorazepam** (Ativan®***). Those used as antiepileptic drugs include: diazepam, **clonazepam** (Klonopin®****), and **nitrazepam**. Benzodiazepines used as hypnotics include **flurazepam** (Dalmane®*****), **temazepam** (Restoril®******), **triazolam** (Halcion®*******), and **quazepam** (Doral®********). Additionally, all of these drugs have muscle relaxant properties, but diazepam is probably most commonly used for this purpose.

There is another major class of drugs that act as positive allosteric modulators of the GABA$_A$ chloride channel. These are the barbiturates such as **phenobarbital**, **pentobarbital**, and **secobarbital**. The barbiturates are widely used as hypnotic agents (sleeping pills) and as adjuncts to anesthetics during surgery. Moreover, some barbiturates find important use as antiepileptic drugs (e.g., phenobarbital and **primidone**). Barbiturates bind to a different site on the chloride channel than do the benzodiazepines, and they increase the duration of channel open time rather than the frequency of opening.

GABA$_B$ receptors also mediate inhibition in the nervous system through the action of G-proteins and second messengers. **Baclofen** (Lioresal®*********) is a GABA$_B$ receptor agonist that has long been used to treat spasticity in patients with multiple sclerosis or other neurological diseases.

Drugs That Block GABA Degradation

There are a whole host of compounds used experimentally to block GABA-T, but only one of these is used clinically, gamma vinyl-GABA or **vigabatrin**, which is used as an antiepileptic drug in Europe and should soon be approved for use in the United States.[83] Vigabatrin is an irreversible GABA transaminase inhibitor that has been shown to be of value in some drug-refractory epileptic patients. **Valproic acid** (Depakene®**********) has also been shown to elevate brain GABA levels by inhibiting GABA-T and also by increasing GABA synthesis. Valproic acid is used to treat a variety of seizure types, including absence and generalized tonic-clonic. Whether the action of valproic acid in epilepsy is due primarily to an enhancement of the action of GABA is not known, because it has another important effect that is probably responsible for its effect in tonic-clonic seizures; namely, it blocks sodium channels in a frequency- and voltage-dependent fashion.[83]

Drugs That Inhibit GABAergic Neurotransmission

Drugs That Block GABA Receptors

There are several GABA antagonists available for experimental use. However, because all the GABA$_A$ antagonists are convulsants, they have no clinical use at the present time. The classical GABA$_A$ antagonist is **bicuculline**, but **picrotoxin** is also an antagonist. **Saclofen** and **phaclofen** are GABA$_B$ antagonists that are being used in experimental animals to help deduce the functional importance of the GABA$_B$ receptor. There is also a group of experimental compounds that bind to the benzodiazepine binding site on the chloride channel and cause a reduction in the effectiveness of GABA. These latter compounds, of which **beta-carboline-3-carboxylic acid** (and other beta carbolines) is an example, are called *inverse agonists*.

---

* Registered Trademark of Wyeth–Ayerst Laboratories, Philadelphia, Pennsylvania.
** Registered Trademark of The Upjohn Company, Kalamazoo, Michigan.
*** Registered Trademark of Wyeth–Ayerst Laboratories, Philadelphia, Pennsylvania.
**** Registered Trademark of Roche Laboratories, Nutley, New Jersey.
***** Registered Trademark of Roche Products, Inc., Manati, Puerto Rico.
****** Registered Trademark of Sandoz Pharmaceuticals Corp., East Hanover, New Jersey.
******* Registered Trademark of The Upjohn Company, Kalamazoo, Michigan.
******** Registered Trademark of Wallace Laboratories, Cranbury, New Jersey.
********* Registered Trademark of Geigy Pharmaceuticals, Ardsley, New York.
********** Registered Trademark of Abbott Laboratories, North Chicago, Illinois.

Clearly, the GABA antagonists and the inverse benzodiazepine agonists are pro-convulsant and have no clinical use in medicine.

GLYCINE

Glycine has the simplest chemical structure of any amino acid and it is not an essential component of the diet. It is believed to function as a neurotransmitter in spinal cord interneurons (e.g., Renshaw cell) and perhaps in the brainstem.[5] Like GABAergic synapses, all of the glycinergic synapses appear to be inhibitory. The inhibition also seems to be mediated through a ligand-gated chloride channel which, as indicated above, places these receptors in a common family with the nicotinic ACh, GABA$_A$, and glutamate receptors.

The anatomical distribution of glycinergic neurons has not been extensively mapped; however, the concentrations of glycine found in the spinal cord (dorsal and ventral horn), medulla, and pons are higher than in other CNS regions. Neuronal pathways suggested to be glycinergic include spinal interneurons, reticulospinal projections from the raphe and reticular formation, brainstem afferents to the substantia nigra, cerebellar golgi cells, and retinal amacrine cells.[59]

Synthesis, Storage, Release, and Inactivation of Glycine

Glycine is synthesized from glucose via the glycolytic pathway to produce 3-phosphoglycerate and 3-phosphoserine which forms *serine*. Serine, the immediate precursor of glycine, is converted to glycine by the enzyme serine hydroxymethyltransferase (SHMT). Radioactive tracer studies show that most of the glycine in the brain is made from serine.[62] Serine hydroxymethyltransferase requires tetrahydrofolate, pyridoxal phosphate, and manganese ion for activity.[60]

Glycine appears to be abundant in the CNS, and it is not clear what, if any, factors are rate limiting in the overall synthesis. Moreover, it is not clear whether neurons utilizing glycine as a neurotransmitter must synthesize it *de novo* or whether they accumulate existing glycine.[5] SHMT is inhibited by pyridoxal phosphate inhibitors which also interfere with GABA synthesis and degradation.

Whether glycine is stored in and released from vesicles remains somewhat controversial, as noted above for GABA. Nevertheless, recent evidence indicates that glycine (like GABA and glutamate) is taken up into synaptic vesicles by an Na$^+$-independent mechanism involving a low-affinity uptake system.[84]

The evidence suggests that glycine uptake (like that of GABA and glutamate) is driven by an electrochemical proton gradient, generated by an ATP-dependent proton pump (ATPase) located in the synaptic vesicle membrane. Kish et al.[84] have found that the glycine vesicle transporter has a different substrate specificity from that of the GABA uptake system and a different regional distribution in the brain, suggesting they are in separate neurons. The likelihood that there is both vesicular and cytoplasmic release of glycine as there appears to be for GABA (see above) remains very high.

A sodium-dependent, high-affinity uptake of glycine has been demonstrated in tissue slices and synaptosomes isolated from the spinal cord and brainstem of rats and is presumed to be the method of neurotransmitter inactivation.[85-87] There appears to be both a high-affinity and a low-affinity uptake system in glycinergic neurons.[61] Like GABA, glycine is taken up into glial cells as well as neurons.

Glycine Receptors

As indicated above, the glycine receptor is a member of a superfamily of ligand-gated ion channels where the ligand binding site and the ion channel are in the same molecule. In this regard, the glycine receptor, like that of the nicotinic ACh and GABA$_A$ receptors, has been classified as an ionotropic receptor.[59] The glycine receptor has been purified using affinity chromatography[88] and cloned.[89] It is a glycoprotein with two polypeptide subunits called alpha (48 kDa) and beta (58 kDa).

These polypeptides have four membrane-spanning hydrophobic regions (like the nicotinic ACh and $GABA_A$ receptors), and it is believed that three alpha and two beta subunits are responsible for forming the ion channel.[88] One hydrophobic region of each subunit (probably M2) is believed to contribute to the walls of the chloride channel.

Strychnine is the classical glycine antagonist, and radioactive strychnine was originally used to map the distribution of glycine receptors in the CNS. The strychnine binding site is on the 48-kDa subunit, which is where glycine also binds.[88]

Glycine also has an action at a strychnine-insensitive receptor that has been linked to the NMDA (*N*-methyl-D-aspartate) excitatory amino acid receptor (see below).[60] This is a high-affinity site that appears to increase the action of glutamate at its NMDA receptor.[90]

This strychnine-insensitive glycine binding site has a widespread distribution in the brain and seems to be similar to that of the NMDA receptors. Thus glycine, in submicromolar concentrations, appears to enhance the action of excitant amino acid neurotransmitters and may even be necessary.[90] It appears to enhance excitant amino acid action by binding to a site within the channel and producing an allosteric modification. In this regard, it appears to be analogous to the interaction between the GABA receptor and the benzodiazepine binding site. The strychnine-insensitive glycine binding site also appears to have an endogenous antagonist. The tryptophan metabolite, kynurenic acid, is an antagonist of the glycine binding site on the NMDA receptor. However, 7-chlorokynurenic acid is a more selective and more potent antagonist and is now being widely used to study this glycine receptor.[90]

Clinically Useful Drugs Which Alter Glycinergic Neurotransmission

At the present time, there are no clinically available drugs whose mechanism of action is mediated through glycinergic neurotransmission. However, there is an experimental drug called **milacemide** that is believed to increase glycine levels in the brain and is being tested as an anticonvulsant agent in experimental animals. Thus, we may have drugs available to enhance glycinergic neurotransmission in the future.

As far as antagonists are concerned, **strychnine**, which is a convulsant drug, was once used to treat a variety of disorders besides being a potent poison. This agent no longer finds any medical use. As indicated above, glycine appears to also bind to a site on the NMDA receptor (the so-called strychnine-insensitive receptor) to enhance the excitatory effects of glutamate or aspartate (see below). Thus, at this site, glycine is pro-convulsant. At the present time, there is considerable interest among drug companies to explore the use of strychnine-insensitive glycine antagonists (e.g., 7-chlorokynurenic acid) as potential antiepileptic drugs, and it is conceivable that we will see such agents available in the future.

L-GLUTAMIC ACID AND/OR L-ASPARTIC ACID

L-glutamic acid (glutamate) and L-aspartic acid (aspartate) are excitatory amino acid neurotransmitters (also called *excitant amino acids* [EAA's]). Glutamate is found in higher concentrations than any other free amino acid in the CNS, being three or four times higher than aspartate and six times higher than GABA.[60] The excitant amino acid neurotransmitters are the subject of intense current investigation, in part, because of their abundance and importance in so many neural pathways and, in part, because of studies implicating them in such pathological conditions as epilepsy, postanoxic cell loss, and neurotoxicity. It has been suggested that the vast majority of the synapses in the mammalian brain use an excitatory amino acid (EAA) as their neurotransmitter.[91]

So, glutamatergic and aspartatergic neurons are found throughout the CNS. There are, however, some specific pathways that have been mapped using lesion and biochemical analyses. These include the well-known cortico-striate pathway from the cerebral cortex to the striatum as well as many other corticofugal pathways.[59] In addition, the perforant pathway, from the entorhinal cortex to the dentate gyrus of the hippocampus, contains a heavy glutamatergic component as do the Schaffer collaterals from CA3 to CA1 of hippocampus.[59] The dorsal horn of the spinal cord has a high concentration of EAA, which disappears after cutting the primary sensory afferents, indicating that glutamate and aspartate are important neurotransmitters of the primary afferents.

Synthesis, Storage, Release, and Inactivation of EAA's

Glutamate and aspartate are nonessential amino acids that do not cross the blood-brain barrier. Therefore, they must be synthesized in the brain.[60] However, unlike most other neurotransmitters, the synthesis of glutamate and aspartate is far from straightforward. This problem arises, in part, because glutamate plays many roles in the brain and is available from many sources. For example, in addition to its neurotransmitter role, it is an important component of protein and peptide (e.g., glutathione) synthesis.[92] It also functions as an amino group acceptor to detoxify ammonia in the brain and it is the immediate precursor of GABA for GABA synthesis. Glutamate and aspartate can be synthesized from several sources, but it is not always clear which one contributes most to the neurotransmitter pool.[5]

Some investigators have suggested that the main pathways contributing to the transmitter pool of glutamate are from glucose via the Krebs cycle intermediates or from glutamine by the enzyme glutaminase (in the mitochondria). Although both glucose and glutamine are readily converted to glutamate, the pool derived from glutamine is preferentially released,[62] suggesting that this may be more important. However, *in vivo* studies using ^{14}C-glucose and ^{14}C-glutamine showed that released glutamate was derived equally from glucose and glutamine.[93]

Most evidence indicates that aspartate is also derived equally from glucose and glutamine. The various routes of synthesis are shown in Figure 4.11. Some authors have suggested that the transmitter pool may utilize glutamate (and aspartate) from several sources and that the critical factor is the transmitter-storing vesicle that can take it up irrespective of its source.[60] Glial cells probably also play a role in the synthesis of glutamate.[94] These cells can actively accumulate glutamate by a sodium-dependent process and convert the glutamate to glutamine by the enzyme glutamine synthetase. The glutamine can diffuse out of glial cells and into glutamatergic terminals where it is converted back to glutamate by glutaminase.

There has been some controversy over whether glutamate and aspartate are stored in and released from synaptic vesicles. However, recent evidence indicates that vesicles do serve as storage organelles for EAA's, just as they do for other transmitters.[92,95] Glutamate is released from synaptosomes in a Ca^{2+}-dependent manner and is derived from a noncytosolic compartment.[67] Thus, the finding that glutamate can be taken up and stored in synaptic vesicles and that its calcium-dependent release from synaptosomes is from a noncytoplasmic compartment has led many investigators to favor the view that release occurs by exocytosis. At present, the view that glutamate is released from neurons by exocytosis has considerable support. Whether aspartate is released by a similar mechanism is questionable since its uptake into vesicles has not been demonstrated.[95]

High-affinity uptake is believed to be responsible for terminating the synaptic actions of glutamate and aspartate. The transporter involved in terminating the actions of EAA's is a sodium-dependent, high-affinity transporter found in synaptosomes and brain slices which does not distinguish between L-glutamate, L-aspartate, and D-aspartate.[92,96,97] This transporter has an uneven regional distribution in the brain consistent with a role in neurotransmission.

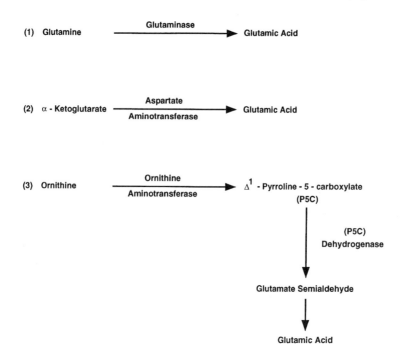

FIGURE 4.11 Synthetic pathways responsible for the formation of glutamic acid (glutamate) in the brain.

However, glial cells also possess a high-affinity uptake for glutamate and aspartate which is believed to play an important role in terminating the action of the EAA neurotransmitters following their release from nerve endings, as was discussed above for GABA. Indeed, it has been shown that some glial cells possess receptors for glutamate which, when activated, lead to a transient increase in intracellular calcium (i.e., a Ca^{2+} wave) which may pass from one glial cell to another and function as a form of intercellular communication.[98] The significance of this type of cellular communication in the brain is not yet clear.

Excitatory Amino Acid Neurotransmitter Receptors

The EAA receptors (i.e., receptors for glutamate and aspartate) have been actively investigated over the last eight years and are now among the most vigorously targeted areas by drug companies seeking new compounds for epilepsy, stroke, and degenerative brain disease. Five distinct EAA receptors have been identified. These include 1) the NMDA receptor (which is the most thoroughly studied and has four or five modulatory sites), 2) the kainate receptor, 3) the quisqualate (now called AMPA) receptor (which may represent the most common nonvoltage-dependent EAA receptor in the brain and may be codistributed with the NMDA receptor), 4) the L-AP4 receptor which seems to be a presynaptic autoreceptor on glutamate neurons, and 5) the ACPD receptor (which is the only EAA receptor that is metabotropic and linked to phosphatidyl inositol metabolism via a G-protein).[91]

Except for the ACPD receptor, all the EAA receptors are believed to be ligand-gated ion channels in the same family as the nicotinic ACh receptor, the $GABA_A$ receptor, and the glycine receptor. Of the ligand-gated EAA receptor channels, the NMDA receptor is unique in that it is voltage dependent, requiring some depolarization of the membrane to remove a Mg^{++} block within the ion channel.[60] The NMDA receptor also has several functional subcomponents with discrete binding domains which make it similar to the $GABA_A$-benzodiazepine receptor complex.[91]

In this regard, glycine has a binding site on the NMDA receptor and has been shown to facilitate the excitatory action of NMDA receptor agonists.[91,99] The glycine binding site has often been referred to as a *strychnine-insensitive glycine binding site* (discussed above). Thus, glycine appears to have important influences on EAA neurotransmission, and there are now some selective antagonists for this glycine site (e.g., 7-chlorokynurinate).

The agonist binding site on the NMDA receptor has several selective competitive antagonists (e.g., 2-amino-5-phosphonovalerate or AP5, 2-amino-7-heptanoate or AP7, and 2-carboxypiperazin propyl-1-phosphonic acid or CPP). In addition, some noncompetitive antagonists of the NMDA receptor have been discovered. These apparently bind to a site within the ion channel to inhibit neurotransmission. The latter compounds include such drugs as phencyclidine (PCP), ketamine, and MK-801 (dizocilpine).[91,100]

The EAA receptors (especially the NMDA receptor) are believed to be important in learning and memory (see Chapter 9), which is believed to be mediated through their role in long-term potentiation (LTP).[60] Indeed, the NMDA receptor may be the primary receptor responsible for LTP. The distribution of the NMDA and non-NMDA glutamate (AMPA and kainate) receptors has been extensively mapped in the rat brain using radioactive ligands and autoradiography.[91]

However, excessive amounts of EAA's in the brain are believed to be responsible for excitotoxicity (leading to neuronal death) and seizures. The latter effect has led to the interest in EAA antagonists in neuropathological states such as those following stroke.[91] The excitatory amino acids have also been shown to play a role in posttraumatic brain injury,[101] and the neuropathology may be due to the excitotoxic effects of EAA's released after injury.

The first EAA receptors to be cloned and characterized were the non-NMDA receptors.[102] None of the early cloned receptors were sensitive to NMDA, but were sensitive to kainate, AMPA, quisqualate, and glutamate. Like other ligand-gated ion channels, these receptors have four hydrophobic regions that are believed to be the membrane-spanning domains. It was suggested that these are part of a family of AMPA receptors and that kainate and AMPA receptors overlap.

In 1991, cloning of the genes for the NMDA receptor was finally achieved by two groups.[103,104] The molecular neurobiology of glutamate receptors has recently been reviewed.[105]

Clinically Useful Drugs Which Alter Excitant Amino Acid Neurotransmission

Drugs That Enhance the Action of Glutamate/Aspartate

Basically, there are no clinically useful drugs that are known to enhance the action of excitant amino acids. Indeed, those that are available for experimental studies in animals (e.g., **glutamate, kainate, ibotenic acid**, etc.) are all convulsants which also cause excitotoxic lesions of neuronal cell bodies. Whether agents that selectively enhance LTP in the hippocampus can be developed without the danger of killing neurons remains to be determined.

Drugs Which Inhibit the Action of Glutamate/Aspartate

Several glutamate receptor antagonists are available for experimental work in animals and some of these have been described above but, again, none are available for clinical use at the present time. These drugs are of interest for treating such disorders as epilepsy, postischemic brain syndrome, and posttraumatic brain injury. Moreover, such drugs are believed to have some potential in various neurodegenerative diseases such as Huntington's chorea, Alzheimer's disease, Friedreich's ataxia, and stroke. Thus, a great deal of research time and money has been, and continues to be, invested in developing effective EAA antagonists. One disappointing aspect of this work has been the psychoticlike side effects that have accompanied the testing of some NMDA antagonists in humans.

It is of interest to note that the widely used drug **dextromethorphan** (marketed as a cough suppressant) has been shown to antagonize experimental seizures in animals and has been found to be an NMDA antagonist.[106-108]

PEPTIDE NEUROTRANSMITTERS

Until 1960, acetylcholine and the monoamines were the only well-recognized neurotransmitters. Then came GABA and the amino acids in the 1960's and 1970's. The amine and amino acid neurotransmitters are sometimes referred to as the *classical* neurotransmitters. However, within the last 20 years, there has been an explosion in the number of candidate neurotransmitters, due largely to the discovery of various peptides that may function as neurotransmitters or neuromodulators. Many of the neuroactive peptides were first discovered as hormones and were then found to also be present in neurons within the CNS. Another common finding was that many of the neuroactive peptides were also found in the gut where they served as gastrointestinal hormones (e.g., cholecystokinin).

Although one finds that the peptide neurotransmitters are not classified in any consistent manner, a common approach used by authors is based on localization. For example, peptide neurotransmitters have been grouped into the following categories: 1) the gut-brain peptides, 2) the pituitary peptides, and 3) the hypothalamic-releasing hormones.[109]

There are far too many candidate peptide neurotransmitters to cover here. Moreover, there are no clinically useful drugs to affect their action, except in the case of the opioid peptides, which mediate their effects through the receptors on which morphine and other potent narcotic analgesics act. Therefore, we will restrict this discussion to the opioid peptides.

However, substance P is also of interest because it was the first peptide neurotransmitter isolated from horse gut and brain by Euler and Gaddam,[110] although it was 40 years later before its structure was determined. Substance P is of interest because, while there are no clinically available drugs to modify its action, it appears to be the neurotransmitter of primary sensory afferent fibers carrying pain sensation (i.e., C-fibers) and it can be released from such nerve terminals by the active ingredient in chili peppers (i.e., capsaicin).[111-113] Moreover, neurons containing opioid peptides appear to synapse on the terminals of substance P containing neurons in the dorsal horn of the spinal cord. Substance P is one of a group of interesting peptides known as *tachykinins* for which three receptors have been cloned and new antagonists are being developed. Cooper, Bloom, and Roth[5] provide a review of further information on this subject.

Opioid Peptides as Neurotransmitters

The first discovered opioid peptides were the pentapeptides (containing five amino acids), leucine-enkephalin and methionine-enkephalin, which were isolated by Hughes et al.[114] We now have three separate families of opioid peptides, each derived from a separate gene family.[115] These include 1) the enkephalins (pentapeptides derived from a pro-enkephalin precursor), 2) the endorphins (e.g., β-endorphin, a 31-amino-acid-containing peptide derived from pro-opiomelanocortin or POMC), and 3) the dynorphins (8- to 13-amino-acid-containing peptides derived from a pro-dynorphin precursor).

Extensive maps of the enkephalin, endorphin, and dynorphin-containing neurons in the rat brain have been obtained using immunocytochemistry, but these will be only briefly described here (see Khachaturian, Lewis, Schafer, and Watson[116] for more detail). In general, the enkephalinergic neurons are short interneurons widely distributed throughout the neuraxis. A high density of enkephalinergic neurons is found in the basal ganglia, cerebral cortex, amygdala, hippocampus, and in such brainstem areas as the periaqueductal gray, interpeduncular nucleus, parabrachial nucleus (concerned with respiration), and the nucleus tractus solitarius, as well as in the dorsal horn of the spinal cord.

The dynorphin-like immunoreactivity follows the distribution of the enkephalinergic neurons fairly closely and also appears to be found mostly in short local neurons rather than in long projection fibers. Thus, the enkephalin and dynorphin systems appear to be anatomically contiguous. The endorphin-containing neurons are, however, different in that they tend to be long projection neurons which arise from the arcuate nucleus of the hypothalamus. Another area containing a high density of endorphin (POMC) containing cell bodies is the pituitary gland from which β-endorphin is presumably released into the blood. However, the precursor of β-endorphin, POMC, is also the precursor for adrenocorticotropic hormone (ACTH) and melanocyte-stimulating hormone (α-MSH). Thus, depending on where this large peptide is cleaved by enzymes, one gets different biologically active peptides. It is little wonder, then, that the endorphins are intimately related to the endocrine system and are apparently released during stress.

Synthesis, Storage, Release, and Inactivation of Opioid Peptides

The synthesis of any peptide involves transcription of the information in the genetic code of DNA (the gene) into messenger RNA (mRNA) and the translation of the message in mRNA into the appropriate sequence of amino acids in the peptide chain to form a functionally important peptide or protein. A detailed description of protein synthesis is clearly beyond the scope of this chapter, and the reader is referred to a basic textbook of biochemistry for more detail.

As indicated above, there are three families of opioid peptides derived from different genes which lead to the synthesis of precursor proteins from which the neuroactive peptide is cleaved by the action of enzymes. Thus, pro-enkephalin, pro-dynorphin, or pro-opiomelanocortin (POMC) can be synthesized in the cell body of a cell that expresses these genes.

After the peptide precursors are formed, they are usually sent to the golgi apparatus where they are packaged into membrane-bound vesicles and then transported to the nerve terminals by axoplasmic transport. At the axon terminal, the opioid peptides are stored in vesicles from which they are released by exocytosis.[59] However, the mechanisms of peptide packaging, storage, and release are poorly understood at the present time. It is important to note that peptides cannot be synthesized at nerve terminals and must be made in the cell body and transported to the terminal for release, making them much more expensive in terms of energy expenditure.

Once the opioid or any other neuroactive peptide is released from a neuron, it is apparently degraded by peptidases (enzymes) and cannot be recaptured by reuptake. Thus, utilization of peptides is less efficient than that for the classical neurotransmitters and is, again, a more energy-expensive process. Moreover, once they are used, it will take a significantly longer time to replace them at the nerve terminal than it does for the classical transmitters.[59,117]

Another interesting aspect of peptide neurotransmitters is that they appear to be co-stored in neurons with other neurotransmitters, either other peptides or the classical neurotransmitters. Examples of a classical transmitter coexisting in a neuron with a peptide include: 1) serotonin and substance P, 2) dopamine and cholecystokinin, and 3) acetylcholine together with vasoactive intestinal polypeptide (VIP). In some neurons, the classical transmitter and the peptide may even be stored within the same vesicle (e.g., 5-HT and substance P).[117]

Opioid Receptors

Opioid receptors were known to exist long before the discovery of the opioid peptides. Indeed, it was the discovery of opioid receptors using radioactive ligands that led to the search for the endogenous peptides by Hughes and Kosterlitz.[109] The distribution of opioid receptors was mapped before the distribution of the peptides. The opioid receptors are now divided into three main subtypes: 1) mu (μ) receptors, 2) delta (δ) receptors, and 3) kappa (κ) receptors], although some authors include the sigma (σ) receptors as a fourth subtype.

Mu receptors appear to be the primary receptors involved in mediating analgesia and, therefore, have a high affinity for morphine and related drugs. The endorphins have a higher affinity for mu receptors than for any other opiate receptor. Indeed, the rank-order potency of agonists for opioids binding to the mu receptor is β-endorphin > morphine > met-enkephalin > leu-enkephalin.

The mu receptor is believed to be a 65-kDa protein with a widespread distribution in the CNS.[118] The density of mu receptors is high in striatum, amygdala, cortex, periaqueductal gray regions of midbrain, and thalamus.[119] Mu receptors are also found in the periphery. The mu receptor appears to be a G-protein linked receptor that is negatively coupled with cAMP (i.e., a G_i protein) and is involved in mediating hyperpolarization by opening K^+ channels.[119]

The use of mu agonists can alleviate the opiate withdrawal syndrome. Beta-endorphin is probably the naturally occurring ligand for the mu receptor, although morphine and its analogues appear to mediate most of their effects through the mu receptor. Naloxone is a potent antagonist of the mu opioid receptor.

The delta receptor binds leu-enkephalin with a greater affinity than met-enkephalin, β-endorphin, or morphine. Thus, the enkephalins are believed to be the natural ligands for the delta receptor.[118] The distribution of δ-receptors corresponds closely to the distribution of enkephalin neurons and, like the mu receptors, are linked to adenylate cyclase in a negative fashion via a G_i protein.[118] **Naloxone** is a less potent antagonist at delta receptors than it is at mu receptors so that higher concentrations of naloxone are required. The delta receptor was finally successfully cloned late in 1992 and, as predicted, was found to be similar to other G-protein linked receptors.[120]

The kappa opioid receptors bind ketocyclazocine with high affinity. The latter compound, along with **pentazocine, bremazocine**, and **butorphanol**, is a kappa receptor agonist. The density of kappa receptors is highest in the spinal cord and brainstem and the dynorphins are believed to be the naturally occurring agonists for these receptors. Naloxone can act as an antagonist at kappa receptors, but it is less potent than at mu receptors. Kappa agonists cannot alleviate the symptoms of opioid withdrawal. However, stimulation of kappa receptors can alleviate pain, especially viscerally mediated chemical pain.[118]

Clinically Useful Drugs Which Alter Opioid Neurotransmission

Drugs Used to Enhance Neurotransmission

Opioid Agonists

A comprehensive discussion of the pharmacology of opioid agonists and antagonists has been provided by Jaffe and Martin[115] and is beyond the scope of this chapter. The agonists are the only available drugs for enhancing opioidergic neurotransmission. These are the narcotic analgesics used to treat severe pain such as that occurring postoperatively. **Morphine** is the prototypical drug in this class and has been around since 1806. It is a natural constituent of opium powder, but can now be made in the chemistry laboratory. **Meperidine** (Demerol®*) is a synthetic analogue of morphine widely used in hospitals for postoperative pain. Both of these are primarily mu agonists, but also have some agonist activity at delta and kappa receptors. **Codeine**, the *O*-methyl analogue of morphine, has similar properties, but is a weaker agonist. Indeed, codeine is metabolized to morphine in the body. **Pentazocine** (Talwin®**) is a kappa agonist and a mu antagonist and **butorphanol** (Stadol®***) has similar properties. Pentazocine was originally marketed as a nonnarcotic analgesic, but this error was

---

* Registered Trademark of Sanofi Winthrop Pharmaceuticals, New York, New York.
** Registered Trademark of Sanofi Winthrop Pharmaceuticals, New York, New York.
*** Registered Trademark of Mead Johnson Laboratories, Princeton, New Jersey.

eventually corrected when it was found to be addicting. **Buprenorphine** (Buprenex®*) is a partial mu agonist and a kappa antagonist. The latter drugs are sometimes referred to as *mixed agonist-antagonists*.

Opioid analgesics have many side effects, not the least of which is respiratory depression, which can kill the patient in overdose. These drugs are also very useful to suppress the cough reflex and are commonly added to cough mixtures (syrups).

Drugs That Inhibit Opioidergic Neurotransmission

Opioid Antagonists

Naloxone (Narcan®***) is a pure opioid antagonist that is used to treat life-threatening overdoses of opioid analgesics. It functions as an antagonist at mu, delta, and kappa receptors, but must be given by injection. The administration of 0.4 to 0.8 mg intravenously or intramuscularly can reverse the effects of mu opioid agonists in humans and will precipitate a withdrawal syndrome in addicted individuals.[115] **Naltrexone** (Trexan®****) is also a pure narcotic antagonist with greater oral efficacy and a longer duration of action allowing it to be administered orally.

SUMMARY

The preceding pages provide considerable detail concerning the process of neurotransmission in the nervous system. It is clear that this is the major form of communication between neurons and the principal site of controlling neuronal function. It is also clear that neurotransmission is the principal target for drugs that affect the nervous system. Although it is impossible to provide a concise summary of the broad array of topics covered in this chapter, the editors felt that some type of summary of the clinically relevant drugs showing the neurotransmitters through which they exert their action would be useful for the busy practitioner and I fully agree. Therefore, an appendix has been provided to summarize these relationships and to give the reader a quick mechanism for linking the drugs to the neurotransmitters. It should be noted, however, that in the interest of space we have only included those drugs discussed in this chapter. Although they represent some of the more popular ones in use today, they are by no means the only ones available. Practitioners of rehabilitation as well as other specialties in medicine must be aware that pharmacology is a constantly changing field with new drugs being introduced every day. It is hoped that this chapter also provides a foundation that will allow the reader to appreciate and understand the mechanism of action of new (undiscovered) drugs that will be introduced in the future.

EDITORS' SUMMARIZING NOTE

While this chapter represents a challenge to nearly every level of readership, the information contained herein allows for insight into rationale for pharmacological intervention, successes and failures, and complications of treatment. The chapter is best absorbed after, perhaps, the third or fourth review and will serve, it is hoped, as a reference tool for the practicing clinical team attempting pharmacological augmentation of medical and rehabilitative treatment for the traumatically brain-injured population.

---

* Registered Trademark of Reckitt & Colman Pharmaceuticals, Inc., Richmond, Virginia.
** Registered Trademark of DuPont Multi–Source Products, Garden City, New York.
*** Registered Trademark of DuPont, Wilmington, Delaware.

REFERENCES

1. Werman, R., Criteria for identification of a central nervous system transmitter, *Comp. Biochem. Physiol.*, 18, 745, 1966.

2. Snyder, S. H. and Bredt, D. S., Biological roles of nitric oxide, *Sci. Am.,* 266, 68, 1992.

3. Lefkowitz, R. J., Hoffman, B. B., and Taylor, P., Neurohumoral transmission: The autonomic and somatic motor nervous systems, in *The Pharmacological Basis of Therapeutics*, Gilman, A. G., Rall, T. W., Nies, A. S., and Taylor, P., Eds., Pergamon Press, New York, 1990, 84.

4. Blusztajn, J. K. and Wurtman, R. J., Choline and cholinergic neurons, *Science*, 221, 614, 1983.

5. Cooper, J. R., Bloom, F. E., and Roth, R. H., *The Biochemical Basis of Neuropharmacology*, 6th edition, Oxford University Press, New York, 1991.

6. Collier, B., Kwok, Y. N., and Welner, S. A., Increased acetylcholine synthesis and release following presynaptic activity in a sympathetic ganglion, *J. Neurochem.*, 40, 91, 1983.

7. Johns, C. A., Greenwald, B. S., Mohs, R. C., and Davis, K. L., The cholinergic treatment strategy in aging and senile dementia, *Psychopharmacol. Bull.*, 19, 185, 1983.

8. Wurtman, R. J., Choline metabolism as a basis for the selective vulnerability of cholinergic neurons, *Trends Neurosci.,* 15, 117, 1992.

9. Koshimura, S., Miwa, S., Lee, K., Hayashi, H., Hasegawa, H., Hamahata, K., Fujiwara, M., Kimura, M., and Itokawa, V., Effects of choline administration on *in vivo* release and biosynthesis of acetylcholine in the rat striatum as studied by in vivo brain microdialysis, *J. Neurochem.*, 54, 533, 1990.

10. Johnson, D. A., Ulus, I. H., and Wurtman, R. J., Caffeine potentiates the enhancement by choline of striatal acetylcholine release, *Life Sci.*, 51, 1597, 1992.

11. Taylor, P. and Brown, J. H., Acetylcholine, in *Basic Neurochemistry*, Siegel, G., Agranoff, B., Albers, R. W., and Molinoff, P., Eds., Raven Press, New York, 1989, 203.

12. Marshall, I. G. and Parsons, S. M., The vesicular acetylcholine transport system, *Trends Neurosci.,* 4, 174, 1987.

13. Dale, H. H., The action of certain esters and ethers of choline, and their relation to muscarine, *J. Pharmacol. Exp. Ther.*, 6, 147, 1914.

14. Browning, R. A., Overview of neurotransmission: Relationship to the action of antiepileptic drugs, in *Drugs for Control of Epilepsy: Actions on Neuronal Networks Involved in Seizure Disorders*, Faingold, C. L. and Fromm, G., Eds., CRC Press, Boca Raton, FL, 1992, 23.

15. Beani, L., Bianchi, C., Nilsson, L., Nordberg, A., Romanelli, L., and Sivilotti, L., The effect of nicotine and cystisine on 3H-acetylcholine release from cortical slices of guinea pig brain, *Arch. Pharmacol.*, 139, 323, 1985.

16. Richard, J., Araujo, D. M., and Quirion, R., Modulation of cortical acetylcholine release by cholinergic agents in an *in vivo* dialysis study, *Soc. Neurosci. Abst.*, 15, 1197, 1989.

17. Hulme, E. C., Birdsall, N. J. M., and Buckley, N. J., Muscarinic receptor subtypes, *Ann. Rev. Pharmacol. Toxicol.*, 30, 633, 1990.

18. Lapchak, P. A., Araujo, D. M., Quirion, R., and Collier, B., Binding sites for [3H] AF-DX 116 and effect of AF-DX 116 on endogenous acetylcholine release from rat brain slices, *Brain Res.*, 496, 285, 1989.

19. Turski, L., Ikonomidou, C., Turski, W. A., Bortolutto, Z. A., and Cavalheiro, E. A., Review: Cholinergic mechanisms and epileptogenesis. The seizures induced by pilocarpine, *Synapse*, 3, 154, 1989.

20. Taylor, P., Cholinergic agonists, in *Goodman and Gilman's The Pharmacological Basis of Therapeutics*, 8th edition, Gilman, A. G., Rall, T. W., Nies, A. S., and Taylor, P., Eds., Pergamon Press, New York, 1990, 122.

21. Clark, W. G., Brater, D. C., and Johnson, A. R., *Medical Pharmacology*, 13th edition, Mosby Year Book, St. Louis, 1992, 123.

22. Falck, B., Hillarp, N. A., Thieme, G., and Torp, A., Fluorescence of catecholamines and related compounds condensed with formaldehyde, *J. Histochem. Cytochem.*, 10, 348, 1962.

23. Moore, R. Y. and Bloom, F. E., Central catecholamine neuron systems: Anatomy and physiology of the norepinephrine and epinephrine systems, *Ann. Rev. Neurosci.*, 2, 113, 1979.

24. Weiner, N. and Molinoff, P. B., Catecholamines, in *Basic Neurochemistry*, 4th edition, Agranoff, B. W., Albers, R. W., and Molinoff, P.-B., Eds., Raven Press, New York, 1989, 233.

25. Bogdanski, D. F., Norepinephrine uptake dependent upon apparent Mg^{++}-ATPase activity and proton transport in storage vesicles in axoplasm, *Synapse*, 2, 424, 1988.

26. Graham, D. and Langer, S. Z., Minireview: Advances in sodium-ion coupled biogenic amine transporters, *Life Sci.*, 51, 631, 1992.

27. O'Dowd, B. F., Lefkowitz, R. J., and Caron, M. G., Structure of the adrenergic and related receptors, *Ann. Rev. Neurosci.*, 12, 67, 1989.

28. Minneman, K. P., 1-Adrenergic receptor subtypes, inositol phosphates, and sources of cell Ca^{2+}, *Pharmacol. Rev.*, 40, 87, 1988.

29. Baldessarini, R. J., Drugs and the treatment of psychiatric disorders, in *The Pharmacological Basis of Therapeutics*, Gilman, A. G., Rall, T. W., Nies, A. S., and Taylor, P., Eds., Pergamon Press, New York, 1990, 383.

30. Bakhit, C., Morgan, M. E., Peat, M. A., and Gibb, J. W., Long-term effects of methamphetamine on the synthesis and metabolism of 5-hydroxytryptamine in various regions of the rat brain, *Neuropharmacology*, 20, 1135, 1981.

31. Ricaurte, G. A., Schuster, C. R., and Seiden, L. S., Long-term effects of repeated methylamphetamine administration on dopamine and serotonin neurons in the rat brain: A regional study, *Brain Res.*, 193, 153, 1980.

32. Ricaurte, G. A., Seiden, L. S., and Schuster, C. R., Further evidence that amphetamine produces long-lasting dopamine neurochemical deficits by destroying dopamine nerve fibers, *Brain Res.*, 303, 359, 1984.

33. Axt, K. and Molliver, M. E., Immunocytochemical evidence for methamphetamine-induced serotonergic axon loss in the rat brain, *Synapse*, 9, 302, 1991.

34. Giros, B. and Caron, M. G., Molecular characteristics of the dopamine transporter, *Trends Pharmacol. Sci.*, 4, 43, 1993.

35. Creese, I., Sibley, D. R., and Leff, S. E., Agonist interactions with dopamine receptors: Focus on radioligand-binding studies, *Fed. Proc.*, 43, 2779, 1984.

36. Sokoloff, P., Giros, B., Martres, M. P., Bouthenet, M. L., and Schwartz, J. C., Molecular cloning and characterization of a novel dopamine receptor (D3) as a target for neuroleptics, *Nature*, 347, 146, 1990.

37. Van Tol, H. H. M., Bunzow, J. R., Guan, H., Sunahara, R. K., Seeman, P., Niznik, H. B., and Civelli, O., Cloning of the gene for a human dopamine D4 receptor with high affinity for the antipsychotic clozapine, *Nature*, 350, 610, 1991.

38. O'Dowd, B. F., Structures of dopamine receptors, *J. Neurochem.*, 60, 804, 1993.

39. Seeman, P. and Van Tol, H. H. Dopamine receptor pharmacology, *Trends Pharmacol. Sci.*, 15, 264, 1994.

40. Uhl, G., Blum, K., Noble, E., and Smith S., Substance abuse vulnerability and the D2 receptor gene, *Trends Neurosci.*, 16, 83, 1993.

41. Lal, S., Merbitz, C. P., and Grip, J. C., Modification of function in head-injured patients with sinemet, *Brain Injury*, 2, 225, 1988.

42. Eames, P., The use of sinemet and bromocriptine, *Brain Injury*, 3, 319, 1989.

43. Kaakkola, S. and Wurtman, R. J., Effects of catechol-o-methyltransferase inhibitors and L-3, 4, dihydroxy phenylalanine on extracellular dopamine in rat striatum, *J. Neurochem.*, 60, 137, 1993.

44. Dahlstrom, A. and Fuxe, K., A method for the demonstration of monoamine containing nerve fibers in the central nervous system, *Acta Physiol. Scand.*, 60, 293, 1964.

45. Molliver, M. E., Serotonergic neuronal systems: What their anatomic organization tells us about function, *J. Clin. Psychopharmacol.*, 7, 35, 1987.

46. Gershon, M. D., Biochemistry and physiology of serotonergic transmission, in *Handbook of Physiology — The Nervous System I*, Brookhart, J. M., Mountcastle, V., and Kandel, E., Eds., American Physiological Society, Washington, DC, 1977, 573.

47. Wurtman, R. J., Hefti, F., and Melamed, E., Precursor control of neurotransmitter synthesis, *Pharmacol. Rev.*, 32, 315, 1981.

48. Green, J. P., Histamine and serotonin, in *Basic Neurochemistry*, Siegel, G. J., Agranoff, B. W., Alberts, R. W., and Molinoff, P. B., Eds., Raven Press, New York, 1989, 253.

49. Sanders-Bush, E. and Martin, L. L., Storage and release of serotonin, in *Biology of Serotonergic Transmission*, Osborne, N. N., Ed., Wiley, New York, 1982, 95.

50. Halaris, A. E. and Freedman, D. X., Vesicular and juxtavesicular serotonin: Effect of lysergic acid diethylamide and reserpine, *J. Pharmacol. Exp. Ther.*, 203, 575, 1977.

51. Maynert, E. W., Levi, R., and deLorenzo, A. J. D., The presence of norepinephrine and 5-HT in vesicles from disrupted nerve-ending particles, *J. Pharmacol. Exp. Ther.*, 144, 385, 1964.

52. Adell, A., Sarna, G. S., Hutson, P. H., and Curzon, G., An in vivo dialysis and behavioural study of the release of 5-HT by p-chloroamphetamine in reserpine-treated rats, *Br. J. Pharmacol.*, 97, 206, 1989.

53. Kuhn, D. M., Wolf, W. A., and Youdim, B. H., Review: Serotonin neurochemistry revisited: A new look at some old axioms, *Neurochem. Int.*, 8, 141, 1986.

54. Reinhard, J. F. and Wurtman, R., Relation between brain 5-HIAA levels and the release of serotonin into brain synapses, *Life Sci.*, 21, 1741, 1977.

55. Schmidt, A. W. and Peroutka, J., 5-hydroxytryptamine receptor "families", *FASEB J.*, 3, 2242, 1989.

56. Richardson, B. P. and Engel, G., The pharmacology and function of 5-HT3 receptors, *Trends Neurosci.*, 9, 424, 1986.

57. Sumatriptan for migraine, in *Med. Lett.*, 34, 91, 1992.

58. Ferrari, M. D. and Saxena, P. R., Clinical and experimental aspects of sumatriptan in humans, *Trends Pharmacol. Sci.*, 14, 129, 1993.

59. McGeer, P. L., Eccles, J. C., and McGeer, E. G., *Molecular Neurobiology of the Mammalian Brain*, 2nd edition, Plenum Press, New York, 1987.

60. McGeer, P. L. and McGeer, E. G., Amino acid neurotransmitters, in *Basic Neurochemistry*, Siegel, G., Agranoff, B., Albers, R. W., and Molinoff, P., Eds., Raven Press, New York, 1989, 331.

61. Obata, K., Biochemistry and physiology of amino acids neurotransmitters, in *Handbook of Physiology — The Nervous System I*, Brookhart, J. M., Mountcastle, V., and Kandel, E., Eds., American Physiological Society, Washington, DC, 1977, 625.

62. Bradford, H. E., *Chemical Neurobiology*, W. H. Freeman & Co., New York, 1986.

63. Meldrum, B., GABA and other amino acids, in *Antiepileptic Drugs, Handbook of Experimental Pharmacology*, Volume 74, Frey, H. H. and Janz, D., Eds., Springer-Verlag, Berlin, 1985, 153.

64. Martin, D. L. and Rimvall, K., Regulation of g-aminobutyric acid synthesis in the brain, *J. Neurochem.*, 60, 395, 1993.

65. Tobin, A., Molecular biological approaches to the synthesis and action of GABA, *Semin. Neurosci.*, 3, 183, 1991.

66. Kaufman, D. L. and Tobin, A. J., Glutamate decarboxylase and autoimmunity in insulin-dependent diabetes, *Trends Pharmacol. Sci.*, 14, 107, 1993.

67. Nicholls, D. G., Short review: Release of glutamate aspartate, and g-aminobutyric acid from isolated nerve terminals, *J. Neurochem.*, 52, 331, 1989.

68. Angel, I., Fleissner, A., and Seifert, R., Synaptic vesicles from hog brain: Their isolation and coupling between synthesis and uptake of GABA by GAD, *Neurochem. Int.*, 5, 697, 1983.

69. Shira, T. S. and Nicholls, D. G., GABA can be released exocytotically from guinea-pig cerebrocortical synaptosomes, *J. Neurochem.*, 49, 261, 1987.

70. Fykse, E. M., Christensen, H., and Fonnum, F., Comparison of the properties of g-aminobutyric acid and L-glutamate uptake into synaptic vesicles isolated from rat brain, *J. Neurochem.*, 52, 946, 1989.

71. De Belleroche, J. S. and Bradford, H. F., On the site of origin of transmitter amino acids released by depolarization of nerve terminals in vitro, *J. Neurochem.*, 29, 335, 1977.

72. Bernath, S. and Zigmond, M. J., Characterization of [3H]-GABA release from striatal slices: Evidence for a calcium-independent process via the GABA uptake system, *Neuroscience*, 27, 563, 1988.

73. Erecinska, M., Wantonsky, D., and Wilson, D. F., Aspartate transport in synaptosomes from rat brain, *J. Biol. Chem.*, 258, 9069, 1983.

74. Wheeler, D. D. and Hollingsworth, R. G., A model of GABA transport by cortical synaptosomes from the Long-Evans rat, *J. Neurosci. Res.*, 4, 266, 1979.

75. Erecinska, M., The neurotransmitter amino acid transport systems: A new outlook on an old problem, *Biochem. Pharmacol.*, 36, 3547, 1987.

76. Barnard, E. A., Darlison, M. G., and Seeburg, P., Molecular biology of the $GABA_A$ receptor: The receptor/channel superfamily, *Trends Neurosci.*, 10, 502, 1987.

77. Iversen, L. L. and Kelly, J. S., Uptake and metabolism of g-aminobutyric acid by neurons and glial cells, *Biochem. Pharmacol.*, 24, 933, 1975.

78. Guastella, J., Nelson, N., Nelson, H., Czyzyk, L., Keynan, S., Miedel, M. C., Davidson, N., Lester, H. A., and Kanner, B. I., Cloning and expression of a rat brain GABA transporter, *Science*, 249, 1303, 1990.

79. Olsen, R. W. and Tobin, A. J., Molecular biology of $GABA_A$ receptors, *FASEB J.*, 4, 1469, 1990.

80. Sieghart, W., $GABA_A$ receptors: Ligand-gated Cl-ion channels modulated by multiple drug-binding sites, *Trends Pharmacol. Sci.*, 13, 446, 1992.

81. Matsumoto, R. R., GABA receptors: Are cellular differences reflected in function? *Brain Res. Rev.*, 14, 203, 1989.

82. Bowery, N., $GABA_B$ receptors and their significance in mammalian pharmacology, *Trends Pharmacol. Sci.*, 10, 401, 1989.

83. Rogawski, M. A. and Porter, R. J., Antiepileptic drugs: Pharmacological mechanisms and clinical efficacy with consideration of promising developmental stage compounds, *Pharmacol. Rev.*, 42, 223, 1990.

84. Kish, P. E., Fischer-Bovenkerk, C., and Veda, T., Active transport of g-aminobutyric acid and glycine into synaptic vesicles, *Proc. Natl. Acad. Sci.*, 86, 3877, 1989.

85. Johnston, G. A. R. and Iversen, L. L., Glycine uptake in rat central nervous system slices and homogenates: Evidence for different uptake systems in spinal cord and cerebral cortex, *J. Neurochem.*, 18, 1951, 1971.

86. Neal, M. J., The uptake of [14C] glycine by slices of mammalian spinal cord, *J. Physiol.*, 215, 103, 1971.

87. Logan, W. J. and Snyder, S. H., High affinity uptake system for glycine, glutamic acid and aspartic acids in synaptosomes of rat central nervous tissues, *Brain Res.*, 42, 413, 1972.

88. Langosch, D., Thomas L., and Betz, H., Conserved quaternary structure of ligand-gated ion channels: The postsynaptic glycine receptor is a pentamer, *Proc. Natl. Acad. Sci.*, 85, 7394, 1988.

89. Greeningloh, G., Rienitz, A., Schmitt, B., Methfessel, C., Zensen, M., Beyreuther, K., Gundelfinger, E. D., and Betz, H., The strychnine-binding subunit of the glycine receptor shows homology with nicotinic acetylcholine receptors, *Nature*, 328, 215, 1987.

90. Thomson, A. M., Glycine modulation of the NMDA receptor/channel complex, *Trends Neurosci.*, 12, 349, 1989.

91. Monaghan, D. T., Bridges, R. J., and Cotman, C. W., The excitatory amino acid receptors: Their classes, pharmacology, and distinct properties in the function of the central nervous system, *Ann. Rev. Pharmacol. Toxicol.,* 29, 365, 1989.

92. Fonnum, F., Glutamate: A neurotransmitter in mammalian brain, *J. Neurochem.,* 42, 1, 1984.

93. Ward, H. W., Thank, C. M., and Bradford, H. F., Glutamine and glucose as precursors of transmitter amino acids: *Ex vivo* studies, *J. Neurochem.,* 40, 855, 1983.

94. Robinson, M. B. and Coyle, J. T., Glutamate and related acidic excitatory neurotransmitters: From basic science to clinical application, *FASEB J.,* 1, 446, 1987.

95. Maycox, P. R., Hell, J. W., and Jahn, R., Amino acid neurotransmission: Spotlight on synaptic vesicles, *Trends Neurosci.,* 13, 83, 1990.

96. Balcar, V. J. and Johnston, G. A. R., The structural specificity of the high affinity uptake of L-glutamate and L-aspartate by rat brain slices, *J. Neurochem.,* 19, 2657, 1972.

97. Snyder, S. H., Young, A. B., Bennett, J. P., and Mulder, A. H., Synaptic biochemistry of amino acids, *Fed. Proc.,* 32, 2039, 1973.

98. Cornell-Bell, A. H., Finkbeiner, S. M., Cooper, M. S., and Smith, S. J., Glutamate induces calcium waves in cultured astrocytes: Long-range glial signaling, *Science,* 247, 470, 1990.

99. Lehmann, J., Randle, J. C. R., and Reynolds, I. J., Meeting report: Excitatory amino acid receptors, *Trends Pharmacol. Sci.,* 11, 1, 1990.

100. Watkins, J. C., Krogsgaard-Larsen, P., and Honore, T., Structure-activity relationships in the development of excitatory amino acid receptor agonists and competitive antagonists, *Trends Pharmacol. Sci.,* 11, 25, 1990.

101. Faden, A. I., Demediuk, P., Panter, S. S., and Vink, R., The role of excitatory amino acids and NMDA receptors in traumatic brain injury, *Science,* 244, 798, 1989.

102. Wada, K., Dechesne, C. J., Shimasaki, S., King, R. G., Kusano, K., Buonanno, A., Hampson, D.-R., Banner, C., Wenthold, R. J., and Nakatani, Y., Sequence and expression of a frog brain complementary DNA encoding a kainate-binding protein, *Nature,* 342, 684, 1989.

103. Moriyoshi, K., Masu, M., Ishii, T., Shigemoto, R., Mizuno, N., and Nakanishi, S., Molecular cloning and characterization of the rat NMDA receptor, *Nature,* 354, 31, 1991.

104. Kumar, K. N., Tilacaratne, N., Johnson, P. S., Allen, A. E., and Michaelis, E. K., Cloning of cDNA for the glutamate-binding subunit of an NMDA receptor complex, *Nature,* 354, 70, 1991.

105. Gasic, G. P. and Hollmann, M., Molecular neurobiology of glutamate receptors, *Ann. Rev. Physiol.,* 54, 507, 1992.

106. Faingold, C. L. and Meldrum, B. S., Excitant amino acids in epilepsy, in *Generalized Epilepsy: Cellular, Molecular and Pharmacological Approach,* Avoli, M., Gloor, P., Kostopoulos, P., and Naquet, R., Eds., Birkhauser, Boston, 1990, 102.

107. Feeser, H. R., Kadis, J. L., and Prince, D. A., Dextromethorphan, a common antitussive reduces kindled amygdala seizures in the rat, *Neurosci. Lett.,* 86, 340, 1988.

108. Leander, J. D., Rathbon, R. C., and Zimmerman, D. M., Anticonvulsant effects of phencyclidine-like drugs: Relation to N-methyl-D-aspartic acid antagonism, *Brain Res.,* 454, 368, 1988.

109. Snyder, S. H., Brain peptides as neurotransmitters, *Science,* 209, 976, 1980.

110. Euler, U. S., An unidentified depressor substance in certain tissue extracts, Von and Gaddam, J. H., *J. Physiol.,* 72, 74, 1931.

111. Krieger, D. T. and Martin, J. B., Brain peptides, Part 1, *N. Engl. J. Med.,* 304, 876, 1981.

112. Krieger, D. T. and Martin, J. B., Brain peptides, Part 2, *N. Engl. J. Med.,* 304, 944, 1981.

113. Otsuka, M. and Yanagisawa, M., Does substance P act as a pain transmitter? *Trends Pharmacol. Sci.,* 8, 506, 1987.

114. Hughes, J., Smith, T. W., Kosterlitz, H. W., Fothergill, L. A., Morgan, B. A., and Morris, H. R., Identification of two related pentapeptides from the brain with potent opiate agonist activity, *Nature,* 258, 577, 1975.

115. Jaffe, J. H. and Martin, W. R., Opioid analgesics and antagonists, in *Goodman and Gilman's The Pharmacological Basis of Therapeutics,* Gilman, A. G., Rall, T. W., Nies, A. S., and Taylor, P., Eds., Pergamon Press, New York, 1990, 485.

116. Khachaturian, H., Lewis, M. E., Schafer, M. K. H., and Watson, S. J., Anatomy of the CNS opioid systems, *Trends Neurosci.,* 8, 111, 1985.

117. Krieger, D. T., Brain peptides: What, where and why? *Science,* 222, 975, 1983.

118. Simon, E. J., Opioid receptors and endogenous opioid peptides, *Med. Res. Rev.,* 11, 357, 1991.

119. Civelli, O., Machida, C., Bunzow, J., Albert, P., Hanneman, E., Salon, J., Bidlack, J., and Grandy, D., The next frontier in the molecular biology of the opioid system: The opioid receptors, *Molec. Neurobiol.,* 1, 373, 1987.

120. Evans, C. J., Keith, D. E., Jr., Morrison, H., Magendzo, K., and Edwards, R. H., Cloning of a delta opioid receptor by functional expression, *Science,* 258, 1952, 1992.

Appendix: Summary of Relationship Between Therapeutically-Used Drugs and Various Neurotransmitters

Drug Name	Brand Name[a]	Neurotransmitter	Receptor	Drug Action
alpha-methyltyrosine	Metyrosine	Dopamine; NE	—	Blocks synthesis of dopamine and NE
acebutolol	Sectral	NE	Beta-1	Beta-1 receptor blocker
acetylcholine	Miochol (ophthalmic)	ACh	Nicotinic and muscarinic-cholinergic	Agonist for muscarinic and nicotinic receptors
albuterol	Proventil	Epinephrine (hormone)	Beta-2	Beta-2 receptor agonist
alprazolam	Xanax	GABA	Benzodiazepine — $GABA_A$ complex	Agonist for benzodiazepine receptor
amantadine	Symmetrel	Dopamine	—	Increases release and blocks reuptake of dopamine
amphetamine	Obetrol	Dopamine; NE	—	Increases release and blocks reuptake of NE and dopamine
apomorphine	Apomorphine HCl	Dopamine	D-1 and D-2 dopamine	Agonist for D-1 and D-2 receptors
atenolol	Tenormin	NE	Beta-1	Blocks beta-1 receptors
atropine	Atropine Sulfate	ACh	Muscarinic-cholinergic	Blocks muscarinic receptors
baclofen	Lioresal	GABA	$GABA_B$	Agonist for $GABA_B$ receptors
benztropine	Cogentin	ACh	Muscarinic-cholinergic	Blocks muscarinic receptors
bethanechol	Urecholine	ACh	Cholinergic-muscarinic	Agonist for muscarinic receptor
bretylium	Bretylium Tosylate	NE	—	Blocks release of NE
bromocriptine	Parlodel	Dopamine	Dopamine (D-1, D-2, etc.)	Nonselective dopamine receptor agonist
buprenorphine	Buprenex	β-endorphin; enkephalin	Opioid (mu)	Partial agonist for mu receptor and a kappa antagonist
buspirone	BuSpar	Serotonin (5-HT)	$5\text{-}HT_{1a}$	Partial agonist for $5\text{-}HT_{1a}$ receptor
butorphanol	Stadol	β-endorphin; enkephalin	Opioid (kappa)	Kappa agonist and mu antagonist
capsaicin	Zostrix-HP	Substance P	—	Depletes C-fibers (pain fibers) of Substance P; used as topical analgesic
carbachol	Isopto Carbachol	ACh	Muscarinic-cholinergic, nicotinic-cholinergic	Muscarinic and nicotinic agonist
cimetidine	Tagamet	Histamine (not covered in chapter)	H_2 histamine receptors	H_2 blocker
clomipramine	Anafranil	Serotonin	—	Blocks serotonin reuptake
clonazepam	Klonopin	GABA	Benzodiazepine-$GABA_A$ complex	Facilitates action of GABA
clonidine	Catapres	NE	Alpha-2	Alpha-2 agonist
clozapine	Clozaril	Dopamine	Dopamine D_4	D_4 antagonist
cocaine	Cocaine HCl	NE, dopamine	—	Blocks reuptake of NE and dopamine
d-tubocurarine	Tubocurarine chloride	ACh	Nicotinic-cholinergic	Nicotinic receptor blocker
desipramine	Norpramin	NE	—	Blocks NE reuptake

Drug	Trade name	Neurotransmitter	Receptor	Action
dextroamphetamine	Dexedrine	NE; dopamine	—	Increases release of NE and dopamine and blocks reuptake
dextromethorphan	Found in many cough syrups (e.g., Robitussin-DM)	Glutamate	NMDA	Blocks glutamate NMDA receptor
diazepam	Valium	GABA	Benzodiazepine-GABA$_A$ complex	Agonist for benzodiazepine receptor
disulfiram	Antabuse	NE	—	Blocks synthesis of NE
edrophonium	Tensilon	ACh	—	Cholinesterase inhibitor; prevents degradation of ACh
esmolol	Brevibloc	NE	B$_1$	Blocks B$_1$ receptor
fenfluramine	Pondamin	Serotonin	—	Increases the release of serotonin
fluoxetine	Prozac	Serotonin	—	Blocks reuptake of serotonin
flurazepam	Dalmane	GABA	Benzodiazepine-GABA$_A$ complex	Facilitates the action of GABA
gallamine	Flaxedil	ACh	Nicotinic-cholinergic	Blocks nicotinic receptors at neuromuscular junction
guanabenz	Wytensin	NE	Alpha-2	Alpha-2 agonist
guanadrel	Hylorel	NE	—	Blocks the release of NE
guanethidine	Ismelin	NE	—	Blocks the release of NE
guanfacine	Tenex	NE	Alpha-2	Alpha-2 agonist
ipratropium	Atrovent	ACh	Muscarinic-cholinergic	Muscarinic blocker
isocarboxazid	Marplan	NE; dopamine; serotonin	—	Inhibits degradative enzyme (monoamine oxidase)
isoproterenol	Isuprel	NE, epinephrine	B$_1$ and B$_2$	Agonist for all beta receptors
ketamine	Ketalar	Glutamate	NMDA	Noncompetitive blocker of NMDA receptor
L-dopa and carbidopa	Sinemet	Dopamine	—	Increases synthesis of dopamine
levodopa	Larodopa	Dopamine	—	Increases synthesis of dopamine
lorazepam	Ativan	GABA	Benzodiazepine-GABA$_A$ complex	Agonist for benzodiazepine receptor
maprotiline	Ludiomil	NE	—	NE reuptake inhibitor
mecamylamine	Inversine	ACh	Nicotinic-cholinergic	Blocks neuronal nicotinic receptors
meperidine	Demerol	β-endorphin; enkephalin	Opioid (mu)	Agonist for mu opioid receptors
metaproterenol	Metaprel	NE, epinephrine	Beta-2	Selective agonist for beta-2 receptor
metaraminol	Aramine	NE	Alpha-1	Agonist for alpha-1 receptors
methacholine	Provocholine	ACh	Muscarinic-cholinergic	Agonist for muscarinic receptors
methamphetamine	Desoxyn	NE and dopamine	—	Increases release of NE and dopamine
methoxamine	Vasoxyl	NE	Alpha-1	Agonist for alpha-1 receptor
methylphenidate	Ritalin	Dopamine and NE	—	Increases release of dopamine and NE
methysergide	Sansert	Serotonin	Serotonin	Nonselective serotonin receptor blocker
metoclopramide[b]	Reglan	Dopamine; serotonin	Dopamine D-2; 5-HT$_3$	Blocks dopamine D-2 and 5-HT$_3$ receptors

Appendix: Summary of Relationship Between Therapeutically-Used Drugs and Various Neurotransmitters (continued)

Drug Name	Brand Name[a]	Neurotransmitter	Receptor	Drug Action
metoprolol	Lopressor	NE	Beta-1	Blocks beta-1 receptors
morphine	Morphine Sulfate	β-endorphin	Mu opioid	Agonist for mu receptor
naloxone	Narcan	β-endorphin; enkephalin	Opioid	Nonselective opioid receptor blocker
naltrexone	Trexan	β-endorphin; enkephalin	Opioid	Nonselective opioid receptor blocker
neostigmine	Prostigmin	ACh	—	Blocks degradation of ACh by cholinesterase
nicotine	Nicoderm (patch); Nicorette (gum)	ACh	Nicotinic-cholinergic	Agonist for nicotinic receptor
nitrazepam	Mogadon	GABA	Benzodiazepine-GABA$_A$ complex	Agonist for benzodiazepine receptor
norepinephrine	Levophed	NE	Alpha-1, alpha-2, beta-1	Agonist for adrenergic receptors
nortriptyline	Aventyl	NE	—	Blocks reuptake of NE
ondansetron	Zofran	Serotonin	5-HT$_3$	Blocks 5-HT$_3$ receptor
oxazepam	Serax	GABA	Benzodiazepine-GABA$_A$ complex	Agonist for benzodiazepine receptor
pancuronium	Pavulon	ACh	Nicotinic-cholinergic (at neuromuscular junction)	Blocks nicotinic receptor
pentazocine	Talwin	β-endorphin; enkephalin	Mu opioid; kappa opioid	Mu antagonist; kappa agonist
pentobarbital	Nembutal	GABA	GABA$_A$	Facilitates action of GABA
pergolide	Permax	Dopamine	Dopamine D-1 and D-2	Agonist for D-1 and D-2 receptors
phenelzine	Nardil	NE; dopamine; serotonin	—	Blocks monoamine oxidase to prevent degradation of monoamine transmitters
phenobarbital	Luminal	GABA	GABA$_A$	Facilitates action of GABA
phenylephrine	Neo-Synephrine	NE	Alpha-1	Alpha-1 agonist
phenoxybenzamine	Dibenzyline	NE	Alpha-1, alpha-2	Irreversibly blocks alpha-1 and alpha-2 receptors
phentolamine	Regitine	NE	Alpha-1, alpha-2	Reversibly blocks alpha-1 and alpha-2 receptors
physostigmine	Eserine Sulfate	ACh	—	Blocks enzymatic breakdown of ACh
pilocarpine	Pilocarpine HCl	ACh	Muscarinic-cholinergic	Muscarinic agonist
pindolol	VisKen	NE	Beta-1 and beta-2	Blocks beta adrenergic receptors
pirenzepine	Gastrozepine	ACh	M-1 muscarinic	Blocks M-1 receptors
prazosin	Minipress	NE	Alpha-1	Blocks alpha-1 receptor
primidone	Mysoline	GABA	GABA$_A$	Facilitates action of GABA
prochlorperazine	Compazine	Dopamine	Dopamine D-1 and D-2	Blocks D-1 and D-2 receptors

propranolol	Inderal	NE	Beta-1 and beta-2	Blocks beta-1 and beta-2 receptors
protriptyline	Vivactil	NE	—	Blocks reuptake of NE
pyridostigmine	Mestinon	ACh	—	Blocks enzymatic breakdown of ACh
quazepam	Doral	GABA	Benzodiazepine-GABA$_A$ complex	Agonist for benzodiazepine receptor
reserpine	Serpasil	NE; dopamine; serotonin	—	Blocks storage of monoamine transmitter and depletes nerves
scopolamine (hyoscine)	Isopto Hyoscine	ACh	Muscarinic-cholinergic	Muscarinic blocker
secobarbital	Seconal	GABA	GABA$_A$	Facilitates action of GABA$_A$
selegiline	Eldepryl	Dopamine	—	Inhibits monoamine oxidase Type B which degrades dopamine
sotalol	Betapace	NE	Beta-1 and beta-2	Beta-1 and beta-2 blocker
succinylcholine	Anectine	ACh	Nicotinic-cholinergic (at neuromuscular junction)	Nicotinic receptor blocker
sumatriptan	Imitrex	Serotonin	5-HT$_{1D}$	Agonist for 5-HT$_{1D}$ receptors
tacrine	Cognex	ACh	Nicotinic and muscarinic cholinergic	Cholinesterase inhibitor; partial agonist at muscarinic receptors
temazepam	Restoril	GABA	Benzodiazepine-GABA$_A$ complex	Agonist for benzodiazepine receptor
terazosin	Hytrin	NE	Alpha-1	Alpha-1 blocker
terbutaline	Brethine	NE; epinephrine	Beta-2	Agonist at beta-2 receptor
tranylcypromine	Parnate	NE; serotonin; dopamine	—	Inhibits degradation of monoamines by MAO
triazolam	Halcion	GABA	Benzodiazepine-GABA$_A$ complex	Agonist for benzodiazepine receptor
trimethaphan	Arfonad	ACh	Nicotinic-cholinergic (at autonomic ganglia)	Blocks nicotinic receptor
valproic acid	Depakene	GABA	GABA	Increases synthesis and blocks degradation of GABA
vecuronium	Norcuron	ACh	Nicotinic-cholinergic (at neuromuscular junction)	Blocks nicotinic receptor

Note: ACh, acetylcholine; GABA, gamma aminobutyric acid; 5-HT, 5-hydroxytryptamine; NE, norepinephrine; NMDA, N-methyl-D-aspartate.

a Includes only one example of a brand name.

b See Table 4.4 for other dopamine receptor antagonists.

5

Heterotopic Ossification in Traumatic Brain Injury

Douglas E. Garland

CONTENTS

As a patient presents at an emergency room with multiple trauma, the injuries which are life threatening tend to receive the greatest attention. Often, orthopedic injuries are monitored while the patient's overall medical stability is achieved and some degree of neurological stability or improvement is realized. While orthopedic issues are usually of secondary importance in these early stages of treatment, they can develop to primary areas of concern once the patient has moved through acute medical management and becomes appropriate for rehabilitative efforts. Much has been learned in recent years regarding the prevention and treatment of orthopedic injuries associated with traumatic brain injury (TBI). The development of untoward orthopedic complications, such as contractures or the transformation of soft tissues to osseous ones, following TBI is painful for the patient, limits functional gains which can be realized by the patient, and can be exceedingly expensive to treat. In the past, patients who were unfortunate enough to develop osseous transformation were subjected to vigorous range of motion and/or poorly timed, though well-intentioned, surgeries for excision of the offending tissues, only to experience re-growth of those tissues. Early on, there were no pharmacological solutions to develop for this problem, and overall the degree of understanding in the field concerning osseous transformation from soft tissue was poor. This chapter is provided for the purpose of reviewing the variables which seem to impact the development of heterotopic ossification, its prevalence and frequency of occurrence at specific body locations, and its diagnosis and treatment options.

HETEROTOPIC OSSIFICATION

The designation *heterotopic ossification* (HO) is preferred to such terms as *ectopic ossification* or *paraosteoarthropathy* when discussing the formation of new bone around joints as a consequence of traumatic brain injury (TBI). *Heterotopic* refers to the occurrence of bone in more than one location. Microscopically, the bone is a true "ossific" process arising *de novo* to new bone formation rather than calcification of soft tissue. Heterotopic ossification associated with TBI is labeled *neurogenic HO*.

The majority of HO associated with TBI is around joints, although it may also occur in the thigh. Neurogenic HO is commonly para-articular and usually occurs in a single plane around a joint, although it may occur in multiple sites. The bone itself lies within a well-defined tissue plane and usually does not involve the joint capsule or muscles. Patients exhibiting marked spasticity, especially extensor rigidity, are the most likely to develop this bone. Multiple sites are common in patients with marked spasticity. The HO frequently forms in the vicinity of the spastic musculature. The position of the extremity often permits early prediction of the future location of the HO. It is uncommon for a patient with only cognitive dysfunction to develop neurogenic HO.

GENETICS AND PATIENT PREDISPOSITION

Strong evidence for some type of genetic predisposition to HO formation comes from the hereditary disorder fibrodysplasia ossificans progressiva (FOP).[1] FOP is inherited as an autosomal dominant trait with full penetrance and variable expression. It is a disorder of connective tissue with skeletal malformations and HO. The natural history of HO from FOP has similarities to the natural history of HO from other causes, especially neurogenic HO. Although the majority of cases of FOP-associated HO are spontaneous, some cases also occur after trauma. A predilection of HO for certain locations (i.e., the axial musculature and proximal limbs) that is similar in both traumatic and neurogenic HO is documented. Heterotopic ossification frequently recurs after surgical resection. Recurrence is also noted after resection of neurogenic HO and occasionally after traumatic HO resection.

The association of human leukocyte antigens (HLA's) with neurogenic HO has been noted. An increased prevalence of HLA-B18 and HLA-B27 antigens has been reported in patients with HO in comparison to normal subjects.[2,3] However, follow-up studies from other centers have not confirmed these findings, and this system does not appear capable of predicting susceptibility to HO.[4-6]

PREVALENCE AND ONSET

The reported prevalence varies for most types of HO, but much of this difference may be the result of methodology and institutional variations. The type of center (acute care vs. rehabili-tation) and the type of patient (with hemiplegia, paraplegia, or quadriplegia) influence the incidence. Methodology also affects study outcomes. Prospective vs. retrospective studies, whole-body radiographs vs. hip only, and six-month vs. one-year follow-ups have the potential to influence final data.

The prevalence of clinically significant HO, that which limits joint motion, as opposed to HO of purely academic interest, or that which is solely a radiographic observation, is similar when studies from similar institutions and methodologies are compared. The most commonly reported prevalence of clinically significant HO is 10 to 20%.[7-10] Joint ankylosis occurs in less than 10% of the lesions.

DIAGNOSIS

Physical Examination

Limited joint motion is the most common physical finding and, frequently, the earliest sign of HO. An increase in spasticity usually occurs. Joint erythema or warmth occasionally requires differentiation from a septic joint. Lower limb swelling may mimic thrombophlebitis. The most common symptom of HO is pain. An increase in pain, spasticity, or muscle guarding should alert the examiner to the impending onset of HO.

Serum Alkaline Phosphatase Determination

Early reports on HO failed to associate elevated serum alkaline phosphatase (SAP) levels. However, follow-up studies have demonstrated that elevated levels of SAP are present with clinically significant HO. SAP levels begin to rise, although remaining in the normal range, within two weeks of injury.[11] Elevated levels may occur by three weeks, and the duration of persistently high titers averages five months. The majority of patients who develop clinically significant HO about the hip will have an elevated SAP level. This may not be true at the elbow where small amounts of HO may decrease motion. SAP titers do not correlate with inactivity, peak activity, or number of HO lesions. SAP determination is nonspecific and not absolute, but it may constitute the earliest and, certainly, the most convenient and inexpensive laboratory test for early detection of HO. Many patients are in intensive care units and cannot undergo special studies. Medicinal treatment may be initiated solely on the basis of SAP elevation if fractures are not present.

Radionuclide Bone Imaging

Radionuclide bone imaging (RNBI) became effective as a diagnostic tool in the late 1960's and early 1970's. Early bone scan techniques employed injection of technetium-99m polyphosphate with follow-up scans obtained approximately four to five hours after injection. Presently, the "three-phase" bone scan is the best method for early detection, as well as confirmation, of HO.[12] This test involves injection of Tc-labeled methylene diphosphonate followed by imaging in three phases:

> Phase I: A dynamic blood flow study with frequent photoscans during one-minute frame
> Phase II: A static scan for blood pool after the completion of phase I
> Phase III: A two- to four-hour bone scan to determine the amount of the labeled radionuclide in bone

The first two phases are the most sensitive for early detection of HO and may show abnormal results within two to four weeks after TBI. The period of positive uptake in Phases I and II with a negative Phase III may range from two to four weeks. Likewise, Phase III may be positive up to four weeks before HO is observed radiographically.

A large prospective, or even retrospective, study of the RNBI Phase III evaluation of HO is not available. Correlation of RNBI with evolution of radiographic features has not been performed. The majority of bone scans return to baseline within seven to twelve months, while a slowly downward activity occurs in many of the remainder of the scans. A few scans remain fully active during the first year. The RNBI may become reactivated after a quiescent period.

Quantitative radionuclide bone scans compare the ratio of uptake in normal ossification vs. HO. Since HO uptake decreases with time, it is assumed that serial decreases or a steady state in the ratio of uptake between normal and heterotopic bone indicates HO maturity. It is proposed that the incidence of recurrence of HO is decreased after resection if HO is removed during a radionuclide steady state. Unfortunately, this premise has not been adequately verified in a large homogeneous series. Our large surgical resection series demonstrated that this steady state was not a predictor of recurrence.[13] Patients with persistent active scans predictably had recurrence, whereas patients with baseline scans not uncommonly had recurrence. Consequently, it seems that neither the natural history of HO nor treatment guidelines based on RNBI activity have been adequately established.

Radiography

Before RNBI became available, radiographs provided confirmatory evidence of HO. Although plain films may detect HO as early as three weeks after injury, radiographic detection is usually not confirmatory until two months after the stimulus.

Radiographs offer other benefits. They identify the site of HO at the joint and are an easy, inexpensive, and reliable method for evaluation of treatment. Radiographs permit evaluation of maturation of HO, especially when coupled with results of SAP determinations and physical examination (decrease in spasticity).

Computed Tomography

The precise role of computed tomography (CT) scanning as a clinical tool for diagnosis and a measure of maturation of HO is not established.[14] Computed tomography may aid in preoperative surgical planning. Multiple sites of HO at a joint may be more readily delineated by CT. CT scan more clearly defines HO and its relation to muscle, vessel, and nerve.

LOCATION

Our retrospective review of 496 patients revealed 57 patients (11%) with 100 joints involved with neurogenic HO.[15] Thirty of the patients had single joint involvement, while 27 patients had multiple joint involvement. The ratio of the involved male and female patients was similar to the ratio of male to female in the total population. This is significant since some people suggest that, based on spinal cord injury (SCI) patients wherein female HO is uncommon, HO is a disease of males. Eighty-one of the involved joints were located on spastic extremities. We think the other extremities may have been previously spastic but had no spasticity at transfer to our unit.

The 11% incidence may not indicate the true incidence. A routine radiographic survey of major joints was not undertaken. Only clinically significant HO, in a joint associated with pain and decreased range of motion, was detected. Although the series was consecutive, the population was selected. Patients with mild head injuries are not transferred to our unit. The incidence of HO in these patients may be low or may occur in a mild, clinically insignificant form. Patients with severe neurologic involvement are frequently not candidates for rehabilitation and are not transferred to our unit. The incidence in this group, as well as the amount of HO, may be increased.

Hip

Forty-four hips developed HO in 33 patients. Three main locations were detected. The site of HO could frequently be predicted from the abnormal posture of the extremity. Occasionally, HO developed in more than one plane.

Heterotopic bone anterior to the hip may result in swelling of the thigh with a palpable and visual mass (Figure 5.1-A). The lower extremity often assumes a mildly reflexed position with external rotation of the leg. The massive amount of HO present in SCI patients at this location is seldom observed in TBI patients.

HO occurring posterior to the hip may be associated with hip flexion contractures. This location of HO may not result in great limitation of motion.

The most common location of HO at the hip was the inferomedial location (Figure 5.2-A). HO, in this location, is frequently associated with adductor spasticity. Ankylosis is uncommon unless the patient had a severe neurologic insult. Some loss of hip flexion and extension normally occurs. If a large amount of HO is present, adduction range is compromised due to a mechanical block.

Elbow

Two sites of HO generally occur in the elbow, although HO may form in any or all planes, especially in the traumatized elbow. HO anterior to the elbow is often associated with flexor spasticity, as noted in the hemiplegic limb (Figure 5.3-A). If ankylosis results, the bone usually bridges the distal humerus and proximal radius.

New bone occurring posteriorly at the elbow is often associated with extensor posturing (rigidity). Since extensor rigidity resolves with neurologic improvement, the elbow may assume a more flexed position at the time ankylosis is occurring. This explains the paradox of posterior HO in a normal, hemiplegic, or flexed extremity. Ankylosis most commonly occurs posteriorly at the elbow. Ankylosis is usually between the distal humerus and olecranon.

Shoulder

The rate of occurrence is similar to the elbow. The new bone is generally located inferomedial to the joint. The shoulder position is internal rotation and adduction. Ankylosis is uncommon unless the patient sustains a severe neurologic insult.

Knee

HO about the knee and the quadriceps muscle is uncommon. It may appear anywhere in the distal thigh or about the knee.

NATURAL HISTORY

The natural history of HO is defined through radiographs and not frequently emphasized.[16-18] The natural radiographic history is similar and predictable in the majority of patients. It also closely parallels the elevation of SAP level and the presence of spasticity.

Our retrospective review of 23 TBI patients who underwent resection of HO at an average of 28 months after injury allowed classification of patients from I to V according to their neurologic recovery. Class I patients had near-normal neurologic recovery, whereas Class V patients had severe cognitive deficits and spasticity. Class I patients rarely had recurrence after resection. In contrast, every Class V patient had recurrence regardless of the site of HO. Radiographic progression subsided by six months, and SAP

A

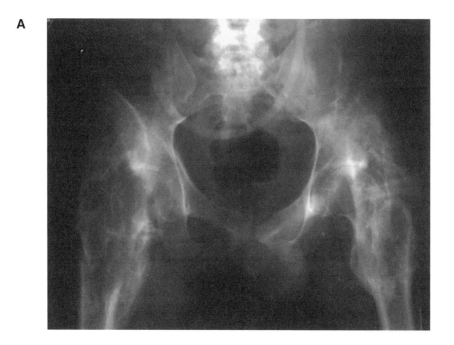

B

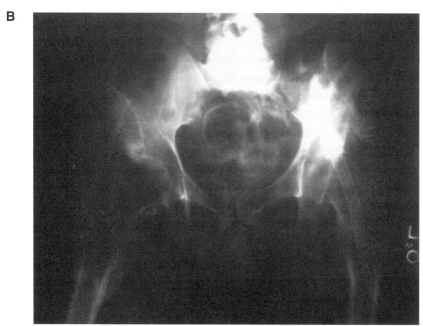

FIGURE 5.1   Anteroposterior (AP) radiograph of hips. (A) The HO is located anteriorly and is causing ankylosis. (B) The HO was resected $1^1/_2$ years after TBI. The patient was neurologically Class II. Radiation was used as a postoperative prophylaxis. No bone recurred.

levels and RNBI activity were normal, or significantly decreasing, in patients who made an early, normal neurologic recovery (Class I). Patients with severe motor compromise had larger amounts of HO. This HO progressed, in some instances, for more than one year, with elevated SAP levels for two years or longer and, occasionally, persistent activity on RNBI.[13]

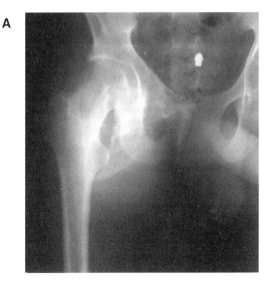

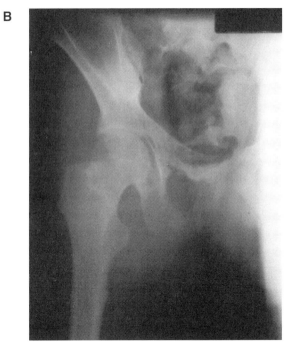

FIGURE 5.2 AP radiograph of the right hip. (A) The HO is located inferomedially. Flexion-extension range is only mildly compromised, but no adduction is present and abduction is limited. Ambulation was perceived by the patient as abnormal. (B) The HO was resected at two years after TBI. The patient was neurologically Class II. Radiation was used as a postoperative prophylaxis. No bone recurred and gait returned to near normal.

TREATMENT

HO runs a gamut from being undetected, and therefore untreated, to having a poor response to all treatment modalities. Some patients with minimal HO require no specific treatment, whereas others may require physical therapy, medicine, manipulation, surgical excision, or all of these. The majority of patients with HO maintain functional joint motion with standard physical therapies, medicines, and, occasionally, forceful manipulations. A small group require surgery, with some developing recurrence after surgery.

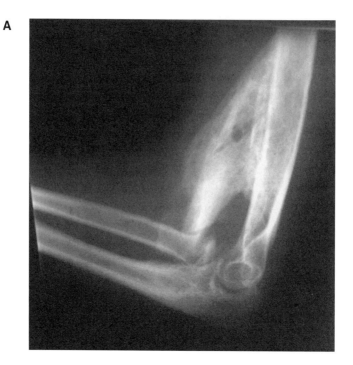

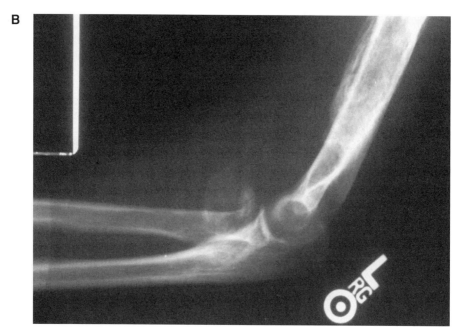

FIGURE 5.3   Lateral radiographs of the left elbow. (A) The HO is located anteriorly and causing ankylosis. (B) The HO was resected at $1^{1}/_{2}$ years after TBI. The patient was neurologically Class II. Radiation was used as a postoperative prophylaxis. No bone recurred and full flexion-extension range was obtained.

Medical treatment, including radiation, is used prophylactically in two general situations: (1) to prevent HO formation after the primary insult, and (2) to prevent recurrence of HO after surgical resection.

Ethylhydroxybisphosphonate (Etidronate Disodium)

In the early 1960's, research with polyphosphates and their inhibitory activity on calcium phosphate precipitation led to evaluation of bisphosphonates, most specifically ethylhydroxybisphosphonate (EHDP), for similar effects. Definitive studies demonstrated that bisphosphonates inhibited the precipitation of calcium phosphate from clear solutions, delayed aggregation of apatite crystals into layer clusters, blocked the transformation of amorphous calcium phosphate into hydroxyapatite, and delayed dissolution of crystals. All effects seemed related to their affinity for hydroxyapatite. The ability of EHDP to inhibit experimental soft tissue ossification, as well as normal mineralization of bone, led to the clinical use of EHDP to prevent HO.[19,20]

Clinical research has not irrefutably proved or disproved its effectiveness, but no study has been able to prove absolute arrest of HO when the studies are subjected to strict scientific scrutiny.[7,12,21] Other authors have stated that EHDP is not effective in preventing HO.

The desired response to EHDP is dictated by the proper dosage and duration of treatment. Simplistically speaking, EHDP prevents conversion of the amorphous calcium phosphate compounds into hydroxyapatite crystals, which is one of the final stages of bone formation. Since the majority of HO evolves radiographically over a period of six months, it is concluded that EHDP should generally be given over this six-month span.[16-18] Lower EHDP doses are adequate to inhibit crystal resorption, but they are less effective in inhibiting crystal growth. The 20-mg/kg dosage is necessary to prevent HO formation. Treatment for this duration and at this dosage should prevent HO lesions in the majority of patients and also decrease the incidence of the so-called rebound calcification. Prolonged treatment with EHDP produces undesirable side effects such as long bone fractures in dogs.[22] Therefore, dosages of 20 mg/kg for longer than six months' duration may not be warranted, and continued treatment may be deleterious. EHDP will not be effective for the persistent neurologically compromised patient regardless of dosages and duration of treatment.

Quantitative histomorphometry demonstrates an increased number of osteoclasts, as well as osteoblasts, in the HO lesion compared to normal bone.[23] EHDP, at a much lower dosage than that necessary for the inhibition of ossification, interrupts osteoclastic function but does not destroy the osteoclasts. They eventually recover full function but over a prolonged period. The impairment of osteoclast function is extremely undesirable. Resorption is the final aspect of HO maturation and involves partial or even complete resolution of the HO lesion. With cessation of treatment, the osteoid may ossify immediately, yet the resorptive capability remains impaired until osteoclastic function returns. This may influence the rebound phenomenon as well as resorption. The effect of EHDP on osteoclasts, the recovery or rebound phase, the length of treatment, patient compliance, and the cost of the medication may eventually contribute to the selection of another drug for treatment of HO.

Indomethacin

Dahl is generally credited with demonstrating the prophylactic effects of indomethacin on HO formation after total hip replacement.[24] Other studies have verified its effectiveness.[25,26] The ability of indomethacin to inhibit prostaglandin synthetase is proposed as the primary mechanism for HO prevention, although many effects on bone formation are known. Prostaglandins are mediators of inflammation, and part of indomethacin's effect is inhibition of the inflammatory response or suppression of mesenchymal cell proliferation. Indomethacin dosage is 25 mg, three times a day for six weeks, after total hip replacement. Ibuprofen and aspirin may also be effective when used in a similar fashion. The effectiveness and the duration of treatment of nonsteroidal, anti-inflammatory drugs (NSAID's) to prevent HO in the neurologic patient have not been established.

Radiation

The ability of radiation to inhibit bone growth has been known by radiotherapists for years. Irradiation prevents conversion of precursor cells to bone-forming cells. Early reports of irradiation in the treatment of myositis ossificans were often anecdotal. Now it appears that 1000 rads or less, immediately after total hip replacement, is effective in preventing HO.[27,28] The location of HO formation in the neurologic patient cannot be predicted. Because radiation is relatively ineffective once HO is detected, its use in prevention and early treatment of initial neurogenic HO may be limited.

Forceful Manipulation

The role of ranging joints involved with HO for maintenance or increasing joint motion is controversial. Some authors have suggested that ranging increases the amount of HO, whereas others have reported beneficial gains or maintenance of joint motion. A review of patients who underwent forceful manipulation under anesthesia demonstrated its usefulness in maintaining motion in most patients and actually increasing motion in others.[29] Traumatic brain injury patients frequently have spasticity, intolerance to pain, and voluntary muscle guarding. Consequently, anesthesia is usually required for manipulation. Examination under anesthesia allows differentiation of spasticity and true ankylosis. If spasticity is determined to be a major factor, treatment may also be directed towards it.

Large increases in motion are sometimes achieved under anesthesia, but motion may be gradually lost thereafter. If neurologic improvement continues, joint manipulation may be repeated as necessary. If the patient remains at a low level of neurologic recovery, repeated manipulations are not beneficial. We have not manipulated a joint more than three times. Final arc of motion is closely related to the amount of neurologic recovery. Twenty-three of 28 joints (82%) gained motion with anesthesia. Eighteen joints (64%) maintained or gained further motion with rehabilitation. Review of the radiographs did not reveal an exacerbation of the ossific process.

Surgery

Surgery is indicated for joint mobility, limb positioning, or sitting. Various operative procedures have been described.[13,17,18,30] Precise timing for surgery is mentioned infrequently but is determined in respect to the quiescent state, indicated by normal SAP levels, mature radiographic appearance, and baseline RNBI. Postoperative complications are common when compared to standard orthopedic procedures.

The natural history of neurologic recovery is the best indicator for time of surgical excision, recurrence, and functional outcome. The majority of motor recovery occurs by $1^1/_2$ years and resection should be considered at that time. Excision in the patient with a rapid neurologic recovery may be undertaken earlier when alkaline phosphatase is normal and no spasticity is present. Surgery should be delayed longer than $1^1/_2$ years if the motor recovery is prolonged (Figures 5.1-A, B; 5.2-A, B; 5.3-A, B). Recurrence is common in the presence of normal or abnormal laboratory values in the neurologically compromised patient, and delaying excision because of abnormal laboratory values is not warranted. Surgery is indicated for limb positioning in the neurologically compromised patient.

No currently available studies have defined the role of medical prophylaxis after resection. The stimulus to form HO has subsided in the normal recovery group and medical prophylaxis may not be necessary for these patients. Since the neurologically compromised patient continues to form HO after resection, present prophylaxis methods seem inadequate. A mildly to moderately neurologically compromised patient should respond to prophylaxis after resection.

REFERENCES

1. Connor, J. M. and Evans, D. A. P., Fibroplasia ossificans progressiva. The clinical features and natural history of 34 patients, *J. Bone Jt. Surg.,* 64B, 76, 1982.
2. Larson, J. M., Michalski, J. P., Collacott, E. A., Eltoral, D., McCombs, C. C., and Madorsky, J. B., Increased prevalence of HLA-B27 in patients with ectopic ossification following traumatic spinal cord injury, *Rheumatol. Rehabil.,* 20, 193, 1981.
3. Minare, P., Betuel, H., Girard, R., and Pilonchery, G., Neurologic injuries, paraosteoarthropathies, and human leukocyte antigens, *Arch. Phys. Med. Rehabil.,* 61, 214, 1980.
4. Garland, D. E., Alday, B., and Venos, K. G., Heterotopic ossification and HLA antigens, *Arch. Phys. Med. Rehabil.,* 65, 5531, 1984.
5. Hunter, T., Dubo, H. I. C., Hildahl, C. R., Smith, N. J., and Schroeder, M. L., Histocompatibility antigens in patients with spinal cord injury or cerebral damage complicated by heterotopic ossification, *Rheumatol. Rehabil.,* 19, 97, 1980.
6. Weiss, S., Grosswasser, A., Ohri, A., Mizrachi, Y., Orgad, S., Efter, T., and Gazit, E., Histocompatibility (HLA) antigens in heterotopic ossification associated with neurological injury, *J. Rheumatol.,* 6, 88, 1979.
7. Garland, D. E., Alday, B., Venos, K. G., and Vogt, J. C., Diphosphonate treatment for heterotopic ossification in spinal cord injury patients, *Clin. Orthop.,* 176, 197, 1983.
8. Mendelson, L., Grosswasser, Z., Najenson, T., Sandback, U., and Solzi, P., Periarticular new bone formation in patients suffering from severe head injuries, *Scand. J. Rehabil. Med.,* 7, 141, 1975.
9. Mielants, H., Vanhove, E., deNeels, J., and Veys, E., Clinical survey of and pathogenic approach to para-articular ossifications in long-term coma, *Acta Orthop. Scand.,* 46, 190, 1975.
10. Sazbon, L., Najenson, T., Tartakovsky, M., Becker, E., and Grosswasser, Z., Wide-spread peri-articular new bone formation in long-term comatose patients, *J. Bone Jt. Surg.,* 63B, 120, 1981.
11. Orzel, J. A. and Rudd, T. G., Heterotopic bone formation: Clinical, laboratory, and imaging correlation, *J. Nucl. Med.,* 26, 125, 1985.
12. Freed, J. H., Hahn, H., Menter, M. D., and Dillion, T., The use of the three-phase bone scan in the early diagnosis of heterotopic ossification (HO) and in the evaluation of didronel therapy, *Paraplegia,* 20, 208, 1982.
13. Garland, D. E., Hanscom, D. A., Keenan, M. A., Smith, C., and Moore, T., Resection of heterotopic ossification in the adult with head trauma, *J. Bone Jt. Surg.,* 67A, 1261, 1985.
14. Bressler, E., Marn, C., Gore, R., and Hendrix, R., Evaluation of ectopic bone by CT, *Am. J. Radiol.,* 148, 931, 1987.
15. Garland, D. E., Blum, C. E., and Waters, R. L., Periarticular heterotopic ossification in head injured adults: Incidence and location, *J. Bone Jt. Surg.,* 62A, 1143, 1980.
16. Garland, D. E., Clinical observations on fractures and heterotopic ossification in the spinal cord and traumatic brain injured populations, *Clin. Orthop.,* 233, 86, 1988.
17. Garland, D. E., A clinical perspective of common forms of acquired heterotopic ossification, *Clin. Orthop.,* 263, 13, 1991.
18. Garland, D. E., Surgical approaches for resection of heterotopic ossification in traumatic brain-injured adults, *Clin. Orthop.,* 263, 59, 1991.
19. Fleisch, H., Diphosphonates: History and mechanisms of action, *Bone,* 3, 279, 1981.
20. Russell, R. G. G. and Smith, R., Diphosphonates — Experimental and clinical aspects, *J. Bone Jt. Surg.,* 55B, 66, 1973.
21. Spielman, G., Gennarelli, T. A., and Rogers, C. R., Disodium etidronate: Its role in preventing heterotopic ossification in severe head injury, *Arch. Phys. Med. Rehabil.,* 64, 539, 1983.
22. Flora, L., Hassing, G. S., Cloyd, G. G., Parfitt, A. M., and Villanueva, A. R., The long-term skeletal effects of EHDP in dogs, *Bone,* 3, 289, 1981.
23. Puzas, J. E., Miller, M. D., and Rosier, R. N., Pathologic bone formation, *Clin. Orthop.,* 245, 269, 1989.
24. Ritter, M. A. and Gioe, T. J., The effect of indomethacin on para-articular ectopic ossification following total hip arthroplasty, *Clin. Orthop.,* 167, 113, 1982.
25. Kjaersgaard-Andersen, P. and Schmidt, S. A., Indomethacin for prevention of ectopic ossification after hip arthroplasty, *Acta Orthop. Scand.,* 57, 12, 1986.
26. Schmidt, S. A., Kjaersgaard-Anderson, P., Pederson, N. W., Kristensen, S. S., Pederson, P., and Neilsen, J. B., The use of indomethacin to prevent the formation of heterotopic bone after total hip replacement, *J. Bone Jt. Surg.,* 70A, 834, 1988.
27. Ayers, D. G., Evarts, C. M., and Parkinson, J. R., The prevention of heterotopic ossification in high-risk patients by low-dose radiation therapy after total hip arthroplasty, *J. Bone Jt. Surg.,* 68AA, 1423, 1986.
28. Coventry, M. B. and Scanton, P. W., Use of radiation to discourage ectopic bone, *J. Bone Jt. Surg.,* 63A, 201, 1982.
29. Garland, D. E., Razza, B. E., and Waters, R. L., Forceful joint manipulation in head-injured adults with heterotopic ossification, *Clin. Orthop.,* 169, 133, 1982.
30. Roberts, J. B. and Pankratz, D. G., Surgical treatment of heterotopic ossification at the elbow following long-term coma, *J. Bone Jt. Surg.,* 61A, 760, 1979.

6

Vestibular Dysfunction After Traumatic Brain Injury: Evaluation and Management

Peter S. Roland and Erik Otto

CONTENTS

0-8493-9463-5/95/$0.00+$.50
© 1995 by CRC Press Inc.

Vestibular injury is frequently overlooked in the diagnostic evaluation of the traumatically brain-injured individual. Many of the patients we see in our postacute setting have never been formally evaluated for vestibular dysfunction. Yet an important percentage of these patients suffer from vestibular dysfunction. The complaint of vertigo is not the only symptom of vestibular injury. Other symptoms may include decreased ability to balance, visual complaints (double vision, blurriness), or nausea. Complaints that may or may not be symptoms of vestibular injury per se, but often accompany a vestibular lesion after a head injury, are headache, irritability, oversensitivity to sounds and/or lights, and decreased attention and concentration span. These symptoms are often seen as a psychological response following a head injury and not related to organic damage. In addition to the vestibular and associated complaints, there is the issue of litigation that can cloud the mind of the patient and caregiver alike. Only following a complete evaluation can the process of treatment begin. Treatment may include exercise, medication, and/or a surgical procedure. Finally, when complete rehabilitation is not expected, the role of a counselor can be crucial in dealing with adjustment to disability. This process should also include patient education about the extent of the lesion and its consequences. Patient education is critical to help bring under control a process that otherwise might lead to a degree of disability not warranted by the lesion itself.

Recovery from head injury is now recognized to be a complex process which progresses over many months. The patient recovering from a head injury is frequently afflicted with more than a single area of difficulty or dysfunction. Many of these areas are the focus of specific chapters in this volume. Such problem areas frequently cross disciplinary boundaries and, in practical clinical situations, symptoms outside the specialty area of the primary caregiver may receive less-than-adequate attention. Comprehensive care is, therefore, improved when the post-head-injury patient is served by a multidisciplinary team whose efforts are orchestrated by a designated coordinator.

Review of the literature suggests that dizziness or disequilibrium following a head injury represents an area which requires considerably more attention and postinjury rehabilitation than it has received to date.

DEMOGRAPHICS

Although previous investigations are few in number, the evidence presented by available studies[1,2] argues powerfully that postconcussive balance disturbance is the primary cause of very substantial morbidity and long-term disability. Indeed, Healy[1] asserted that cochlear and vestibular dysfunction represent the largest group of delayed complications of head injury.

Berman and Fredrickson[3] evaluated 321 head injury patients within the Canadian Workman's Compensation System. Forty percent (40%) of this group complained of postinjury vertigo and, of those complaining of vertigo, fifty percent (50%) had objective electronystagmographic (ENG) findings of organic dysfunction. When the 140 patients with complaints of vertigo were evaluated five years after injury, only fourteen percent (14%) had returned to their preaccident or equivalent work. Forty-six percent (46%) of this group had not returned to any work at all. Vertigo, together with headache, was of prime importance in determining long-term work status. Although no long-term studies exist for U.S. populations, since social, cultural, and compensation variables are quite similar, it seems reasonable to extrapolate these results to the United States.

Rantanen et al.[4] evaluated 41 patients within several days of head injury. Sixty percent (60%) complained of vertigo. When eye movement was evaluated by physical examination alone (even with Frenzel lenses), only twenty percent (20%) had observable nystagmus. However, when electronystagmography (ENG) was performed with eyes closed, nystagmus was detectable in over sixty percent (60%). Elimination of "visual fixation" by eye closure releases pathological nystagmoid eye movement in a significant percentage of injured people, and Rantanen et al.[4] emphasize that formal ENG evaluation is important in the objective evaluation of postinjury patients complaining of dizziness.

Saito et al.[5] evaluated 22 patients who complained of dizziness after head injury. All had positional nystagmus on ENG. Eleven had ENG findings suggestive of central nervous system injury. Of the eleven patients with ENG findings suggestive of CNS injury, only four recovered in two months or less and four were still unrecovered after three months. Patients with ENG indicators of peripheral vestibular dysfunction recovered much more quickly. By differentiating between central and peripheral pathology, ENG was helpful in establishing a prognosis.

Tuohimaa[6] carefully studied 82 patients who had sustained only "mild" head injuries (duration of unconsciousness less than two hours or not at all) and compared them to a matched control group. Seventy-eight percent (78%) of the postinjury patients complained of vertigo. Central ENG disturbances were observed immediately after injury in sixty percent (60%) of the patients, but the incidence fell to twelve percent (12%) at six months postinjury. The incidence of persistent central ENG changes increased with increasing age of the post-head-injury patient. Tuohimaa's group of patients demonstrated a dramatic impairment of the ability to suppress nystagmus by deliberate visual fixation. He argues that diminished fixation suppression indicates that reduced central inhibition is a frequent consequence of mild head injury. The incidence of both spontaneous and positional nystagmus was significantly higher in mild head injury patients immediately after injury than in normal controls.

Grimm et al.[7] studied 102 patients with mild craniocervical trauma who experienced positional vertigo. This group displayed a set of symptoms often referred to as *postconcussion* syndrome. Over ninety-five percent (95%) of these patients suffered from disequilibrium and seventy percent (70%) from vertigo. Headache, memory loss, tinnitus, nausea, confusion, clumsiness, alteration of subjective visual perception, and stiff neck were all present in over fifty percent (50%) of this group of patients. Their conclusion that all of these patients had a perilymphatic fistula is highly controversial, but their work does highlight the importance of balance disturbance in patients with even mild head injury. Moreover, they have documented well the pattern of characteristic symptomatology found so frequently after head injury.

Vertaineu and Karjalaineu[8] examined 199 children after blunt head trauma. Fifty percent (50%) had positional or spontaneous nystagmus and fifty percent (50%) had central ENG disturbances. The incidence of abnormalities dropped rapidly after two to eight years, but was somewhat higher in the peripheral group (18%) than in the central group (12%). Clinically, when compared to adults, a much lower percentage of these children (1.5%) remained symptomatic at two to eight years.

Evatar et al.[9] evaluated 22 children aged six to eighteen years for posttraumatic vertigo. Children with hearing loss were excluded. Five pathologically distinct etiologies were identified, including posttraumatic migraine (5), seizure disorders (4), postconcussion syndrome (4), whiplash injury (4), and posttraumatic neurosis (5). Their work emphasizes the variety of processes which can produce posttraumatic disequilibrium and emphasizes the value of objective ENG testing in distinguishing among various etiologies.

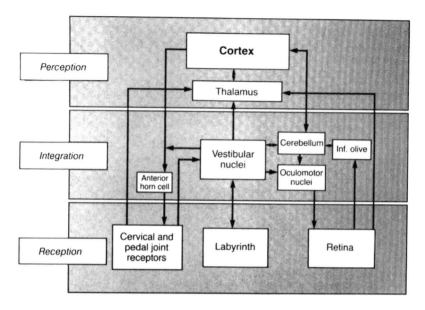

FIGURE 6.1 Conceptual schema of the vestibular system. This subdivides the various components of the vestibular system into a vertically oriented hierarchy with receptor organs at the bottom and perception at the top. Lateral organization distinguishes between various different receptors at lower levels and brainstem nuclei at higher levels. A fully functional vestibular system requires coordination and integration of sensory receptor information. Plasticity of the vestibular system arises from the fact that deficiencies in information provided by receptors can be compensated for at the integrative or perceptive level by reorganizing input from residual receptors. (Reprinted by permission from Brown, J. J., A systematic approach to the dizzy patient, *Diagnost. Neurotol. Neurol. Clin.,* 8(2), 210, 1990.)

ANATOMY AND PHYSIOLOGY OF THE VESTIBULAR SYSTEM

The anatomy of the vestibular system is complex and, especially in its ramifications within the central nervous system, poorly understood. Anatomically speaking, one may divide the vestibular system into four parts: 1) the peripheral vestibular end-organ enclosed within the bony labyrinthine capsule, 2) the vestibular nerve, 3) the brainstem vestibular nuclei together with their vestibulo-ocular, vestibulo-cerebellar, and vestibulo-spinal radiations and feedback loops, and 4) vestibular cortex (Figure 6.1).

Vestibular End Organ

The *labyrinth* (inner ear) consists of a folded, fluid-filled tube (membranous labyrinth or endolymphatic space) which lies within the bony labyrinthine capsule. The membranous labyrinth is suspended in, and cushioned by, a second fluid compartment (perilymphatic space). Anteriorly within the bony labyrinth is the spiral-shaped cochlea, the organ of hearing. Posteriorly are the three semicircular canals. Between the cochlea and semicircular canals is a central chamber, the vestibule, which contains the utricle and saccule (Figures 6.1 and 6.2).

The two inner fluids are chemically distinct. Endolymph (like intracellular fluid) contains a relatively high concentration of potassium and a relatively low concentration of sodium. Perilymph (like extracellular fluid) contains much sodium but relatively little potassium. The difference in electrolyte composition between these two fluids is essential in maintenance of the resting electrical potential, which is critical for normal functioning of the receptor cells.

The composition of endolymph is thought to be regulated by a vascular structure within the lateral wall of the endolymphatic duct called the *stria vascularis*. The production and composition of endolymph may, therefore, be altered by conditions and substances that alter blood flow, vascular permeability, or systemic fluid balance. Perilymph is, at least partially, an

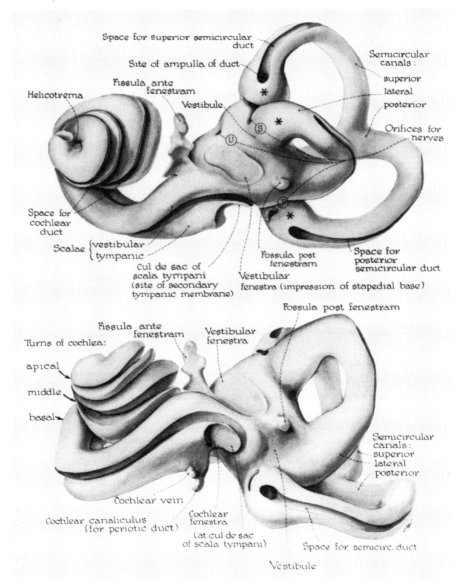

FIGURE 6.2 The labyrinth is seen from the lateral position (top view) and from below (bottom view). The bony labyrinth has been opened to show the position of the membranous endolymphatic duct. The appropriate structures are labeled. Asterisks indicate the cupular dilatations of the semicircular canals. S, saccule; U, utricle. (Reprinted by permission from Lindemann, H. H., *Studies on the Morphology of Sensory Regions of the Vestibular Apparatus*, Springer-Verlag, New York, 1969.)

ultrafiltrate of spinal fluid. The perilymphatic space is connected with the subarachnoid cerebrospinal fluid space via the cochlear aqueduct. Changes within the subarachnoid space may alter the perilymphatic compartment. Increased intracranial pressure produced by disease or by straining may be transmitted to the perilymphatic space and produce chronic or acute perilymphatic hypertension. Chemicals, toxins, and viral and bacterial infectious agents may all pass from the cerebrospinal fluid to the perilymph via the cochlear aqueduct.

Alterations in the chemical composition, relative volumes, or mixing of the inner ear fluids may incapacitate both the vestibular and hearing end-organ. Depending upon the anatomic extent and severity of the alteration, various combinations of balance disturbance, hearing loss, aural fullness, and tinnitus may result.

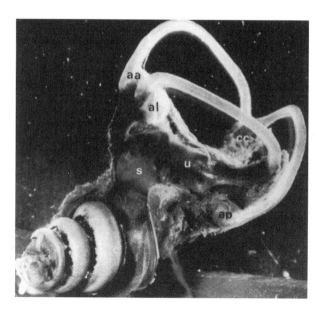

FIGURE 6.3 This is an actual microdissection. The bone has been completely removed leaving only the membranous endolymphatic duct system. The microdissection is oriented in approximately the same position as the top drawing in Figure 6.2. AA = cupula of the superior canal; AL = cupula of the lateral semicircular canal; AP = cupula of the posterior semicircular canal; CC = crus communis; U = utricle; S = saccule; C = cochlea. (Reprinted with permission from Lindemann, H. H., *Studies on the Morphology of Sensory Regions of the Vestibular Apparatus*, Springer-Verlag, New York, 1969.)

The common sensory receptor within the inner ear is the *hair cell*. Its function is to translate fluid motion into a pattern of neuronal electrical discharge. The labyrinthine fluids first translate both head acceleration and sound waves into fluid movement. Movement of fluid across the stereocilia of receptor hair cells deflects the stereocilia and changes the resting rate of discharge in the nerve attached to the hair cell (Figure 6.3). Movement in one direction may increase the rate of discharge, and movement in the opposite direction may decrease the rate of discharge. It is this change in rate of neuronal activity which is processed by the central nervous system into conscious and subconscious information about spatial orientation and sound.

The vestibular end-organ consists of five separate structures, each with its own specialized sensory epithelium. The three semicircular canals are at right angles to each other — one in the horizontal, one in the sagittal, and one in the coronal plane. The receptor organ of the semicircular canals is the crista ampullaris (Figures 6.1 and 6.2). Each crista consists of a group of hair cells, the stereocilia of which protrude into a dilated portion of the membranous labyrinth called the *ampulla*. The stereocilia of the hair cells are embedded in a gelatinous matrix that fills the ampulla (Figure 6.4). Head acceleration in the plane of the semicircular canals results in the bending of stereocilia due to inertial lag in the movement of endolymph. The same "bending" event occurs when head movement is stopped because the endolymph will "keep going" for a few milliseconds after the head comes to a complete rest. The semicircular canals, therefore, respond exclusively to angular acceleration. They do not respond to constant velocity — only to changes in velocity. This distinction is important. Once constant velocity is achieved, the sense of motion is eliminated. A pilot in a rolling airplane may, absent of visual clues, lose all sense of rotation if the rotation continues at constant velocity for more than a few seconds.

The saccule and utricle are the two otolithic end-organs. They sense linear acceleration and static tilt. They are gravity sensitive and maintain the ability to distinguish "up" from "down". Each otolithic end-organ consists of an outpouching of the endolymphatic duct, on one wall of which rests a collection of hair cells called the *macula*. The hair cells are covered with a

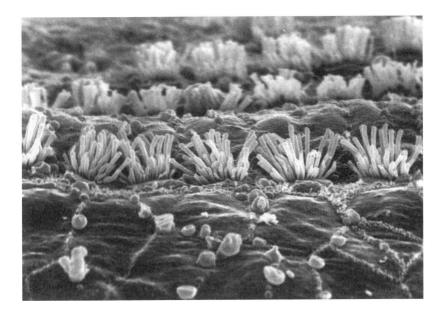

FIGURE 6.4 This is a scanning electron micrograph of the stereocilia from the cochlear hair cells. (Photomicrograph courtesy of C. Gary Wright, Ph.D.)

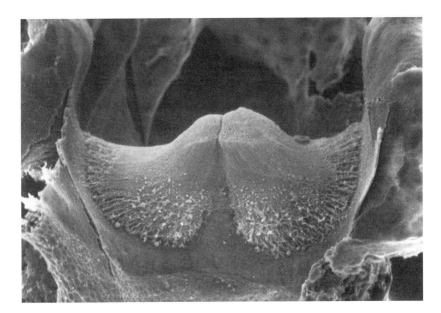

FIGURE 6.5 The open cupula of a semicircular canal reveals the gelatinous matrix out of which hair cells protrude. (Photomicrograph courtesy of C. Gary Wright, Ph.D.)

gelatinous matrix in which are embedded crystals of calcium carbonate called *otoconia* (Figure 6.5). The otoconia (Figure 6.6) are acted upon by gravitational forces as well as linear acceleration. A change in head position alters the direction in which the otoconia are pulled by gravity and bends the stereocilia of the macular hair cells in that direction. Thus, any change in head position produces a sense of head movement. Since resting head position produces constant otoconial displacement and stereociliar "bending," the otolithic organs are also sensitive to static "tilt" and help maintain orientation to "up and down".

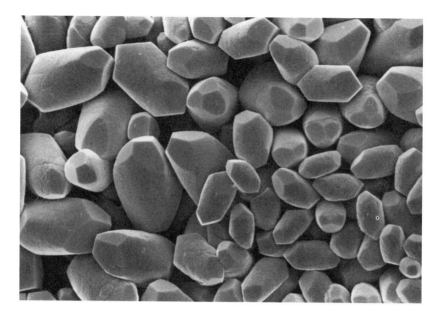

FIGURE 6.6   Scanning electron micrograph of calcium carbonate otoconia. (Photomicrograph courtesy of C. Gary Wright, Ph.D.)

Vestibular Nerve

Information from the vestibular labyrinth is carried to the brainstem by the vestibular nerve. The superior vestibular nerve carries fibers originating from the superior and horizontal semicircular canals, utricle, and a small portion of the saccule. The inferior vestibular nerve carries fibers originating from the posterior semicircular canal and from most of the saccule. Within the internal auditory canal, the superior and inferior vestibular nerves join together, first with each other, and then with the auditory nerve, and form a single cochleovestibular nerve. The facial nerve also travels through the temporal bone within the internal auditory canal in close proximity to the vestibular and auditory nerves. The vestibulocochlear nerve crosses the subarachnoid spinal fluid space to the brainstem where the vestibular fibers synapse within the vestibular nuclei. The anterior inferior cerebellar artery, or one of its branches, is often closely associated with the vestibulocochlear nerve, either within the internal auditory canal or within the subarachnoid space between the temporal bone and the brainstem.

The Central Vestibular System

The first-order vestibular neurons which constitute the vestibular nerves synapse with one or more of the four brainstem vestibular nuclei. The neurons from one labyrinth will often synapse within the vestibular nuclei on both sides of the head, thus providing bilateral representation of the vestibular system even at the brainstem level. The wide-ranging ramifications of the vestibular system within the central nervous system are very complex and poorly understood. Four principal areas can then be conceptually distinguished, even if they cannot always be precisely anatomically delineated: vestibulo-ocular, vestibulo-spinal, vestibulo-cerebellar, and vestibulo-cortical.

Vestibulo-ocular connections form the basis of the vestibulo-ocular reflex (VOR).[10-12] Each semicircular canal has an elaborate pattern of both direct and indirect synaptic connections to the ocular motor nuclei that control eye movements. The vestibular nuclei on each side are connected to the ocular motor nuclei of both eyes in such a way that stimulation of each semicircular canal can produce eye movements in the plane of that canal, i.e., stimulation of the horizontal semicircular canal can produce horizontal eye movement. These complicated connections are responsible for the production of nystagmus. Stimulation of one labyrinth produces slow movement of the eyes in the opposite direction from the direction of head movement and of roughly equal magnitude. Eye movement continues until a predetermined amount of lateral deviation is reached. Ocular centers within the brain are able to recognize that no further eye movement is appropriate. In order to prevent "pinning" of the eyes in extreme lateral gaze, the eyes are returned to the neutral "straight ahead" position from which lateral deviation can begin again. The eye movement perceived by an observer, therefore, is of slow lateral deviation followed by a very "quick" return movement which, in turn, is followed by another slow movement phase. The rapid return phase is a *saccade*. Saccades are the mechanism of eye movement utilized during volitional change of focus when we "look around". Saccades may occur with speeds of up to 800 degrees per second. During each saccade, reflex brainstem activity suppresses vision so that the visual field is prevented from constant "jumping". Since the fast phase of nystagmus is a saccade, vision is suppressed as it occurs. Since this is not true of the "slow" phase which is controlled by the labyrinth, some patients will complain that their visual field "jumps" in the direction opposite to slow phase when they have nystagmus. Since the slow phase of nystagmus is about equal to, but in the opposite direction of, head movement, it appears to be a mechanism which reflexively permits retention of visual fixation during head movement or when falling.

Vestibulo-Cerebellar

There are extensive direct and indirect descending (efferent) and ascending (afferent) pathways between the midline cerebellar nuclei (principally the vermis and fastigial nucleus) and the brainstem vestibular nuclei and associated integrative centers. These extensive connections permit precise modulation of equilibrium both at rest and during complex body movements. Since most of the pathways discussed have a pattern of inhibitory connections as complex as the excitatory ones, brainstem centers subserving the vestibular system are capable of making very fine discriminations and executing highly precise adjustments of movement and balance.

Cortical Projections

The vestibular system (via the thalamus) projects onto the superior temporal gyrus near the auditory cortex. Stimulation of this cortical area can produce a sense of movement often described as "spinning". Input from proprioceptive and visual centers is integrated to produce the final conscious "sensation". Occasionally, epileptiform discharges or neoplasms produce "vertigo" by direct stimulation of these areas of cerebral cortex.

PATHOPHYSIOLOGY: SPECIFIC DISEASE PROCESSES

While the pathophysiologic mechanisms of posttraumatic vertigo are frequently obscure, several specific injuries with reasonably well described mechanisms are recognized.

Temporal Bone Fracture

Because the largest portion of the skull base is made up of the temporal bone, most basilar skull fractures involve some portion of the temporal bone. Such fractures are loosely categorized into two types — longitudinal and transverse. Longitudinal fractures are more common and, fortunately, are accompanied by low incidence of fracture into the labyrinthine capsule and facial nerve paralysis. Transverse temporal bone fractures are less common (5 to 10% of temporal bone fractures) but are much more likely to fracture into the labyrinthine capsule despite the fact that the labyrinthine bone is the hardest bone found anywhere within the

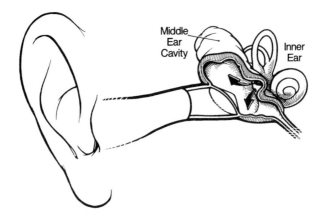

FIGURE 6.7 Diagrammatic representation of a perilymphatic fistula. Perilymph can escape from either the oval window (upper arrow) or round window (lower arrow). Since the amount of fluid is extraordinarily small, the patient has no subjective sense of fluid within his middle ear space.

human body.[13] When fracture lines extend into the labyrinthine capsule, complete ipsilateral hearing loss and total ablation of ipsilateral vestibular function is the rule. If normal vestibular function is retained in the contralateral ear, then, following several days of overwhelming rotational vertigo with nausea and vomiting, normal functioning will likely return. The rate of improvement depends on the presence or absence of associated injuries and on the age of the injured subject. Younger patients recover at a much faster rate than older patients. An individual in his twenties may be expected to be able to ambulate unassisted in three to four days. He may be able to resume fairly demanding activities like bicycle riding and ladder climbing in three to four weeks. (Ultimately, clinical recovery in this age group is usually complete, although subtle testing will continue to uncover abnormalities of the vestibular system.) The pattern of recovery will be quite different in more elderly persons. It will be slower. A person who is in his sixties or seventies may not be able to ambulate unassisted for several weeks and may be able to perform demanding tasks only after several months. Recovery of fine balance skills may never be complete in the older person. Although vestibular rehabilitation therapy will hasten recovery in the younger individual, many younger patients will do well without a formal rehabilitation program. The outcome in persons over age 40, even if the vestibular loss is an isolated disability, may depend critically on the early implementation of a comprehensive, individualized rehabilitation program. This may also be so in younger patients if the vestibular injury is accompanied by other motor, sensory, or neurologic deficits.

Perilymphatic Fistulas

Head injury may produce rupture of the membranes which seal the inner ear and prevent escape of perilymphatic fluid into the middle ear space (Figure 6.7). When perilymph is removed from the labyrinth, inner ear function is degraded. A combination of otologic symptoms may result, and symptoms may fluctuate in complex ways that are difficult for the patient to explain. In obvious cases, trauma is accompanied (or followed within a few minutes) by rapid, severe hearing loss, loud roaring tinnitus, and severe rotational vertigo. Vertigo is often incapacitating and accompanied by visceral autonomic symptoms (sweating, pallor, nausea, vomiting). Even cursory examination will demonstrate marked instability and nystagmus. Audiometric evaluation reveals sensorineural hearing loss. Platform posturography will confirm disequilibrium with a vestibular pattern, and the platform fistula test will be positive. Vertigo and, to a lesser degree, tinnitus and hearing loss are sometimes exacerbated by straining or Valsalva's maneuver. Repair of the fistula by grafting the round and oval windows often produces immediate and complete elimination of vertigo. Infrequently, hearing will be improved as well.

Unfortunately, many perilymphatic fistulas do not manifest themselves in this straightforward manner.[7,14] Onset of symptoms may be delayed for several days, or the acute phase may be masked by more serious injuries in other areas. Rotational vertigo may be entirely absent and disequilibrium may be mild, vague, and episodic. Hearing loss, tinnitus, and aural fullness may come and go unpredictably. Such protean and elusive symptomatology has led to controversy. Opinions differ widely among credible otologists about how frequently perilymphatic fistulas occur, what types of injuries and forces produce them, and what sort of ancillary symptoms (headache, concentration defects, phobias, and impaired mentation) accompany them. Although one might hope that middle ear exploration could resolve this controversy by establishing the actual frequency with which perilymphatic fistulas occur, it has not. The average human inner ear contains only 0.07 cc (70 µl) of perilymph and, therefore, even relatively rapid leaks will, in absolute terms, be quite small. Even with magnification, leaks involving only five to ten percent (5 to 10%) of the perilymph will be difficult to see in an operative field where local anesthetics have been injected, irrigating fluids have been used, and where there is even minimal bleeding.

Because no reliable method of proving the absence or presence of perilymphatic fistula is yet available, reliable incidence and prevalence figures do not exist. At the present time, considerable effort at the national level is being expended to clarify the perilymphatic fistula controversy but, at this time, it remains unresolved.

Posttraumatic Ménière's Syndrome

In 1861, Prosper Ménière[15] described a syndrome of episodic rotational vertigo accompanied by tinnitus and fluctuating neurosensory hearing loss. A sense of aural fullness or pressure is now also considered an important part of this syndrome. Attacks generally last 15 to 100 minutes and are followed by several hours of asthenia, nausea, and disequilibrium. When no cause (i.e., syphilis, acoustic tumor, or viral labyrinthitis) can be established, the syndrome is idiopathic and may be termed *Ménière's disease.* Histopathologic evidence demonstrates that this syndrome arises as a consequence of excess amounts of endolymph which produce distension of the endolymphatic space. Both Ménière's syndrome and perilymph fistula share a common factor — the ratio of endolymph to perilymph is altered in the same direction (relative excess of endolymph compared to perilymph), although, in Ménière's, it results from excess endolymph whereas, in perilymph fistula, it results from loss of perilymph. While in their typical or classical presentations, these conditions are clinically separable, in their atypical manifestations, they are indistinguishable. Ménière's disease may, like perilymph fistula, manifest as a highly variable and changing combination of aural fullness, disequilibrium, hearing loss, and tinnitus. No physical finding, laboratory test, radiographic or audiometric study can definitively separate these two conditions. Although uncommon, the development of Ménière's syndrome after traumatic brain injury (posttraumatic Ménière's syndrome) is well established and not rare.[16] It usually appears weeks or months (perhaps even years) after the original injury. Diagnosis depends on history, documentation of fluctuating neurosensory hearing loss, positive electrocochleography, and/or positive dehydration audiometry and electrocochleography.

Treatment for Ménière's syndrome, whether idiopathic or posttraumatic, should begin with attempted medical management. Surgical intervention should be limited to patients who fail aggressive medical therapy. Rigorous adherence to a salt-restricted diet (2000 mg daily) and diuretic therapy are the mainstays of medical treatment. A vestibular suppressant should be added during symptomatic periods. If aggressive medical management is inadequate or poorly tolerated, then consideration should be given to one of the many surgical options available.

Cupulolithiasis

Traumatic injury may dislodge otoconia from the macula of the saccule or utricle. A loose otolith may "roll around" within the membranous labyrinth and produce vertiginous symptoms associated with positional changes and/or head movement. Classically, rolling from side to side while in the supine position (i.e., in bed), propels the displaced otolith into the posterior semicircular canal and produces a specific positional vertigo termed *benign paroxysmal positional vertigo* (BPPV).[14] BPPV constitutes a specific pathophysiologic entity with characteristic ENG findings and should not be confused with benign positional vertigo from other causes. BPPV can be diagnosed during physical examination if the Dix-Hallpike maneuver is performed. For Dix-Hallpike testing, the patient starts in the sitting position. He is then rapidly moved into a supine position with head turned to the side.[12] When this maneuver is performed to the affected side, vertigo and nystagmus will be induced after a latency of a few seconds and will continue for 15 to 40 seconds, after which it will disappear. The nystagmus is away from the undermost ear. If the patient is returned rapidly to the sitting position, the nystagmus may reappear (again, with a brief latency), beating, this time, in the opposite direction. The response fatigues quickly and repeated Dix-Hallpike maneuvers will eliminate the phenomenon within a few repetitions at most. ENG evaluation is always helpful and frequently essential in clarifying and documenting these classic characteristics.

Fortunately, otoconia generally reabsorb within a few weeks to a few months after release from the otolithic membrane. Only rarely do symptoms persist beyond eight to twelve months. When they do, surgical section of the posterior ampullary nerve or complete vestibular nerve section is curative. Vestibular rehabilitation may promote accommodation and hasten resolution of symptoms.

Labyrinthine Concussion

Labyrinthine concussion is an imprecise term which subsumes a variety of symptoms, complaints, and, possibly, etiologies. Generally, it is assumed that the injury arises from bleeding within the labyrinthine capsule, but mechanical membrane disruption caused by acceleration and deceleration effects may also occur.[13,14] Diagnosis depends on detecting objective vestibular abnormalities in the vestibular laboratory. ENG testing is most frequently helpful, and pathologic positional nystagmus is the most common abnormality. Unilateral weakness on ENG testing occurs less commonly, but is compelling when identified. Platform posturography showing reduced function with a vestibular pattern is confirmatory. Sinusoidal harmonic acceleration may show asymmetry with or without phase lag depending on the extent of the injury and the degree of compensation.

Symptoms may include vertigo and disequilibrium with or without hearing loss, tinnitus, or aural fullness. Recovery depends upon the extent of the injury and the presence or absence of associated abnormalities. Often, recovery is complete within a few weeks. When recovery is slow, vestibular rehabilitation can hasten its arrival and often improve the final outcome. If unilateral weakness can be demonstrated on ENG, consideration should be given to surgical ablation of the injured labyrinthine end-organ.

Posttraumatic Vascular Loop

From time to time, head injury may displace one of the posterior fossa intracranial vessels and cause it to come to rest against the eighth cranial nerve in the cerebello-pontine angle. Generally, the anterior inferior cerebellar artery or one of its branches is involved. Vascular compression of the cochleovestibular nerve produces a characteristic syndrome. The afflicted individual is overwhelmed by an almost constant, severe positional vertigo often associated with visceral symptoms. While actual severity may vary over a fairly wide range, the patient is frequently not able to function. Motion usually results in marked exacerbation of symptoms.

Unilateral tinnitus and hearing loss may accompany the vestibular symptoms but are frequently absent. Diagnosis depends on the presence of typical abnormalities seen during auditory brainstem response audiometry (ABR). Specifically, changes in interpeak latency suggestive of cochlear-vestibular nerve pathology will be noted. Radiographic demonstration of the juxtaposition of the nerve to the vessel is helpful but not essential. When present, surgical decompression is curative.

Cervical Vertigo

Since cervical position sense receptors and muscle stretch receptors provide information to the central nervous system about the orientation of the head in space, musculoskeletal abnormalities of the neck and cervical spine may result in "dizzy" sensations.[17-20] Most commonly, myofascial pain dysfunction syndromes involving either the lateral or posterior cervical muscles are responsible. Since cervical proprioception is not the most important sensory modality subserving equilibrium, disorders of the cervical musculoskeletal system usually produce symptomatology that is relatively mild. Patients typically complain of a vague disquiet and uneasiness about their balance. They resist free movement and frequently use support structures (walls, handrails, etc.). "Spinning" is not experienced and falls do not, in fact, occur, although the patient is ever fearful that he *will* fall. Frequent headaches occur commonly. Physical examination will generally detect muscle spasms and tenderness. Tenderness is frequently focal and of the "trigger point" variety.[21] Common focal points are the spinous process of the seventh cervical vertebrae and along the posterior nuchal line, where the posterior cervical muscles insert into the periosteum of the skull or at the insertion of the sternocleidomastoid and splenius capitis muscles into the mastoid tip. Aggressive physical therapy, exercises, and anti-inflammatory medications must be combined regularly for several weeks in order to achieve relief.

Central Vertigo

Dizziness and disequilibrium originating within the nervous system and not from the labyrinth or eighth nerve is a relatively common component of posttraumatic head injury. Vertigo which arises within the CNS itself is accompanied more often by other cranial neuropathies and neurologic deficits than is peripheral vertigo. Dysarthria, dysphagia, ocular motor deficits, numbness and tingling in the extremities, and focal motor weakness are common.[13,17,22-26] A significant number of these individuals have been severely injured so that they have been in prolonged coma. Many have significant long-tract signs.

Involvement of the cerebellum produces "dizziness" and disequilibrium only in the standing position and when attempting to walk. Subjective rotational vertigo is notably absent. Ambulation, however, may be severely impaired and is no better with eyes open than with eyes closed. Nystagmus will also be as vigorous with eyes open as with eyes closed. Indeed, nystagmus may be so pronounced as to be apparent from several feet away but, when queried, the patient will often deny subjective vertigo.

Frequently, disorders of balance are recognized relatively late in the rehabilitation of these individuals. Early in treatment, other injuries are more apparent and need to be addressed more urgently. As consciousness returns, mentation improves, motor weakness resolves, and efforts can be directed toward beginning ambulation and resuming normal activities. It may be when such retraining is begun and proceeds poorly that balance disturbance is first recognized.

The pathophysiology of central balance disturbance remains unclear. Punctate hemorrhage and degeneration within the vestibular nuclei of head-injured guinea pigs have been demonstrated.[13] Much evidence of central involvement comes from ENG evaluation. Many investigators have shown a high incidence of central ENG findings in the head-injured population. Tuohimaa[6] has argued cogently that ENG findings imply that vestibular dysfunction may be the result of impaired cortical inhibition and not solely the result of disruption of brainstem nuclei or pathways. Subjective vertigo from stimulation or injury to the temporal cortical projections of the vestibular system is uncommon but may occur as a component of a seizure disorder.

There are no medical or surgical methods for managing central vestibular injury. Indeed, the presence of a central component is frequently cited as a cause for the reduced effectiveness of eighth nerve section in head-injury patients even when a clear-cut peripheral component is present. Vestibular rehabilitation will continue to be the mainstay of treatment for patients who have a significant central component, but medical and surgical treatment may be of significant ancillary assistance when there is a concomitant peripheral vestibular injury.

CLINICAL EVALUATION

History

An adequate history is frequently the key to both diagnosis and management of vestibular disorders. This can be a difficult undertaking in the individual recovering from brain injury. However, every effort should be made to elicit as much information as possible, even though this may be taxing to the evaluator.

Patient's History

Questions about premorbid leisure activities can give important information regarding physical impairment, including vestibular injury. Did the patient return to sports and leisure after his injury and, if not, why not? Are there any close relatives or friends who are able to substantiate this information?

Does the patient's direct family report any changes regarding the patient's participation in the family circle? Specifically, are there complaints of balance (i.e., in darkness or with leisure activities)? Has the patient become less physically active at all? Are there any complaints of visual or auditory overstimulation that can be associated with a vestibular lesion?

When balance dysfunction is present, it should first be established whether the patient suffers from a subjective sense of vertigo or disequilibrium. Individuals with central dysfunction and cerebellar disorders, although clearly impaired by balance dysfunction, may have no associated sense of disequilibrium or vertigo. When present, such sensations are frequently referred to as feeling *dizzy*. It is astonishing how frequently this term may remain unclarified and ill-defined even though treatment persists for months. It is critical to clarify, in as much detail as possible, what the individual means by the term *dizzy*. Often the patient will protest that he is unable to further elucidate the experience but, if pressed, this is almost never the case and important information can almost always be obtained with perseverance. *Vertigo* is a technical term which refers to the illusion of movement when no movement is, in fact, present. The most obvious example of such a sensation is the sense of rotation when one is still. However, a sense that one is falling when one is not falling, or the sense that one is "veering" when one is not, also constitutes an illusion of movement when none is present. These sensations are appropriately subsumed under the term *vertigo*. It will turn out that a goodly number of patients do not have an illusion of movement even when they use the term *dizzy*. Such patients may be referring to a sense of lightheadedness, giddiness, a vague feeling of nausea, a sense that they are walking on air, a feeling of being "closed in", weakness, disorientation, or a general sense of "confusion".

After clarifying the character of the dizzy sensation, it is crucial to determine if the sensation is invariably present or present only episodically. If present episodically, how frequently and for how long it persists are important data to be gathered. Whether the symptoms are always of the same severity needs to be ascertained and, if the severity is variable, a search for exacerbating or remitting factors needs to be made. The relationship of the symptoms to movement is crucial. Many patients have their symptoms only in certain head or body positions, or the act of moving into certain positions precipitates symptomatic episodes. The patient should be questioned about whether there is any relation between his symptoms and diet, exercise, or situational stress. One should determine if the symptoms are reliably reproduced in a given place. Individuals suffering from anxiety disorders, for example, will frequently have their symptoms very reliably "place associated". They may experience symptoms in open places or closed places or in church or in the car. When symptoms are closely linked to a specific place or situation, organic vestibular dysfunction is improbable. On the other hand, certain types of visual stimuli will reliably produce symptoms in patients with vestibular disease. Complex geometric patterns and rapid movement in the peripheral visual field are two such common stimuli. A surprising number of patients will complain of disequilibrium when shopping in the grocery store because of the rapid movement of the high, grocery-laden shelves in their peripheral visual field as they move down the aisle.

A search for associated symptoms should be made. The patient must be carefully queried as to the presence or absence of dysarthria, dysphagia, visual change, numbness or tingling in the extremities or around the mouth, and focal motor weakness. He should be questioned about the presence or absence of headache and syncopal episodes.

Physical Examination

A complete neurotologic examination must be performed. It should start with close examination of the external auditory canals and tympanic membranes. Such an examination will not only determine the stigmata of temporal bone fracture or serious head injury but also the more mundane findings of middle ear effusion, cholesteatoma, or tympanic membrane perforation. It must always be remembered that the traumatically brain-injured individual is not immune to the commonplace afflictions of everyday life. The pneumatic otoscope should be utilized in order to assure adequate tympanic membrane mobility. A complete cranial nerve examination is mandatory. Eye movement abnormalities should be noted prominently because they will affect interpretation of the electronystagmogram. Similarly, evaluation of the facial nerve must be compulsive because it travels so closely with the vestibular nerve that it is an invaluable localizing sign. Evaluation of hearing is compelling for the same reasons and should include Rinne and Weber tests as well as a complete audiometric battery. Abnormalities of the lower cranial nerves, including swallowing dysfunction and disorders of voice, may indicate significant brainstem injury.

Coordination is evaluated using standard tests of cerebellar function, such as the fingertip-to-nose test, the tests for dysdiadochokinesia and rebound phenomenon which are performed for the upper extremities, and the heel-shin maneuver for the lower extremities.

Cerebellar ataxia in gait comprises a widened base of support, an irregular step length, and weaving from side to side. Vestibular dysfunction can also result in an ataxic gait quite similar to the one described above but does not result in positive cerebellar tests.

Gait and station should be evaluated using the Romberg test and tandem gait as well as heel-and-toe walking. A severely disabled individual might not be able to perform some of these tests and these tests will have to be omitted in such cases.

Clinical Testing

Clinical evaluation of head-injury patients suspected of vestibular dysfunction will have to go beyond the administration of a few clinical tests as, in addition to the suspected vestibular dysfunction, other symptoms of CNS injury might compromise overall physical functioning. Also, clinical vestibular tests are not pathognomonic for specific lesions, but indicators. Additionally, the vestibular patient will not always be able to clearly discuss or communicate the changes that are a result of the vestibular injury.

TABLE 6.1 Mat Rolling — An Effective General Technique for Desensitization

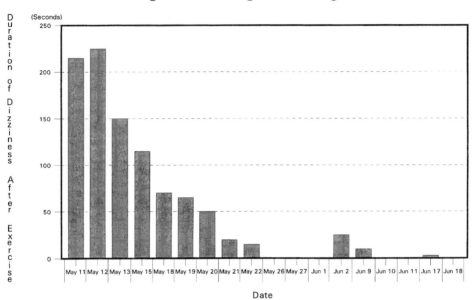

Rolling Left and Right x5 Lengths on Mat

Note: The patient is asked to roll back and forth along a mat. The duration of dizziness after exercise is then measured. This patient's graph shows progressive improvement over a period of two weeks.

The evaluation of a brain-injured individual comprises, next to taking the patient's history, a number of standard tests of range of motion, muscle strength, and cardiorespiratory conditioning. In addition, we evaluate coordination, weight bearing, weight shift with rolling, quadruped crawling and crawling on the knees, balance in standing, balance during ambulation, and more complex balance activities, reflexes, and sensation.

Preambulatory Activities

Rolling on a ten-foot-long, floor-placed exercise mat for a number of repetitions (usually five times left and right) regularly provokes dizziness to the extent that clients spontaneously stop the activity with complaints of dizziness and/or nausea (Table 6.1).

This response can be seen as vestibular sensitivity toward angular repetitious movement without lower extremity weight bearing. Such sensitivity can be a result of general deconditioning or be the first clinical sign of vestibular pathology.

Balance

A total of 14 balance tests are used to evaluate the spectrum from simple static balance to complex dynamic balance (Table 6.2-A and B). Balance can be affected by a vestibular deficit but also by generalized weakness, dyscoordination, spasticity, rigidity, decreased vision, or lack of sensation.

A vestibular deficit can be expected when any of the following indicators of vestibular involvement are present:

TABLE 6.2-A Clinical Balance Testing — Test and Score Sheet

Static and Dynamic Balance
Test List

Static balance	Attempts	Score
1. Romberg, eyes open	1 2 3 4 5	secs
2. Romberg, eyes closed	1 2 3 4 5	secs
3. One foot balance left, eyes open	1 2 3 4 5	secs
4. One foot balance right, eyes open	1 2 3 4 5	secs
5. Sharpened Romberg, eyes open, left foot posterior	1 2 3 4 5	secs
6. Sharpened Romberg, eyes open, right foot posterior	1 2 3 4 5	secs
Dynamic balance		
7. Heel toe ambulation, 50 feet, eyes open, straight line	(errors)	feet
8. Balance beam forward, 50 feet, eyes open	(errors)	feet
9. Balance beam backward, 50 feet eyes open	(errors)	feet
10. Hop both feet, times 10, maintain one rhythm	1 2 3 4 5	reps
11. Hop left foot only, times 10, maintain one rhythm	1 2 3 4 5	reps
12. Hop right foot only, times 10, maintain one rhythm	1 2 3 4 5	reps
13. Jump rope, times 10, maintain one rhythm, jump both feet	1 2 3 4 5	reps
14. Jump alternately on 10 inch elevation, maintain one rhythm, times 20	1 2 3 4 5	secs

NOTES: _____

_____

_____

1. Difficulty with any balance task that either limits or excludes vision. Example of the first is walking backwards on a balance beam; example of the latter, the classic Romberg test with eyes closed. Vestibular patients rely heavily on visual input to compensate for the loss of (reliable) vestibular information. When this is denied in a testing situation, they score poorly.

2. Difficulty with postural adjustment with static balance tests such as one foot balance or the sharpened Romberg test. The tests require a period of 30 seconds for a normal score. Normal subjects can adjust smoothly to balance disturbance. Vestibular patients can perceive gravitational effects sometimes but not accurately and therefore overcorrect, ultimately leading to a loss of balance or excessive weaving.

3. Difficulty with complex, repetitious dynamic balance tasks. An example is hopping ten times on both feet. Vestibular patients have difficulty with this test because of poor gaze stabilization, or because they are unable to make the quick postural adjustment necessary to maintain balance.

Clinical Vestibular Testing

Clinical vestibular testing can be divided into two categories — functional testing and provocation of specific deficits. Provocation of specific deficits can be done if the patient's history indicates a specific lesion. A good example is the Dix-Hallpike maneuver done when a patient's complaints are suspect for benign paroxysmal positional vertigo. Routinely, we

TABLE 6.2-B Clinical Balance Testing — Explanation of Test Procedure

How the balance test is performed

Static balance

Tests 1–6: Client is tested barefoot on a wooden, circular (25″ diameter) surface and needs to stay in one place. Five attempts are given; only the best effort is entered. A normal score is 30 seconds.

Tests 1–2: A comfortable base of support, chosen by client, on the support surface.

Dynamic balance

Tests 7–9: Client is instructed to perform each of the tasks at leisurely pace, barefoot.

Test 7: Mistakes are counted and entered. A mistake is stepping out of the straight line or not placing the feet heel to toe.

Tests 8–9: Client is instructed to walk forward (8)/backward (9) on a 4″ wide beam. Heel to toe placement is not necessary. A mistake is when client steps off the beam. Total number of mistakes is entered. We use a 10′ long, 4″ wide beam. He/she travels the beam ×5 forward/backward.

Tests 10–14: These are the most complex of this test. Tests 10-13 are performed on the floor. Client is allowed to hop "around", as long as a sequence of 10 repetitions is maintained. Five attempts are given with the best result being entered.

Test 14: One foot is placed on the floor, the other on a 10″ high support surface (e.g., first step of exercise stairs of physical therapy department). Client is instructed to alternate this foot placement while jumping straight up, again for a sequence of 10 smooth repetitions.

These tests move from simple to complex balance tasks. The more complex balance tasks are sometimes too strenuous for deconditioned clients. The therapist needs to be attentive to this and can stop the test when necessary. An explanation can be entered at the bottom of the score card in the "Notes" section. Testing is repeated one month following therapy. Therapy excludes any of the tests used for evaluation to avoid "teaching the test".

Testing is performed in a quiet corner of the gym. Movement in the client's visual field should be excluded, as it might interfere with performance.

---

perform two functional vestibular tests, discussed below. If either is positive, a vestibular lesion should be suspected.[27,28]

Unterberger test — The patient is asked to take 50 steps in place with the eyes closed. A positive test is turning to either side more than 45 degrees. The patient will turn to the side of the lesion.[29]

Babinski-Weil test — The patient is asked to walk five steps forward and backward five times with the eyes closed, maintaining an imaginary straight line. A positive outcome is seen when the patient constantly drifts to the affected side walking forward and away from that side walking backward.

Functional vestibular testing is done while the patient listens to music through headphones to prevent spatial orientation through environmental sounds.

None of our tests are pathognomonic for a type of vestibular lesion or localization of a lesion, but the entire evaluation can give strong indicators necessitating further laboratory evaluation. We frequently request a vestibular evaluation performed by a neurotologist or otolaryngologist specializing in vestibular dysfunction.

Laboratory Evaluation

Auditory Testing

Because the vestibular system and auditory system are so closely interrelated (at the level of the labyrinth, the eighth cranial nerve, and within the brainstem), complete audiometric testing is essential in the evaluation of any patient with balance disturbance. This should include a formal audiogram which tests pure tone reception at octave intervals from 125 Hz (cycles per second) to 8000 Hz. Both air conduction and bone conduction should be tested. Speech discrimination scores should be obtained and the speech reception threshold measured. If inconsistent or ambiguous information is developed within the pure tone audiogram or speech testing, this information should be confirmed or expanded using auditory brainstem response audiometry (ABR).[30] The initial pure tone evaluation should be accompanied by immittance testing, which measures not only tympanic membrane compliance, but also assists in identification of ossicular disarticulation and assesses the stapedius reflex at several frequencies. Stapedius reflex testing is sensitive to a variety of different sorts of retrocochlear pathology. Abnormalities of stapedius reflex testing, if not explained by known difficulties, should be considered indications for further evaluation with auditory brainstem response audiometry or radiographic imaging. Based on the history and the pure tone audiogram, further evaluation with electrocochleography, vestibular testing, middle latency response evaluation, or central auditory testing can be considered.[24,31,32] The results of auditory testing should be consistent with the results of tuning fork tests as determined in the physical examination. If there are inconsistencies between these test results, these inconsistencies need to be resolved.

The Electronystagmogram

Nystagmus is the only sign on physical examination uniquely linked to the vestibular system. Therefore, the electronystagmogram plays a crucial and pivotal role in evaluating the vestibular system. The electronystagmogram offers a number of advantages. First and foremost, it is capable of detecting nystagmus with eyes closed. The vast majority of peripheral nystagmus is effectively suppressed by visual fixation and will not be apparent to the examiner with the patient's eyes open. Frenzel lenses are thick, 20-diopter lenses used to assist in the detection of nystagmus on physical examination. These lenses make the detection of pathologically significant nystagmus easier in two ways. First, they prevent visual fixation by the patient since they make it virtually impossible to see anything but light. Second, they magnify the cornea and iris when the examiner views the patient's globe through the Frenzel glasses. Frenzel lenses will permit the detection of clinically significant nystagmus which would be otherwise inapparent. But even with Frenzel lenses, about half of pathologically significant nystagmus will be missed.[33,34]

The electronystagmogram is capable of detecting subtle abnormalities of both volitional and reflex eye movement controlled at the brainstem and even higher levels. These abnormalities cannot be detected by any other method. Their detection can be the most significant and easily documented evidence for brainstem dysfunction.

An additional advantage to electronystagmography is the ability of this testing method to test each labyrinthine end-organ separately. No other clinical test of vestibular function permits unequivocal isolation of one labyrinth from its contralateral partner.

The electronystagmography produces a permanent objective record of labyrinthine function. Such a record can be reviewed months or years after it was made and compared with new tracings to determine the evolution of a pathological process or to document improvement.

There are some disadvantages to ENG. The stimulus is not physiologic and stimulus intensity is subject to a variety of variables only partially under the examiner's control. These include the shape and nature of the external auditory canal, the size of the tympanic cavity, and the thickness and position of the tympanic membrane. The test requires a compulsive and meticulous examiner who is willing to recalibrate his equipment before every examination, remove any cerumen impeding the flow of air or water into the canal, and assure good contact between the electrodes and the skin. A first-rate ENG technician will also interact with the patient in a tactful, compassionate, and sympathetic fashion. Not only is this an intrinsically desirable end in itself but it will also encourage maximum effort from the patient and procure the most consistent and reliable tracings.

Electronystagmography requires relatively intact extraocular muscle function. Thus, individuals with certain intrinsic abnormalities of the extraocular muscles or paresis of cranial nerves III, IV, or VI may generate tracings that are uninterpretable.

Electronystagmography is, perhaps, more properly termed *electro-oculography* (EOG). Although generally used to measure and detect nystagmus in the evaluation of individuals with vertigo, the test actually measures the movement of the globe within the orbit. The positively charged cornea and the negatively charged retina together create a dipole whose movement can be detected when electrodes are placed around the orbits. The testing apparatus is calibrated so that eye deviations to the right produce an upward deflection and eye deviations to the left produce a downward deviation of the pen. In the vertical channel, upward eye movements create an upward deviation of the pen, and downward movements, a downward deviation of the pen. The system is calibrated so that each degree of eye movement produces a one-millimeter deflection of the pen. The system needs to be recalibrated before each test.

The complete electronystagmogram consists of a set of seven different subtests:

1. Saccade test
2. Gaze test
3. Tracking test
4. Optokinetic test
5. Positional test
6. Dix-Hallpike maneuver
7. Bithermal caloric test

The saccade test is usually done first because the system can be calibrated at the same time the test is performed. With lights on, the patient is instructed to look back and forth between two spots located on the wall directly in front of him without moving his head. An arbitrary distance of about six feet is selected so that the patient's eyes move about 20 degrees in the horizontal and vertical plane as he looks back and forth, as directed, between spots. The spots on the wall are then selected to produce a 20-millimeter pen deflection. The speed and accuracy with which these movements are produced is inspected and measured. Normal individuals can perform this test with great rapidity and with very high degrees of accuracy. Brainstem dysfunction produces well-recognized abnormalities, including systematic "overshoot" and "undershoot". These abnormalities may occur in one or both directions of gaze.

Gaze testing is performed by having the patient look straight ahead and then 30 degrees to the right, left, up, and down. Gaze in these positions is maintained for at least 20 seconds with eyes open, then an additional 20 seconds with eyes closed. Any nystagmus present during these sustained eye deviations is recorded. Gaze nystagmus can arise from both central and peripheral vestibular pathology as well as a consequence of normal variations such as endpoint nystagmus or congenital nystagmus (Figure 6.8). Frequently, one can distinguish between various etiologies by carefully examining the eye position in which the nystagmus occurs and the morphology of typical nystagmoid beats. Nystagmus which occurs with eyes open and disappears with eyes closed is reliably attributed to central nervous system pathology.

Sinusoidal tracking or pursuit testing is also performed in a lighted room. The patient is asked simply to visually track an object moving back and forth in front of his visual field. This may be a ball suspended on a string from the ceiling or a sophisticated computer-driven light bar. Normal individuals can track such sinusoidal motions with amazing accuracy. A variety of possible abnormalities can be detected (Figure 6.9). Certain of these are characteristic of central nervous system (particularly brainstem) pathology and others may simply represent the superimposition of peripherally induced nystagmus on the tracing.

Optokinetic testing is performed by moving a series of alternating black and white stripes in front of the patient's visual field. This reliably induces nystagmus in normal individuals. Typically, the stripes are moved first to the right and then to the left in front of the patient's visual fields at 20 and then 40 degrees per second. Comparisons are made between the resulting tracings. Several possible abnormalities can occur. Optokinetic nystagmus can be effectively and

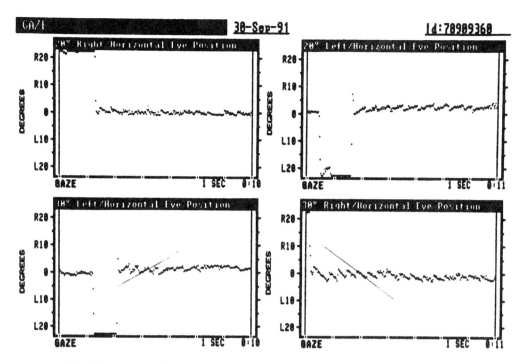

FIGURE 6.8 Gaze nystagmus is present in all gaze positions. It is most obvious in the 30-degree left and right deviations (lower tracings) than in the upper 20-degree eye deviation tracings.

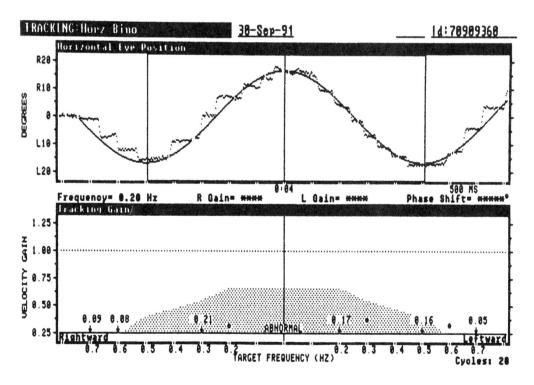

FIGURE 6.9 Horizontal tracking is illustrated in this computerized electronystagmographic tracing. Most subjects can follow a sinusoidal pattern very accurately. This patient follows it in a steplike, "saccadic" fashion which is usually pathognomonic for central nervous system pathology.

normally induced in one direction but not in the other. Occasionally, the system breaks down under stress, and individuals whose optokinetic nystagmus is normal at lower speeds produce abnormal optokinetic nystagmus when the speed is increased. Virtually all abnormalities of optokinetic testing arise from central pathology, most commonly within the brainstem.

Positional testing is important not only to document pathological eye movements in patients whose chief complaint is positional nystagmus, but also because abnormal test results occur in individuals who complain of nonpositionally related disequilibrium and vertigo. The test is performed by examining electronystagmographic tracings produced in four positions — with the patient sitting up looking straight ahead, with the patient lying supine looking straight ahead, with the right ear down, and with the left ear down. Not only does the tracing need to be examined for the presence of nystagmus produced in one position or another but, in patients with preexisting spontaneous nystagmus, a record needs to be carefully examined to see if positional changes produce any alteration in the underlying nystagmus pattern. A large variety of different patterns of positional nystagmus have been detected. These include direction-fixed and direction-changing varieties. Among direction-changing varieties are those which beat consistently away from the ground (ageotropic) and those which beat consistently toward the ground (geotropic). Although direction-fixed nystagmus is more characteristic of peripheral disorders and direction-changing more characteristic of central disorders, so many exceptions to these rules have been identified that it is not possible to make definitive statements about the etiologic significance of particular positional patterns.[35-37] An exception is the individual in whom the direction of the nystagmus changes while in a single head position. Such a pattern is invariably associated with central nervous system pathology.

An objective record of fistula testing can be made using the electronystagmogram and the impedance bridge. In order to accomplish this, the immittance probe is placed into first one ear and then the other. The pressure in the external auditory canal is varied between +200 and –200 millimeters of mercury. The electronystagmogram is then examined for induced nystagmus. Each ear is tested separately. A positive test result is identified by the production of nystagmus associated with a change in pressure on the tympanic membrane. In some cases, the nystagmus can seem to change direction as the pressure changes from positive to negative. One would expect that the patient's subjective symptoms of vertigo, with or without nausea, would be induced during the presence of nystagmoid eye movements in positive tests. The results of the ENG fistula test can then be compared (when available) to platform fistula test results.[11,24,38]

Dix-Hallpike testing is a test of position*ing* nystagmus. In this test, the patient is rapidly moved from a sitting position to the supine position with first the right ear and then the left ear down. The test is specifically designed to identify benign paroxysmal positional nystagmus. The test is positive when, after latency of 10 to 15 seconds, bursts of horizonto-rotary nystagmus lasting 20 to 30 seconds are observed. The response fatigues rapidly so that, when the maneuver is repeated, the response will be much less vigorous. Usually, several repetitions in rapid succession are sufficient to eliminate any detectable response whatsoever. Positive Dix-Hallpike testing is classically associated with cupulolithiasis. Cupulolithiasis is a common consequence of blunt head injury. Since the response fatigues rapidly, Dix-Hallpike testing should precede other forms of positional testing. If it follows conventional positional testing, the expected response may actually have been inadvertently "fatigued out" by the previous positioning maneuvers.

Bithermal caloric examination permits quantification of the "strength" of the response obtained from each labyrinth separately. Although the strength of the bithermal caloric response is generally assumed to represent the activity of the individual labyrinth as a whole, it is important to remember that, in actuality, only the horizontal semicircular canal is stimulated. Careful evaluation of patients and comparison of electronystagmographic and sinusoidal harmonic acceleration (SHA) responses clearly demonstrate that it is possible to have residual function in the superior and posterior semicircular canals even when no response can be generated using bithermal caloric testing in the horizontal canal.

The test depends on the production of convection currents within the horizontal semicircular canal. Warmed and cooled air or water is systematically irrigated through the external auditory canal. This produces a raising or lowering of the temperature of the tympanic membrane and produces a temperature change within the middle ear space. As air is cooled or heated in the middle ear space, that portion of the horizontal semicircular canal which protrudes effectively into the middle ear space is also cooled or warmed. Since the nonexposed portions of this canal do not suffer the same temperature change, convection currents are produced within the endolymphatic space of the horizontal semicircular canal. This fluid movement will produce cupular deflection, discharges within the vestibular nerve, and nystagmus which can be measured. Thermal stimuli reliably produce nystagmus in a specific direction. Cold water will produce nystagmus with its fast component away from the irrigated ear. Warm stimuli, on the other hand, will produce nystagmus with the fast component toward the stimulated ear. A useful mnemonic for these relationships is COWS (Cold Opposite Warm Same). The simplest clinical application of this principle is seen in the utilization of ice water caloric examination which can be performed at the bedside or in the emergency department. Ice water calorics are performed by putting 10 to 20 cc of ice water into the external auditory canal. This will produce an extremely vigorous response in normal individuals with easily detected gross nystagmus away from the irrigated ear. Unfortunately, nausea and vomiting often accompany such intense stimulation. The vigorous response produced by ice water caloric examination is poorly accepted by patients and, therefore, current testing protocols use stimuli which produce a less violent response. When water is used, the temperature is usually adjusted to 30°C for the cool irrigation and 44°C for the warm irrigation. If air is chosen as the stimulating medium, then temperatures of 24°C and 50°C are generally utilized. Understanding the mechanics of the test makes it obvious that certain types of ear pathology invalidate or change test results. An individual with a unilateral tympanic perforation can be expected to have a much more vigorous response on the perforated side than on the intact side because the irrigant will pass through the perforation and stimulate the horizontal semicircular canal directly. Individuals with stenoses, mass lesions, or other types of obstruction of the external auditory canal can be expected to produce little or no response on the affected side. This, however, does not mean that the examination should not be performed. It means that the interpreter must be aware of the condition and make his interpretation in light of the existing pathologic process. Should, for example, an individual have no response in an ear with a perforated tympanic membrane, the perforation does not invalidate the pathological finding. Indeed, the presence of the perforation makes one even more secure that this labyrinth lacks appropriate physiologic function.

Normal individuals produce a fairly typical nystagmus response to caloric irrigation. There is generally a latency of 20 to 30 seconds followed by the onset of nystagmus which rapidly peaks in intensity at 60 to 90 seconds. The response then gradually diminishes over the next three to four minutes. In order to compare one labyrinth to the other, it is crucial that comparisons of nystagmoid response be made between peak responses for each irrigation. This is done by examining the tracing and picking out the strongest beats on each irrigation. Three or four of these beats should be measured and then averaged in order to obtain a typical "peak" response. The magnitude of the response is quantified in terms of *eye speed* in degrees per second. One should note that this is a different measurement than the assessment of *total amplitude* of the response. Very large deviations can be obtained at slow speeds. A variety of calculations can then be made to assess labyrinthine integrity. The most useful measurement is that which detects unilateral weakness (UW). This measurement compares the total response from the right ear to the total response from the left ear using the formula below when all of the responses are measured in degrees per second:

$$\frac{(RW + RC) - (LC + LW)}{(RW + RC + LC + LW)} \times 100 = \text{Percent Unilateral Weakness (UW)}$$

Using this formula, negative values indicate weakness on the right and positive values indicate weakness on the left. Convention dictates that the weakness is expressed according to the weaker side in absolute magnitude (i.e., one would say that there is a left unilateral weakness of 28%).

Most practitioners utilize a twenty percent (20%) difference between ears as the threshold for abnormality. Some examiners, however, use a more stringent twenty-five percent (25%) or thirty percent (30%) difference.

In addition to evaluating the strength of an individual labyrinth, one can also compare the total strength of all beats in one direction to all the beats in another (i.e., one can compare the strengths of right-beating nystagmus to that of left-beating nystagmus). In order to make such a calculation, one uses the following formula:.

$$\frac{(RW + LC) - (RC + LW)}{(RW + LC + RC + LW)} \times 100 = \text{Percent Directional Preponderance (DP)}$$

When there is an apparent preference for the eyes to beat in the right or left direction, this is referred to as a *directional preponderance*. As a general rule, directional preponderances are a reflection of spontaneous nystagmus. Although directional preponderances can occur in the absence of spontaneous nystagmus, one should be suspicious that there has been some technical error in the irrigations whenever directional preponderance occurs in the absence of spontaneous nystagmus.

The significance of directional preponderance when not associated with spontaneous nystagmus remains unclear and, for that reason, some evaluators do not make this calculation.

An important part of the caloric examination is the test for visual fixation suppression. At some point, when the induced nystagmoid response is still brisk, the patient should be asked to open his eyes. Eye opening should produce a marked reduction in the intensity of nystagmus (Figure 6.10). Indeed, the strength of the response should be reduced by at least sixty percent (60%). When this is not the case, central nervous system pathology is implied.

Computed Sinusoidal Harmonic Acceleration

An alternative method of assessing the vestibulo-ocular reflex (VOR) utilizes a motorized chair to produce a back and forth (sinusoidal) movement (Figure 6.11). In response to such movement, the vestibulo-ocular reflex will induce compensatory eye movements in the opposite direction to body movement. These eye movements can be measured and compared to the rotational stimulus. Since the stimulus which initiates the vestibulo-ocular reflex is, in this case, mechanically generated by a chair in which the patient sits, it can be very precisely and accurately controlled. One advantage of sinusoidal harmonic acceleration is that the stimulus can be determined with much greater precision than can the thermal effects utilized to generate a caloric response in conventional electronystagmography. An additional advantage of slow harmonic acceleration is that the stimulus is physiologic. That is, the sort of rotational movement used to generate a response in the vestibulo-ocular reflex arc is qualitatively and quantitatively like many of the stimuli encountered in everyday movement. Generally speaking, most movements performed during ambulation are a bit quicker but, certainly, the stimuli used to generate a response utilizing the motorized chair are basically normal. This same characteristic (of providing a physiologic stimulus) which constitutes a principal advantage of SHA is also responsible for one of its principal disadvantages compared to conventional ENG. By necessity, both labyrinths are stimulated simultaneously and it is not possible to collect data from one side alone.

The patient is tested at five separate rotational speeds measured in cycles per second (Hertz). Typical speeds are one hundredth (0.01 Hz), two hundredths (0.02 Hz), four hundredths (0.04 Hz), eight hundredths (0.08 Hz), and sixteen hundredths (0.16 Hz) of a rotation

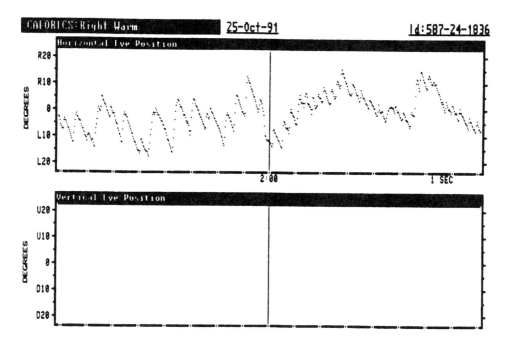

FIGURE 6.10 Electronystagmographic tracing taken from a patient with a central nervous system tumor. The right warm caloric is shown. At the vertical bar in the middle of the tracing, the patient was asked to open his eyes and fixate on a mark on the wall. Visual fixation produced only very slight decrease in the velocity of his nystagmus. Failure of visual fixation is a reliable sign of central nervous system pathology.

per second. Three separate characteristics of the VOR response are determined for each frequency of rotation.[34,39-41]

Phase

It is reasonably appropriate and much easier to understand phase relationships as synonymous with latency. Because the SHA uses a rotational stimulus, it happens that relationships usually characterized as latency can be appropriately described as phase relationships. Suffice it to say that abnormalities of phase (latency) represent changes in how long after the start of the stimulus the compensatory eye movement occurs. It so happens in SHA (as in many other neuro-diagnostic tests) that changes in latency are relatively reliable and sensitive indicators of pathological disturbance of function and most peripheral vestibular disorders (i.e., severe viral labyrinthitis, Ménière's disease, traumatic ablation, etc.) have been associated with abnormalities of phase. It is quite typical, in these cases, for the phase abnormality to be more pronounced at lower frequencies and to return toward normal at the higher frequencies. In fact, if phase abnormalities are the same or worse at higher frequencies, then central dysfunction should be suspected. The data is presented by comparing the patient's response to established norms. As a rule, any response more than two standard deviations from normal is considered pathologic. Once injury has occurred, phase generally remains abnormal indefinitely. Adaptation and compensation do not eliminate phase abnormalities.

Gain

Another parameter of the vestibulo-ocular reflex evaluated at each frequency during SHA is the magnitude of the induced eye movement compared to the magnitude of the rotational stimulus. This comparison is referred to as *gain*. If the eye movements induced by a given rotation (in degrees per second) were exactly the same as the magnitude of the chair rotation

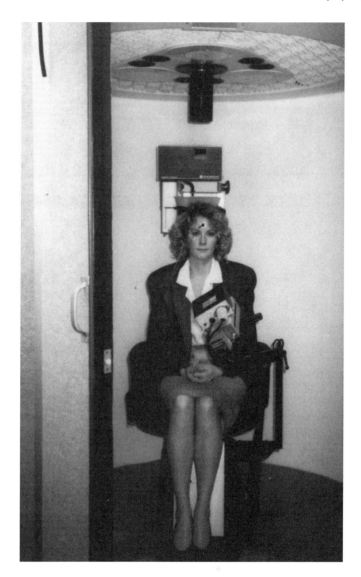

FIGURE 6.11 A rotational chair. The subject is seated in the chair and is seen through the open door. With the door closed, the patient will be in complete darkness. The subject can be monitored from outside the booth by infrared photography. Electrodes are placed in the appropriate positions for monitoring of the induced vestibulo-ocular reflex. (Photograph courtesy of Stacy Riddick.)

(in degrees per second), the gain would be said to be 1.0. If the induced eye movements were twice as large as the initial movement of the chair, the gain would be 2.0 and, if they were half as large, the gain would be 0.5. Not surprisingly, the amount of gain depends on the velocity of rotation. Very slow rotational movements induce relatively small eye movements and typical gains for 0.01 Hz stimuli are 0.5. As the speed of rotation increases, the amount of eye movement similarly increases. It increases faster than the rotational speed so that at 0.16 Hz, normal gains are in the 0.7 range.

Patients with bilateral vestibular weakness have abnormal gains and, generally speaking, the abnormality is more pronounced at the lower frequencies. As the frequency of rotation is increased, the amount of gain tends to return toward normal, even in patients with bilateral vestibular hypofunction. When gain is very low, there is insufficient vestibular input to provide meaningful data and, with very low gains, one should not interpret abnormalities of phase or symmetry. Low gains will occasionally occur in response to acute labyrinthine lesions when the cerebellum deliberately suppresses output from the vestibular nuclei; however, very low gains are more frequently a consequence of chronic bilateral vestibular weakness. Patients with central vertigo will occasionally show increased gain due to the absence of descending inhibition.

Symmetry

Asymmetric responses are a manifestation of directional preponderance or "bias". That is to say, if there is asymmetry to the right, right-beating nystagmus is always greater than left-beating, regardless of the stimulus. The most obvious examples are situations in which there is spontaneous nystagmus to one side. If the patient, at rest, has ten degrees of right-beating nystagmus, then his right-beating responses to rotational stimuli will be enhanced by ten degrees per second but his left-beating responses will be reduced by ten degrees per second. Thus, when examining the response to rotational stimuli, it appears that the individual's eyes "prefer" to beat toward the right. Acute peripheral lesions frequently have significant asymmetries associated with them. If the lesion is peripheral, then one would expect a phase abnormality to be apparent as well. With classic unilateral vestibular injury, marked phase and symmetry abnormalities are present during the first several weeks or months. With the passage of time and the development of compensation, the asymmetry tends to disappear but the phase lag will remain. Some types of central disorders will have variable low-level asymmetries associated with them (Figure 6.12).

Rotatory chair testing has a number of advantages that make it a useful addition to the armamentarium of vestibular testing:

1. The stimulus is precisely controlled and physiologic.
2. The test is quite sensitive and very repeatable. Test variability is minimized.
3. It produces an objective, quantified assessment of vestibular function.
4. In many cases, elimination of asymmetry can document compensation and adaptation.
5. Generally speaking, it is well accepted by patients and produces less subjective discomfort than electronystagmography.

There are some disadvantages associated with SHA:

1. Both labyrinths are stimulated simultaneously.
2. The test is relatively expensive and requires fixed equipment installation.
3. It was initially thought that asymmetry data could not be utilized to identify the side of lesion.

Recently, Mohammed Hamid[42] has documented convincingly that asymmetry is reliably toward the side of the lesion when *phase abnormalities are present*. In the absence of phase abnormalities, asymmetry has no localizing value whatsoever. If additional centers are able to confirm this observation, then the role for SHA testing will be considerably enhanced.

Dynamic Platform Posturography

The development of dynamic platform posturography has been an important addition to the armamentarium in evaluating individuals with disorders of balance (Figure 6.13). The use of dynamic platform posturography directly assesses the individual's ability to maintain his balance in a variety of circumstances. It is thus capable of assessing not only vestibular function but also contributions to balance from the visual and proprioceptive systems. Dynamic platform posturography assesses changes in the subject's center of gravity (COG) in response to a variety of stimuli in different test conditions. Movement of the center of gravity around a fixed point is termed *sway*. Sway can be measured in both the anterior-posterior and

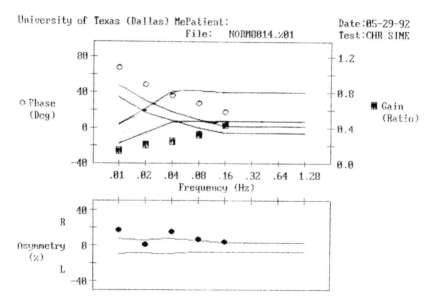

FIGURE 6.12 Summary of diagnostic information obtained from sinusoidal harmonic acceleration. In this patient, there is a significant phase lag. The circles are shown above the lines showing that they are significantly outside the usual standard deviation. In the bottom graph, one can see a mild asymmetry to the right. However, the small squares indicating gain on the upper tracing are below two standard deviations from the norm indicating a bilateral weakness. In the face of such reduced gain, it is not possible to accurately interpret phase or symmetry changes. This is from a patient after head injury with significant reduced bilateral vestibular function. ENG evaluation showed no response to warm or cold water irrigations bilaterally.

in the lateral planes. Excessive sway can occur at rest in a variety of circumstances but occurs most frequently in response to deliberate perturbations.[43-45]

Sensory Organization Testing

The amount of sway produced in response to six different situations is recorded. The different test conditions are designed either to eliminate information normally utilized in maintaining equilibrium or to subvert the system by providing inaccurate information. Movement of the patient's center of gravity is assessed in the following situations:

Sensory Test Condition 1 — The patient stands on the platform with eyes open.

Sensory Test Condition 2 — The patient stands on the platform but his eyes are closed. This test condition eliminates vision as a source of information in maintaining balance.

Sensory Test Condition 3 — The patient stands on the platform with eyes open; however, when the patient sways, the amount of movement he makes is exactly compensated for and mimicked by the movement of the visual surround. He will stay exactly the same distance from the visual surround regardless of what movement his body makes. Thus, vision will provide inaccurate information as to where he is in space relative to his visual surround. In short, in this test condition, the patient's visual system will "lie" to him. This is a more stressful situation than the mere absence of visual information produced in Sensory Test Condition 2. This condition is termed *sway referenced vision* (i.e., the visual surround is "referenced" to the amount of sway the patient has).

Sensory Test Condition 4 — The patient stands on the platform with eyes open. Each swaying motion the patient produces is now exactly compensated for by a similar movement in the platform on which he is standing. This is a condition analogous to Sensory Test Condition 3 except that, in this condition, it is the patient's lower extremity proprioceptive system that is "lying" to him. This is referred to as *sway referenced support*.

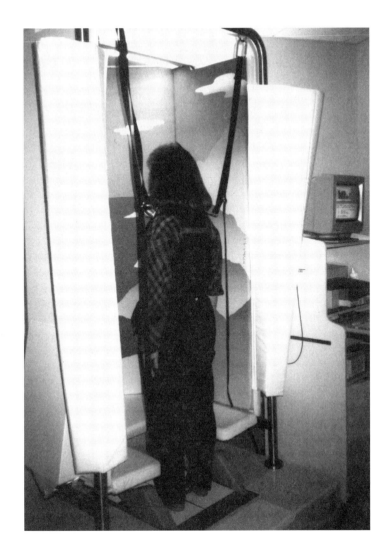

FIGURE 6.13 NeuroCom®* dynamic platform posturography. The patient is standing on a moveable platform within the visual surround. Safety straps prevent injury from falling. Sway is monitored in response to a variety of different sensory test conditions. (*Registered Trademark for NeuroCom International, Inc., Clackamas, Oregon.)

Sensory Test Condition 5 — This condition is exactly the same as Sensory Test Condition 4. There is sway referenced support but the patient is asked to keep his eyes closed. This functionally produces a situation where the patient's lower extremities are lying to him and his visual system is providing no helpful information. Theoretically, his balance is now dependent on vestibular function.

Sensory Test Condition 6 — The patient stands on the platform with eyes open but both vision and support are sway referenced. That is to say, each sway excursion is matched both by compensatory movement in the platform and in the visual surround. Thus, both the patient's visual and proprioceptive systems are "lying" to him. In this condition, balance is determined solely by the intact vestibular system which must overcome false information from the visual and proprioceptive systems.

If the patient does not perform well during the first trial, he is allowed two additional chances in which to improve his performance. "Learning" is frequent and many patients will be able to develop a normal response given two or three tries. However, if the patient's center of gravity shows abnormal excursions (i.e., sway) when compared to statistical norms, he is considered to have "failed" that test condition.

As it turns out, different types of pathology produce different patterns of dysfunction on dynamic platform posturography. Not surprisingly, vestibular disorders are reliably associated with very poor performance in Conditions 5 and 6 when compensatory mechanisms are crippled by the test conditions. Patients who are overly dependent on vision tend to perform very poorly in Conditions 3 and 6. Patients who are visually dependent and also have vestibular abnormalities tend to do poorly on Conditions 3, 5, and 6. If Conditions 4, 5, and 6 are abnormal, it suggests that the patient is quite dependent on somatosensory input to maintain balance. Additional combinations and patterns can be correlated with different sorts of abnormalities. Patients with functional disorders or patients who are malingering frequently produce as bad or worse results on the easier conditions as on the harder ones.

An important contribution of dynamic platform posturography is the ability of this test to determine what sort of "strategy" the patient is utilizing to recover his balance. While standing still, the platform is suddenly "jerked" and the patient's response is assessed. Several forward and several backward perturbations ("jerks") are evaluated. Well-functioning, normal individuals tend to move their center of gravity around their ankles in response to impending disequilibrium. The use of movement about the hips or "hip strategy" is maladaptive and counterproductive. Fortunately, vestibular rehabilitation may be able to redirect the patient's efforts and reorient his strategy from hip to a more effective ankle strategy.

In addition to assessing the sensory modalities utilized to maintain and correct balance, dynamic platform posturography is able to partially characterize the motor response generated after perturbations. The length of time it takes for the muscle response to occur is measured and called *latency*. In actual clinical situations, it turns out that abnormalities of latency are almost always associated with extravestibular CNS pathology. The strength "symmetry" is measured. This simply assesses the amount of strength utilized in each leg to retain balance. In normal persons, equal amounts of strength will be utilized in each leg in the process of balance recovery. Once again, in the absence of obvious peripheral or orthopedic problems (i.e., peripheral muscle atrophy, unilateral hip disease, etc.), abnormalities of symmetry also reflect central nervous system disorders. The size of the response is also measured. If minor induced external perturbations produce very large compensatory excursions, large sway oscillations are induced.

Dynamic platform posturography is useful not only in diagnosis but also in the assessment of risk and in rehabilitation. Not surprisingly, patients who perform poorly on platform posturography are at greater risk for falling than patients who perform normally. Specific pattern abnormalities in sensory organization and movement coordination testing correlate even more closely with risk for falling.

An understanding of what sort of compensatory mechanisms the patient is using in response to balance perturbations can be helpful in guiding vestibular rehabilitation therapy. Patients who are overly dependent on vision can be given tasks to enhance their ability to utilize vestibular and proprioceptive information. Persons utilizing a maladaptive hip strategy, for example, can be redirected to a more appropriate ankle strategy (Figure 6.14).

Platform Fistula Testing

Dynamic platform posturography can be used to generate a sensitive test for perilymphatic fistula. In this test, pressure is applied to the external auditory canal. This increase or decrease (i.e., "negative" pressure) is transmitted to the tympanic membrane, middle ear space, and, if

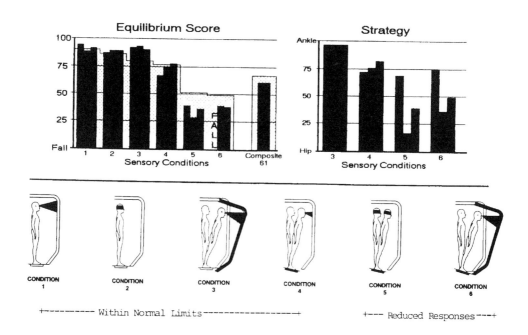

Movement Coordination Test

Symmetry:	Within normal limits
Latency:	Within normal limits
Amplitude Scaling:	Grossly within normal limits
Adaptation:	Patient is able to adapt

INTERPRETATION/RECOMMENDATION:

Reduced responses on conditions 5 and 6 are consistent with a deficiency in the vestibular system.

FIGURE 6.14 Six different sensory organization test conditions are monitored and the patient's performance compared with statistically valid norms. A typical summary form is illustrated here. This patient had an acute unilateral vestibular lesion resulting in a very poor performance in sensory organization test Conditions 5 and 6.

a fistula is present, the inner ear. When perilymphatic fistula is present, abnormal sway will be generated by these pressure changes. Using the acoustics impedance bridge to quantify changes in external auditory canal pressure and the dynamic platform to quantify both anterior posterior and lateral sway in response to such pressure changes, a sensitive assessment for perilymphatic fistula can be developed. Several studies have demonstrated that patients with positive platform pressure testing have a high likelihood of suffering from a perilymphatic fistula.

VESTIBULAR REHABILITATION

The clinical rehabilitation process of the brain-injured individual can be much more complicated than the rehabilitation of an individual suffering from vestibular dysfunction only.

Cognitive impairment with decreased attention span, inability to concentrate, and poor frustration tolerance can discourage the patient as well as the therapist.

In addition, our patients present with a wide spectrum of central neurological impairments, affecting different subsystems of the central nervous system. These impairments demonstrate themselves with symptoms of upper motor neuron lesion (spasticity, weakness), rigidity, and dyscoordination.

Given these complicated circumstances added to the vestibular dysfunction, the task at hand is very difficult at least. It is necessary to develop a treatment philosophy and to explain this philosophy to the patient each time circumstance dictates the need for more comprehension or motivation.

Vestibular rehabilitation depends on two important characteristics of the vestibular system — redundancy and plasticity.[23] Redundancy occurs principally at the receptor level. That is to say, there are several sensory systems which process information about the body's position in space and relay that information to the central nervous system. These include the vestibular system, the visual system, muscle stretch and position sense receptors in the lower extremity, and muscle stretch and position sense receptors in the cervical area. The last two are generally subsumed under the single heading of the somatosensory or proprioceptive system but, in fact, they often function quite independently of each other. The visual and vestibular systems are themselves redundant in the sense that the system has two separate sides. When information from one side is eliminated, the system can function using the intact contralateral side alone. Data received from all of the available sensory receptors is initially processed in the brainstem where decisions are made on a reflex basis. Details of this process remain obscure, but it appears that most of the processing is done in, or close to, the vestibular nuclei with significant input from both the cerebellar nuclei and descending cortical projections. The ability of sensory receptor information to be evaluated, emphasized, de-emphasized, or changed at this level is the principal feature of the vestibular system allowing for progressive modification or "plasticity".[46]

One way plasticity can be achieved is by the systematic "substitution" of sensory input from one receptor cell system for another. For example, individuals with bilateral vestibular weakness come to utilize visual information more intensively for maintenance of balance and equilibrium. *Habituation* is an additional mechanism for compensation although its exact physiologic basis remains unclear. Despite its elusive electroneurophysiologic basis, it is clear that constant exposure to situations which produce unpleasant and counterproductive stimulation will reduce or eliminate the unpleasant response.

An instructive example of neuroplasticity is the central nervous system's response to acute unilateral labyrinthine ablation. In the circumstance of abrupt and devastating injury to one inner ear (i.e., temporal bone fracture), the afflicted individual will immediately experience rapid, violent rotation with massive visceral autonomic outflow producing intense diaphoresis, weakness, nausea, and vomiting. This effect is a consequence of asymmetry at the level of the vestibular nuclei. Vestibular nuclei connected to the intact labyrinth are continuing to receive normal sensory input and continue to respond in an appropriate way. Cells in the vestibular nuclei connected to the affected side now no longer receive stimulation from the ablated labyrinth and are "silent". Initial adaptation to this injury occurs within several hours to a couple of days and consists of marked inhibition of those cells still connected to the intact labyrinth. Control of this process occurs in the cerebellum and is accomplished via afferent cerebello-bulbar fibers. This response has been termed the *cerebellar clamp* because it diminishes activity in normally functioning vestibular cells.[47,48] By reducing function in the normal intact cells, the level of imbalance between the nonfunctioning cells and the intact cells is reduced and the symptoms of disequilibrium, nausea, vomiting, and rotational vertigo are reduced. This response has been documented in acute vestibular lesions using sinusoidal harmonic acceleration where, occasionally, within a day or two after ablative vestibular procedures, a marked decrease in gain can be documented on SHA testing. Over time, those vestibular nuclei originally connected to the now nonfunctioning labyrinth will develop a spontaneous rate of discharge. As spontaneous activity develops in these neurons, inhibition of the "clamped" normal vestibular nerve cells by the cerebellum is reduced. As the individual regains normal activity and as he is exposed to situations challenging the vestibular system, he will slowly regain normal function. This series of events is an excellent example of neuroplasticity in the vestibular system.[49,50]

Data from patients and animals with acute unilateral vestibular ablation as well as from other types of studies suggest that "relearning" is an important characteristic of vestibular compensation. Stressing the system by having the individual engage in activities which produce disorienting or discomforting symptoms is an important stimulus for compensation and rehabilitation.

Vestibular rehabilitation capitalizes on the natural plasticity of the vestibular system.[51] A good vestibular rehabilitation program should both extend and accelerate the normal process of physiologic adaptation to injury.

Because of the wide variety of possible separate injuries and the almost infinite possible combinations of different sorts of injuries, we believe that each vestibular rehabilitation program needs to be specifically tailored to a particular individual's needs. This is particularly true when dealing with post-head-injury patients because they will almost always have significant concomitant deficits outside the vestibular system. We believe that this is best accomplished by a physical or occupational therapist who has made a special study and gained experience in managing vestibular injuries. Such an individual will be best qualified to create programs which take into consideration all of the patient's deficits and all of his potential assets.

Propaedeutic to developing a program for rehabilitation, the vestibular rehabilitation therapist needs to make his own assessment.[46,52] At first glance, this would appear to be redundant but, in fact, it is not. The assessment made by the rehabilitation expert will not only review the history, physical, and laboratory findings already obtained by physicians and other healthcare professionals but will make a detailed assessment of specific situations which induce vertigo (i.e., elevators, crowded stores, driving), assess the severity on a quantitative scale, and do a detailed assessment of the affect of both position and position*ing*. As many as 20 separate positions and movements can be separately assessed, and each position or movement can be rated for intensity, duration, and presence of nystagmus and/or dizziness. The patient's history and type of complaint dictate how much positional testing is required. A separate evaluation of eye, head coordination, and gaze stabilization is made as well as a separate and detailed assessment of postural control, both in the sitting and standing positions. Gait is evaluated separately.

Whenever making an assessment for vestibular rehabilitation, it is important to determine whether there are other areas of difficulty outside the vestibular system which may affect rehabilitative strategies. This is clearly especially important in the post-head-injury area.

A complete evaluation of the musculoskeletal system needs to be made in order to determine whether there are any coexisting difficulties or deficits. Reduction in strength is common in the post-head-injury patient. Such reduced muscle strength may be secondary to muscle atrophy from coma or inactivity or may be secondary to direct neural injury. It may, therefore, be generalized or affect only a specific body part. Reduced range of motion should be determined. Range of motion is frequently reduced in the extremities secondary to orthopedic extremity injuries and may then be limited to a specific body part. Many patients will have associated back injuries. The effect of cervical spine injuries, especially, needs to be taken into consideration. Patients with significant cervical spine injuries will either have had surgery or prolonged periods of neck immobilization. Many, if not all, of these patients will have a disordered somatosensory feedback from cervical muscle stretch and joint position sense receptors.

The presence of pain will frequently limit movement. The nature of the pain, its severity, what movements provoke it, and which positions relieve it all need to be detailed as part of the initial assessment.

Some musculoskeletal abnormalities, especially those involving the cervical spine and neck musculature, may actually be secondary to the vestibular disorder itself. Individuals prone to vertigo and disequilibrium will limit head and trunk movements in order to avoid symptoms. Over time, these limitations of movement may cease to be volitional and require specific consideration.

The presence or absence of associated neurological injuries also needs to be addressed. Such injuries may limit or prohibit motor control. These abnormalities may be subtle and manifested only on sophisticated testing as increased response latencies or may be quite blatant in the form of spasticity or paralysis. Such disorders may arise out of injury to either the peripheral or central nervous system. Special note should be made of injuries to the extraocular muscle system. Inability to appropriately move and position the eyes may have a significant effect on balance and equilibrium and, certainly, can be expected to complicate a proposed program of vestibular rehabilitation.

Additionally, and perhaps particularly important in post-head injuries, is injury to the cortical, subcortical, and brainstem areas. Such injuries may produce abnormalities of sensory selection, gaze control, and perceived stability. It is probable that some of the abnormal oculovestibular reflex (production of vertigo secondary to repetitive rapid movement in the visual field) seen in post-head-injury patients also occurs at this level. Oftentimes, sophisticated neuropsychiatric testing will have documented abnormalities of memory, perception, and cognitive processing which are frequently associated with post-head-injury cortical dysfunction.

Any or all of the above associated difficulties may contribute to the patient's symptomatology and require specific and special consideration when a vestibular rehabilitation program is being designed.[53,54] Clearly, individuals with significant associated visual deficits will need management different from those who have associated spastic hemiparesis. Many patients requiring vestibular therapy, and especially the post-head-injury patient will have suffered significant deconditioning and require directed programs to improve both muscle strength and general aerobic conditioning.

The process of rehabilitation consists of three parts:

1. Desensitizing the affected vestibular apparatus (habituation)
2. Balance retraining
3. Cardiorespiratory training, or conditioning

Before we start this process, we explain the necessity of each part to our patient.

Desensitization (Habituation)

Peripheral lesions produce hypersensitivity to movement, with dizziness and nausea as common complaints. Patients are particularly sensitive to specific angular or linear acceleration and deceleration.[55] Desensitization is accomplished by giving the patient a variety of positional exercises designed to reproduce his vertiginous symptoms. These are repeated twice daily for 10 to 15 minutes until the symptoms are ameliorated. The simplest (though often effective) habituation exercises are those first used by Cawthorne.[56] We still use them today (Table 6.3). A variety of more sophisticated techniques are also used.[47,57-59] It is important to explain to the patient that, in order to get less sensitive to these complaints, it is necessary to provoke them. With repetition of the prescribed exercise, sensitivity to these movements will subside (Table 6.1).

TABLE 6.3 Cawthorne Head Exercises

Begin in a sitting position —
   Lie flat on your back
   Roll to the left side
   Roll to the right side
   Back flat
   Sit up
Now stand —
   Turn to the right
   Turn to the left
Sit again —
   Put your nose on your left knee
   Place your right ear on your right shoulder
   Nose to right knee
   Left ear on left shoulder
While sitting —
   Turn your head counter-clockwise
   Now turn it clockwise
   Repeat while bending forward
   Repeat while going from sitting to an erect standing position
   Repeat as you move your head forward
   Repeat as you move your head backward
In a sitting position —
   Hang your head between your legs, turning to the left
   Sit up
   Hang your head turning to the right
   Sit up
   Hang your head in the middle between your legs
   Sit up

Note: Cawthorne head exercises have been used since the 1940's as effective treatment for vertigo and disequilibrium. The patient is asked to select the six exercises from the above list which provoke the most severe symptoms. He is asked to perform these six selected exercises for ten minutes twice a day.

Graphs are used to illustrate progress over a period of time. They are good tools for motivation for the patient and give the clinician information regarding the effectiveness of the program.

Balance Retraining

Balance retraining with any vestibular lesion will always start at a level that the patient is independently able to perform. It is very important to stress the issue of independence with rehabilitative exercise as this will build confidence.

Repetition of the balance exercise, during the session as well as for an agreed period of time after the session, also helps build confidence because the exercise will become easier to perform and can be performed more quickly.

Simplicity of design will enhance both repetition and independence. Obstacle courses are good exercise but, in the beginning of the rehabilitation process, they may increase the patient's sense of frustration rather than his feeling of accomplishment.

Functionality of the exercise is important; nothing will frustrate the balance-impaired subject more than exercise that has no bearing in daily life. And, realistically, do we improve a person's ability to balance if we teach him to stand on one leg?

The treatment approach with balance retraining is not identical for peripheral or central lesions; however, the philosophy remains the same. The difference is that we expose our centrally affected patients to the same exercise longer during a treatment session and for a longer period of time — the time necessary until they can move to more complex balance activities.

Central Vestibular Lesions

These are hard to deal with as they do not respond to desensitization exercises as described in the above group. Central vestibular pathology gives rise to complaints that cannot be specifically provoked by certain movements or positions but forms a more steady ingredient in the activities of daily life of a patient.[54,59,60]

A diagnosed central lesion does, therefore, require a somewhat different approach. The diagnosis "central lesion" does not exclude the possibility of adaptation of the central nervous system. The expectation, however, is that rehabilitation will be less complete and will usually take a longer period of time.

We still implement a program based on angular and linear acceleration and deceleration, but we use more repetitions per session, usually at a lower speed, and maintain the program for a period of six to twelve weeks. Cardiorespiratory endurance training (see further in this chapter) is even more crucial to these patients than with the above described group, as physical reconditioning will enhance self-confidence and esteem, which will impart overall motivation.

The effects of such an approach are:

1. A decrease in vestibular symptoms
2. An increase in self-confidence
3. Becoming more physically active

Cervical Vertigo

This is a condition where the complaint of dizziness is related to posterior or lateral cervical myofascial pain dysfunction syndrome, i.e., decreased range of motion of the cervical spine with pain. The proper approach here is to deal with the orthopedic dysfunction first; that is, first treat the pain and impaired motion.

Cardiorespiratory Endurance Training or Conditioning

The vestibular-impaired patient experiences difficulty with balance or nausea and dizziness when moving about and, therefore, becomes less active, no matter the premorbid lifestyle. As a consequence, all our patients experience deconditioning and sometimes undesirable weight gain as a result.

Ideally, we start our patients on the Schwinn Air-Dyne® bicycle with a modified Cooper test to get baseline information on the level of conditioning. This stationary bike provides a gentle form of exercise which rarely triggers vestibular complaints. We encourage our patients to maintain a pace that will elevate their heart rate to a level appropriate for their sex and age group (target heart rate). Resting heart rate, postexercise heart rates (immediately after stopping and five minutes thereafter), and resting blood pressure are monitored (Figure 6.15).

Not all our patients can be motivated to participate in such a rigorous exercise routine and they are asked to participate in another form of endurance exercise. Most patients can be motivated to participate in some form of cardiorespiratory training, and it is best to engage the patient in a form of training that has his or her full motivation because it will increase the possibility of overall success of the rehabilitation process.

Therefore, in addition to the use of the Schwinn Air-Dyne® bicycle, we use treadmills, swimming pools, walking groups, stairclimbers, or anything else that will increase the activity level of our vestibular patients.

A number of variables will influence the outcome. First and foremost is compliance. Our current program of vestibular rehabilitation requires the patient to spend 15 minutes twice a

---

Cardiorespiratory Endurance

Clearance for Fitness Program Obtained:
    From _____(M.D.) Date _____

Resting Blood Pressure: _____

Resting Heart Rate: _____

Target Heart Rate for M/F_____ Age_____
    Formula   Men   205 - 1/2 age x .8
                  Women   220 - age x .8

12 Minute Cooper Air-Dyne Bicycle:
    Distance _____
    Post Exercise Heart Rate_____
    5 Minute Recuperating Heart Rate_____

Fitness Category:

FIGURE 6.15 The above cardiorespiratory endurance table is used on a weekly basis to evaluate cardiovascular fitness improvements.

day in specifically directed exercises which are advanced on a weekly or biweekly basis. We believe a typical program will require eight to twelve weeks. Poor compliance is common in individuals with multiple deficits and they generally do less well. Poor compliance may result because the patient has had serious central nervous injury which impairs motivation and cognition or because he has associated musculoskeletal or sensory injuries which make it impossible for him to perform the most helpful sorts of exercises. In many of these patients, two to three rehabilitation programs will be in progress simultaneously which may overwhelm the patient's ability. Individuals with central dysfunction improve at a much slower rate and may never achieve the same improvement as those who have peripheral receptor level disorders. Age is another variable which works against rapid recovery.

There is objective evidence to support the usefulness of vestibular rehabilitation. Telian et al. have evaluated the outcome in 98 patients with a variety of different vestibular problems.[59,61] Some patients were excluded because of disease process but all had to meet one of the following criteria: 1) positional or motion-provoked vertigo, 2) abnormalities of SOT or abnormal recovery strategies, and 3) abnormal chair/ENG findings. After a 10- to 15-week program performed at home, eighty-seven percent (87%) of patients reported significant subjective improvement and eighty-three percent (83%) had objective improvement in disability ratings. Thirty-one percent (31%) of the patients were completely asymptomatic at the time a follow-up evaluation was performed. Ten percent (10%) were worse. Half of these had unequivocal progressive unilateral vestibular injuries and underwent deafferentation surgical procedures.

In summary, vestibular rehabilitation is an effective way of utilizing the central nervous system's natural plasticity to compensate for vestibular dysfunction. Specifically, it is useful to improve postural and balance control, eliminate vertigo and disequilibrium, and reduce the effects of visually provoked stimuli. While most patients achieve improvement, only about one third achieve complete elimination of symptomatology. It is useful to present these techniques to the patient as methods for managing and controlling symptoms rather than eliminating them. Vestibular rehabilitation needs to be integrated into an overall plan which takes into consideration all of the patient's deficits as well as his assets and abilities. Those therapists whose priority is improvement in balance and elimination of vertigo need constantly to coordinate with the patient's multidisciplinary team leader to achieve a maximally effective overall rehabilitation strategy for the posttraumatically brain-injured individual.

ACKNOWLEDGMENT

Both authors extend their thanks and appreciation to Mrs. Reta Ramirez, who worked many hours in the preparation of this manuscript.

REFERENCES

1. Healy, G. B., Hearing loss and vertigo secondary to head injury, *N. Engl. J. Med.,* 306, 1029, 1982.
2. Pearson, B. W. and Barber, H. O., Head injury: Some otoneurologic sequelae, *Arch. Otolaryngol.,* 97, 81, 1973.
3. Berman, J. M. and Fredrickson, J. M., Vertigo after head injury: A five year follow-up, *J. Otolaryngol.,* 7, 237, 1976.
4. Rantanen, T., Aantaa, E., Salmiualli, A., and Meurman, O. H., Audiometric and electronystagmographic studies of patients with traumatic skull injuries, *Acta Otolaryngol. Suppl.,* 229, 256, 1967.
5. Saito, V., Ishikawa, T., Makiyama, Y., Hasegawa, M., Shigihora, S., Yasukata, J., Ighayama, E., and Tomita, H., Neurological study of positional vertigo caused by head injury, *Auris, Nasus, Larynx,* B Suppl., 69, 1986.
6. Tuohimaa, D., Vestibular disturbance after acute mild head injury, *Acta Otolaryngol. Suppl.,* 359, 7, 1978.
7. Grimm, R. J., Hemenway, W. G., LeBray, P., and Black, F. O., The perilymph fistula defined in mild head trauma, *Acta Otolaryngol. Suppl.,* 464, 1, 1989.
8. Vertaineu, E. and Karjalaineu, S., Vestibular disorders following head injury in children, *J. Pediatr. Otolaryngol.,* 9, 135, 1985.
9. Evatar, M., Bergtraum, M., and Randel, R. M., Post traumatic vertigo in children: A diagnostic approach, *Pediatr. Neurol.,* 2, 61, 1986.
10. Baloh, R. W. and Honrubia, V., *Clinical Neurophysiology of the Vestibular System,* 2nd edition, F. A. Davis, Philadelphia, 1990.
11. Barber, H. O. and Stockwell, C. W., *Manual of Electronystagmography,* 2nd edition, C. V. Mosby Company, St. Louis, MO, 1980.
12. Stockwell, C. W., *ENG Workbook,* Pro-Ed, Austin, TX, 1983.
13. Olsson, J. E., Blunt trauma of the temporal bone, presentation to the American Academy of Otolaryngology-Head and Neck Surgery Meeting, Washington, DC, 1986.
14. Hughes, G. B., *Textbook of Clinical Otology,* Chapter 18, Thieme-Stratton, New York, 1988.
15. Ménière, P., Congestions cérébrales apoplectiformes, *Gaz. Med. Paris,* 16, 55, 1861.
16. Clark, S. K. and Rees, T. S., Post-traumatic endolymphatic hydrops, *Arch. Otolaryngol.,* 103, 725, 1977.
17. Barber, H. O. and Sharpe, J. A., *Vestibular Disorders,* Year Book Medical Publishers, Chicago, 1988.
18. Chester, J. B., Whiplash, postural control, and the inner ear, *Spine,* 16, 716, 1991.
19. Hinoki, M., Vertigo due to whiplash injury: A neurotologic approach, *Acta Laryngol. Suppl.,* 418, 9, 1985.
20. Pfaltz, C. R., Vertigo in disorders of the neck, in *Vertigo,* Dix, M. R. and Hood, J. D., Eds., John Wiley & Sons, New York, 1984.
21. Travell, J. G. and Simons, D. G., *Myofascial Pain and Dysfunction: The Trigger Point Manual,* Williams & Wilkins, Baltimore, 1983.
22. Baloh, R. W., *The Essentials of Neurotology,* Chapters 5–7, 9, F. A. Davis, Philadelphia, 1984.
23. Brown, J. J., A systematic approach to the dizzy patient, *Neurol. Clin.,* 8, 209, 1991.
24. DeWeese, D. D., Differential diagnosis of dizziness and vertigo, in *Otolaryngology,* 3rd edition, Paparella, M. M., Shumrick, D. D., Gluckman, J. L., and Meyerhoff, W. L., Eds., W. B. Saunders, Philadelphia, 1991.
25. Rudge, P., Central causes of vertigo, in *Vertigo,* Dix, M. R. and Hood, J. D., Eds., John Wiley & Sons, New York, 1984, 321.
26. Vesterhauge, S., Clinical diagnosis of vestibular disorders, *Acta Otolaryngol. Suppl.,* 469, 114, 1988.
27. Hickey, S. A., Ford, G. R., Buckley, J. G., and Fitzgerald O'Connor, A. F., Unterberger stepping test: A useful indicator of peripheral vestibular dysfunction? *J. Laryngol. Otol.,* 104, 599, 1990.
28. Theunissen, E. J. J. M., Huygen, P. L. M., Folgering, H. T. H., and Nicolasen, M. G. M., The velocity step test, *Acta Otolaryngol. Suppl.,* 460, 104, 1988.
29. Moffat, D. A., Harries, M. L., Baguley, D. M., and Hardy, D. G., Unterberger's stepping test in acoustic neuroma, *J. Laryngol. Otol.,* 103, 839, 1989.
30. Glasscock, M. E., Jackson, C. G., and Josey, A. F., *The ABR Handbook: Auditory Brainstem Response,* Thieme Medical Publishers, Inc., New York, 1987.

31. Ruth, R., Lambert, P., and Ferraro, J., Electrocochleography: Methods and clinical applications, *Am. J. Otol.,* Suppl., 9, 1, 1988.
32. Vermeersch, H., Meyerhoff, W. L., and Boothby, R., Diagnosis and management of hearing loss, in *Vertigo*, W. B. Saunders, Philadelphia, 1985, 105.
33. Coats, A. C., Electronystagmography, *Physiological Measures of the Audio-Vestibular System*, Academic Press, New York, 1975, 37.
34. Jacobson, G. P. and Newman, C. W., Rotational testing, *Semin. Hear.,* 12, 199, 1991.
35. Baloh, R. W., Konrad, H. R., and Honrubia, V., Vestibulo-ocular function in patients with cerebellar atrophy, *Neurology*, 25, 160, 1975.
36. Baloh, R. W., Honrubia, V., and Jacobsen, K., Benign positional vertigo: Clinical and oculographic features in 240 cases, *Neurology*, 37, 371, 1987.
37. Barber, H. O., Positional nystagmus especially after head injury, *Laryngoscope*, 79, 891, 1964.
38. Shepard, N. T. and Telian, S. A., Balance disorders, in *Diagnostic Audiology*, Jacobson, J. T. and Northern, J. L., Eds., Pro-Ed, Austin, TX, 1991.
39. Baloh, R. W., Honrubia, V., Yee, R. E., and Jacobson, K. M., Rotational testing: An overview, in *Vestibular Disorders*, Barber, H. O. and Sharpe, J. A., Eds., Year Book Medical Publishers, Chicago, 1988, 117.
40. Cyr, D. G., Moore, G. F., and Moller, C. G., Clinical application of computerized dynamic posturography, *ENTechnol.*, September Suppl., 36, 1988.
41. Hirsh, B. E., Computed sinusoidal harmonic acceleration, *Ear Hear.,* 7, 198, 1986.
42. Hamid, M. A., Determining side of vestibular dysfunction with rotary chair testing, *Otolaryngol. Head Neck Surg.,* 105, 40, 1991.
43. Balzer, G. K., Clinical contributions of dynamic platform posturography, *Semin. Hear.,* 12, 238, 1991.
44. Hunter, L. L. and Balzer, G. K., Overview and introduction to dynamic platform posturography, *Semin. Hear.,* 12, 226, 1991.
45. Mirka, A. and Black, F. O., Clinical application of dynamic posturography for evaluating sensory integration and vestibular dysfunction, *Neurol. Clin.,* 8, 351, 1990.
46. Dix, M. R., Rehabilitation of vertigo, in *Vertigo*, Dix, M. R. and Hood, J. D., Eds., John Wiley & Sons, New York, 1984.
47. Katsarkas, A., Electronystagmographic (ENG) findings in paroxysmal positional vertigo (PPV) as a sign of vestibular dysfunction, *Acta Otolaryngol.*, III, 193, 1991.
48. McCabe, B. F., Vestibular physiology: Its clinical application in understanding the dizzy patient, *Otolaryngology*, 3rd edition, W. B. Saunders, Philadelphia, 1991, 911.
49. Dichgans, J., Bizzi, E., Morasso, P., and Tagliasco, V., Mechanisms underlying recovery of eye-head coordination following bilateral labyrinthectomy in monkeys, *Exp. Brain Res.,* 18, 548, 1973.
50. Fetter, M. and Zee, D. S., Recovery from unilateral labyrinthectomy in the rhesus monkey, *J. Neurophysiol.,* 59, 370, 1988.
51. Norré, M. E., Rationale of rehabilitation treatment for vertigo, *Am. J. Otolaryngol.,* 8, 31, 1987.
52. Herdman, S. J., Assessment and treatment of balance disorders in the vestibular-deficient patient, in *Balance*, Duncan, P. W., Ed., Proceeding of the APTA Forum, American Physical Therapy Association, Alexandria, VA, 1990.
53. Shumway-Cook, A. and Horak, F. B., Rehabilitation: An exercise approach to managing symptoms of vestibular dysfunction, *Semin. Hear.,* 10, 196, 1989.
54. Shumway-Cook, A. and Horak, F. B., Rehabilitation strategies for patients with vestibular deficits, *Neurol. Clin.,* 8, 441, 1990.
55. Norré, M. E., Treatment of unilateral vestibular hypofunction, in *Otoneurology*, Oosterveld, W. J., Ed., John Wiley & Sons, Ltd., New York, 1984, 23.
56. Cawthorne, T., Positional nystagmus, *Ann. Otol. Rhinol. Laryngol.*, 63, 481, 1954.
57. Brandt, T. and Daroff, R. B., Physical therapy for benign paroxysmal positional vertigo, *Arch. Otolaryngol.,* 106, 484, 1980.
58. Hecker, H. C., Haug, C. O., and Herdon, J. W., Treatment of the vertiginous patient using Cawthorne's vestibular exercises, *Laryngoscope*, 84, 2065, 1974.
59. Telian, S. A., Shepard, N. T., Smith-Wheelock, M., and Kemink, J. L., Habituation therapy for chronic vestibular dysfunction: Preliminary results, *Otolaryngol. Head Neck Surg.,* 103, 89, 1990.
60. Norré, M. E. and Beckers, A. M., Vestibular habituation training, *Arch. Otolaryngol. Head Neck Surg.,* 114, 883, 1988.
61. Shepard, N. T., Telian, S. A., and Smith-Wheelock, M., Habituation and balance retraining therapy, *Neurol. Clin.,* 8, 459, 1990.

7

Visual Dysfunction Following Traumatic Brain Injury

Ronald L. Morton

CONTENTS

INTRODUCTION

Individuals sustaining traumatic brain injury (TBI) often sustain other injuries in tandem with injury to the brain. Injuries involving the face, neck, back, torso, and extremities are commonly associated with TBI. Frequently, these injuries are readily diagnosed and treated, as they are easily evidenced when the patient presents at the emergency room.

Less obvious injuries, however, can be overlooked during lifesaving endeavors, in particular those involving systems which are more difficult to thoroughly evaluate, such as the vestibular or visual systems. This chapter focuses on deficits commonly observed in the visual systems of TBI patients. The purpose of the chapter is to provide a review of the neuroanatomy of vision and illustrate the relation of visual perceptual and visual motor deficits commonly observed following TBI to neuroanatomical structures. Visual system dysfunction following TBI is fairly common and can be quite subtle or relatively frank. The visual system has not been long regarded as one which can respond to treatments that are other than compensatory (i.e., lenses) or surgical in nature. That the visual system can respond to treatments which impact visual perceptual and/or visual motor skills is a relatively recent concept as applied to acquired neurological damage. The visual system functions as a primary sensory receptor for

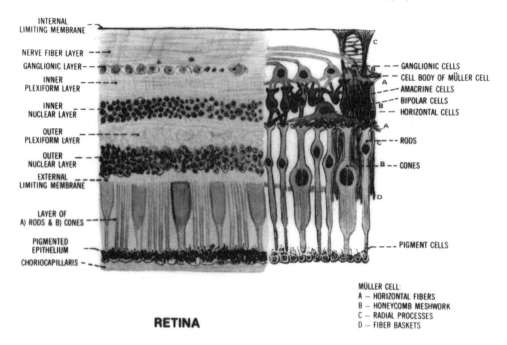

INTERNAL
LIMITING MEMBRANE

NERVE FIBER LAYER

GANGLIONIC LAYER

INNER
PLEXIFORM LAYER

INNER
NUCLEAR LAYER

OUTER
PLEXIFORM LAYER

OUTER
NUCLEAR LAYER

EXTERNAL
LIMITING MEMBRANE

LAYER OF
A) RODS & B) CONES

PIGMENTED
EPITHELIUM

CHORIOCAPILLARIS

GANGLIONIC CELLS
CELL BODY OF MÜLLER CELL
AMACRINE CELLS
BIPOLAR CELLS
HORIZONTAL CELLS

RODS

CONES

PIGMENT CELLS

RETINA

MÜLLER CELL:
A — HORIZONTAL FIBERS
B — HONEYCOMB MESHWORK
C — RADIAL PROCESSES
D — FIBER BASKETS

FIGURE 7.1   Eye anatomy. (Reprinted with permission from *The Eye* (chart), W. Jacobson, Jr. (Ed.). Copyright 1979, 1981, 1986 by Anatomical Chart Co., Skokie, IL.)

motor, social, cognitive, communicative, and emotive functions. As such, the visual system is therefore highly integrated with many neural functions other than simply "sight". Visual system disorders, then, require a fair amount of attention in the person with TBI and should be considered an integral part of the rehabilitation program. Remediation of visual perceptual and visual motor disorders can enhance function in all of the aforementioned areas as well as reduce the likelihood of reinjury and enhance maximal functional improvement.

ANATOMICAL CONSIDERATIONS

Retina

To begin, it is important that the reader have an understanding of the intricacies of visual anatomy. The organization of the visual system is crucial to an understanding of potential visual system deficits following traumatic brain injury. In order to fully appreciate the complexities of the visual system, one must recognize that visual integration is not just a cortical process; rather, visual integration begins peripherally in the visual receptor fields of the retinas.[1]

The fact that visual processing starts in the retina may seem strange until it is recalled that the eye is actually an outpouching of the brain from early in embryological development.[2,3] Figure 7.1 depicts the organization of the photoreceptors, bipolar cells, and ganglion cells. Photoreceptors, when stimulated, pass information to adjacent bipolar cells, which, in turn, differentially affect firing of the ganglion cells. Linear and cross connections of ganglion and adjacent bipolar cells are demonstrated by the fact that the adjacent bipolar cells increase the firing rate of ganglion cells when certain conditions are met.

For example, if a spot of light lands on one photoreceptor while adjacent photoreceptors remain unilluminated, the stimulated photoreceptor will fire at a higher rate compared to the rate at which it will fire when all surrounding photoreceptors are simultaneously illuminated. These patterns of illuminated and nonilluminated photoreceptors were referred to by Werblin and Dowling[4] as *on-center* and *off-surround* groups.

On-center and off-surround groups may be joined in such combinations as to form units sensitive to stimuli in the environment of particular spatial orientations. These include, for example, vertical, horizontal, and diagonal lines or edges. Stimuli which are thus organized are relayed to the cortex via the optic tract. The processing of visual stimuli continues, via the optic tract, to be further processed in the lateral geniculate bodies, the occipital cortex, and associated cortices receiving radiations from the primary occipital areas.

As a normal individual gazes upon an object, the image is registered simultaneously in both the right and left retina. Each retina, however, is situated slightly differently in orientation to the object, thus producing a slightly different image to the brain from each retina.[5] This can be demonstrated by gazing at an object and alternately closing one eye, then the other. The object appears to "move" due to the fact that the image registered is different because of the distance separating the eyes and the slight difference in angular orientation of each eye to the object. Stereopsis, which is the ability to visualize the dimension of depth, arises from the fusing of these two separate images by the sensory system[5] and, consequently, plays a major role in several visual perceptual skills.

Optic Tract Organization and Lesion Characteristics

Organization of the optic tract is interesting and of great importance in determinating the site of lesion from visual deficits presented. Lesions at different points in the optic tract will be demonstrated by pathognomonic visual deficits.[3] In the days prior to CT scanning and magnetic resonance imaging (MRI), the localization of injury was dependent upon knowledge of anatomical relationships. Knowing the proximity of motor and sensory pathways adjacent to the visual pathways allowed determination of site of lesion based upon the constellation of signs and symptoms. Localization of the site of lesion or injury can assist in further diagnosis, determination of etiology, and likely systemic sequelae.

Each retina must direct its information toward the cortex and does so via the optic nerve. The information passes from the ganglion cells, located in each retina, posteriorly via the optic nerve to the optic chiasm. Figure 7.2 illustrates how, at the optic chiasm, right and left visual spaces are segregated, with the contribution of each hemi-retina passed to a single corresponding lateral geniculate body, the specific thalamic relay nucleus for the visual pathway.[6] Right visual space images upon the nasal retina of the right eye and the temporal retina of the left eye. At the chiasm, the optic fibers of the nasal retina of the right eye cross to the left to join the optic fibers of the temporal retina of the left eye. The temporal fibers of the left eye continue uncrossed in the optic tract, beyond the chiasm, and find their way to the lateral geniculate body on the left. Thus, the left lateral geniculate body receives information from the right visual space from both eyes.

Information from the upper retinal fibers (nasal crossed, temporal uncrossed) passes through the corresponding lateral geniculate body and continues in a portion of the optic tract known as the *geniculocalcarine tract* until it projects to the primary visual cortex (cuneate gyrus, area 17) of the occipital lobe.[7] The geniculocalcarine tract courses through the parietal lobe, and a lesion involving the geniculocalcarine tract on the right would result in an inferior contralateral quadrantanopsia (Figure 7.2, Item 9).

Information from the nasal lower retina, however, after crossing over at the optic chiasm to join the temporal lower retinal fibers, leaves the lateral geniculate body and courses into the temporal lobe (Figure 7.3) in a band of fibers known as *Meyer's loop*.[7] These fibers terminate in the lingual gyrus of the occipital lobe. A lesion involving Meyer's loop on the right would cause a contralateral left superior quadrantanopsia (Figure 7.2, Item 10).

Bitemporal hemianopsia (Figure 7.2, Item 4), for example, results from a lesion which involves the optic chiasm — in particular the fibers which cross from the nasal field of each retina, serving temporal visual space — to the lateral geniculate body of the contralateral side of the brain. Pituitary hormone dysfunction may be associated with this visual system deficit

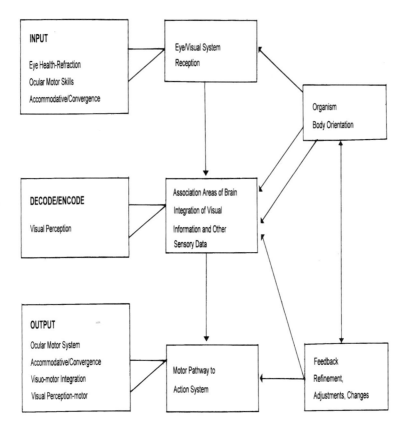

FIGURE 7.2 Visual pathway and resultant field defects. (Reprinted with permission from Jones, L.T., Reeh, M.J., Wirtschafter, J.D.: *Ophthalmic Anatomy: A Manual With Some Clinical Application*, San Francisco, American Academy of Ophthalmology, 1970, Figure 9, p 176.)

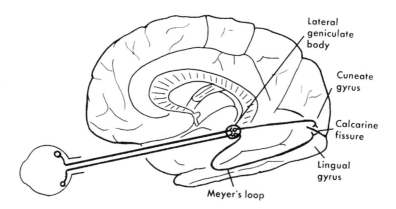

FIGURE 7.3 Meyer's loop. (Reprinted with permission from *Medical Neurobiology: Neuroanatomical and Neurophysiological Principles Basic to Clinical Neuroscience* (2nd ed.) (p. 287) by W. D. Willis and R. G. Grossman. Copyright 1977 by C. V. Mosby Company.)

due to the proximity of the optic chiasm to the pituitary gland. Binasal hemianopsia (Figure 7.2, Item 5), on the other hand, would implicate a lesion of the lateral aspects of the optic chiasm, involving the uncrossed temporal fibers from the nasal fields of each retina. In this instance, carotid disease may be involved.

TABLE 7.1 Cranial Nerve Innervation

Cranial nerve	Muscle innervated	Brainstem nucleus
III	Pupilloconstrictor and ciliary muscles	Edinger-Westphal
	Superior, inferior, and medial rectus	Oculomotor
	Inferior oblique	
	Levator palpebrae	
IV	Superior oblique	Trochlear
VI	Lateral rectus	Abducens

The primary visual cortex is made up of the region of the cortex immediately surrounding the calcarine fissure, extending anteriorly toward the splenium of the corpus callosum.[8] This area is known as the *calcarine cortex*. Lesions involving selective portions of the calcarine fissure and occipital pole can likewise present with specific visual field defects. Figure 7.2 depicts an occipital-pole-lesion-induced central scotoma (Item 12). A lesion at the midportion of the calcarine fissure or of fibers to this area would result in a contralateral homonymous hemianopsia with macular sparing (Item 13). Lastly, a lesion involving the anterior portion of the calcarine fissure will result in a contralateral temporal crescentic field deficit (Item 14).

Oculomotor and Brainstem Organization

Discussion of the visual system must include a review of the ocular motor system and its innervation. Oculomotor deficits following brain injury can result in misalignment of the eyes which, in turn, may be reported by the patient as double vision, blurred vision, impaired eye/hand coordination, impaired tracking during reading, and so on. Misalignment of the eyes can also lead to cortical image suppression with resultant perceptual deficits which will impact therapeutic performance, balance, coordination, and safety.

The six extrinsic muscles of the eye[9] are innervated by three cranial nerves, as listed in Table 7.1. Cranial nerve III is responsible for innervation of the superior rectus, inferior rectus, medial rectus, and inferior oblique. The superior rectus rotates the eye upward when the eye is abducted; however, when the eye is adducted, this muscle moves the superior part of the eye toward the medial wall of the orbit (intorsion). The medial rectus rotates the eye nasally. The inferior rectus rotates the eye downward when the eye is in abduction and extorts the eye when in adduction. The inferior oblique elevates the eye when the eye is adducted and extorts the eye during abduction.

Cranial nerve IV innervates the superior oblique, which is responsible for eye depression during eye adduction and intorts the eye during abduction. Cranial nerve VI innervates the lateral rectus, which produces temporally directed rotation of the eye.

The nuclei of cranial nerves III, IV, and VI are found in the brainstem ranging from the midbrain to the pons.[10] Figure 7.4 shows the nuclei of cranial nerve III located inferior to the superior colliculus and lateral to midline on either side. The axons innervating the four extrinsic muscles of the eye innervate ipsilateral muscles, except for the superior rectus, which may project contralaterally.[1]

The nucleus of cranial nerve IV is located below the inferior colliculus. Innervation of the superior oblique muscles is contralateral in nature. Finally, the cranial nerve VI nucleus is located in the pons. Its axons remain ipsilateral, as they innervate the lateral rectus muscles.

These three cranial nerves are interrelational in function. The medial longitudinal fasciculus (MLF) comprises the major projection system allowing such interrelation.[1] Vestibular projections influencing eye movement connect to these cranial nerves via the MLF and account for a good portion of the MLF. The vestibular projections arise mainly from the

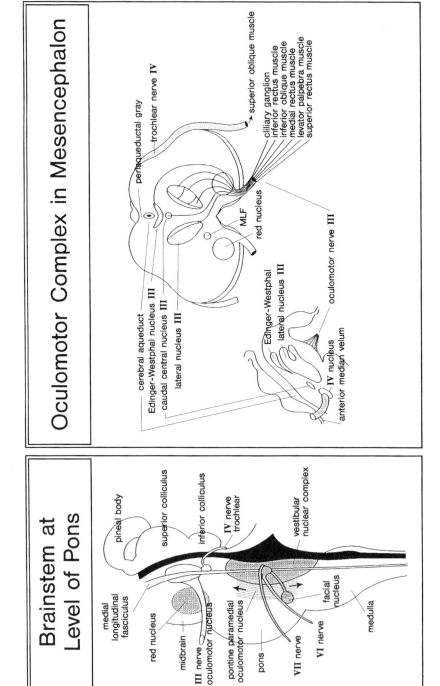

FIGURE 7.4   Brainstem and nuclei and oculomotor complex in mesencephalon cutaneous.

superior and medial vestibular nuclei. These interconnections, between vestibular and ocular nuclei, are responsible for coordination of head/eye movements and the production of nystagmus following vestibular overstimulation.

Cranial nerves III, IV, and VI receive afferents from the retina, the frontal and occipital lobes, the vestibular nuclei, and the superior colliculus. There may be reticular projections as well.[1]

Perhaps the most common oculomotor dysfunction seen is that of esophoria. In this condition, the lateral rectus of one eye is weakened, presumably due to injury to the corresponding cranial nerve VI nucleus or pathway. These patients may report blurred or double vision, though they may also accommodate to misaligned images via cortical suppression of the image from one eye. Careful evaluation of these patients may turn up additional subtle impairments of other extrinsic muscle innervations. Suffice it to say that innervational deficits resulting in complete or partial motor paralysis of the corresponding extrinsic muscle(s) are prevalent following TBI and require careful delineation and treatment.

Pupillary Responses

Pupil size is modulated by both the sympathetic nervous system with its dilator fibers and the parasympathetic system with its constrictor fibers. Pupils are normally of equal size, but differences of less than 1 mm may be present in as much as 20% of the normal population. Pathologic anisocoria is caused by lesions either of the sympathetic or parasympathetic pathways or by local iris disease, such as tumors or scar adhesions.

Sympathetic impulses to the eye originate in the hypothalamus. They are transmitted along the spinal cord, synapsing in the lateral grey columns. They exit the cord via preganglionic fibers at C8 to T2 and travel upward in the sympathetic chain to synapse in the superior cervical ganglia, lying at the level of C1 and C2. Nonmyelinated, postganglionic fibers form a plexus around the common carotid artery with vasomotor fibers to the face and the external carotid artery. The internal carotid artery carries sympathetic nerves through the cavernous sinus where the fibers join the nasociliary branch of the fifth nerve. From the nasociliary nerve, they travel into the eye to the radial dilator muscle fibers in the pupils, resulting in dilation.

Parasympathetic preganglionic axons originate in the Edinger-Westphal nucleus of the third cranial nerve (medulla), where they produce a simultaneous and bilateral response in each third nerve through intraneuronal connections. The parasympathetic preganglionic axons run forward in the third nerve and pass through the inferior division of the anterior aspect of the cavernous sinus to the ciliary ganglion for synapse on their way via the short ciliary nerves into the annular constrictor pupillary fibers. The output of the Edinger-Westphal nucleus represents the summation of the input from both the right and left eye via a certain set of the ganglion cells, some of which cross in the chiasm, along with the other visual fibers through the optic tract and lateral geniculate body on their way to synapse at the Edinger-Westphal nucleus.

This summation, at the Edinger-Westphal nucleus, allows one to elicit a relative afferent pupillary defect — a different pupil size in response to a monocle light stimulus. This reaction is caused by an asymmetry of conduction in the afferent visual system, either at the retina or optic nerve, specifically in the area anterior to the lateral geniculate body. To illustrate, when a traumatic optic atrophy causes the loss of a significant number of ganglion cell axons, the conduction of a light stimulus to the Edinger-Westphal nucleus is diminished and a larger pupil will result (i.e., 5 mm) rather than the small pupil resultant from full stimulation (i.e., 3 mm). Therefore, as a light is swung[11] from the normal side, with 3-mm pupils in both eyes, to the affected side, the pupils will dilate to 5 mm.

Visual Fields

An understanding of visual field integrity is of key importance in accurate diagnosis of visual deficits and their neurological correlates in the TBI patient.[12] Visual field is measured in degrees, and the center of fixation is used as a zero referent. Visual field extends to approximately 90 degrees in all directions. Decreasing sensitivity is found the farther out the stimulus is from center. Targets in the less sensitive periphery must be larger and brighter to be seen.

Two types of measurement devices are available for delineation of visual fields. Devices can be categorized as *kinetic* or *static* dependent upon whether the stimulus moves or is stationary. The Goldmann Perimeter is a kinetic device in which the stimulus presented is a spot of light of specific size and intensity which is moved toward the center of fixation until the patient reports seeing it. The Humphrey Perimeter is a static device which measures visual field by increasing the brightness of a spot at a fixed location until the patient sees it. These two devices have been demonstrated to be fairly accurate and reliable in tests of both a neurologically and nonneurologically impaired population. Goldmann fields have been shown to be 97% reliable, while Humphrey fields were 91% reliable.[13]

Diplopia fields are evaluated using the Goldmann Perimeter. The patient is not patched as they would be for peripheral field testing. The patient is positioned at the machine so that the fixation light is aligned between the patient's eyes. A light is introduced. The patient follows this light, from center outward, and informs the examiner when it breaks into a double image. Thus, a specific map of the patient's diplopia is made and can be tracked as treatment progresses. It should be noted that the vast majority of diplopia can be accounted for as a result of acquired paresis or palsy of one or more of the extraocular muscles.[14]

Visual fields can also be evaluated by "confrontation" which requires no elaborate devices. Confrontation testing is performed by movement of the examiner's finger, or a red bottle cap, slowly into the patient's visual field, with central visual fixation, until the stimulus is viewed. While not a precise system of measurement, confrontation testing can reliably demonstrate certain visual field deficits in the absence of more elaborate testing.[14] Fading of the color red in the field periphery can be an early sign of visual field depression.

EXAMINATION

Examination of the TBI patient should first establish best corrected visual acuity, if at all possible. This can be difficult to establish due to problems the patient may have in cooperating with the evaluation. Communication problems may be lessened by using the services of a speech pathologist or family member familiar with the communication deficits of a given patient.

The face should be examined for lacerations, scars, or foreign bodies. Check the lids for position, remembering that cranial nerve III is responsible for palpebral elevation and cranial nerve VII for closure via the orbicularis muscles.[15] These motor systems should be evaluated for weakness. Skin sensation should be checked in distributions of cranial nerve V (Figure 7.5), possibly manifesting as anesthesia or abnormal sensation as well as associated motor functions which can manifest as paresis of mastication.[16] Head and neck positioning should be carefully evaluated as compensatory head tilts are quite common due to diplopia and the patient's attempt to compensate for same.[5]

Ocular Examination

Examination of the anterior structures of the eye is facilitated by magnification and illumination ranging from penlight and bifocals to slit-lamp examination. Slit-lamp examination allows greater detail to be viewed as well as better assessment of the depth of any foreign body lodging or scar tissue. The anterior chamber, thus examined, may show blood or inflammatory debris.

Examination of the pupil can provide clues as to the integrity of cranial and optic nerve functions. The responsiveness of a pupil to light and accommodative stimuli can provide information regarding the integrity of the pupillary nerve fibers between the lateral geniculate body, the Edinger-Westphal nucleus (part of the nucleus of cranial nerve III in the medulla of

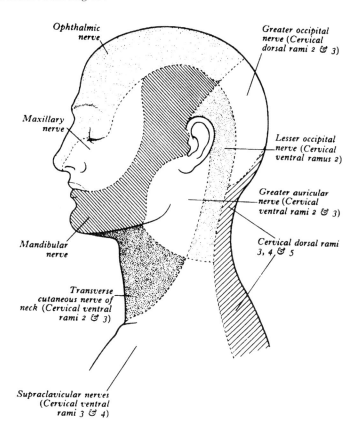

FIGURE 7.5 Distribution of cranial nerve V. (Reprinted with permission from *Gray's Anatomy* (35th ed.) by R. Warwick and P. L. Williams. Copyright 1973 by Churchill Livingstone.)

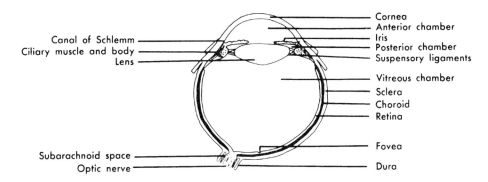

FIGURE 7.6 Major components of the human eye. (Reprinted with permission from *Medical Neurobiology: Neuroanatomical and Neurophysiological Principles Basic to Clinical Neuroscience* (2nd ed.) (p. 282) by W. D. Willis and R. G. Grossman. Copyright 1977 by C. V. Mosby.)

the brainstem), and the sympathetic and parasympathetic nerves which innervate the dilators and constrictors of the pupil. Thus, a relative afferent pupillary defect (APD) may imply optic nerve lesion, traumatic vascular insult, an inflammatory process, or multiple sclerosis.

As shown in Figure 7.6, behind the pupil is the lens.[1] The lens may be affected by trauma in a number of ways. These include penetration by a foreign body, laceration of the globe, blunt trauma to the globe, electrical injury, chemical injury, or concussion. Any of these injuries can result in a loss of lens clarity and result in cataract formation. Cataracts may

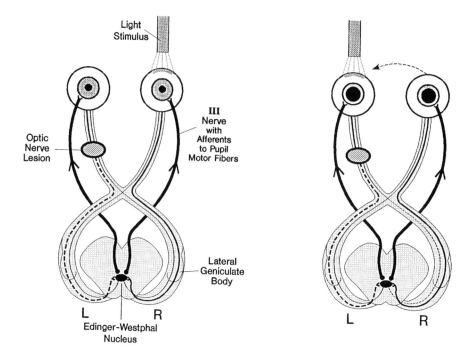

FIGURE 7.7   Anatomy of pupillary defect.

become dense enough to significantly limit visual acuity and may interfere with the rehabilitative process. In this circumstance, surgical intervention may be required. It is important to note that cataract formation can be accelerated by some tranquilizers or steroids.

Opacities of the ocular media, such as a dense cataract, are usually not sufficient to produce an APD. However, very dense vitreous hemorrhage or dense amblyopia may be sufficient, although it is usually indicative of pathologic lesion in the afferent visual system. This can be correlated with an asymmetric loss of visual field, central acuity, color saturation, or subjective brightness. It should be noted, also, that monocular diplopia can arise from media opacities which cause splitting of the image.[5]

The diagram in Figure 7.7 shows that the intact right eye causes more firings of the central nucleus with light stimulating that side. As the light stimulus is moved to the left side, relatively less stimulus is received at the nucleus, resulting in less tone at the constrictor fibers. The result is a larger pupillary aperture. Thus, as the light stimulus is moved from the intact right eye to the affected left eye, the pupils will dilate as the swinging flashlight crosses to the affected side. This is called a *positive swinging flashlight test* or a *left Marcus-Gunn pupil*. This is an apparent paradox, with a pupil dilating as it is struck by light, as the light moves from the position determined by the intact right side (i.e., a 3-mm pupil) to the affected left side (i.e., a 5-mm pupil).

Trauma may extend to the posterior segment of the eye. As such, injuries can include retinal breaks, tears, or detachment in which the retina separates from its underlying supportive tissues, losing function, and ultimately causing wrinkling and scarring. Hemorrhage may occur and it is possible for there to be contusion to the optic nerve itself.

Extraocular Motility: Peripheral and Central Dysfunction

The extraocular muscles of the eye are responsible for aligning the eyes, enabling them to be pointed at the same object, and for moving the eyes to different positions of gaze in a manner which allows the continuous perception of a single image. The movement of each eye is managed by six muscles and controlled by three cranial nerves. Therefore, between the two eyes, there are twelve muscles and six cranial nerves involved. Any of these muscles or nerves can be adversely affected following injury, resulting in interference with the alignment and tracking of the eyes. Injuries such as direct contusion to the orbit or fracture of the orbit can cause injury to the muscle or nerve complex. Mechanical entrapment of a muscle can occur, or bony fragments from an orbital fracture can impinge upon cranial nerves.

The course of the cranial nerves from the brainstem to the orbit makes them subject to contusion injuries. In particular, cranial nerve VI exits from the ventral side of the brainstem and ascends the bone along the base of the skull. It enters the superior orbital fissure of the orbit on its way to the lateral rectus muscle. Cranial nerve IV exits from the dorsal side of the brainstem and sweeps around to the sides. It also passes through the superior orbital fissure to innervate the superior oblique. Blunt head trauma, with the associated violent shaking of the brain, can cause the dura along the dorsal aspect of the brain to impinge on the nerve as it exits and crosses the dorsum of the brain. The result is a fourth nerve palsy which manifests in the patient as the inability to rotate the eye downward during adduction and a loss of intortion during abduction.

In addition to lesions which can affect individual cranial nerves and muscles, resulting in misalignment, there is also coordination which occurs between various cranial nerve motor nuclei in a tract in the brainstem known as the *medial longitudinal fasciculus* (MLF). The MLF serves as a coordination and integration center between the third, fourth, and sixth cranial nerve motor nuclei. As an example, when an individual who is looking straight ahead wishes to turn his/her gaze to the right, several things must happen in a coordinated fashion. First, the firing rate of the right lateral rectus muscle via the sixth motor nucleus must increase as must the firing rate for the left medial rectus muscle, mediated by the third motor nucleus on the left side. At the same time, a relative inhibition or decrease in the firing rate of the right medial rectus muscle and the left lateral rectus muscle must occur, leading to a deviation of the eyes to the right. A lesion in the brainstem involving the MLF would interfere with the coordination of these four motor nuclei, and coordination of eye and/or head movements might subsequently be impaired.

Eye movements must be coordinated with changes in head position or acceleration of the body in any plane which might stimulate the vestibular apparatus. The vestibular apparatus is mediated through the eighth cranial nerve which has projections into the lateral gaze center located adjacent to the sixth motor nucleus on the ipsilateral side. The right horizontal gaze center fires directly into the adjacent right sixth motor nerve nucleus for its contribution to conjugate deviation of the eyes.

This can be contrasted to a request for a volitional turning of the eyes to the right. Compliance with such a request would require involvement of the left frontal premotor area which feeds posteriorly in the white tracts and projects to the right horizontal gaze center. Consequently, an injury to the frontal lobe or its conduction path to the horizontal gaze center could adversely affect the ability of a patient to voluntarily turn the eyes from one side to the other. At the same time, vestibular input to the lateral gaze center may remain intact. The doll's head maneuver, wherein the head is rotated by the examiner to one side and the normal response is such that the eyes deviate to the opposite side, can be utilized to test the integrity of pathways from the vestibular nuclei to the lateral gaze center.

Horizontal and vertical gaze systems are located in different anatomical locations and tend to function independently of each other (Figure 7.8). Therefore, each should be examined separately to check for impairment. Also, it is important to note if a patient can hold steady gaze in the primary or eccentric positions in the presence of any type of nystagmus.

Horizontal gaze palsy with an inability to make a conjugate ocular movement to one side may result from either pontine or supranuclear lesions. Evaluation by the doll's head maneuver or caloric stimulation[14] to the external auditory meatus allows differentiation of a lower pontine lesion from one of the supranuclear pathways which would cause a loss of saccadic

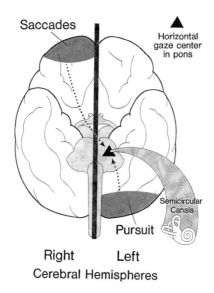

FIGURE 7.8   Inputs to horizontal gaze center.

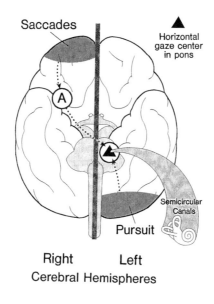

FIGURE 7.9   Supranuclear lesion.

gaze in the direction opposite the site of Lesion A (Figure 7.9). Input from the intact hemisphere causes ocular deviation toward the site of the lesion. If the patient is unable to look toward that gaze direction by either a voluntary or tracking movement, but can deviate the eyes to the involved side during a doll's head rotation, this demonstrates that the lower pontine reflexes are intact and that the lesion is in the supranuclear pathway.

The vertical gaze centers are divided above and below the aqueduct of Sylvius anterior to the motor nuclei of cranial nerve III. The vertical gaze centers can also be selectively injured. Damage to the dorsal vertical nerve nucleus will affect the ability to initiate upgaze beyond midline, allowing horizontal gaze to be preserved with smooth pursuits and saccades intact (Parinaud's syndrome).

Vertical gaze palsies caused by a lesion in the area of the upper midbrain in the area of the superior colliculus can result in three signs known, collectively, as *Parinaud's syndrome* or *dorsal midbrain syndrome*. This is composed of a loss of vertical gaze ability and pupillary light reflex, with preservation of near reflex and the presence of an eye movement disorder called *convergence retraction nystagmus*. Convergence retraction nystagmus is triggered by an upward saccade, either voluntary or in response to a downward rotating optokinetic drum, which causes simultaneous firing of both the medial and lateral rectus muscles resulting in convergence and retraction of globes into the orbit. Examination of the pupil shows light/near dissociation with normal to mild dilation of pupils and poor or absent light response but, with an accommodative target, the pupil will constrict to a near reaction. A patient with this condition has the ability to make rapid horizontal saccades, but abilities for voluntary up and down gaze are lost and the patient attempts a head posture change to compensate. A doll's head rotation may show that vertical movement can be produced with vestibular input when pontine reflexes are intact and only a supranuclear pathway lesion is present.

Early lesions in the region of the posterior commissure can affect upgaze preferentially, particularly vertical saccades. Lesions can press on the midbrain aqueduct leading to hydrocephalus and papilledema. A lateral extension of such a lesion can involve the optic radiation, while a posterior extension of a lesion can produce ataxia from cerebellar compression. Pineal tumors are the most common of such lesions, although emboli, vasculitis, arteriovenous malformations, or arteriosclerosis may also be causal factors. An upper midbrain CVA by branches from the posterior cerebral artery can also result in impairment of vertical gaze with retraction of both upper eyelids, called *Collier's sign*. These symptoms usually recover over two to three weeks.

As has been stated, ocular deviation or misalignment can result from cranial nerve palsies. Deviation is often initially incomitant, or variable, in different directions of gaze. There is often more deviation in looking to the side of the affected muscle than when looking away from its field of action. This condition may resolve in time with return to normal function or the condition may become more comitant, or even and consistent, in the different fields of gaze. Sequential measurements are used to study the deviation in nine cardinal positions. Via sequential measurements, the examiner can more readily make determinations about whether function is returning to normal or whether deviation is becoming more comitant.

When ocular deviation is relatively even in primary and reading gaze, prisms can be used to optically move the image to compensate for the mechanical misalignment. Press-on prisms can be applied to the patient's glasses resulting in increased comfort and resumption of the ability of the patient to see binocularly. Press-on prisms may be changed at will, unlike ground-in prisms. As the patient's divergence reduces, the amount of prism can also be diminished to maintain alignment and keep fusional vergence drive active as an aid to further rehabilitation.

LEARNING AND VISUAL THERAPY

One model for learning and memory includes repetition. Repetitive use of a synaptic connection causes a broadening and flattening of the endplates with a decrease in resistance across the synaptic gap, and a preference for using that synapse over adjacent pathways that have not been so facilitated.[17] Learning has been shown to affect dendritic spine formation.[18] These concepts are anatomically supportive of many standard teaching methods from repetition of spelling lists and multiplication tables to rehearsing a speech to learn a pattern of words. Coaches use repetition in training athletes to learn certain body positions or sequences of moves.

Repetition may also serve as a foundation for retraining a traumatically brain-injured patient in whom preferred pathways may have been damaged, resulting in an initial inability to perform an old, remembered task. The inherent complexity of the central nervous system may be a blessing in that there seems to be alternate pathways available for bypass of damaged areas and establishment of new circuits or series of synapses that will allow one to perform old tasks in perhaps new ways. Therapy can be thought of as a means of helping to identify some of these previously unused or little used pathways and, through repetition and building upon prior skills, developing new ways of performing old tasks.

Case History 1

A 32-year-old male sustained postconcussion syndrome after being struck in the head by a falling pallet. Initially, he presented with complaints of diplopia and blurry vision. On evaluation, he was noted to have 8 prism diopters of exophoria at near and distance, with some difficulty on upgaze. Cogwheeling of saccades was present. It was noted, on screening and confrontation fields testing, that temporal constriction in the right eye was present. Recommendation was made for saccadic exercises, such as the vertical swinging ball, and convergence exercises. At the next visit, exophoria was decreased to 6 prism diopters and saccades had improved with therapy.

Two months later, exophoria remained about the same and saccades had ceased cogwheeling on left to right gaze and had greatly improved on right to left gaze. The patient continues with vision therapy and has graduated to exercises that are more difficult for him, such as the color bead sorting tray.[19]

Case History 2

A 42-year-old male suffered blunt head trauma from metal pipe. Initially, he presented with complaint of decreased vision. On examination, acuity was correctable to 20/25 in the right eye, 20/20 in the left eye. No strabismus was noted. Saccades were slowed with difficulty moving eyes left to right and slight exophoria on upgaze. Pursuit was jerky. Worth Four-Dot testing revealed partial suppression with left eye. Visual fields, on confrontation, were constricted bilaterally. Recommendations were for pursuit and saccadic exercises and the patient was started on swinging ball exercise.

Two months later, saccades were greatly improved, with almost no cogwheeling. Approximately six months after the initial examination, the patient was started on Ritalin®* for impaired speed of processing. Immediately, he began to complain of more difficulty with tracking and decreased vision. On examination, smooth pursuit had become very jerky as were saccades. Best corrected acuity had decreased to 20/30 in the right eye and 20/40 in the left eye. Three months later, he discontinued Ritalin® and was evaluated two weeks later, noting vision still decreased. Smooth pursuits and saccades were still jerky. Acuity had increased to 20/20 in each eye, with difficulty. Final evaluation was done four months later. Acuity was 20/20 in each eye, best corrected. Smooth pursuits were improved, but still jerky, and suppression was noted in the left eye via Worth Four-Dot testing.

Case History 3

A 31-year-old male suffered a closed head injury with intracerebral hemorrhages after a motor-cycle vs. car accident. Initially, he presented with 20/20 vision, best corrected, bilaterally. Six prism diopters of exophoria with 10 prism diopters of left hyperphoria was noted on primary gaze. There was vertical nystagmus on abduction and large lag on abduction. Smooth pursuits were jerky. Recommendations were for saccadic and smooth pursuit exercises, such as the Marsden ball, color bead sorting tray, and accommodative flexibility exercises. Four diopters of prism were applied to present glasses via press-on prism. Six months later, with prism, exophoria was decreased to 2 prism diopters. Vertical nystagmus had improved, as had saccades. He started the bead sorting tray exercises on a vertical orientation and vertical door jamb reading.[19]

---

* Registered Trademark of CIBA Pharmaceutical Company, Summit, New Jersey.

Most therapy consists of taking a task, breaking it down into smaller steps, teaching, learning, and repeating each one of the steps, and linking them into larger and larger groups until, finally, a more complex behavior can be performed. Since the goal of therapy is to minimize disabilities and maximize abilities, this retraining process is at the heart of the things we do.

We first need to determine what systems or subsystems have been adversely affected, what things a patient is unable to do, what things the patient can do to a limited extent, and devise a means of working from what the patient can do in an additive fashion to allow him to regain as much skill as possible. For example, in treating diplopia, the first temptation might be to simply patch the more severely affected eye to relieve the symptom of diplopia. While this does relieve the immediate symptom, it does very little toward rehabilitation or establishing these alternate pathways that were discussed earlier. Therefore, the act of putting a patch on the eye temporarily blocks the symptom but does not approach a solution to the problem, which is mistracking of the eyes.

A preferred plan would be to determine whether there is any position of gaze in which the patient does not see double. Treatment would incorporate prisms in glasses to move the images into alignment so as to allow the person to continue to use both eyes at the same time. The goal would be to enlarge the area of single vision through a series of training exercises. The exercises encourage the movement of the eyes and stimulate the utilization of existing or new pathways to allow tracking of an object smoothly, or to acquire its fixation and maintain it in good alignment. We may start off by using a large amount of prism in the glasses, perhaps a plastic press-on prism, so that it can be easily changed as the patient improves with time under therapy to keep encouraging the patient to move ahead. The areas of first concern should be primary gaze, straight ahead gaze, and slightly down gaze in a reading position. These may require two different sets of glasses with two different amounts of prism.

Programs of visual therapy require coordination of efforts between the physician and the therapist. The physician conducts serial repetitive measurements to determine baseline alignment and provide comparison to previous measurements to monitor progression. The therapist makes suggestions in consultation with the physician regarding what therapies might best improve the patient's condition, keeping in mind the patient's tolerance, strengths, and any other concomitant difficulties. As long as progress is being made, visual therapy should be encouraged and allowed to proceed.

It may take many months for the damaged neural tracts to repair themselves or for compensation to occur within the neurological system. Nerve repair proceeds at a slow pace. At some point, the ophthalmological measurements may plateau and the patient may show no further progress. Depending upon the nature of the deficit at that time, one may consider surgical intervention to realign the eyes in a more central and aligned position. Visual therapy may play a role in stimulating binocular vision either preoperatively, in preparation for surgery, or postoperatively, in an attempt to stabilize the alignment that has been achieved by mechanical movement of the muscles. Once again, small bits of prism may be utilized to complete the alignment process and then be gradually weaned away as the patient's fusional amplitudes increase over time.

A number of patients have shown rather dramatic improvement in areas that traditional medicine will tell us should not have improved. Some patients, who initially could not tolerate things moving near their heads because it gave them a feeling of extreme discomfort, developed a tolerance for having a ball swinging in a circle around their head as they tracked it back and forth. Other patients needed a program geared specifically to their areas of difficulty such as working from near to far as they changed their fixation. With time and repeated efforts, they developed an increased facility in this regard. Still other patients who had specific difficulties in their saccadic tracking systems were able, with simple repetitive exercises such as door jamb reading, to demonstrate increased facility. This was reported both subjectively, in that they felt they could do the exercises more quickly, more easily, and with less fatigue, and also objectively, in that their examination scores showed improvement over time. It is important to understand that 1) the therapist must realize that the patient can get better, and 2) the patient must be willing to undergo a fairly rigorous and, sometimes, uncomfortable therapeutic process in order to develop the synaptic relays necessary for improved function.

Traumatically brain-injured patients and their rehabilitation are much like patients and rehabilitation in other areas of medicine. The problem must be diagnosed with an understanding of the underlying systems that are involved. A therapeutic plan must be outlined and executed. Progress must be assessed and the plan periodically modified to maximize the results. This is true whether it be antibiotics to treat an infection, setting a broken leg and then checking the alignment by repeated X-ray through the cast, or setting up a diet and exercise plan for a patient following a heart attack.

The idea is to provide an environment in which the patient can get well, encourage him to do so, monitor progress, and keep moving the game ahead. In therapy of the TBI patient, "It ain't over 'til it's over," and the fat lady hasn't yet sung.

REFERENCES

1. Willis, W. D. and Grossman, R. G., *Medical Neurobiology: Neuroanatomical and Neurophysiological Principles Basic to Clinical Neuroscience,* 2nd edition, C. V. Mosby Company, St. Louis, 1977.

2. Cook, C. S., Ozanics, V., and Jakobiec, F. A., Prenatal development of the eye and its adnexa, in Duane's *Foundations of Clinical Ophthalmology,* Volume 1, Revised edition, Tasman, W. and Jaeger, E. A., Eds., J. B. Lippincott, Philadelphia, 1992.

3. Wirtschafter, J. D., Ophthalmic neuroanatomy: The visual pathway, in *Ophthalmic Anatomy: A Manual with Some Clinical Applications,* Jones, L. T., Reeh, M. J., and Wirtschafter, J. D., Eds., American Academy of Ophthalmology and Otolaryngology, Rochester, MN, 1970, 161.

4. Werblin, F. S. and Dowling, J. E., Organization of the retina of the mudpuppy. Necturus maculosus: II. Intracellular recording, *J. Neurophysiol.,* 32, 339, 1969.

5. Neger, R. E., The evaluation of diplopia in head trauma, *J. Head Trauma Rehabil.,* 4, 27, 1989.

6. Jones, L. T., Reeh, M. J., and Wirtschafter, J. D., *Ophthalmic Anatomy: A Manual with Some Clinical Applications,* American Academy of Ophthalmology, Rochester, MN, 1970.

7. Glaser, J. S., Anatomy of the visual sensory system, in Duane's *Clinical Ophthalmology,* Volume 2, Revised edition, Tasman, W. and Jaeger, E. A., Eds., J. B. Lippincott, Philadelphia, 1992[a].

8. Sadun, A. A. and Glaser, J. S., Anatomy of the visual sensory system, in Duane's *Foundations of Clinical Ophthalmology,* Volume 1, Revised edition, Tasman, W. and Jaeger, E. A., Eds., J. B. Lippincott, Philadelphia, 1992.

9. Eggers, H. M., Functional anatomy of the extraocular muscles, in Duane's *Foundations of Clinical Ophthalmology,* Volume 1, Revised edition, Tasman, W. and Jaeger, E. A., Eds., J. B. Lippincott, Philadelphia, 1992.

10. Pedersen, R. A., Abel, L. A., and Troost, B. T., Eye movements, in Duane's *Foundations of Clinical Ophthalmology,* Volume 1, Revised edition, Tasman, W. and Jaeger, E. A., Eds., J. B. Lippincott, Philadelphia, 1992.

11. Levitan, P., Pupillary escape in disease of the retina or optic nerve, *Arch. Ophthalmol.,* 62, 768, 1959.

12. Glaser, J. S. and Goodwin, J. A., Neuro-ophthalmologic examination: The visual sensory system, in Duane's *Clinical Ophthalmology,* Volume 2, Revised edition, Tasman, W. and Jaeger, E. A., Eds., J. B. Lippincott, Philadelphia, 1992.

13. Beck, R. W., Bergstrom, T. J., and Lichter, P. R., The clinical comparison of visual field testing with a new automated perimeter — The Humphrey Field Analyzer and the Goldmann Perimeter, *Ophthalmology,* 92, 77, 1985.

14. Glaser, J. S., Neuro-ophthalmologic examination: General considerations and special techniques, in Duane's *Clinical Ophthalmology,* Volume 2, Revised edition, Tasman, W. and Jaeger, E. A., Eds., J. B. Lippincott, Philadelphia, 1992[b].

15. Smith, C. H. and Beck, R. W., Facial nerve, in Duane's *Foundations of Clinical Ophthalmology,* Volume 1, Revised edition, Tasman, W. and Jaeger, E. A., Eds., J. B. Lippincott, Philadelphia, 1992.

16. Beck, R. W. and Smith, C. H., Trigeminal nerve, in Duane's *Foundations of Clinical Ophthalmology,* Volume 1, Revised edition, Tasman, W. and Jaeger, E. A., Eds., J. B. Lippincott, Philadelphia, 1992.

17. Schubert, D., The possible role of adhesion in synaptic modification, *Trends Neurosci.,* 14, 127, 1991.

18. Black, J. E. and Greenough, W. T., Developmental approaches to the memory process, in *Learning and Memory: A Biological View,* 2nd edition, Martinez, J. L., Jr. and Kesner, R. P., Eds., Academic Press, San Diego, 1991, 61.

19. Richman, J. E. and Cron, M. T., *Guide to Vision Therapy,* Bernell Corp, South Bend, IN, 1988.

8

Rehabilitation and Management of Visual Dysfunction Following Traumatic Brain Injury

Penelope S. Suter

CONTENTS

INTRODUCTION

This chapter surveys the nonsurgical rehabilitative services available to provide effective treatment of brain-injured patients with visual sequelae. It should be a useful reference for those who deal with these patients in intensive rehabilitative environments, as well as for primary care professionals who sometimes find these patients in their care when a rehabilitative hospital or center is not accessible. It may also be useful to vision care providers who are novices in the area of traumatic brain injury (TBI) rehabilitation, as many are, since it is a relatively new field. Many of the therapeutic approaches used with TBI patients were developed for other special needs vision patient populations. For this reason, much of the information provided here is applicable not only to the TBI patient, but also to other patients who have suffered organic insult to the brain. For the same reason, although they may lack specific experience with TBI patients, vision care professionals who practice other forms of visual rehabilitation and vision therapy will often be able to provide appropriate rehabilitation for TBI patients suffering from visual dysfunction.

PHYSICAL SUBSTRATES OF VISION

In the rhesus monkey, which provides an excellent model of the human visual system, more than 50% of the neocortex is involved in visual processing, with approximately 90 intracortical pathways linking at least 19 different cortical areas implicated in visual function.[1] The ganglion cells traveling from the retinae represent approximately 70% of all sensory input fibers to the brain.[2] In addition to multiple subcortical areas (see Chapter 7 in this volume), every lobe of the cortex is involved in visual processing (reviewed by Kaas[3]). The occipital lobe contains primary visual cortex for initial processing of vision as contour, contrast, and depth. The inferior temporal lobe is involved in object identification, the middle temporal area in motion processing, and the parietal lobe in processing for spatial organization and visual attention.[3,4] The frontal eye fields and adjacent areas of the frontal and prefrontal lobes are involved in motor planning and initiation of self-directed eye movements, as well as visual search[5] (Figure 8.1). Considering this, *visual rehabilitation* becomes a sweeping term which ranges from rehabilitation of the eye and surrounding structures, to rehabilitation and management of sensory processing, organization of sensory input from the eye into visual percepts, and use of these percepts to support cognitive or behavioral functions. Visual dysfunction may affect the ability to carry out daily tasks such as reading, driving, walking, and functioning in the workplace. Diagnosis and rehabilitation of the eye, eyelids, extraocular muscles and surrounding bony structure, eye movement and eye teaming disorders, as well as the higher visual functions such as visual perception, spatial organization, and the ability to integrate visual information with other modalities, all fall under the umbrella of visual rehabilitation. Multiple professionals may be involved and considerable networking or case management provides for the most effective care.

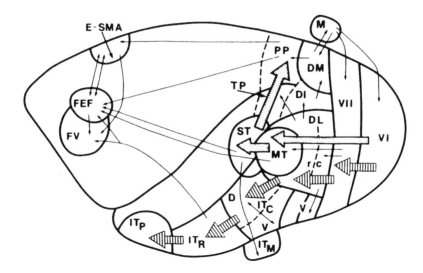

FIGURE 8.1 Areas of visual cortex and some of the ipsilateral cortical connections in visual cortex of the owl monkey. The arrows indicate two major cortical pathways of visual processing. The superior path (dotted arrows) to posterior parietal lobe via the middle temporal area supports "where" processing. The inferior path (hatched arrows) to temporal lobe supports "what" processing. (From Kaas, J. H., Changing concepts of visual cortex organization in primates, In *Neuropsychology of Visual Perception*, Lawrence Erlbaum Associates, Hillsdale, NJ, 1989. With permission.)

THE MULTIDISCIPLINARY APPROACH

Two types of "eye doctors" are frequently required in management of the visual consequences of TBI — the ophthalmologist and the optometrist. In general, their roles may be considered analogous to computer hardware and software repair persons, respectively. The ophthalmologist will often be needed to provide medical/surgical treatment of the "hardware", or anatomical and physiological aspects of the visual system, before the optometrist can provide rehabilitation of the "software", or functional aspects of the visual system.

Ophthalmologists are trained to diagnose and manage damage to the eye and surrounding structures, as well as to diagnose lesions of the visual pathways and ocular motor system. They sometimes prescribe exercises for eye movement disorders which are often performed with the assistance of an occupational therapist. Occasionally, an ophthalmologist will work with an orthoptist, an ophthalmologically trained therapist, to remediate eye teaming disorders such as strabismus. However, ordinarily, ophthalmologists are mostly concerned with providing the medical/surgical support required in early rehabilitation, or for later surgical intervention if spontaneous recovery and therapy fail to produce an acceptable result with a traumatic strabismus.

Neuro-ophthalmologists are ophthalmologists who have specialized in diagnosis and treatment of neurological dysfunction of the visual system. They are more likely to have some experience with rehabilitating the visual software, or application of nonsurgical or pharmacological therapies, than are general ophthalmologists.

Optometrists specializing in vision therapy and/or rehabilitation are trained in diagnosis and nonsurgical treatment of more complex fixation, eye movement or eye teaming (i.e., binocular) disorders, as well as perceptual dysfunctions in the visual system. Usually the treatment of such disorders is performed with the assistance of a vision therapy technician under the doctor's supervision. In an inpatient or rehabilitation center outpatient situation, occupational therapists working under a doctor's supervision or prescription will sometimes assist patients with vision therapy for perceptual and sensorimotor dysfunctions, or less complex eye movement and eye teaming dysfunctions. They may also assist with teaching new living skills to compensate for residual vision deficits.

Optometrists specializing in low vision assessment are trained in prescription of low vision aids for patients with reduced visual acuity, and "field expanders" which may be required for patients with visual field defects. These doctors will often work with or refer to a low vision rehabilitation specialist who can assist in teaching patients new living and mobility skills to cope with their acquired visual deficits.

Vestibular system damage may cause nystagmus, and/or obstruct normal fixation and pursuit. In such a case, referral for vestibular work-up to a professional equipped to perform eye movement recordings for diagnosis and to make rehabilitative recommendations may be helpful. Neuropsychological examination may help to give a broader perspective on visual perceptual dysfunctions. Finally, as with other types of rehabilitation following a TBI, visual rehabilitation may be significantly enhanced by the assistance of a counselor or psychotherapist to assist patients in understanding their new limitations and the need to rehabilitate, as well as managing emotional sequelae which can interfere with effective rehabilitation.

PREVALENCE AND IMPACT OF VISUAL DYSFUNCTION IN TBI PATIENTS

Because of the multifaceted nature of visual dysfunction and the broad distribution of visual functional areas in the brain, many, if not most, TBI patients suffer from some sort of visual dysfunction. Transient changes in refractive error which may last for months or years are common after TBI.[6,7] Accommodative (i.e., focusing) dysfunctions are also common[8] and may interfere with reading, fine depth discriminations, and rehabilitative therapies which are performed at nearpoint. Nearpoint tasks, as well as balance, orientation, mobility, and daily living skills may be affected by field defects and binocular disorders, as well as dysfunctions in visual perception and spatial organization.[7,9] Binocular disorders can cause postural changes as the patient finds ways to either maintain fusion or enhance suppression of one eye by tilting or turning the head and/or torso.

It is often the case with TBI patients that eye care professionals untrained in diagnosing more subtle visual and ocular motor dysfunctions may dismiss patient complaints of headache, dizziness, inability to concentrate, blurred vision, fatigue, light sensitivity, or inability to read as due to emotional or other nonvisual etiologies. While many of these symptoms may have nonvisual causes, a careful assessment of the visual system will often reveal the physiological or perceptual difficulty underlying the patient's complaint.[10] Schlageter et al.[11] found that 71% of TBI patients admitted to an acute rehabilitation center had eye movement or eye teaming dysfunctions. *Therefore, it is important that the TBI patient be examined by an eye/vision care provider who has a special interest in the area of neuro-, rehabilitative, or therapeutic vision care.* See Appendix for a partial list of organizations that can provide educational materials or lists of member doctors who practice in this area.

A literature survey shows some of the types of visual problems encountered. Cohen et al.[12] found convergence insufficiency (i.e., difficulty pulling the eyes inward as is necessary for binocular fixation on near targets) in approximately 40% of both TBI inpatients with recent injuries, and follow-up patients three years postinjury. In the follow-up group, convergence insufficiency was positively correlated with duration of coma, dysphasia, cognitive disturbances, and failure to find placement in nonsupported work situations. Out of 114 patients referred to an ocular motor clinic for visual disturbances following motor vehicle accidents, fourth nerve palsy was noted in 36%, third nerve palsy in 25%, and multiple diagnoses in 25%. Aberrant regeneration was noted in 78% of third nerve palsies.[13] Groswasser et al.[14] found eye movement disturbances related to lesions of the oculomotor, trochlear, and abducens nerves in 19% of severe TBI patients. They also reported bilateral visual field defects in 14% of these patients. The ocular motor defects were associated with poor recovery, as defined by return to work or school. Bilateral visual field defects were more common in the poor recovery group, but this finding was not significant. A 15-year follow-up study of U.S. Vietnam veterans with penetrating head injuries showed that visual field loss and visual memory loss were negatively correlated with return to work.[15] In an assessment of successful vs. unsuccessful TBI clients in a supported employment program, Wehman et al.[16] evaluated the functional limitations of those clients rated "most difficult" and "least difficult" to maintain in an employed situation. The two areas of functional limitations which were significantly different between these groups were visual impairment and fine motor impairment. Najenson et al.[17] found that performance on The Raven Matrices Test — which is heavily loaded for visuospatial performance — was highly correlated with successful performance in the rehabilitated TBI patient's working life.

Lastly, as reviewed by Murray et al.,[18] attentional deficits in TBI patients have recently been considered in terms of information processing models rather than in terms of constructs such as sustained attention or distractibility. They provide evidence for a four-step sequential information processing model[19] in which attentional processes are considered as the sequential stages of 1) feature extraction, 2) identification, 3) response selection, and 4) motor adjustment. Feature extraction and identification are visual system functions. Children who had suffered severe TBI showed significant impairment on complex-choice reaction time tasks designed to test each of these processing areas, as compared to age- and gender-matched controls. Based on these findings, diagnosis and treatment of these primary processing disorders may be the most direct approach to treating attentional disorders in TBI patients.

THERAPEUTIC INTERVENTION: WHAT AND WHY?

Flexibility in the Adult Visual System

The amazing flexibility in modification of the vestibulo-ocular reflex, as well as the visual perceptual apparatus, has been demonstrated in normal adults by application of inverting prisms.[20] Initially, when wearing these prisms, the world appears upside down and backwards, but with continued prism wear, the vestibulo-ocular reflex reverses and the visual perception reverts to normality. Substantial neural plasticity is present in other areas of the adult visual system, as demonstrated by orthoptic therapy remediation of amblyopia and strabismus in adults.[21-23] In the non-TBI population, vision therapy has proven effective for treatment of many visual disorders such as accommodative dysfunctions, eye movement disorders, nonstrabismic binocular dysfunctions such as convergence insufficiency, strabismus, nystagmus, amblyopia, and some visual perceptual disorders in both adults and children.[24-26] Most of these visual disorders may be suddenly acquired with a brain injury.

Remediation of Ocular Motor and Binocular Disorders Following TBI

Vision therapy has also been applied successfully to remediation of vision disorders secondary to brain injury.[27-32] Ron[33] studied six patients with oculomotor dysfunctions resulting from TBI such as saccadic dysmetria and decreased optokinetic nystagmus gain. Both saccades and optokinetic nystagmus normalized more rapidly with training, as compared to control patients, and gains were maintained after cessation of treatment. Convergence insufficiency, as well as strabismus, has also been successfully remediated with vision therapy in brain trauma patients.[28,30,34] In an experiment to test the practicality of applying therapy to vision deficits in a short-term acute care rehabilitation setting, Schlageter et al.[11] failed to show statistically significant improvements from repeated baseline measures on pursuits and saccades in six TBI patients who received between two and six hours of therapy. However, when quality of eye movements was graphed against treatment, the slope increased (showing faster improvement) during therapy for both saccades and pursuits, as compared to the baseline period. Although the occupational therapists and speech pathologists who administered the therapy were trained in a number of therapy techniques for saccades and pursuits, it became apparent during the study that "establishing a hierarchy of progressively more difficult exercises required a significant amount of training",[11] and they may have found even better results had they used staff trained in orthoptic or vision therapy. Because of multiple demands on patient time in the acute care setting, treatment for visual disorders will generally not be completed in this setting. However, progress can be made, and visual dysfunction should be considered when making recommendations for the patient at discharge from acute care.

When surgical intervention is required for remediation of a residual posttraumatic strabismus, patterns of eye movement and teaming must be relearned. Among 92 TBI patients who had extraocular muscle surgery, 50% required more than one surgery, and 30% more than two.[13] Of these patients, 52% had satisfactory outcomes, as defined by a satisfactory field of single binocular vision with tolerable diplopia (i.e., double vision) when shifting gaze to the sides. Another 27% had moderate outcomes, defined as suppression or diplopia with the ability to comfortably ignore one image. Finally, 22% had persistent, troublesome diplopia necessitating occlusion. Their success rates might have been even better had they used functional therapy in conjunction with surgery. Pre- or postsurgical application of therapy can be a useful adjunct to surgery in encouraging fusion, expanding the range of binocular gaze, and eliminating diplopia. Unfortunately, it is common that the professionals who treat strabismus are dichotomized into those practitioners who apply surgery and those who apply functional therapies, without having the two work as a team. Those who apply surgery alone rely on the existing visual system to relearn fusion without any guidance; often, this does not occur. Those who apply therapy alone risk not offering their patients the full range of services to assist in the best possible outcome. As more eye/vision care professionals begin to treat TBI patients, it is hoped an integrated approach will become more widely accepted.

Management of Other Visual Dysfunctions Following TBI

In patients with visual loss as measured by decreased visual acuity or visual field, low vision devices such as magnifiers, special telescopes (some of which may be spectacle mounted), or field expanding devices can be applied. As our population has aged, more research and development has gone into rehabilitation for these types of visual loss, which are frequent sequelae of stroke- and age-related eye disease. Therapy for homonymous hemianopias has been shown to increase speed and breadth of visual search and improve both objective and subjective measures of visual abilities on activities of daily living.[35] Therapy for visual hemifield neglect can be similarly effective.[36]

Therapies for perceptual dysfunctions other than spatial neglect have been previously applied in non-TBI populations by some educators, optometrists, psychologists, and neuropsychologists. Development of computerized therapies for perceptual deficits has made perceptual rehabilitation more accessible and applicable by other therapists, including occupational therapists. As perception is dependent on reception, it is advisable to test for and remediate or manage any sensory visual deficits prior to testing for perceptual dysfunction other than neglect. Present evidence (reviewed by Gianutsos and Matheson[37]) generally supports the efficacy of perceptual therapy following brain injury, although one must be aware that substantial spontaneous recovery occurs during the first six months following the injury.

When to Treat

The timing of therapeutic intervention has been a controversial issue. Some practitioners argue that patients who are diplopic should have visual examinations as soon as possible after they are medically stabilized. Appropriate patching (discussed later) or prism application in the early weeks postinjury can give the patient some relief of symptoms as well as prevent maladaptations which must be trained away later. However, application of either patches or prisms during these early weeks requires frequent reevaluation and adjustment to keep pace with spontaneous resolution of visual defects.

While there is evidence that some visual defects such as muscle palsies and pareses may spontaneously recover up to twelve months postinjury,[38] other evidence shows that, in general, untreated brain-injured persons do not spontaneously recover from binocular disorders such as convergence insufficiency.[12] The decision about when to intervene is most appropriately determined by factors other than the hope of spontaneous recovery.

During the initial three months postinjury, a rapid resolution may occur in many visual defects as edema in the brain diminishes. After this time, although spontaneous resolution may still be ongoing, it is likely to be slower, and unwanted compensatory mechanisms such as suppression set in. Further, in patients who are struggling with such deficits as orientation problems or diplopia, failure to address these difficulties in a timely manner may lead to depression and/or a poor attitude toward rehabilitation when it is finally offered. Patients who are left to their own devices after the acute phase of medical rehabilitation is completed will find ways to survive with remaining deficits — often in ways which are not positive adaptations. Follow-up studies in untreated TBI patients show that they generally do not make continued functional progress, and they may even decline in function over the long run.[37]

Even with the most careful diagnosis, one cannot always tell which patients are going to respond to treatment. In the areas of ocular motor and binocular dysfunction following TBI, reevaluation on a monthly basis can be used to determine whether the patient is making progress. If therapy has been consistent and intensive, and no progress is being made, then compensatory measures should be prescribed. Gianutsos[39] suggests that, in cognitive rehabilitation, intensive rehabilitation with an initial goal of restoration of function should be applied for six months. If no progress is made, then a different approach should be tried. This also seems to be a good rule for visual perceptual rehabilitation, with the modification that some compensatory strategies are often applied immediately to help the patient function while pursuing therapy.

A USEFUL MODEL FOR ORGANIZING VISUAL REHABILITATION

Moore[40] has emphasized the importance of considering functional units in the brain, taking into account contemporary metabolic maps that show brain function, rather than thinking of the brain as it has been mapped in the last century into discrete compartments associated with individual functions. While it is necessary to have an understanding of the neuroanatomy of the visual system in order to help formulate an appropriate diagnosis, "knowing the neurons" does not provide an adequate basis for guiding therapy. It is equally important to have a working model of visual performance to guide rehabilitation efforts and higher order visual testing. Neuropsychological models of information processing, or even of reading, will often begin with a box labeled "visual input" or "sensory input." Exposure to such models may give the nonvision specialist the impression that visual input and its involvement in information processing is discrete and simple enough to fit into such a box. Working without a model of visual processing may encourage attempts to rehabilitate "splinter skills" such as convergence in cases where a more holistic approach is necessary to get the patient reading again or reoriented in space. Many therapy-oriented optometrists use a model of visual processing similar to that developed by Cohen and Rein,[41] shown in Figure 8.2.

Sensory Input/Reception

Visual system input, or reception, is dependent on formation of a focused optical image on the retina, healthy eyes, and healthy, intact pathways to primary visual cortex. Accommodation

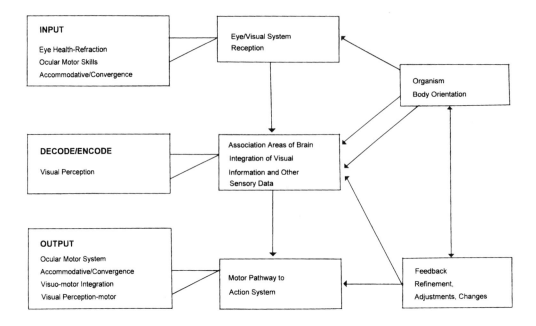

FIGURE 8.2   A model of visual function developed by Cohen and Rein, similar to that used by many optometrists to help guide vision therapy. (From Cohen, A. H. and Rein, L. D., *J. Am. Optom. Assoc.*, 63, 534, 1992. With permission.)

(the internal focusing of the eye mediated by the ciliary muscle) and vergence (the ability to make disjunctive or inward and outward movements of the eyes) are also an important part of getting visual input to the visual cortex without confusion. These two functions are tied together by neural feedback loops. As one expends accommodative effort (trying to focus closer), the accommodative effort drives convergence, pulling the eyes inward. As accommodation is relaxed, the eyes diverge, or relax outward as for viewing distant targets. There is a similar, but lower amplification loop from convergence to accommodation; as one exerts convergence effort, it drives accommodation. It should be obvious that a disruption in the balance between these two interacting systems — accommodative-convergence and convergence-accommodation — can cause serious dysfunction in eye teaming and focusing. There are useful models of such disturbances.[42,43]

Visual reception is also dependent on the ocular motor skills — full range of motion of the extraocular muscles, the ability to fixate the target of regard, track it if desired, or saccade to another target efficiently and accurately. These abilities are dependent on feedback from areas that monitor head and body orientation and movement, as well as those areas that monitor feedback from the ocular motor drivers. Reception ends at primary visual cortex, where the initial binocular combination of input from the two eyes occurs to allow for fusion and stereopsis. The input is processed as color, contour, contrast, and depth.

Perception/Integration

Visual perception and integration are dependent on intact reception, as well as neural communication within visual association areas and pathways between these association areas. Integration is also dependent on pathways to and from association areas mediating other sensory and motor functions. Much of the cerebral cortex is involved in visual processing, with close to 90 intracortical pathways between the visual areas. Therefore, it is important to maintain a holistic model of the functions of this stage of processing so that one can test for and address

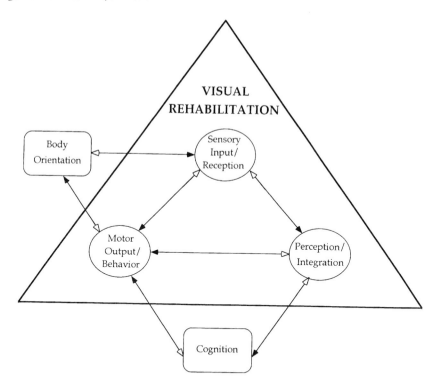

FIGURE 8.3   A modified model for guiding rehabilitation of the visual system. Functions within each processing area (circles) are as delineated in the original model by Cohen and Rein.[41] Visual processes fall within the triangle. Closed head arrows indicate the major direction of information flow. Note that all arrows are bidirectional — information flow is bidirectional in most known pathways in the visual system[1] and other bidirectional influences are explained in text.

functional loss with some guidance from available topographic details of the injury. The major functions of this stage in the model are organization of space and motion, form perception, and object recognition,[41,44] as well as integration of vision with the other senses and motor system input. Interfaces with cognitive processes are not in the original model (Figure 8.2), but should be added at this stage in a bidirectional manner as in the modified model in Figure 8.3. Our percepts feed into cognition, and cognitive processes influence our perceptions.

Two major vision processing pathways proceed forward from the occipital cortex — the "where" pathway to the parietal lobe, and the "what" pathway to the temporal lobe (Figure 8.1). The "where" pathway is first identified anatomically at the lateral geniculate nucleus, where large magnocellular ganglion cells are segregated from the smaller parvocellular ganglion cells. Magno cells are sensitive to large contours, lower contrast, faster temporal frequencies, and are retinotopically distributed more peripherally than parvo cells (reviewed by Bassi and Lehmkuhle[45]). The magno-system is preserved in a relatively segregated manner through primary visual cortex to the middle temporal area for motion processing, and ultimately ends in posterior parietal cortex for cortical processing of object localization and visual attention. Parvo cells subserve focal vision; they transmit more slowly and are more sensitive to high contrast, detailed stimuli. The parvo pathway ultimately traverses to inferior temporal cortex and is involved in object perception (discussed later).

In addition to the magno pathway, an extrageniculate, midbrain visual system[46,47] processes information from both the retina and striate cortex to organize orientation in ambient space. Organization of space and motion by both the cortical magno system and the midbrain "ambient" system requires interpretation of reception from substrates reporting body orientation as well as from the ocular motor drivers in order to ascertain the spatial location of objects in relation to ourselves. This analysis allows us to determine whether we are moving, the external stimulus is moving, or some combination of both.

Feedback from both accommodation and convergence helps localize objects in depth.[48] Form perception and object recognition require figure-ground segregation, form constancy, visual closure, and some processing of spatial relationships. These functions interact with visual reception in that the ability to perform these functions may be limited by field loss or degraded visual acuity, contrast sensitivity, or fixation.

Cross modality integration is dependent on intact pathways to and from the neural substrates mediating the other senses, as well as cortical processing to make matches between them. Object perception includes integration of all our sensory information about the object with the visual input.

Motor Output/Behavior

Organization of body movements in relation to visual targets is mediated most directly by the posterior parietal areas and angular gyrus. Three major pathways connect these areas with the motor areas — one via intracortical connections, one via the basal ganglia, and one via the cerebellum.[20] Individual functions of these three pathways are not well understood.

The percepts of our visual world that we construct during reception and perception are used to guide further motor activity, both in the visual system and in visually guided motor activity such as mobility or eye-hand coordination. These percepts direct our ocular motor activity and eye pointing. They influence the frontal lobe areas which generate "voluntary" eye movements so that we may regard objects at will, rather than in a purely stimulus-driven manner. In short, these visual percepts and the cognitive activity dependent on them are the foundations for much of the everyday behavior of a sighted person.

ASSESSMENT AND REHABILITATION OF THE VISUAL SYSTEM

Assessment and Rehabilitation of Sensory Input/Reception

In the rehabilitation setting, testing and treatment of visual dysfunction has traditionally centered on the higher order perceptual disorders, tending to ignore reception.[46] It is important to keep in mind that many of the higher order visual abilities are dependent on sensory input and ocular motor functions involved in reception.

Eye Movements

Eye movements can be classified into those which shift the direction of gaze (i.e., saccades, smooth pursuits, and vergences) and those which hold the direction of gaze steady (i.e., the vestibular-driven, optokinetic and fixation mechanisms).[49] Vergences are discussed below under binocular disorders. Optokinetic nystagmus (OKN) may be used in testing and therapy for other visual dysfunctions, but deficits in OKN are not generally considered and rehabilitated in the TBI population as visual deficits. This may be because detection of deficits in OKN requires more sophisticated eye movement monitoring than is available in most vision practices.

Saccades

Saccades are the fast eye movements one makes to change the object of fixation without moving the head; the eyes seem to jump from one target to another. They are the movements that take us from word to word in reading and from object to object in driving. Saccades during reading may be affected in a "bottom up" manner, i.e., the eye movement controllers (see Chapter 7 in this volume) have been damaged, or in a "top down" manner, i.e., the ability to comprehend text has been damaged causing more regressions and less accurate fixations due to poor guesses about what is coming next.[50] Patients with acquired primary saccadic dysmetria (i.e., saccades that overshoot or undershoot the target) will often complain of slow and inaccurate reading.

Voluntary saccades, which allow us to change our gaze at will, and stimulus-generated or reflexive saccades, where we correct our gaze or saccade to a target that has attracted our gaze, are controlled, in part, by separate brain centers and should be addressed separately. It is also important to assess the ability to *inhibit* saccades to peripheral targets. This may be a function of the fixation mechanism discussed below. Simple observation while the patient makes voluntary saccades between two targets, or reflexive saccades to alternately lit targets, gives a qualitative measure of latency, speed, and accuracy of the saccades. This procedure should be done at least for lateral saccades in right and left gaze orientation. Each eye should be observed independently. Scoring systems for these observations are reviewed by Griffin.[51]

A more quantitative approach which can provide additional data is provided by the Developmental Eye Movement Test (DEM)*. This is a timed test in which the patient must saccade to numbers which are arrayed on a page and name them as quickly as possible. The DEM is a substantial improvement over earlier saccadic tests of this genre in that timed baseline measurements are taken with the patient reading columns of evenly spaced vertical numbers so that difficulties with decoding or verbal expression can be differentiated from difficulty with the ocular motor task. Next, a series of horizontal rows of digits are read. The number of errors and the time required to read all of the digits are combined into separate scores for the vertical and horizontal tasks, with a higher score being slower or less accurate performance. A high ratio of horizontal score/vertical score indicates a saccadic problem. The DEM does not differentiate between difficulties in speed, latency, or accuracy, although error scores give some indication of the latter. Normative data by age is provided for times and error scores on both the vertical and horizontal tasks, as well as the ratio between them.

A variety of instruments have been designed to objectively monitor and record eye movements. These eye movement monitors give the most easily interpreted data, but are less frequently used in the clinical setting due to issues of availability and expense.

Ordinarily, when training saccades, latency, speed, and accuracy are lumped into the same scores; one trains for speed which improves as any one of the three parameters improves. Therapy may start with something as simple as saccading from one penlight to another as they are alternately lit in a dim room, and progress to complex search tasks such as finding the next in a series of letters or numbers scrambled on a page. Instruments such as the Wayne Saccadic Fixator** or the Acuvision*** with various programs for training saccades in combination with eye-hand coordination are both useful and motivational. A number of computer-based programs have also been developed for orthoptic treatment of ocular motor and binocular disorders. If difficulty inhibiting saccades or sustaining fixation is noted, then one can apply therapies such as making saccades only on a designated command, as in the game of Simon Says, to each in a series of targets. The ultimate goal of therapy is to develop fast, accurate saccades, both large and small, which can be sustained and performed with a high degree of automaticity. The latter is tested by adding a cognitive load such as addition or spelling while the patient does a saccadic task. This is an important concept in much of the visual therapy of eye movements. When a cognitive load is added, performance of the ocular motor task will break down in patients who are *allocating excessive resources to what should be, for the most part, an automatic task.* Griffin[51] has written an excellent text for vision care providers interested in learning about vision therapy programming and specific therapeutic techniques.

---

* Developmental Eye Movement Test: Available from Bernell Corporation, South Bend, IN.
** Wayne Saccadic Fixator: Available from Wayne Engineering, Northfield, IL.
*** Acuvision: Available from International Acuvision Systems, Inc., Carlsbad, CA.

Many of these therapy techniques may be prescribed for application by occupational therapists in the rehabilitation setting.

Pursuits

Pursuits are the smooth eye movements used to follow a moving object and hold a clear image of it stationary on the retina. They are complementary to the vestibulo-ocular reflex in holding images stationary on the retina when we are moving. Pursuits are limited in speed to about 30 degrees per second. Attempts to track a faster target cause saccadic intrusions and "cogwheeling" of the movement. Pursuits are usually tested at the same time that the range of extraocular muscle motion in each eye is tested. Simple observation gives qualitative information about the ability to track a target to the full range of motion of each of the extraocular muscles monocularly, and then binocularly. The ability to track should be judged on smoothness, accuracy, stamina, and the ability to track without head movement. As with saccades, a cognitive load may be applied to judge automaticity. Griffin[51] outlines systems for scoring pursuits.

Therapy for pursuits is often combined with extraocular "stretching" exercises relieving restrictions or contractures of the extraocular muscles by following targets to the farthest peripheral directions of gaze possible. These exercises are also important in the initial stages of therapy for binocular disorders. If there is any deficit on monocular testing, extraocular movements are trained monocularly prior to training binocularly so that equal facility is gained with each eye before adding a fusional load to the task.

For most vision therapy, one goal is to make the patient self-monitoring. Pursuit therapy is most effective when patients can be made aware of jerkiness or saccadic intrusions in their pursuits, so that they can try to correct them. Many patients will be able to feel their eyes "jump" when their attention is directed to noticing interruptions in their smooth pursuit. However, in many TBI patients, proprioception from the extraocular muscles seems to be diminished or absent so that they are unable to feel when their eyes jump. In such cases, cues can be added to assist the patient. One technique is to use afterimages to tag the fovea by using a camera flash which has been masked off except for a small central target on which the patient fixates while the flash is triggered. The patient tries to maintain this afterimage on the pursuit target without interruption. A simpler technique, which is sometimes effective, is to have the therapist tell patients every time their eyes jump, until the patients can begin to feel it for themselves.

Various instruments, from rotating discs with targets on them to computer-generated pursuit games, have been designed for facilitating pursuit therapy under both monocular and fused conditions. The ultimate goal of therapy is to be able to sustain smooth pursuits with either or both eyes in all fields of gaze with a high degree of automaticity, and without moving one's head.

Vestibular-Driven Eye Movements

Vestibular-driven eye movements, in particular the vestibulo-ocular reflex (VOR), help hold the visual world steady as we move within it. Patients who do not spontaneously adapt to damage affecting the VOR may complain of oscillopsia, or rhythmic movement of stationary objects. One way to test a VOR problem is to have patients read a nearpoint acuity card while shaking their head side to side. In the case of a VOR dysfunction, the visual acuity will be severely degraded as compared to an acuity taken with the stationary target.[52] While therapy techniques have not been specifically developed for VOR dysfunction, applying the afterimage techniques discussed above with the patient attempting to stabilize the afterimage, initially while sitting still and later with head movements, may give enough extra feedback to assist in recovery. Whether the patient recovers, or learns to adjust to the movement, oscillopsia should be taken into consideration in driving rehabilitation.

Fixation

Fixation, or the act of holding gaze steady on a target, was once thought to be a function of the pursuit system at zero velocity. This may be why fixation itself is seldom evaluated except in relation to strabismic amblyopia. However, recent evidence implicates an independent visual fixation system, perhaps located in the parietal lobe.[49] Disturbances in fixation may be considered in terms of inability to sustain fixation, as well as inability to fixate centrically and steadily. The former can be easily observed by having the patient hold fixation on a target for a minute. The ability to fixate steadily and centrically is only observable with special techniques. The easiest, most objective measure is with a visuoscope, or similarly, an ophthalmoscope with a central target. The examiner looks into the patient's eye with the scope which projects a target onto the retina. Both the anatomy of the posterior pole of the eye and the projected target are viewed simultaneously. The patient is instructed to fixate the target while covering the other eye. The stability of the foveal reflex and centricity with regard to the target are easily observed in this manner. Other methods require reliable subjective feedback. For instance, the Haidinger brush, an entoptic phenomenon which marks the fovea, may be elicited with an instrument such as the Macula Integrity Tester*; the patient fixates a target and reports the location and stability of the Haidinger brush in relation to the fixated target.

In the case of inadequate ability to sustain fixation, the first step is to rule out binocular, accommodative, or other ocular motor dysfunctions that may lead to asthenopia (i.e., eyestrain and/or headache) or discomfort. Such dysfunctions may make extended viewing aversive. They are also remediable, where a primary attention or fixation mechanism dysfunction might not be.

Unsteady and/or eccentric fixation are most typically encountered as developmental phenomena associated with strabismic amblyopia. In this manifestation, they cause decreased visual acuity, but are seldom accompanied by asthenopic symptoms. There is an effective arsenal of therapeutic techniques to routinely remediate developmental eccentric fixation.[23,51] Unfortunately, unsteady fixation which is acquired following TBI may cause asthenopic symptoms, as it may be bilateral rather than unilateral, and it may be more resistant to treatment (see the case report on L. D. later in this chapter). More case reports and research are necessary. As vision care professionals become aware of the need to assess fixation in TBI patients, more data will become available.

Binocular Dysfunction

Accommodation

Accommodative dysfunctions are common in the TBI population.[6] They can cause blur and/or asthenopic symptoms at nearpoint, as well as slow focus change from distance to near and back. *A simple nearpoint acuity test does not rule out an accommodative problem* because it only indicates whether the patient can momentarily hold focus at near. It does not indicate whether patients can sustain that focus, or whether they have any focusing flexibility. Objective techniques, such as nearpoint retinoscopy performed while the patient processes visual information (e.g., reading or active involvement in viewing a picture), give an accurate assessment of the patient's lag of accommodation and ability to sustain accommodation on a nearpoint task. Use of such tools as convex-to-concave lens "flippers" (i.e., devices with two pairs of lenses for viewing — one pair of convex lenses which requires that accommodation relax to clear the target, and one pair of concave lenses which requires accommodative effort to clear the target — set into a holder so that one can "flip" between the pairs of lenses) of various powers can give measurements of facility. These can be used as a subjective test with

---

* Macula Integrity Tester: Available from Bernell Corporation, South Bend, IN.

patients reading small print as they are able to clear it, or as an objective test during retinoscopy. As discussed above, accommodative difficulties can cause convergence dysfunction and convergence difficulties can cause accommodative dysfunction. In many cases, it is impossible to tell which problem is primary.

Typical treatments for accommodative dysfunctions are vision therapy or convex lenses worn either as single vision reading glasses or bifocals. In a prepresbyopic patient, exercises are an effective way to improve the amplitude and facility of accommodation, provided that the innervation subserving the function is somewhat intact. Near-to-far focusing jumps and concave-to-convex lens jumps with nearpoint targets may increase both amplitude and facility. Associated vergence difficulties must be treated in conjunction with the accommodative problem for effective remediation. If rehabilitation of accommodative function is not possible in the young patient, then compensatory convex reading lenses should be prescribed, generally in a bifocal format. Treatment of convergence insufficiency due to the sudden loss of the accommodative-convergence mechanism may be necessary in these patients.

Nonstrabismic Binocular Disorders

Nonstrabismic binocular disorders are those eye-teaming difficulties which do not result in a frank strabismus (eyeturn). Convergence insufficiency — difficulty pulling the eyes inward for near work — may be the most common nonstrabismic binocular finding in TBI patients. *Convergence insufficiency will often be missed by the simple "pushup" or nearpoint of convergence test.* Krohel et al.[34] found that six of 23 TBI patients with convergence insufficiency had a normal nearpoint of convergence, but showed abnormal convergence reserves on prism testing. Prism vergence ranges should be mandatory in the visual evaluation of the TBI patient. Convergence insufficiency can lead to fatigue, headache, tearing, blurred vision, and eyestrain.[34] Often it will cause skipping of words while reading or transpositions when reading digits in numbers as the eyes struggle to converge after each saccade. High exophoria (i.e., nonstrabismic *outward* resting posture of the eyes) is also a common finding in TBI patients. Padula et al.[7] hypothesizes that exodeviations of the eyes following TBI are caused by damage to the midbrain structures which integrate ambient vision and spatial orientation.[47] This would be anatomically consistent with simultaneous damage to the mesencephalic structures involved in convergence control.[12]

Prior to treating any binocular disorder, eye movement and accommodative dysfunctions should be treated insofar as possible. Treatment of exo binocular disorders may include prism in reading or distance lenses, or therapy. One difficulty with putting base-in prism in lenses is that patients may prism adapt over a matter of days or weeks, developing the same phoria through the prisms as they had prior to introduction of the prisms. In such cases, the prescription of base-in prism increases the tonic error in binocular posture — leading some optometrists to argue that "prism is poison." However, in a significant number of patients, base-in prisms provide an immediate reduction of symptoms and the patients do not prism adapt. The difficulty is in determining for which patients this will be the case. In-office, short-term trials may help in this decision. In any case, patients wearing base-in prism in their habitual spectacles should be followed carefully. If they prism adapt, additional prism should not be prescribed.

Besides use of base-in prism, Padula and Shapiro[8] recommend use of bitemporal or binasal occluders (i.e., occluders covering only the temporal portion of both lenses or nasal portion of both lenses, respectively) applied to the patient's habitual spectacles for nonstrabismic visual dysfunctions. They suggest that bitemporal patches may reduce confusion by reducing input from the midbrain ambient vision system when the patient is attempting *focal* tasks such as reading. Binasal patches may be used in an effort to increase patients' awareness of their *ambient* vision while eliminating physiological diplopia (i.e., the normal diplopia for objects in front of or behind the plane of fixation) which may initially cause confusion in the post-TBI patient. They also feel that this encourages reorganization of the midbrain-based ambient visual system which is critical for visuospatial organization and vision during movement.

Vision therapy for poorly compensated exophoria or convergence insufficiency should include fusional exercises to improve the amplitude of and ability to sustain convergence, as well as the speed of reflex fusion. Convex lenses may be used to work fusional convergence through the accommodative-convergence loop. Viewing through the convex lens relaxes accommodative-convergence so that the patient must exert more fusional convergence to avoid diplopia. Prisms can be used for manipulating images, causing the fusional vergence system to respond to the displaced image. Polarized or anaglyphic materials may be used in order to create second- or third-degree fusion targets (i.e., flat fusion or stereoscopic fusion, respectively) which can be manipulated to expand vergence ranges. At the same time, matches are developed between the ocular motor feedback and position-in-space interpretation. Many specialized instruments have been developed for treatment of such binocular disorders. Some of these techniques may be prescribed for application by occupational therapists. Many of these techniques require more experience in vision therapy for effective application, or more extensive instrumentation and, therefore, need to be performed in the vision care setting.

Esophoric (i.e., nonstrabismic *inward* resting posture of the eyes) deviations of binocular vision are less common. This may be due to anatomical considerations, or because esophorias are more difficult to compensate for and are more likely to break down into a strabismus. Poorly compensated esophoria will often cause eyestrain or headache around the eyes or temples. Treatment may include use of convex lenses for near work, base-out prism and vision therapy similar to that described for exodeviations. The same cautions regarding use of prisms apply here — perhaps even more so, as base-out prism is more difficult to remove once the patient has become dependent on it.

Strabismus

In strabismic deviations secondary to TBI, diplopia causes disorientation, and difficulty with spatial judgments, hand-eye coordination, mobility, and reading. Patients will often squint, or assume head turns or tilts in order to try to block one eye or to keep objects in a field of gaze where they are able to fuse. In children, suppression and amblyopia may result. Patients who are diplopic should have a visual examination early in their rehabilitative program. Assessment of refractive status, binocularity, and ocular health do not require verbal communication from the patient. The same objective techniques that one would use to determine these conditions in a four-month-old infant can be applied in the TBI population when necessary. Prisms or patching (as discussed below) can be prescribed to eliminate diplopia so that other ongoing therapies can be more effective. Any time that prisms or patches are prescribed, frequent follow-up is required to keep pace with spontaneous and therapy-related recovery.

Fresnel (flat, stick-on) prisms may be applied in an effort to reestablish fusion at the angle of the deviation. Lenses may also be applied in a therapeutic manner, using the accommodation–convergence relationship to mediate the angle of the deviation. For patients who are able, therapy is then applied as described above for nonstrabismic errors, creating equal, efficient monocular skills, followed by vergence exercises combined with fusion, depth, and spatial localization training. Initial attempts at reestablishing fusion in adjustable instruments or with variable prisms may be met with horror fusionis-like responses where the images from the two eyes will approach each other and then jump to the other side, or may be superimposed, but not fuse into one object with the percept of depth.[53] The prognosis for recovery is best for patients with horizontal strabismus, uncomplicated by vertical deviations. However, vertical deviations will often resolve with therapy, or as therapy is applied to the horizontal component of the strabismus. Residual vertical deviations can often be managed with prism ground into the patient's lenses. Patients who are not able to perform vision therapy for remediation of their strabismus are managed over the long term with patches and prism.

Traditionally, TBI patients have been advised to use constant patching of one eye to resolve diplopia. However, this has undesirable consequences such as loss of peripheral vision on the patched side while patched, and disuse of the patched eye which may lead to suppression and/or diminish the chances of spontaneous recovery of fusion. *Partial* patching to eliminate diplopia or *patching for limited time periods* to facilitate other therapies is more desirable. If patients are unable to access rehabilitative vision care in a timely manner and diplopia is a major problem, patching the eyes on a daily alternating schedule may minimize the detrimental effects of patching until they can access such care.

Partial patches are tailored to the patient's particular deficit and should, when possible, encourage recovery. As discussed above, binasal patches applied to the patient's spectacles allow for a full field of vision while eliminating diplopia. They are a particularly good patching method for treatment of esotropia and may enhance peripheral awareness while encouraging abduction. If the esotropia is unilateral, a single patch may be applied to the nasal portion of the patient's spectacles over the nondeviating eye. This technique encourages abduction of the esotropic eye, as the patient must either abduct that eye or turn his head to view in the visual field ipsilateral to the deviating eye. Exotropic deviations may sometimes be treated with bitemporal patches. Thus, each eye must adduct to view in the contralateral field. However, bitemporal patches *limit peripheral vision* and are not recommended for long-term application. For patients who fuse in some fields of gaze, but have noncomitant strabismic deviations, partial patches may be applied to a portion of one spectacle lens to occlude only the diplopic field of gaze, allowing for fusion most of the time. At the same time, vision therapy should be applied to expand the field of comfortable binocular vision.

Partial patches may be as inexpensive as a piece of translucent tape applied to the patient's spectacle lenses. Cling patches* are also available commercially. These patches, which stick to the lenses electrostatically, may be easily removed for therapy and reapplied. These also come in varying densities to degrade visual acuity to approximately 20/100, 20/200, or 20/400. The less dense patches enhance patient acceptance as they are cosmetically quite good, and can hardly be discerned on the spectacle lenses by outside observers. Binasal, bitemporal, and partial patching may not work well for persons with various types of field defects.

Because most TBI patients with secondary strabismus had normal fusion prior to their injury, their prognosis is good for recovering fusion even if one or more muscles are palsied. Even in apparent paresis of the muscle, recovery can occur, although the prognosis is more guarded. If a horror fusionis-like response is elicited on initial testing, peripheral fusion techniques emphasizing depth and SILO (see below) may be used until the patient is able to fuse more central targets. Antisuppression therapy should not be used on these patients until there is evidence of their ability to attain central fusion.

Suppression

Suppression is the ability to diminish or eliminate the central vision originating from one eye to avoid diplopia. In children, it may lead to development of amblyopia in a unilaterally suppressed eye. Once suppression develops, antisuppression therapies must be applied in order to continue with fusional training.

Suppression may be considered either a blessing or a curse, depending on the goal of rehabilitation. If the goal is to restore central fusion with all of the fine motor and stereoscopic advantages that come with it, then suppression is to be avoided through proper application of prisms, patching, or early application of vision therapy. If spontaneous resolution and three months of intensive vision therapy show no progress at all toward fusion, then perhaps encouraging suppression to develop may be the most effective way of avoiding diplopia.

If the patient cannot learn to successfully fuse or suppress, then a "monovision" refractive correction may be prescribed, where the spectacle or contact lens for one eye is set for near

---

* Cling Patch: Available from Bernell Corporation, South Bend, IN.

work and the other lens is set for distance clarity. This creates one clear image at each distance so that, with practice, the patient learns to easily attend to the clear image, giving a stable referent at each distance.

Decreased Visual Acuity

TBI patients with decreased visual acuity which cannot be improved by refractive means or by increased contrast will generally profit from standard low vision rehabilitation techniques. Unfortunately, the prospect of accepting their limitations and working hard to learn to use the remaining vision in the most efficient manner possible is not as motivating as the prospect of performing other types of therapy to recover lost visual function. This makes low vision rehabilitation a less positive experience for many patients.

Numerous small telescopes have been developed for magnification of distant objects. These may be handheld for stationary viewing, or for spotting and identification. Increased magnification results in reduced visual field. Therefore, telescopes used only for spotting and identification will generally have higher magnification than telescopes used for distance viewing. Telescopes may also be mounted in the top portion of a spectacle lens for frequent spot reference during such tasks as driving and note taking. A slight downward tilt of the head allows access to the telescope.

For nearpoint tasks, aids range from high-powered convex lenses for nearpoint work, allowing the patient to hold reading material closer, to video enhancement of images via closed circuit television. Bar magnifiers may assist the low visual acuity patients in keeping their place during reading. Magnifiers that are handheld or stand-mounted for stability are also frequently used.

One of the difficulties in prescribing for the patient with moderately reduced acuity (20/60 to 20/120) is that many magnifying techniques will slow the process of reading. One must judge whether the patient can be rehabilitated with convex lenses and proper training, or whether a magnifier will be of greater assistance. Trial and error to find the correction with which the patient is most comfortable will be a large part of the decision.

Decreased Contrast Sensitivity

Contrast sensitivity is the ability to discriminate differences in luminance of adjacent areas. Low contrast situations occur in fog, darkness, and when viewing through media opacities in the eye such as cataracts. Reduced contrast sensitivity should be suspected when patients with good visual acuity complain of not seeing well. Neural damage in the visual system may also cause poor contrast sensitivity.[54] Damage to the magno system results in a reduction of contrast sensitivity for middle to low spatial frequency (larger contours). Damage to the parvo system results in loss of contrast sensitivity in detailed targets and may result in decreased visual acuity. Patients with diminished contrast sensitivity in the high frequency range, with decreased visual acuity, may find magnifying low vision aids helpful. Those with diminished contrast sensitivity for middle to low spatial frequencies are not helped by magnification. Printed material for these patients should be good quality and high contrast. In well-lit conditions, contrast-enhancing tints (usually yellow to amber tints that screen out blue light) or overlays may be used. The selection of tint is usually based on the patient's subjective assessment of the quality of their vision. Working with special lighting for specific tasks may be helpful.

Visual Field Loss

Many patients with TBI have resultant visual field loss. Knowledge of visual field defects is important in helping patients adjust their behavior. It is also important for other rehabilitative therapists working with the patient to adjust their therapy, taking the field defect into account.

Field defects may be either absolute, where there is no sensation of light or movement from within the scotoma, or relative, where brighter, larger, or moving stimuli may still be sensed within the scotoma. Assessment may range from simple confrontation testing to tangent screen to automated perimetry with a fixation monitor. Each has advantages and drawbacks. Confrontation testing can be done with no special equipment on patients who are unable to sit as required for the other tests. It gives a gross assessment of the extent of the visual field, in each direction, with each eye; however, it will not reveal scotomas within those boundaries. Tangent screen testing allows the examiner to very closely map small scotomas and islands of vision within the field, which may not be mapped well on an automated perimeter that presents test points in a predetermined pattern. Automated perimeters with fixation monitoring give a relatively reliable measurement against which one may chart change in the visual field through repeated measures across time. However, the testing is often lengthy, taxing both posture and attention.

The most common visual field defect necessitating rehabilitative services is probably homonymous hemianopia. Rehabilitation has mainly been concentrated on recognizing the field defect and working on compensatory scanning patterns, as well as mirror or prism devices, to allow more peripheral areas of the scotoma to be viewed with smaller excursions of the head or eyes. Compensatory visual search into the scotomatous field is found to expand as a result of training, and these gains remain stable over time. Patients with hemianopic field defects who do not receive training do not tend to use adaptive search strategies.[55]

Mirrors can be mounted on spectacle lenses[56,57] or Fresnel prisms with their apices toward the pupil can be added in the peripheral portion of the lens in the scotomatous field(s).[58] These devices move the images that fall in the periphery of the scotomatous field closer to the center of vision. Both of these techniques enhance peripheral awareness because it is easier to view farther into the scotomatous field without head movement, and having the device applied to the spectacles serves as a reminder to do so. Considerable training and motivation are required for successful application of these devices.

For patients with severe visual field constriction, the Fresnel prism technique may be used in all affected fields.[59] Also, field expanders or reverse telescopes may be helpful in occasional sighting for orientation, as when entering a room or locating objects on a table. The Amorphic lens*, which minifies in the horizontal meridian, may be mounted in a spectacle frame and may be useful for expanding the horizontal field during mobility.[57] Distortion and minification when viewing through field expanders make them difficult to use and, again, considerable training and motivation are required.[60]

Perceptual speed and perceptual span, often trained with tachistoscopic techniques, are also important. During mobility, the patient with visual field loss must make more fixations to cover the necessary visual expanse. Perceptual speed and span are also important for reading, as any visual field loss that approaches the midline will tend to slow the reading process. Patients with left field loss may not see the beginnings of longer words and misread them as similar words. They also have difficulty returning to the beginning of the next line. The simplest technique for remediating this problem is to keep a finger at the beginning of the next line down. Typoscopes or rulers may be helpful. Patients with right hemifield loss lose the preview information that allows them to judge the placement of the next saccade and guess at the content of the next word. They also have difficulty judging where to return at the end of a line of print and will often return to the next line too early. A finger or hand, held at the end of the line, serves as an easy marker. These patients may do better to read upside down, or rotate the text 90 degrees and read vertically so that they can preview the text coming up in their sound visual field.[61]

Lastly, there have been reports in the literature of some minor resolution of hemianopia through training with lit targets moving from the scotoma toward the intact visual field and

---

* Amorphic lens: Available from Designs for Vision, Inc., Ronkonkoma, NJ.

scanning into the scotoma.[35,62] These findings have been questioned by Balliet et al.,[63] who were unable to replicate the findings. They bring up valid concerns regarding this controversial issue. However, Balliet et al. used smaller targets in their training than were used in the original studies because the smaller target led to less intrasubject variability. In therapy, variable responses may be the hallmark of recovery. In their desire for scientific reproducibility, Balliet et al. may have thrown away the therapeutic effect. Kerkhoff et al.,[35] in a study which had positive results, used a three-step training procedure which included 1) performing large saccades into the blind field, 2) improving visual search on projected slides, and 3) transfer of both to activities of daily living. With this procedure, they were training skills that the patient needed to acquire, and partial resolution of the scotoma seemed to be an additional gift for some of their patients.

Photophobia

Photophobia (i.e., extreme light sensitivity) is a common aftereffect of head trauma.[64] Patients who have posttraumatic binocular disorders or pupil dilation of one or both eyes may also complain of photophobia. This may be handled with any number of tints in the patient's spectacle lenses — the color and density of which are mainly prescribed for subjective comfort. Photochromic lenses which darken in sunlight and lighten indoors may be helpful, although they do not darken well for driving applications. While eye protection from ultraviolet radiation should be a consideration for everyone, it is even more important to incorporate ultraviolet protection into tinted lenses for patients with mydriatic pupils. In extreme cases of mydriasis, it is sometimes possible to prescribe an opaque custom contact lens with a small transparent pupil to decrease the light entering the eye. However, patients with mydriatic pupils often have dry eyes, and contact lenses would be contraindicated.

Assessment and Rehabilitation of Perception/Integration

Localization and Spatial Vision

There is little information on effects of brain injury on the magno-pathway until it reaches cortex. However, it is known that the large axon diameter of the magno-cells makes them more vulnerable to various types of damage, as in glaucoma and Alzheimer's disease.[45] Disorders of motion perception are rare.[65] Indeed, lesion studies in monkeys show that a lesion in the middle temporal area produces disorders of motion perception, but that most of these disappear within a few days, presumably because the function is taken over by redundant pathways. Damage to the posterior cerebral cortex (usually, right posterior parietal) often results in spatial inattention to the contralateral visual field known as *unilateral spatial neglect* (USN) discussed below.

A number of dysfunctions of reception affect perception of spatial localization and orientation. For instance, we use the feedback from our vergence system to assist us in judging distance. If our eyes are more converged, then the target we are fixating is seen as closer. In persons with good binocularity, this effect, called *SILO* (Smaller In, Larger Out),[66] can be demonstrated by the use of prisms. If one fixates a target and places a base-out prism in front of the eyes, then the images of the target are moved in a convergent direction and the eyes must converge in order to avoid diplopia. The target will be perceived as having moved *In* toward the observer, and will appear *Smaller* than before. Size constancy dictates that objects get larger as they come closer, but since the target has not really moved, the image size on the retina remains unchanged. Therefore, since the vergence system says the object is closer, but the image size remains unchanged, the interpretation must be that the object is now smaller. Base-in prism produces the opposite effect where the eyes diverge, the object appears to move *Out*, away from the observer and appears *Larger*. Due to the roles of accommodation and convergence in depth perception,[48] sudden onset of dysfunctions in accommodation or convergence secondary to TBI can make objects appear closer or farther away than they actually are, effectively collapsing or expanding visual space.

Conversely, feedback from the cortical and/or subcortical spatial processors affect the vergence system. For example, one type of convergence is driven strictly by proximity to an object; targets close to the face make us converge even though we may be viewing through an optical system set at infinity. The TBI patient with a primary visuospatial disturbance will often have inaccurate eye pointing.

As in the model (Figure 8.3), feedback runs both ways, from the binocular system to visuospatial processors and from visuospatial processors to the binocular system. Therefore, the most effective therapy for disorders of spatial perception in depth must take into account the binocular response. Similarly, the most effective treatment for eye teaming will often concentrate not only on achieving the correct motor response, but in creating correct spatial judgments which can be used to guide the motor response.

Other difficulties in spatial organization may be reflected in inability to properly localize objects in relation to ourselves. Egocentric "midline shifts" of varied etiologies have been noted in patients following brain injury. These shifts in midline perception can cause shifts in posture and weight distribution which may cause difficulty with balance and gait. They may also affect eye-hand coordination. Tests used to detect midline shifts include line bisection tasks[67,68] and subjective judgment of when a small object moved laterally or horizontally is directly on the horizontal midline, or level with the eyes.[8] Visual field defects, hemifield visual neglect, disruption of the midbrain ambient visual system, tonic oculomotor imbalance, and imbalances in extraocular proprioception, or efferent copy commands to the extraocular muscles, are all possible causes of midline shift. Tonic oculomotor imbalance is an increased tone in the muscles turning the eyes to the side contralateral to the lesion. During routine testing, it is masked by the fixation mechanism, but it can be elicited by having the patient attempt to look straight ahead in darkness.[69] During development, we learn to maintain position constancy of objects in spite of eye movements by comparing the efferent copy (commands going out to the eye muscles) and proprioceptive information received from the eye muscles, with the movement of the retinal image.[49] As the eyes, extraocular muscles, and separation between the eyes grow and change, slow adjustments in these systems take place. However, in TBI, a sudden change in any one of these systems may occur, changing the perceived location of objects in relation to ourselves.

Therapy for spatial distortions may include therapy for accommodative and convergence disorders as described above, with special emphasis on development of SILO and spatial localization. Lenses and prisms may be applied in either a compensatory manner or for therapy purposes. Spatial and postural effects of these optical devices are thoroughly reviewed by Press.[70] Padula et al.[7] advocates use of small amounts of base-in prism in order to facilitate reorganization of the ambient system by reducing stress on the peripheral fusional system in cases of exophoria. Yoked prisms (i.e., equal amounts of prism in front of each eye with both bases in the same direction — up, down, right, or left) are an effective intervention for many cases of midline shift. These prisms move images of the surrounds in the direction of the apex of the prism for both eyes. Low amounts may be used in a compensatory manner to shift the midline back toward center. More often, large amounts such as 15 prism diopters will be used in therapy to force problem solving and increase flexibility in the sensorimotor system. Activities such as walking or tapping a swinging ball while wearing these prisms involve recalibration and integration of vestibular, proprioceptive, kinesthetic, and extraocular efferent copy systems. This is an extremely effective technique for disrupting habitual patterns in patients who have been unresponsive to more instrument-based therapies so that, with guidance, they can reorganize their visual-motor system in a more adaptive manner. It is important to note that, in an observer with a normal visual system, prism adaptation would be expected to occur with long-term wear. Therapeutically, yoked prisms are only worn for periods extending from a few minutes to a few hours. Presumably, those individuals who experience a long-term compensatory effect wearing yoked prism full-time have visual dysfunctions which preclude prism adaptation to this prescription. This reasoning makes sense in that, if these patients had been able to do the sort of reorganization that prism adaptation requires, they would probably not have sustained an egocentric midline shift.

Unilateral Spatial Neglect

USN is a phenomenon where an entire hemifield (usually the left) is simply unattended, as if a hemianopia existed there. Worse, patients are unaware of the defect. This makes them more prone to accident and more difficult to rehabilitate than the hemianope without neglect. When neglect affects only the visual system, it may easily be mistaken for hemianopia, and indeed often coexists with true hemianopia. Recently, split-brain research has provided evidence that the right hemisphere allocates attention to both visual fields, where the left hemisphere allocates attention to only the contralateral field. This finding in split-brain patients suggests that the right hemisphere allocation of attention to right visual field is probably mediated through subcortical mechanisms.[71] It may also help explain why most cases of neglect are secondary to right brain damage.

Various tests, including drawing, line cancellation, pointing to objects scattered around the room, reading a newspaper article, and line bisection, have been developed to determine the presence of USN. USN may vary in degree and appear on some tests but not others.[72] Inattention may also be differentially distributed along the vertical meridian of the neglected field.[68,73] As reviewed by Kerkhoff et al.,[35] during line bisection tasks, patients with neglect typically transect the line off to the side contralateral to the field defect. Patients with hemianopia generally do the opposite, deviating in the direction of the scotoma. Patients with both are more likely to bisect the line. Compared to patients with hemianopia without USN, patients with USN have even more abnormal scan paths when viewing simple figures, with fewer excursions into the "blind" field.[74]

Clinically, three considerations are important during therapy for USN (N. W. Margolis, Arlington Heights, IL, personal communication). First, the patient must be made aware of the condition. Second, compensatory strategies such as scanning and reading strategies should be taught. Lastly, these strategies must be generalized to both *predictable stimuli*, such as those encountered in reading or walking down a familiar corridor, and to *nonpredictable stimuli*, as encountered in new environments. Gordon et al.[75] present a three-step program for remediation of perceptual deficits in patients with right brain damage. Step 1 is basic scanning training, Step 2 is somatosensory awareness and horizontal size estimation, and Step 3 is complex visual perception training combined with left-to-right visual scanning within these tasks. They present evidence that, with extensive training, these functions generalize to daily living. Gianutsos and Matheson[37] review the literature on perceptual rehabilitation in USN and conclude that, overall, the efficacy of therapeutic intervention is supported. However, studies of solely microcomputer-based scanning therapy have not been shown to generalize.[76,77]

Object Perception

The visual percept we construct from sensory signals supersedes even the concrete sensation of touch. For instance, if an object such as a square of plastic is viewed through a minifying lens and is simultaneously manipulated by the hand (with the hand covered so that it cannot be used as a visual cue), the observer reports the square as being smaller than the real square. This is true whether the method of report is visual, i.e., picking a matching square out of a range of squares of various sizes; visual and tactile, i.e., drawing the square to size; or surprisingly, tactile, i.e., picking a matching square by touch alone.[78]

It has been suggested that, visually, we construct perceptual objects via a two-step process.[79] First preattentive data-driven filtering produces shapes and registers their features, as in reception. Then focal attention is used to select a spatial location and integrate the features registered there into a perceptual object. This is analogous to figure-ground organization, and should be concept-driven processing rather than data- or sensation-driven. Evidence arguing for this feature integration theory comes from the way that stabilized retinal images fade feature by feature rather than in small random parts. Principles at work during the second integration stage may be the Gestalt principles of proximity, good continuation, similarity, closure, and *pragnanz* (i.e., simplicity, regularity, or symmetry) or local vs. global processing. In addition to integrating visual features, object perception includes cross-modality integration — i.e., integrating auditory, tactile, and olfactory sensations with visual information to complete the perceptual object. Spatial orientation, both the ability to process the orientation of external objects (extrapersonal orientation) and the ability to process the orientation of ourselves with regard to other objects (personal orientation), is discussed here, because the treatment modalities are generally more similar to those used with object perception, rather than other spatial dysfunctions. Personal orientation may be supported by the frontal lobe (particularly in the left hemisphere); extrapersonal orientation may be supported by the "where" pathway, particularly the right posterior parietal area.

Assessment and treatment of perceptual/integrative vision must take into account dysfunctions in reception. Multiple tests, with some redundancy, are necessary to differentially diagnose perceptual dysfunction of the visual system. For instance, copy-form tests are useful, and may tell you something about spatial organization, but if the forms are poorly reproduced, you do not know whether this is due to difficulties in reception, perception, visuomotor integration, or fine motor coordination. One must have a battery of tests that probe perceptual functions such as figure-ground discrimination, closure, spatial organization, as well as cross-modality and visual motor integrative functions from different perspectives using different modalities. Usually, visual short-term memory and sequential memory should also be tested. Gianutsos and Matheson[37] reviews most of the available perceptual tests in the literature. For a sample test battery, see Aksionoff and Falk.[80] The perceptual work-up will generally take two to three hours to administer, and may need to be broken up into multiple sessions for TBI patients who fatigue easily.

During therapy, the patient and therapist must constantly keep in mind that it is the *process*, not the final answer, that is important. Where possible, the strategies patients are using to solve a particular problem in therapy should be discussed. This creates awareness of the process, insight for the therapist, and provides the opportunity for the therapist to suggest modifications in the patient's problem-solving strategy. As reviewed by Groffman,[81] perceptual therapies may be considered as falling into a number of treatment modalities: 1) motor activities, 2) manipulatives, 3) instruments, 4) vision therapy, 5) lens therapy, 6) auditory therapy, 7) workbooks, toys, and games, and 8) computers. The modality is tailored to fit the level and perceptual deficit of the patient.

While gross motor activities applied in vision therapy have often been criticized by those not involved in therapy, they are sometimes necessary to create more optimal support for the visual system. The eyes and visual system do not exist in isolation; the eyes are horizontally displaced from each other in the head and the biomechanics are such that they are intended to work with a horizontal disparity in relation to gravity. Tilting the head induces ocular torsion. Gross motor activities are also used for creating visual proprioceptive and visual kinesthetic matches in ambient space. Vision is dominant over touch in the normal visual system. However, in therapy, proprioceptive and kinesthetic feedback can help teach veridical visual perception. In the rehabilitation setting, many therapeutic activities with these two goals can be taken over by physical or occupational therapists.

Manipulatives are objects that can be used on the tabletop so that they can be handled, rotated, rearranged, and examined in a very concrete way. They allow for learning higher order visual concepts such as visual discrimination, form perception, and spatial orientation and organization with very concrete tools. These include blocks and puzzles specifically designed to teach perceptual skills. Other common examples of manipulatives are flannel boards (used with felt shapes of varied sizes and colors), geo boards (i.e., boards with evenly spaced pegs on which designs are made by stretching rubber bands between the pegs), or pegboards which can be used for reproducing patterns with or without rotations in orientation. Manipulatives also provide excellent eye-hand coordination activity. Visual memory and visual sequential memory can be trained with most manipulatives by creating patterns and having the patient try to reproduce them after a brief exposure.

A variety of instruments have been developed for perceptual training. Instrument techniques are varied and seem to provide additional motivation to many patients. An example would be adjustable speed tachistoscopes, which are used to increase visual perceptual speed and span, as well as visual attention and short-term memory. Tachistoscope targets may vary from abstract geometric forms to be copied, to digit strings or words. They are also useful to demonstrate USN or hemifield loss to the patient as, without time to scan, they will only see the portion of the word presented in their intact field.

Application of vision therapy to remediate receptive dysfunction often involves visual perception — both in spatial organization as discussed above, and in that many fusion tasks require figure-ground discrimination. Lens and prism therapy have already been discussed in terms of shifts in the localization and orientation of local surrounds.

Use of the auditory modality can enhance integration of visual and auditory senses. A number of tape and/or record programs are available for development of various perceptual and perceptual-motor skills, including spatial relations, directionality, and visual motor integration.[82]

Many workbooks, toys, and games are available in educational supply stores, including popular activities with hidden pictures or words for figure-ground discrimination and form perception. Worksheets with simple, incomplete figures to be completed by the patient may be used for development of closure, as well as form perception. These tools also help develop eye-hand coordination. They are generally two-dimensional representations, but have the advantage that, once they understand the process, patients may practice unsupervised with worksheets.

With most of the above modalities, the understanding of the *visual* goals, experience, and creativity of the therapist are keys to the success of therapy. However, through development of computer programs, perceptual therapy has become more accessible, and more easily administered by other rehabilitation disciplines such as occupational therapy. Various companies have developed a number of perceptual programs which combine the challenge and motivation of a videogame with good perceptual therapy. Available programs were reviewed by Press[83] in 1987. Although more programs have been marketed since then, many of the same companies are developing them, and Press's review provides an excellent resource for those interested in applying this therapy modality. Computer therapy generally requires the ability to manipulate a joystick or press a limited number of response keys. For patients having motor control problems, this may be easier than using workbooks or manipulatives.

In addition to the above modalities, visualization, or use of visual imagery, has long been considered a useful, high-end, visual perceptual task by therapy-oriented optometrists. Visualization can be used for visual memory enhancement, such as visualizing the spelling of a word, or for spatial relations and spatial organization, for instance, visualizing object rotations or visualizing a map of how to get home from the grocery store. Recent evidence indicates that, in internally constructing visual imagery, we may use many of the same visual representations as in constructing visual percepts from sensory input. Cerebral blood flow studies, as well as studies of adults with brain damage, show correspondence in functional areas used in both real visual tasks and equivalent imagery tasks.[84] Therapy techniques using visual imagery may be as effective for those patients who do not have manipulative abilities, provided that they are effective at using imagery.

Visual Agnosias

Agnosia is the inability to recognize objects by sight. Object recognition deficits may be *apperceptive*, where the perception of the object is faulty, or *associative*, where the object is perceived correctly, but cannot be associated with prior memories or past experience.[85] In apperceptive agnosia, patients might not be able to match similar objects, draw or copy objects or shapes, or name objects by sight. However, if allowed to use tactile input, they could both name and match the object as well as describe its function. Apperceptive agnosia is rare, and is associated with diffuse cerebral damage of the occipital lobes and surrounding areas.

In associative agnosia, objects and shapes can be matched, but the patients are unable to associate them with past experience or function. For instance, they may be able to draw a key that is placed before them, but be unable to name it or describe its function. When allowed to handle the key, they could both name it and relate that it is used to unlock doors. Associative agnosias can be surprisingly specific. The more common types of agnosia include object agnosia, prosopagnosia (i.e., inability to recognize familiar faces), and color agnosia.

Diagnosis of visual agnosias is important in deciding the proper course of treatment, therapy, or compensation. Associative agnosias may be due to lesions in the pathway that connect the visual "what" pathway with memory areas. De Haan et al.[86] have shown that covert recognition of objects and faces may exist in the absence of overt recognition. They suggest that this may provide a foundation for rehabilitation. Sergent and Poncet[87] report some restoration of overt face recognition under specific circumstances in one patient. While, in some cases, restoration of function may be possible, therapy to directly address the agnosia is likely to be a long process and success is not guaranteed. Compensatory strategies, as for low vision/blind patients, may be the best alternative for immediate management of agnosia.

Alexia

An important part of text recognition is the decoding of visual percepts into language. Interruption of visual pathways at the left angular gyrus[88] or splenium[89] prevent this decoding process from occurring, resulting in acquired alexia or inability to read. Most case reports of this dysfunction show some residual reading function. Treatment of alexia using integration strategies and based on the patient's residual reading skills has been successful. Often, a letter-by-letter reading strategy can be employed by these patients, although it severely slows reading. Motor rehearsal, in terms of copying or tracing letters and words, as well as flash card techniques pairing the written with the spoken word, have been applied with some success.

A successful strategy employed with one patient is described by Daniel et al.[88] Initially, the patient spelled words aloud from flash cards, and then said the word (as he recognized the word from auditory spelling). With practice, the patient was able to substitute covert spelling. Continued practice in this manner significantly increased his ability in reading and naming so that he was able to return to work within four months postinjury. At the one year follow-up, reading was still laborious, but the patient was able to read sufficiently to function in his job.

Assessment and Rehabilitation of Motor Output/Behavior

Visually directed motor output includes not only the planning and execution of eye-hand coordination and visually guided movement through space, but also the planning and execution of the next eye movement. As in the model (Figure 8.3), reception affects perception which affects cognition — and both of the latter affect programming of the next eye movement, feeding back into reception (control of binocularity, eye movements, and fixation). This is a flexible, but closed loop.

The Eyes

Most aspects of assessment and rehabilitation of motor output to the eyes have been discussed above in the section Assessment and Rehabilitation of Sensory Input/Reception. The rehabilitation already discussed is generally performed in the vision care setting. Some specific exercises may be prescribed for application by occupational therapists in either in- or outpatient rehabilitation settings.

In addition to the aspects of ocular motor and binocular control which have already been discussed, ocular motor planning and integration with the output controllers to the eyes are involved. Oculomotor gaze apraxia is the inability to execute purposeful eye movements (reviewed by Roberts[85]). Patients with oculomotor gaze apraxia may be differentially affected for various stimuli, e.g. unable to change fixation in response to verbal commands or peripheral visual, auditory, or touch stimuli. This may be exploitable, in that one may be able to practice saccades to a multimodality stimulus and wean out the intact modality. Letter Tracking*, where one underlines rows of letters until a target letter is reached and then circles the target letter, may allow tactile-proprioceptive feedback to help guide eye movements. Treatment here falls into the realms of neuropsychology, occupational therapy, and vision therapy.

Compensatory strategies should be trained at the same time that remediation is attempted. Many compensatory strategies developed for low vision or the blind may be useful. Other strategies that lessen the necessity of looking in a particular location or reduce the need to scan can also be taught. For instance, moving the television away or using a small screen lessens the need to scan the scene in an organized fashion.

The Hands

Eye-hand coordination will be similarly affected by receptive and perceptual problems, as well as by motor planning and integration of percepts with motor output controllers. Mild difficulties in these areas that occur developmentally will often result in "clumsiness" or difficulty with such tasks as producing clear handwriting. More severe dysfunction is described by two terms — *optic ataxia* and *constructional apraxia*.

Optic ataxia is an inability to visually guide the hand toward an object. Differentiating optic ataxia from primary dysfunctions in motor control can be achieved by having the patient touch his index finger on one hand with the index finger on the other. Usually, in optic ataxia, the misreaching occurs for objects in the peripheral field. However, in more severe cases, misreaching will occur for visually fixated objects.[85] For milder cases, training the patient to visually fixate manipulated objects may be all that is required.

Constructional apraxia generally results from lesions of the posterior parietal lobe or the junction between occipital, parietal, and temporal lobes. It may be due to perceptual deficits, more frequently associated with right hemisphere lesions, or motor function deficits, more frequently associated with left hemisphere lesions. Walsh[90] lists differential effects on drawing which may be used to discriminate between perceptual and motor etiologies. For instance, right hemisphere lesions will tend to result in energetic, scattered, or fragmented drawings with a loss of spatial relations and orientation; left hemisphere involvement tends to result in drawings which are spatially intact and coherent, but simplified and laborious, lacking in detail.

Again, treatment here falls into the realms of neuropsychology, occupational therapy, and vision therapy. A multitude of hand-eye coordination activities exist in the literatures. For constructional apraxia, the differentiation should be made as to whether it is primarily perceptual or primarily motor and treatment should emphasize that modality.

---

* Letter Tracking: Available from Academic Therapy Publications, Novato, CA.

The Body

As discussed above, receptive and perceptual dysfunctions can lead to adoption of head tilts or turns and shifts in posture, creating or complicating problems in balance during standing and walking. Patients are often unaware of these postural adjustments and, when asked, will deny any distortion in their percept and, usually, in their posture, even though something as easily noticed as a pronounced head tilt may be present. Testing for binocular dysfunctions and conditions that may contribute to egocentric midline shifts in the vertical and horizontal directions has been discussed.

If a binocular dysfunction exists, the associated postural problems generally resolve as the binocular problem is remediated or when appropriate patching is applied. Treating the binocular difficulty not only relieves the diplopia or intermittent loss of fusion which can cause patients to adopt compensatory head and body postures, it may also involve teaching patients to reorganize their visual space in which the binocular problem has created distortions.

In the case of an egocentric midline shift, the specific etiology is often not diagnosed. Tests for midline shift and/or observing immediate responses to large amounts of yoked prism may be the extent of the diagnostic procedures. The effects of yoked prism on spatial organization and resultant shifts in posture with a normal visual system are well documented (reviewed by Press[70]). Yoked prisms move the images of the ambient surrounds in the direction of the apex of the prism for both eyes. In the normal visual system, this gives a "fun house" effect. It is initially rather disturbing during head movements and walking to have the world shifted to the right or left, or seemingly stretched upward or squashed downward before you. Base-up prism will cause wearers to shift their weight backward onto their heels; base-down prism has the opposite effect causing the wearers to shift weight forward onto the toes. Sometimes these prisms may be prescribed to assist the physical therapist in rehabilitation of standing and walking. Often, with TBI patients, yoked prism applied in one lateral direction will create no noticeable difference, and application in the opposite direction will make them unable to walk as they try to balance against the shift in surrounds. This type of behavior is a good indication that yoked prism therapy or compensatory yoked prism in the patients' spectacle lenses can help normalize their posture and balance, either by reorienting their egocentric midline or by moving the world to match their new one. Patients who veer in one direction while walking may also benefit. Even without a midline shift, yoked prisms used for short therapy periods may be useful in breaking down maladaptive habitual postures which are resistant to treatment.

SUMMARY

The term *visual rehabilitation* is so broad that it often encompasses the services of neuropsychologists, occupational therapists, and psychotherapists, in addition to both ophthalmologists and optometrists and specially trained orthoptists or vision therapy technicians. Visual dysfunction may be caused by damage to any lobe of the brain, as well as midbrain structures. Functional deficits include photophobia, decreased visual acuity or contrast sensitivity, ocular-motor disorders, binocular dysfunction including strabismus, visual field loss, spatial disorientation, unilateral field neglect, other visual perceptual disorders, integration disorders, and problems with visually guided motor planning and motor output.

Visual sequelae are quite commonplace in the TBI patient, but often overlooked. Therefore, once the medical/surgical rehabilitation of the visual system is complete, the issue of functional recovery or compensation must be examined. Vision care specialists who provide other patient populations with orthoptic or vision therapy or low vision services will generally be able to adapt many of their techniques to working with the TBI patient. Treatments often must be innovative and coordinated among the various professionals providing rehabilitative services. Visual sequelae to TBI can affect the patient's ability to perform such varied tasks as reading, walking, and driving. Unrehabilitated functional visual deficits can interfere with other therapies and with the patient's ability to perform activities of daily living, as well as return to work or school.

The neuroanatomy of the visual system is so complex that, in order to provide effective therapy, one must have a working model with which to organize rehabilitation. Such a model is described here. The major components of the model to be considered in diagnosis and therapy are 1) reception/sensory input, 2) perception/integration, and 3) motor output/behavior. This model is circular, in that each component affects the other. Our receptive functions affect perception. Our percepts affect our motor planning and output. Our motor output affects where our bodies are and how we are going to use our eyes next — receptive function. Carefully planned vision therapy or use of lenses and prisms can intervene in any of these areas in a constructive way, or disruptively to break down bad adaptations. Our perceptions also feed into cognition, and our thoughts affect our perceptions. Therefore, reception and perception should be considered when cognitive rehabilitation is in order.

The redundancy of the visual system as well as the flexibility of the visual system — demonstrated by experiments such as adaptation to inverting prisms, together with clinical experience such as therapeutic remediation of strabismus and amblyopia in adults — makes recovery of function a reasonable goal for many visual dysfunctions following TBI. While one cannot always predict which patients will respond to such therapy, it seems inappropriate to offer less if there is a chance of recovery. Where therapy is ineffective at restoring function within a reasonable time frame, there are many compensatory devices and strategies that can be applied — for instance, patching, prisms, or low vision devices and techniques. Even these should be prescribed with an eye toward maximizing function within the limits set by the patient's condition. The area of visual rehabilitation for TBI patients is still in its infancy. However, many visual dysfunctions encountered in TBI patients have been addressed for other special needs populations. The multiple deficits in sensation, speech and/or language, cognition, or motor control encountered in the TBI patient add to the challenge of providing effective vision care.

ILLUSTRATIVE VISUAL CASE STUDIES

Patient C. L.

Patient C. L. was seen for visual evaluation 13 years after TBI sustained in a motor vehicle accident. Her chief complaints at the time of the vision examination were the fact that her eyes rolled back in her head during seizures and she experienced some eyestrain, although her occupational therapist had noted that C. L. complained of headaches and blurred vision after near work.

Examination revealed a convergence insufficiency exotropia (i.e., strabismus when viewing at nearpoint due to inability to converge her eyes). She was diplopic almost constantly when doing tasks within arm's length. When queried about the diplopia, she said that the doctor she saw just after her accident had told her it would go away in time, so she just waited.

Although her phorias were not large (9 prism diopters of exophoria at near), she had almost no elicitable base-out reflex fusion, and abnormal convergence ranges on prism vergence testing with a negative recovery (i.e., once fusion was broken with base-out prism, it required base-in prism to reestablish fusion). Her nearpoint of convergence on push-up testing was 16". Because she had so little fusion response, we were unable to prescribe any outpatient therapy.

C. L. was treated on a daily basis for two weeks, 45 minutes per day, using large fusion targets projected on a wall to attain peripheral fusion and SILO. Instrument (amblyoscope) convergence techniques were also applied. After two weeks, she was fusing well enough at nearpoint that we were able to prescribe convergence exercises for practice with her occupational therapist at the rehabilitation facility. She continued in-office therapy once weekly and made continued progress with this regimen.

Patient T. R.

T. R. was examined four months after a motor vehicle accident, with chief complaints of blur, triplopia at near, and photophobia. Like C. L., he had an intermittent convergence insufficiency exotropia causing diplopia. His near phoria was only 8 prism diopters of exophoria, but like C. L., his nearpoint of convergence was reduced to approximately 16″ and he had negative recoveries on base-out prism vergence testing. His voluntary saccades were hypometric. Additionally, he had an uncorrected astigmatism in one eye causing monocular diplopia.

Unlike C. L., patient T. R. maintained enough responsivity to fusional stimuli that he could do prescribed convergence exercises on a daily basis with the occupational therapist in his rehabilitation facility. Saccadic exercises were also prescribed. Glasses were prescribed to compensate for the astigmatism to relieve the monocular diplopia.

T. R. was checked at three-week intervals. After three months of therapy, his near exophoria had reduced to 6 prism diopters. Base-out fusional ranges were normal and his nearpoint of convergence was 2″, which he could maintain with some effort. His saccades were fast and accurate. He was visually asymptomatic. T. R. was released with ten minutes of daily maintenance convergence exercises to be practiced for three months.

Patient L. D.

L. D. was seen four months postinjury. For financial reasons, she had been unable to access rehabilitative care other than immediate medical management after her injury which included some physical therapy for a broken arm. Just after her injury, she had demonstrated a large left exotropia which resolved spontaneously prior to her first vision evaluation. Her chief complaints at the time of examination were blurred vision, eyestrain, and difficulty with words running together after a few minutes of reading. She had previously been a clerk-typist and never had difficulty with extended near work.

Examination revealed a convergence insufficiency, again with only a small phoria. She also had unsteady centric fixation with the right eye, and unsteady centric-to-nasal fixation with the left. Versions and ductions were jerky. She showed no appreciation of proprioception from her extraocular muscles. Appreciation of SILO was absent.

With weekly visits and approximately 45 minutes of daily home therapy, she made slow but consistent progress with regard to convergence, quality of her eye movements, spatial localization, and SILO involving large peripheral targets. Afterimage techniques helped her regulate her pursuits. She was unable to feel her eyes jump, but she could see the afterimage jump. Intensive work on monocular fixation, including therapies that are often successful in breaking down developmental unsteady or eccentric fixation, did not result in improvement of her unsteady fixation. Also, her convergence insufficiency resolved in an asymmetric manner; in spite of efforts to converge symmetrically or even to train in positions requiring more convergence with the left eye, her left eye had more difficulty converging and she would often assume a rightward head turn if not monitored closely during therapy.

As therapy progressed in this manner, a measurable horizontal midline shift to the left manifested. This was notable both when measured directly and when yoked prisms were applied. Base-right prisms disturbed her very little, base-left prisms made her feel sick and unbalanced. Therapy was discontinued after approximately nine months due to financial restraints. At this time, small amounts of yoked base-right prism were prescribed for habitual wear.

L. D.'s difficulty with words running together, and to some extent, her ability to sustain at nearpoint tasks improved as her convergence improved. However, she still had asthenopic symptoms when reading for more than half an hour, probably due to the midline shift and unstable fixation.

Patient L. N.

L. N. was referred for orthoptic work-up following a strabismus surgery performed in an attempt to lessen his vertical strabismus secondary to head trauma. L. N. had a history of poor fusion prior to the accident (two surgeries for esotropia — one as a child and one as an adult a few years prior). His job involved extensive paperwork with which he was comfortable prior to his injury. He did not experience diplopia prior to the injury. After the injury, he experienced almost constant diplopia in a diagonal direction which was variable in magnitude. The ophthalmologist performed a vertical muscle surgery in hopes that reducing the magnitude of the vertical deviation would allow him to maintain fusion.

At the time of his orthoptic work-up, L. N. reported that the vertical surgery had reduced the magnitude of the deviation, but he was still unable to fuse. He also reported constant fatigue due to his visual status and he was sleeping at least ten hours daily. He was found to be generally esotropic when viewing at near and generally exotropic when viewing distance targets. He also had a noncomitant vertical deviation which he could fuse in far right gaze and which increased in magnitude through primary gaze and leftward. When tested on central fusion targets in the straight-ahead position, his response was similar to horror fusionis — where the targets could be made to approach each other and then would jump to opposite sides, never fusing. When tested with large peripheral targets set at his angle of deviation, he was able to fuse, but could not elicit a proper depth response. He reported a definite perception of depth, but was able to see targets with two disparity levels as interchangeable in terms of which one appeared closer. In real space, L. N. was able to fuse in far right gaze or, with a head tilt, in a small volume of space approximately one meter away, just to the right of midline.

Therapy proceeded from creating equal monocular skills to working on SILO perception with large peripheral targets in different fields of gaze, as well as small central targets in the space where he could fuse. After three months of therapy (one 45-minute session per week in-office and two hours daily at home), he was able to fuse in all but his leftward field of gaze, where he suppressed. He reported appropriate depth with SILO on both peripheral and central fusion targets. He was less fatigued and was not diplopic when working at nearpoint. At this point, he returned to work.

Patient L. R.

Patient L. R. was seen four months postinjury with chief complaints of poor depth perception and difficulty "keeping things level." Examination revealed a mild (approximately 10 prism diopters) right esotropia and a mild left superior rectus palsy which resulted in a noncomitant vertical component to the eyeturn (6 prism diopters in primary gaze, increasing on left gaze). The superior rectus also intorts the eye. Her complaint of difficulty keeping things level probably resulted from a combination of extorsion of the eye and the noncomitancy of the vertical component. Pursuits were jerky. Ductions were full with the right eye and showed a superior temporal restriction with the left eye. Although she appeared to fixate with her left eye during the entire examination, she showed alternating suppression on her stereopsis testing. She also had reduced accommodative amplitude and facility.

Therapy progressed from monocular and biocular (i.e., two eyes seeing, without fusion) skills to antisuppression activities and in-instrument fusion with vertical and base-in vergences. After twelve weekly sessions in-office, with one hour of home therapy daily, her extraocular range of motion was full with each eye, with smooth pursuits. She showed no vertical or horizontal phoria, at distance or near, and she was comfortable with her vision. Therapy was continued for six additional sessions to improve fusional and accommodative flexibility. At her one year progress check, she had maintained all of her visual gains.

Patient B. B.

Patient B. B. was seen for examination four months postinjury. He had no light perception from his right eye due to optic nerve atrophy following his injury. His left eye was healthy and intact.

He presented with decreased acuity (20/80 when reading a vertical column, and 20/30 when reading horizontal lines). He had reduced contrast sensitivity for medium spatial frequencies. He also had a left hemianopia with macular sparing. He had difficulty reading. He watched his feet when walking and tended to veer leftward. Saccades were slow and pursuits were jerky. He had a reduced amplitude of accommodation, and was already wearing a bifocal correction which he found useful. He read at approximately 8″ from his eyes for the additional magnification.

B. B. was aware that he had a field defect, but did little to compensate for it. The physical therapists had already taught him to use a staff on the blind side, both for physical support and to protect that side. However, like most hemianopes, he did not scan toward the affected side. During tachistoscopic procedures, he generally missed the first few letters or digits and he initially had poor perceptual speed and span. On line bisection tasks, he transected the line at the center or contralateral to the blind field. This is the expected performance for a patient with hemianopia combined with USN, rather than just a hemianopic defect. On some other tasks, his performance was consistent with a mild case of neglect. For instance, when instructed to scan a wall for target figures, he would scan from right (his intact field) to left. When asked to scan again from left to right, he would become argumentative, stating that he *always* scanned left to right, and then would proceed to scan from right to left again. He showed few other indications of neglect. Copied forms were complete. On "crossing out" tasks, he generally covered the entire page, always starting from right to left, but was careful to reach the left margin of the page.

Therapy began with monocular skills and tachistoscopic procedures for perceptual speed and span. These skills improved rapidly with therapy. Peripheral awareness techniques for expanding awareness within his intact field were applied with good success. B. B.'s overall reading speed improved along with his saccadic speed, perceptual span, and perceptual speed.

A number of techniques were applied for making B. B. more aware of space within his blind field. Some of these met with more success than others. He rejected application of Fresnel prism, saying he would rather move his eyes farther without the prism. He actively participated in both tabletop and wall-projected scanning activities, trying to adopt an efficient scanning pattern moving from far left in his blind field, rightward. However, initially, these activities did not seem to generalize outside of the therapy room. He was able to adopt a scanning pattern while walking. He looked left on every fourth step, which helped him walk without deviating leftward. However, after six weeks of therapy, he still walked slowly and remained very dependent on his staff. At the time of this writing, he continues in therapy emphasizing scanning in nonpredictable situations. It is expected that he will be able to learn to scan automatically, with little interruption imposed by addition of cognitive tasks.

ACKNOWLEDGMENTS

I would like to thank Drs. Neil Margolis, Marie Marrone, and Sydney Groffman for reviewing the manuscript and for their helpful comments, Lorna Frost for library assistance, and especially, Dr. Steve Suter for his helpful review and care of baby Andrew so that this manuscript could be completed.

REFERENCES

1. Van Essen, D. C., Functional organization of primate visual cortex, in *Cerebral Cortex: Vol. 3, Visual Cortex*, Peters, A. and Jones, E. G., Eds., Plenum Press, New York, 1985, Chap 7.
2. Padula, W. V., Ed., Vision: The process, in *A Behavioral Vision Approach for Persons with Physical Disabilities*, Optometric Extension Program Foundation, Inc., Santa Ana, CA, 1988, Chap. 1.
3. Kaas, J. H., Changing concepts of visual cortex organization in primates, in *Neuropsychology of Visual Perception*, Brown, J. W., Ed., Lawrence Erlbaum Associates, Hillsdale, NJ, 1989, Chap. 1.
4. Mishkin, M., Ungerleider, L. G., and Macko, K. A., Object vision and spatial vision: Two cortical pathways, *Trends Neurosci.*, 6, 414, 1983.

5. Stuss, D. T. and Benson, D. F., Neuropsychological studies of the frontal lobes, *Psychol. Bull.*, 95, 3, 1984.

6. Cobb, S., An interview with Vincent Vicci, O. D., in *OEP Vision Therapist, Vol. 35, Working with the Brain Injured*, Barber, A., Ed., Optometric Extension Program, Santa Ana, CA, 1993, Chap. 2.

7. Padula, W. V., Shapiro, J. B., and Jasin, P., Head injury causing post trauma vision syndrome, *N. Engl. J. Optom.*, Dec/Winter, 16, 1988.

8. Padula, W. V. and Shapiro, J., Post-trauma vision syndrome caused by head injury, in *A Behavioral Vision Approach for Persons with Physical Disabilities*, Padula, W. V., Ed., Optometric Extension Program Foundation, Inc., Santa Ana, CA, 1988, Chap 14.

9. Freeman, C. F. and Rudge, N. B., Cerebrovascular accident and the orthoptist, *Br. Orthop. J.*, 45, 8, 1988.

10. Roca, P. D., Ocular manifestations of whiplash injuries, *Ann. Ophthalmol.*, 4, 63, 1972.

11. Schlageter, K., Gray, B., Hall, K., Shaw, R., and Sammet, R., Incidence and treatment of visual dysfunction in traumatic brain injury, *Brain Injury*, 7, 439, 1993.

12. Cohen, M., Groswasser, Z., Barchadski, R., and Appel, A., Convergence insufficiency in brain-injured patients, *Brain Injury*, 3, 187, 1989.

13. Fitzsimons, F. and Fells, P., Ocular motility problems following road traffic accidents, *Br. Orthop. J.*, 46, 40, 1989.

14. Groswasser, Z., Cohen, M., and Blankstein, E., Polytrauma associated with traumatic brain injury: Incidence, nature, and impact on rehabilitation outcome, *Brain Injury*, 4, 161, 1990.

15. Schwab, K., Grafman, J., Salazar, A. M., and Kraft, J., Residual impairments and work status 15 years after penetrating head injury: Report from the Vietnam head injury study, *Neurology*, 43, 95, 1993.

16. Wehman, P., Kregel, J., Sherron, P., Nguyen, S., Kreutzer, J., Fry, R., and Zasler, N., Critical factors associated with the successful supported employment placement of patients with severe traumatic brain injury, *Brain Injury*, 7, 31, 1993.

17. Najenson, T., Groswasser, Z., Mendelson, L., and Hackett, P., Rehabilitation outcome of brain damaged patients after severe head injury, *Int. Rehabil. Med.*, 2, 17, 1980.

18. Murray, R., Shum, D., and McFarland, K., Attentional deficits in head-injured children: An information processing analysis, *Brain Cognit.*, 18, 99, 1992.

19. Shum, D. H., McFarland, K., Bain, J. D., and Humphreys, M. S., Effects of closed-head injury upon attentional processes: An information-processing stage analysis, *J. Clin. Exp. Neuropsychol.*, 12, 247, 1990.

20. Glickstein, M., Cortical visual areas and the visual guidance of movement, in *Vision and Visual Dysfunction, Vol. 13, Vision and Visual Dyslexia*, Stein, J. F., Ed., CRC Press, Boca Raton, FL, 1991, Chap. 1.

21. Etting, G. L., Strabismus therapy in private practice: Cure rates after three months of therapy, *J. Am. Optom. Assoc.*, 49, 1367, 1978.

22. Selenow, A. and Ciuffreda, K. J., Vision function recovery during orthoptic therapy in an adult esotropic amblyope, *J. Am. Optom. Assoc.*, 57, 132, 1986.

23. Garzia, R. P., Efficacy of vision therapy in amblyopia: A literature review, *Am. J. Optom. Physiol. Opt.*, 64, 393, 1987.

24. Flax, N. and Duckman, R. H., Orthoptic treatment of strabismus, *J. Am. Optom. Assoc.*, 49, 1353, 1978.

25. Suchoff, I. B. and Petito, G. T., The efficacy of visual therapy: Accommodative disorders and non-strabismic anomalies of binocular vision, *J. Am. Optom. Assoc.*, 57, 119, 1986.

26. The 1986/87 Future of Visual Development/Performance Task Force, The efficacy of optometric vision therapy, *J. Am. Optom. Assoc.*, 59, 95, 1988.

27. Cohen, A. H., Visual rehabilitation of a stroke patient, *J. Am. Optom. Assoc.*, 49, 831, 1978.

28. Cohen, A. H. and Soden, R., An optometric approach to the rehabilitation of the stroke patient, *J. Am. Optom. Assoc.*, 52, 795, 1981.

29. Gianutsos, R., Ramsey, G., and Perlin, R., Rehabilitative optometric services for survivors of acquired brain injury, *Arch. Phys. Med. Rehabil.*, 69, 573, 1988.

30. Berne, S. A., Visual therapy for the traumatic brain-injured, *J. Optom. Vision Dev.*, 21, 13, 1990.

31. Wagenaar, R. C., Van Wieringen, P. C. W., Netelenbos, J. B., Meijer, O. G., and Kuik, D. J., The transfer of scanning training effects in visual inattention after stroke: Five single-case studies, *Disabil. Rehabil.*, 14, 51, 1992.

32. Kerkhoff, G. and Stögerer, E., Recovery of fusional convergence after systematic practice, *Brain Injury*, 8, 15, 1994.

33. Ron, S., Plastic changes in eye movements of patients with traumatic brain injury, in *Progress in Oculomotor Research*, Fuchs, A. F. and Becker, W., Eds., Elsevier, New York, 1981, p. 233.

34. Krohel, G. B., Kristan, R. W., Simon, J. W., and Barrows, N. A., Posttraumatic convergence insufficiency, *Ann. Ophthalmol.*, 18, 101, 1986.

35. Kerkhoff, G., Münßinger, U., and Meier, E. K., Neurovisual rehabilitation in cerebral blindness, *Arch. Neurol.*, 51, 474, 1994.

36. Zoccolotti, P., Guariglia, C., Pizzamiglio, L., Judica, A., Razzano, C., and Pantano, P., Good recovery in visual scanning in a patient with persistent anosagnosia, *Int. J. Neurosci.*, 62, 93, 1992.

37. Gianutsos, R. and Matheson, P., The rehabilitation of visual perceptual disorders attributable to brain injury, in *Neuropsychological Rehabilitation,* Meier, M. J., Benton, A. L., and Diller, L., Eds., The Guilford Press, New York, 1987, Chap. 10.
38. Mazow, M. L. and Tang, R., Strabismus associated with head and facial trauma, *Am. Orthop. J.*, 32, 31, 1982.
39. Gianutsos, R., Cognitive rehabilitation: A neuropsychological speciality comes of age, *Brain Injury*, 5, 353, 1991.
40. Moore, J. C., Recovery potentials following CNS lesions: A brief historical perspective in relation to modern research data on neuroplasticity, *Am. J. Occup. Ther.*, 40, 459, 1986.
41. Cohen, A. H. and Rein, L. D., The effect of head trauma on the visual system: The doctor of optometry as a member of the rehabilitation team, *J. Am. Optom. Assoc.*, 63, 530, 1992.
42. Schor, C., Imbalanced adaptation of accommodation and vergence produces opposite extremes of the AC/A and CA/C ratios, *Am. J. Ophthalmic Physiol. Opt.*, 65, 341, 1988.
43. Schor, C., Influence of accommodative and vergence adaptation on binocular motor disorders, *Am. J. Ophthalmic Physiol. Opt.*, 65, 464, 1988.
44. Finkel, L. J. and Sajda, P., Constructing visual perception, *Am. Sci.*, 82, 224, 1994.
45. Bassi, C. J. and Lehmkuhle, S., Clinical implications of parallel visual pathways, *J. Am. Optom. Assoc.*, 61, 98, 1990.
46. Warren, M., Identification of visual scanning deficits in adults after cerebrovascular accident, *Am. J. Occup. Ther.*, 44, 391, 1990.
47. Trevarthen, C. and Sperry, R. W., Perceptual unity of the ambient visual field in human commissurotomy patients, *Brain*, 96, 547, 1973.
48. Morrison, J. D. and Whiteside, T. C., Binocular cues in the perception of distance of a point source of light, *Perception*, 13, 555, 1984.
49. Leigh, R. J. and Zee, D. S., *The Neurology of Eye Movements*, 2nd edition, F. A. Davis Company, Philadelphia, 1991, Chap. 1.
50. Rayner, K. and Pollatsek, A., *The Psychology of Reading*, Prentice-Hall Inc., Englewood Cliffs, NJ, 1989, Chap. 11.
51. Griffin, J. R., *Binocular Anomalies: Procedures for Vision Therapy*, 2nd edition, Professional Press Books, Fairchild Publications, New York, 1982.
52. Burde, R. M., Savino, P. J., and Trobe, J. D., *Clinical Decisions in Neuro-Ophthalmology*, 2nd edition, Mosby Year Book, Inc., St. Louis, 1992.
53. London, R. and Scott, S. H., Sensory fusion disruption syndrome, *J. Am. Optom. Assoc.*, 58, 544, 1987.
54. Kupersmith, M. J., Siegel, I. M., and Carr, R. E., Subtle disturbances of vision with compressive lesions of the anterior visual pathway measured by contrast sensitivity, *Ophthalmology*, 89, 68, 1982.
55. Kerkhoff, G., Münßinger, U., Haaf, E., Eberle-Strauss, G., and Stögerer, E., Rehabilitation of homonymous scotomata in patients with postgeniculate damage of the visual system: Saccadic compensation training, *Restor. Neurol. Neurosci.*, 4, 245, 1992.
56. Nooney, T. W., Jr., Partial visual rehabilitation of hemianopic patients, *Am. J. Optom. Physiol. Opt.*, 63, 382, 1986.
57. Weiss, N. J., Remediation of peripheral visual field defects in low vision patients, in *Problems in Optometry, Vol. 4, Patient and Practice Management in Low Vision*, Cole, R. G. and Rosenthal, B. P., Eds., J. B. Lippincott Co., Philadelphia, 1992, Chap. 4.
58. Perlin, R. R. and Dziadul, J., Fresnel prisms for field enhancement of patients with constricted or hemianopic visual fields, *J. Am. Optom. Assoc.*, 62, 58, 1991.
59. Hoeft, W. W., The management of visual field defect through low vision aids, *J. Am. Optom. Assoc.*, 51, 863, 1980.
60. Drasdo, N. and Murray, I. J., A pilot study on the use of visual field expanders, *Br. J. Physiol. Opt.*, 32, 22, 1978.
61. Prokopich, L. and Pace, R., Visual rehabilitation in homonymous hemianopia due to cerebral vascular accident, *J. Vision Rehabil.*, 3, 29, 1989.
62. Zihl, J. and von Cramon, D., Restitution of visual field in patients with damage to the geniculostriate visual pathway, *Hum. Neurobiol.*, 1, 5, 1982.
63. Balliet, R., Blood, K. M.,, and Bach-y-Rita, P., Visual field rehabilitation in the cortically blind, *J. Neurol. Neurosurg. Psychiatry*, 48, 1113, 1985.
64. Bohnen, N., Twijnstra, A., Wijnen, G., and Jolles, J., Recovery from visual and acoustic hyperaesthesia after mild head injury in relation to patterns of behavioral dysfunction, *J. Neurol. Neurosurg. Psychiatry*, 55, 222, 1992.
65. Husain, M., Visuospatial and visuomotor functions of the posterior parietal lobe, in *Vision and Visual Dysfunction, Vol. 13, Vision and Visual Dyslexia*, Stein, J. F., Ed., CRC Press, Boca Raton, FL, 1991, Chap. 2.

66. Borish, I. M., *Clinical Refraction*, 3rd edition, The Professional Press, Inc., Chicago, 1975, Chap 30.

67. Halligan, P. W. and Marshall, J. C., Two techniques for the assessment of line bisection in visuo-spatial neglect: A single case study, *J. Neurol. Neurosurg. Psychiatry,* 52, 1300, 1989.

68. Kerkhoff, G., Displacement of the egocentric visual midline in altitudinal postchiasmatic scotomata, *Neuropsychologia*, 31, 261, 1993.

69. De Renzi, E., Oculomotor disturbances in hemispheric disease, in *Neuropsychology of Eye Movements*, Johnston, C. W. and Pirozzolo, F. J., Eds., Lawrence Erlbaum Associates, Hillsdale, NJ, 1988, p. 177.

70. Press, L. J., Lenses and behavior, *J. Optom. Vision Dev.*, 21, 5, 1990.

71. Mangun, G. R., Hillyard, S. A., Luck, S. J., Handy, T., Plager, R., Clark, V. P., Loftus, W., and Gazzaniga, M. S., Monitoring the visual world: Hemispheric asymmetries and subcortical processes in attention, *J. Cognit. Neurosci.*, 6, 267, 1994.

72. Stone, S. P., Halligan, P. W., and Greenwood, R. J., The incidence of neglect phenomena and related disorders in patients with an acute right or left hemisphere stroke, *Age Ageing,* 22, 46, 1993.

73. Halligan, P. W. and Marshall, J. C., Is neglect (only) lateral? A quadrant analysis of line cancellation, *J. Clin. Exp. Neuropsychol.*, 11, 793, 1989.

74. Ishiai, S., Furukawa, T., and Tsukagoshi, H., Eye-fixation patterns in homonymous hemianopia and unilateral spatial neglect, *Neuropsychologia*, 25, 675, 1987.

75. Gordon, W. A., Hibbard, M. R., Egelko, S., Diller, L., Shaver M. S., Lieberman, A., and Ragnarsson, K., Perceptual remediation in patients with right brain damage: A comprehensive program, *Arch. Phys. Med. Rehabil.*, 66, 353, 1985.

76. Robertson, I. H., Gray, J. M., Pentland, B., and Waite, L. J., Microcomputer-based rehabilitation for unilateral left visual neglect: A randomized controlled trial, *Arch. Phys. Med. Rehabil.*, 71, 663, 1990.

77. Ross, F. L., The use of computers in occupational therapy for visual-scanning training, *Am. J. Occup. Ther.*, 46, 314, 1992.

78. Rock, I. and Harris, C. S., Vision and touch, in *Perception: Mechanisms and Models*, Scientific American Inc., San Francisco, 1972, p. 269.

79. Coren, S. and Ward, L. M., *Sensation and Perception*, 3rd edition, Harcourt Brace Jovanovich, San Diego, 1989, Chap. 11.

80. Aksionoff, E. B. and Falk, N. S., The differential diagnosis of perceptual deficits in traumatic brain injury patients, *J. Am. Optom. Assoc.*, 63, 554, 1992.

81. Groffman, S., Treatment of visual perceptual disorders, *Pract. Optom.*, 4, 76, 1993.

82. Groffman, S. and Press, L. J., Computerized perceptual therapy programs: Part I, *Optometric Extension Program Curriculum II*, 61, 387, 1989.

83. Press, L. J., Computers and vision therapy programs, *Optometric Extension Program Curriculum II*, 60, 29, 1987.

84. Farah, M. J., Is visual imagery really visual? Overlooked evidence from neuropsychology, *Psychol. Rev.*, 95, 307, 1988.

85. Roberts, S. P., Visual disorders of higher cortical function, *J. Am. Optom. Assoc.*, 63, 723, 1992.

86. De Haan, E. H. F., Young, A. W., and Newcombe, F., Covert and overt recognition in prosopagnosia, *Brain*, 114, 2575, 1991.

87. Sergent, J. and Poncet, M., From covert to overt recognition of faces in a prosopagnosic patient, *Brain*, 113, 989, 1990.

88. Daniel, M. S., Bolter, J. F., and Long, C. J., Remediation of alexia without agraphia: A case study, *Brain Injury*, 6, 529, 1992.

89. Trobe, J. R. and Bauer, R. M., Seeing but not recognizing, *Surv. Ophthalmol.*, 30, 328, 1986.

90. Walsh, K., *Neuropsychology: A Clinical Approach*, 2nd edition, Churchill Livingstone, New York, 1987.

APPENDIX

Organizations to contact for information regarding orthoptic or vision therapy, or referral to member doctors who may provide or prescribe therapy:

College of Optometry in Vision Development
P.O. Box 285
Chula Vista, CA 91912-0285

Neuro-Optometric Rehabilitation Association
P. O. Box 904
Cranford, NJ 07016

Optometric Extension Program Foundation, Inc
2912 South Daimler St.
Santa Ana, CA 92705

9

Neurophysiological Substrates of Learning

Robert P. Lehr, Jr.

CONTENTS

INTRODUCTION

The purpose of this chapter is to acquaint the reader with neurophysiological substrates subserving learning. The chapter will review recent advances in neuroscience, portraying significant forces at work in neurotransmission. Familiar concepts of learning will be associated with their neurophysiological counterparts so that the reader may gain an appreciation for the actual impact of rehabilitation upon the central nervous system. It is hoped that professionals in the fields of rehabilitation will come to reflect these issues in the manner in which they choose to undertake rehabilitative therapies as well as in their choice of rehabilitative therapies.

Successful rehabilitation of the traumatically brain-injured patient (TBI) requires that the individual relearn old skills or develop new skills, whether they be in cognitive areas or in motor performance. Health care professionals, physical therapists, occupational therapists, and clinical psychologists have known for a long time that success, defined as improvement of the patient, comes from long hours of repetitive activity. The repetitive activity of rehabilitation is similar to the long process of development of the original skills that we learned between the infant and the adult years. The long hours that the traumatically brain-injured patient engages in repetitive activity is sometimes viewed as less acceptable because everyone wants rapid results. However, learning is not a rapid process; it takes time.

Learning is a process we are discovering more about each day. Recent work, as we will show, has found that there is a physical basis in the central nervous system for the changes that we attribute to learning. These changes take place at the very foundation of the structure of the brain, in the neurons and their synapses (see Chapter 4 of this volume for a basic description of a synapse).

These discoveries are based on work in experimental animals such as the California snail, *Aplysia*, and isolated preparations of mammalian hippocampus, and the changes are unequivocal. These changes involve the number of active synapses, the amount of transmitter released,

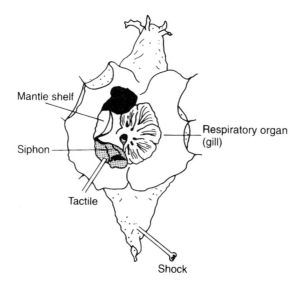

FIGURE 9.1   California snail. *Aplysia.* (Reprinted by permission of the publisher from Chapter 65 by Eric R. Kandel, *Principles of Neural Science, Third Edition*, Eric R. Kandel, James H. Schwartz, and Thomas M. Jessell (Eds.), p. 1010. Copyright 1991 by Elsevier Science Publishing Co., Inc.)

and the tightness of the synaptic junction. This research may provide insight into the cellular and molecular basis for the changes the therapists have seen in their patients' behavior following extended therapy. In addition, it is hoped that the insights gained from looking at this research will expand the practicing therapist's horizon and perhaps assist in the development of new therapies.

Neurons and their synapses, as an anatomical substrate for a physiological basis of learning, had its theoretical origin in the work of Hebb.[1] Hebb suggested that it was changes in the neurons and particularly the synapse that would eventually be shown to provide a physical basis for what is described as learning. He suggested that there would be observable changes in the neurons or their synapses and went on to elaborate on what form the total system might take.[2] Hebb's theories postulated that the behavior changes that an organism makes to the influences of the environment would be reflected in the changes in the synapses in the central nervous system.

Hebb's hypothesis has been largely substantiated in the more recent work of other neurobiologists. A series of experiments by Bailey and Chen,[3] in *Aplysia*, demonstrated that there are physical changes in the synapses of the neurons in the central nervous system during learning. Of course, the learning was in a very simple form, but it provided direct evidence of the plastic nature of the specific synaptic substrate. Kandel[4] followed with more extensive experiments and has provided us with a broad perspective on additional concepts in learning.

The form of learning first investigated in the *Aplysia* was simple habituation. This is characterized by the reduced response to a presentation of a novel stimulation. The *Aplysia* is a small mollusk that has a respiratory organ called the gill, and a mantle shelf which protrudes as a siphon (Figure 9.1).

When a stimulus is applied to the siphon, the snail responds by reflex withdrawal of its gill, mantle, and tail. This motor response to a sensory input is characteristic of all reflex actions. A greatly simplified neuronal circuit of the *Aplysia* nervous system is represented in Figure 9.2.

HABITUATION

This circuit provides the basis for the normal reflex withdrawal of the gill, mantle, and tail to the presentation of the novel stimulus. This is a normal reflex and is used to expel seawater

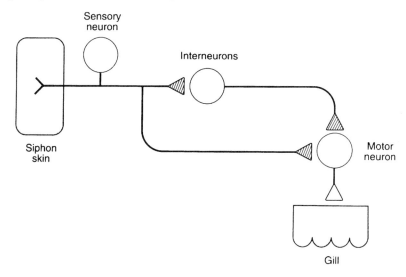

FIGURE 9.2   Simplified neuronal circuit of *Aplysia* nervous system. (Reprinted by permission of the publisher from Chapter 65 by Eric R. Kandel, *Principles of Neural Science, Third Edition*, Eric R. Kandel, James H. Schwartz, and Thomas M. Jessell (Eds.), p. 1010. Copyright 1991 by Elsevier Science Publishing Co., Inc.)

and waste in the normal life of the organism. With repeated stimulation to the siphon, there is a depression of the reflex response. The decreased response is characterized by a decrease in synaptic transmission from the sensory neurons to the interneurons and motor neurons in the reflex circuit. Measurable differences have been shown in the amount of transmitter released. There is a decreased ability of transmitter vesicles to be mobilized into the active zone so as to be available for release. These changes may last for many minutes and are known as *short-term habituation.*

If the stimulation is continued over several training sessions, then, upon sacrifice of the organism, an actual reduction is seen in the number of synapses that are present. The changes that result are physical changes at the cellular level and are a reflection of the response to the environment. These observable changes are described as long-term habituation.

An example of habituation in humans might be the awareness of a constant noise in the environment which is ignored over time as attention is focused on other things. Another example is the pressure we feel on a body part as we first sit down and, after a short period, we ignore the feeling of pressure in that part of the body.

SENSITIZATION

On the other hand, if one looks at the process of sensitization, a slightly more complex learning, the effect is one of enhancement of the reflex response after the presentation of a strong stimulation. Following the strong stimulation, there is a tendency to pay attention to all other stimulations by the organism. This type of learning involves an additional neuronal circuit. An interneuron is interspersed between the sensory and motor loop of the reflex. If one looks at the reflex synaptic area, an increase in connectivity is seen between the neurons. In addition, there is an increase in the size of the synaptic zone and the number of vesicles in the active zone.[3] One of the transmitters which has been identified as playing a key role in sensitization is serotonin, a transmitter that is found in mammalian brains (see Chapter 4 of this volume).

The neurons in the reflex circuit (Figure 9.3) have demonstrated that they have a "memory" of what has happened to them. It has been further demonstrated that the synapse becomes modified and is more adherent. There seems to be a tighter connection due to an increased deposition of glycoproteins in the synaptic cleft.

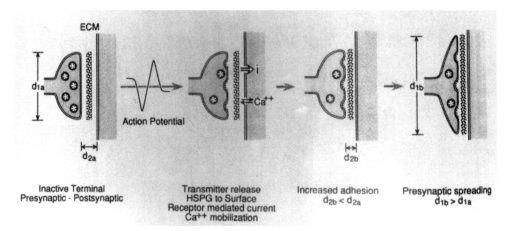

FIGURE 9.3   Schematic model for adhesion-mediated changes associated with synaptic modification. The hatched
area between cells represents the extracellular matric (ECM). (Reprinted by permission of the
publisher from "The possible role of adhesion in synaptic modification" by David Schubert, *Trends
Neurosci.,* 14(12), 128. Copyright 1991 by Elsevier Science Publishing Co., Inc.)

These changes in the presynaptic neurons occur following strong stimulus and can last for
several minutes. This is called *short-term sensitization.*

Long-term sensitization also occurs. Following several training sessions of repeated sensiti-
zations, the neurons undergo physical changes that are a graded extension of what occurred in
the short-term sensitization. This long-term sensitization is often referred to as *long-term
facilitation.* In this process, the repeated strong stimulations cause the synthesis of two new
proteins. The first protein acts on the second messenger component to strengthen the short-term
mechanism and the second to promote the growth of new synapses. The motor neuron responds
by increased dendritic growth to accommodate the increased synapses from the presynaptic
neuron.[4] The animal shows long-term memory for this nonassociative behavioral modification
(long-term sensitization), and the accompanying synaptic plasticity can last a very long time.[5]

This synaptic plasticity of increased axonal sproutings, increased transmitters, and corre-
spondent dendritic field expansion is accompanied by changes in the surrounding tissue. There
is an increase in the glial cell components, as well as the vascular supply to the region. These
changes occur rapidly and have been identified to take place within ten to fifteen minutes.[6] The
potential for the development of new pathways for new behaviors can occur rapidly and,
therefore, the therapist must be ready to reinforce the target behavior when it occurs.

This increased connectivity of the synapse is what might be called the foundation of a habit
or a repeated expected behavior. As we repeat an activity, such as in a therapy setting, we
increase the effectiveness of the desired action.

Work from Kandel's group has shown that there are acquisition stages of the simple forms
of learning. In infant *Aplysia*, there is an order of development as the organism matures. The
infant *Aplysia* is first capable of only habituation. Later, dishabituation is added to the learning
mechanism and finally sensitization. This sequence of development of learning strategies
indicates that the concept of learning is one that builds on previously developed mechanisms
and is not complete at birth. This understanding lends support to the foundations of some
therapies of rehabilitation[7] that suggest a hierarchy exists in the development of the individual
and successful therapy must be carried out in the same order.

TYPES OF LEARNING

Habituation and sensitization are types of nonassociative learning. They are related to learning
the properties of the stimulus. There can also be types of nonassociative learning that are more

complex where the association is not obvious. Kupfermann[8] suggests that perception of sensory facts and imitation learning, such as language acquisition, are probably of this type.

Associative learning can take many different forms. Kupfermann[8] has suggested that the best way to classify them is on the basis of the experimental paradigms used to study them: classical conditioning and operant conditioning. These categories have also found useful clinical application, as we shall see. In associative learning, the organism learns to predict the relation between two presented stimuli.

In classical conditioning, the conditioned stimulus, that stimulation that has been previously incapable of producing a response, is paired with a response that can be considered to be a reinforcement. When these closely paired stimuli are consistently administered together, the organism links them together and is able to predict the relation between them. An example is a tone that precedes a shock to the leg of a rat that results in leg withdrawal (unconditioned response) to the tone (the conditioned stimulus). Eventually, the tone alone will produce the leg withdrawal without the shock.

Established conditioned responses may decrease in probability of occurrence if the conditioned stimulus is presented without the unconditioned stimulus. This is known as *extinction*. The attempt here is to break the relationship between the two, such as breaking a habit! This form of unlearning is just as important to the survival of the organism as the initial learning. This makes the organism adaptable to the environment, whether it be a snail or a human. In therapy, the effort is to not offer reward and reinforcement for behaviors that are undesirable. On the other hand, if a desired behavior is carried out, immediate reinforcement is demanded to solidify the synaptic connections.

Operant conditioning is the other class of associative learning. Operant conditioning may also be called trial and error learning. Again, the organism is learning a predictive relation between two events. The best known experiment is carried out by placing a hungry rat in a box, with the rat, upon pressing the lever, to receive a reward of food. The reward of food reinforces the action of the lever press and the organism learns the relation.

Conditioned and operant learning were at first thought to operate by totally different mechanisms. The advances in our understanding of the cellular mechanisms now show that they are closely related at the synaptic level. In conditioned learning, the response is evoked by a specific stimulus, whereas, in operant learning, the stimulus or relation is not specific, but the association is linked. At the synaptic level, the two types of learning are based on the same mechanisms. The timing of the stimuli is important in conditioned learning, as is the reinforcement in operant learning. In both cases, the organism learns to predict relations.

The establishment of relations between two events has been attributed to the role played by a part of the brain known as the *hippocampus*.[4] This phylogenetically older structure is found on the medial surface of the base of the brain. Recent work has shown that there is increased activity in the hippocampus as the organism acquires associations between visual stimuli and tactile spatial responses. The cells in particular parts of the hippocampus respond to repeated stimulation with an increased facilitation of the excitatory synaptic potentials in the postsynaptic hippocampal neurons which can last for hours, weeks, or months. This activity is called *long-term potentiation* (LTP).

LTP experiments provided the first direct evidence in mammals for Hebb's rule. This rule states that, when an axon of Cell A excites Cell B and repeatedly takes part in firing it, some growth processes or metabolic changes take place in one or both cells so that A's efficiency as one of the cells firing B is increased. This increased activity acts as a continuing reminder that the cell has been active in a particular relationship, and further, closely related or associated events will now activate more neurons. It is the richness of the interactions initiated by the activity of the hippocampus that might account for the relating of events we see in associative learning.

The hippocampus may act like a center for distribution of diverse incoming stimuli of an event. Our presence at a party with all the other people, decorations, smells, conversations, and sounds are filtered through the hippocampus and spun out through the internal circuitry to all parts of the cerebral cortex where associations may be made. This is an essential component of memory and recall and forms the basis of learning. It is interesting to note that deterioration in Alzheimer's disease takes place first in the region of the hippocampus.[9]

Baddeley[10] has suggested a model for the understanding of hippocampal involvement in the process of working memory, which we suggest is similar to what is described above as the association of events. There are three components of his model: (1) a central executive, most likely a component of the hippocampus; (2) a visuospatial sketch pad, a neural pathway connecting components of the occipital lobe for visual association and the parietal lobe for tactile sensation; and (3) a phonological loop, a component of the auditory modality in the temporal lobe and components of the parietal lobe.

These three components of Baddeley's model can account for the role the hippocampus plays in associating events. These associations, as we have seen, probably are based on the long-term potentiation that is characteristic of some of the hippocampal neurons. This ability of the hippocampus to be influenced by multiple inputs may account for the role that a rich, multiple therapy environment plays in successful rehabilitation.

PLASTICITY OF THE NERVOUS SYSTEM

Kandel[4] summarizes the current evidence for the ability of the cerebral cortex to be modified by experience. It has been shown that, during development, certain portions of the visual pathway may be modified during a critical period. But beyond these specialized critical periods, research in experimental animals has shown that injury and loss of function in an extremity results in the alteration of the receptive areas of the cerebral cortex. Again, the evidence supports the changes on the cellular level as reflecting the changes in the periphery or the environment.

Kaplan[11] has conducted experiments and reviewed other literature that confirms the plasticity of the adult mammalian brain. Kaplan's arguments suggest that the "enriched environment" of the rehabilitation plan provides for maintaining and/or enhancing the remaining neural plasticity for cognitive and musculoskeletal functions. The real benefit from this enriched environment may be in its effect on the considerable changes that take place within the brain. These environmental enhancements can provide the proper stimulations for the enhancement of the synaptic connectivity, as shown by Kandel[4] and Kupfermann.[8]

Black and Greenough[12] have suggested that the brain demonstrates a neural plasticity to changes in the environment. They have described two types: experience-expectant plasticity and experience-dependent plasticity. Experience-expectant plasticity occurs during development and is an overproduction of synapses in the sensory systems. During these periods of overproduction, the organism is prepared to respond to the stimulation provided by the environment to reinforce those experience-related synapses that are functionally significant. This suggests the role of the neurons in the sensitive periods of development of the sensory systems.

Experience-dependent plasticity occurs later in development in response to the changes that take place in the environment and is not dependent on the overproduction of synapses. Instead, this is the synaptogenesis that occurs in learning and is the response of the neurons to the stimulations of the environment.

Additional support for the effect that stimulation has on learning has been shown in infant rats by Kevine and Alpert.[13] Their experiments showed that the stimulation provided by the handling of infant rats increased the myelination in the cortex, defined on the basis of total brain cholesterol. Myelin formation is essential for the full functioning of the nervous system.

The stimulation of the developing or recovering neurons accelerates the development of myelin and thus improves the opportunities for improvement in functioning.

IMPORTANCE OF DEVELOPMENTAL NEUROBIOLOGY IN UNDERSTANDING THE BASIS FOR REHABILITATION

One additional concept from the underlying basic sciences is necessary for our understanding of the therapies utilized for the traumatically brain-injured and that is the sequence of development of the organism. Every organism undergoes a sequential development as it matures.

Certain basic events must precede more complex events. "One must crawl before one can walk" is an old adage. Its basis in reality is that the long neuronal pathways and peripheral nerves must be myelinated before the leg muscles become functional for walking. However, the alternating movements of the shoulder and hips in crawling provide the necessary stimulation for the increase in the neuronal connectivity.

The basic locomotor pattern in the midbrain is stimulated and the movement pattern enhanced. This is the basis for the therapies found effective in the treatment of the learning disabled and multihandicapped children. The building of higher level activity on the basic structures is a primary tenet of many physical and occupational therapies.[7,14]

The concept of building higher levels of functional activity on lower levels applies to other areas of rehabilitation as well. In the cognitive area, one develops simple concepts and then adds to them. We are first able to describe objects using very simple descriptions of color, size, and shape. We move on to descriptions of their usefulness and, eventually, to the features of the object, allowing use of the object for other extended purposes (see Chapter 12 of this volume). It has been suggested that the foundations of language are built from simple foundations to higher structures. The distinctive features of the language, such as vowels and later changes to consonants, are built progressively into identifiable sounds with meaning. This development of higher structures in language seems to follow the pattern of the embryological development of the brain.[15] The ability to develop concepts as we mature intellectually is a function of the richness of the connectivities we are able to make. In a similar manner, the rehabilitation process must assure that the foundations are established on which further progress might be imposed.

In the traumatically brain-injured patient, the injury may damage areas of the brain that control functional behaviors that are built on more basic behaviors. Therapy directed at the basic levels prior to the higher or more complex functional behaviors will lead to a more successful rehabilitation.[16]

Ebbesson[17] has postulated that the evolutionary development of the mammalian brain is based on a parsimony of the expansion of the function of previously existing structures. As the brain developed through the species, it utilized existing connectivities to develop new functional areas. This is similar to the mechanisms described for the neuronal basis of learning in which new synapses utilize existing pathways (see above), only this occurs over eons of time. Once again, the foundations that we see have their basis in the neurons of the brain.

In addition, Ebbesson[17] has demonstrated that experimental lesions in animals result in the sprouting of neuronal processes. These new sprouts follow a pattern that mimics the history of the development of that species. This implies that the initial sprouting efforts of the neuron are directed to the basic patterns and later sprouts will be directed to the functioning structures of the existing organism.

The sprouting that occurs after injury suggests the experience-expectant plasticity described above and perhaps offers an explanation for the unexpected improvement seen in some patients. The axonal growth may be a function of the genetically released stimulation and, coupled with the dendritic branching from the stimulation of the learning environment, results in the experience-dependent plasticity.

Therapy should take advantage of the multiple sprouting and direct therapies at the target behavior so as to increase the possibility of capturing the early sprouts for functional activity. The sooner therapies can begin after medical stability, the greater the opportunities for success.

That ontogeny, the development of the individual organism, recapitulates phylogeny, the evolution of the species, is an old concept that grew to be suspect. Based on new work, such as that by Ebbesson[17] and others, it is now considered that the developments of the individual and the species show parallels rather than direct duplications. Understanding these developmental aspects gives us an approach for the therapies that are utilized. The work in experimental animals should guide our activities as we approach the traumatically brain-injured population.

SUMMARY

Rehabilitation of the traumatically brain-injured population is based partially on a learning process. The therapies undertaken are directed at maximizing the remaining functions and developing new functional capacities. In either case, the direction of the activities should be toward increasing useful activities and decreasing undesired behaviors. As we have seen, these behaviors and activities are based on neuronal connectivities.

The joint efforts of the therapist and patient in the long hours of repetitive activity are directed on building simple basic foundations on which later, more complex activities can be overlaid. These therapeutic activities can be directed at the musculoskeletal activities for movement or to the cognitive areas for development of functional conceptualization. It is the constant stimulation provided by the rich rehabilitation environment that opens new possibilities for enhancing the synaptic connectivities in the central nervous system.

The long-term potentiation in the hippocampus, and possibly other parts of the brain, provides the neuronal foundations for the association of stimuli. The repetitive use of the synaptic junctions strengthens the pathways for those desired behaviors. Those therapies that have been shown to be successful in other injured populations can now be applied to the traumatically brain-injured population with renewed confidence. The confidence comes from the rapidly expanding literature on new discoveries in learning — discoveries that are based on the very foundation of the structure of the brain, the neuron, and the synapse.

REFERENCES

1. Hebb, D. O., *The Organization of Behavior*, John Wiley & Sons, New York, 1949.
2. Sejnowski, T. J. and Tesauro, G., The Hebb rule for synaptic plasticity: Algorithms and implementations, in *Neural Models of Plasticity*, Burn, J. H. and Berry, W. O., Eds., Academic Press, San Diego, 1989, 94.
3. Bailey, C. H. and Chen, M., Morphological basis of long-term habituation and sensitization, *Aplysia Sci.,* 220, 91, 1983.
4. Kandel, E. R., Cellular mechanisms of learning and the biological basis of individuality, in *Principles of Neural Science,* 3rd edition, Kandel, E. R., Schwartz, J. H., and Jessell, T. M., Eds., Elsevier, New York, 1991, 1009.
5. Levitan, I. B. and Kaczmarek, L. K., *The Neuron, Cell and Molecular Biology*, Oxford University Press, New York, 1991.
6. Chang, F.-L. F. and Greenough, W. T., Transient and enduring morphological correlates of synaptic activity and efficacy changes in the rat hippocampal slice, *Brain Res.,* 309, 35, 1984.
7. Bobath, B., The treatment of neuromuscular disorders by imposing patterns of coordination, *Physiotherapy,* 55, 18, 1969.
8. Kupfermann, I., Learning and memory, in *Principles of Neural Science,* 3rd edition, Kandel, E. R., Schwartz, J. H., and Jessell, T. M., Eds., Elsevier, New York, 1991, 997.
9. Selkoe, D. J., Amyloid protein and Alzheimer's disease, *Sci. Am.,* 265, 68, 1991.
10. Baddeley, A., Working memory, *Science*, 255, 556, 1992.
11. Kaplan, M. S., Plasticity after brain lesions: Contemporary concepts, *Arch. Phys. Med. Rehabil.,* 69, 984, 1988.

12. Black, J. E. and Greenough, W. T., Developmental approaches to the memory process, in *Learning and Memory: A Biological View*, 2nd edition, Martinez, J. L. and Kesner, R. P., Eds., Academic Press, New York, 1991.
13. Kevine, S. and Alpert, M., Differential maturation of the central nervous system as a function of early experience, *Arch. Gen. Psychiatry,* 1, 403, 1959.
14. Ayers, A. J., *Sensory Integration and Learning Disorders*, Western Psychological Services, Los Angeles, 1972.
15. Ashley, M. J. and Lehr, R. P., Embryological considerations of distinctive feature theory, *Folia Phoniatr.,* 43, 93, 1991.
16. Carr, J. H. and Shepard, R. B., *Physiotherapy in Disorders of the Brain: A Clinical Guide*, William Heinemann Medical Books Limited, London, 1980.
17. Ebbesson, S. O. E., The parcellation theory and its relation to interspecific variability in brain organization, evolutionary and ontogenetic development, and neuronal plasticity, *Cell Tissue Res.*, 213, 179, 1980.

10

The Use of Applied Behavior Analysis in Traumatic Brain Injury Rehabilitation

Craig S. Persel and Chris H. Persel

CONTENTS

0-8493-9463-5/95/$0.00+$.50

INTRODUCTION

The issue of maladaptive behavior as an associated sequela of traumatic brain injury (TBI) is one of the most important aspects in brain injury rehabilitation, since behavior disorders often represent a significant barrier to effective rehabilitation.[1] Changes in personality and behavior are also familiar consequences of TBI.[2,3] In the acute stages of recovery from TBI, it is common for a person to exhibit a variety of behavior disorders.[4] Such behavioral disturbances are considered by many to be a phase of normal recovery of cognition.[5,6] When these behaviors continue past acute recovery, however, and begin to form standard patterns of interaction with others, genuine concern is warranted. Behavior disorders are disturbing to families, disruptive to therapy, and can jeopardize client safety.[7] Thus, effective behavior analysis can be a powerful tool for teaching people more appropriate ways of interacting with their environment.

    The purpose of this chapter is to clearly illustrate and simplify the concepts, techniques, and uses of applied behavior analysis with those suffering from traumatic brain injury. Although it is assumed that the reader has some basic understanding and/or experience with applied behavior analysis, difficult technical terms have been avoided wherever possible. When only technical jargon will suffice to effectively explain or label a particular concept or method, the term is defined.

In keeping with the more practical nature of this chapter, a couple of areas related to applied behavior analysis will not be covered. First, single-subject research design will not be discussed. Although single-subject research is important to the scientific advancement of applied behavior analysis, we feel that it requires special attention that is beyond the scope of this chapter. Second, there will be no instruction for measuring interrater reliability. Although substantiating agreement between independent observers is important in determining reliability of data, like single-subject research design, it falls within the boundaries of research and not necessarily the practical application of behavior technology. Collecting interrater data is also a very time-consuming and expensive procedure and not one to which most rehabilitation facilities are willing to devote resources.

What you will find in this chapter are the tools necessary to organize and carry out effective behavior programming for people with traumatic brain injury. The person with traumatic brain injury represents a special challenge to rehabilitation professionals and family members. Maladaptive behavior is only one facet of a complex neurobehavioral picture. Cognitive, physical, and emotional changes resulting from brain injury must be taken into consideration in the overall behavioral treatment of the client with TBI. Behavioral treatment does not work alone. Behavioral programming is most effective when it is integrated with a comprehensive rehabilitation program. For example, as a client's information processing skills increase, so does the ability to deal with cognitively challenging situations. As adjustment to disability improves, the client becomes better equipped to face the loss of functional ability. As motor and perceptual skills develop, so does the opportunity to live more independently. Behavior programs provide a "metastructure" within which the various therapeutic disciplines are carried out.

The challenge is to rehabilitate people with traumatic brain injury in the least restrictive setting possible.[8] It is hoped this chapter will provide therapists, educators, family members, and other involved people with the materials and methods necessary to help clients with traumatic brain injury regain their highest level of independence.

THE BRAIN-BEHAVIOR RELATIONSHIP

As many readers know, traumatic brain injury can have many serious consequences. Physical, cognitive-communicative, functional, and psychological skills can be severely affected. Common areas of physical deficit are ambulation, balance and coordination, fine motor skills, strength, and endurance.[9] Cognitive deficits can encompass language and communication, information processing, memory, and perceptual skills.[10] Functional skills such as hygiene and grooming, dressing, and money management, to name but a few, are usually affected.[11] A person's psychological status is also stressed. Depression, anxiety, adjustment to disability, and sexuality issues are frequently encountered by people with TBI.[12] Any or all of these difficulties may bear directly on the behavior of a client. Recent studies have even linked cognitive recovery with the degree of psychopathology.[13] Compound these with medical issues, such as location of damage, severity of injury, seizure disorders, preinjury characteristics of personality, intelligence and learning style, and a complex neurobehavioral picture is created.

Brain injury can occur in a number of ways. Traumatic brain injuries, as opposed to stroke, Alzheimer's, Parkinson's, etc., typically result from accidents in which the head impacts an object (e.g., windshield, ground). This is the most common type of traumatic brain injury. However, other brain injuries, such as those caused by insufficient oxygen (e.g., cardiac arrest, near drowning), poisoning (e.g., toxic fumes), or infection (e.g., encephalitis) can cause similar deficits.[14,15] Many of the most severely behaviorally involved clients we have worked with over the years were injured in these "less common" ways

Mild traumatic brain injury (MTBI), another important category of brain injury, is characterized by one or more of the following symptoms: a brief loss of consciousness, loss of memory immediately before or after the injury, any alteration in mental state at the time of the accident, or focal neurological deficits.[16] In many MTBI cases, the person is only dazed, yet continues to endure chronic functional consequences.[17] Some people suffer long-term effects known as *postconcussion syndrome* (PCS).[18] Persons suffering from PCS can experience subtle, yet significant, changes in cognition and personality[19] and even experience seizurelike symptoms.[20]

All of these brain injuries will influence behavior. The relationship between the brain and behavior is very complex and beyond the scope of this chapter to review comprehensively; however, it is important for those involved in behavior programming to have at least a rudimentary understanding of this association because of its significant, underlying effect on behavior. Problems such as denial, apathy, emotional lability, impulsivity, frustration intolerance, lack of insight, inflexibility, perseveration, confabulation, lack of initiation, poor judgment and reasoning, and decreased social skills can often be linked to specific areas of brain damage.[21]

To begin with, most TBI's result in widespread damage to the brain. This is because the brain is "bounced" and "twisted" inside the skull during the impact of an accident. Nerve cells are torn from one another in what is known as *diffuse axonal injury.*[22] Localized damage also occurs when the brain is forced against the skull during the acceleration-deceleration phase of an accident. The brain stem, limbic system, frontal lobe, and temporal lobes are particularly vulnerable in this type of injury.

The brain stem is located at the base of the brain near bony areas. Aside from regulating basic arousal and vegetative functions, the brain stem is involved in attention and, thus, short-term memory skills. Deficits to these areas can lead to disorientation, frustration, and anger. The limbic system, higher up in the brain, is associated with emotions and affect. Disorders of the limbic system can result in explosive rage.[23,24] Connected to the limbic system are the temporal lobes, involved in many cognitive skills such as memory, language, and sequencing. Damage to the temporal lobes or seizures in this region have been associated with a number of behavioral disorders.[25] The frontal lobe is almost always injured due to its size (taking up 29% of total cortical space) and its susceptibility of location near the front of the cranium.[26] The frontal lobe, like the temporal lobes, is involved in many cognitive functions. It is also considered our emotional control center and home of the personality.[27] Damage to this area, resulting in what is sometimes called *frontal lobe syndrome,* can result in decreased judgment and increased impulsivity, irritability, and aggression.[28]

MEDICATION

It is now widely recognized that pharmacological intervention for behavioral disorders with the postacute client with TBI is not necessarily the treatment of choice. It is much more desirable to implement behavior programs that manipulate the environment and help the client develop self-control.[29] Many medications used in the past, or with other populations to combat behavior problems, may elicit more agitation from the traumatically brain-injured person or confuse them at a time when attention and arousal are often already problematic.[30] Recent studies have indicated that disorientation, which can be compounded by medications, is closely related to both physical and verbal aggression with the traumatically brain injured.[31] Although some medications, such as haloperidol, amantadine, and propranolol, have proven useful in treating behavior problems in the early stages of recovery from TBI,[32-34] the brain-injured person may experience more cognitive confusion and react with increased agitation. The use of stimulants, such as methylphenidate, to reduce behavior problems has shown mixed results.[35-36] This is not to say that medications should never be used, but there should be careful monitoring of the interactive effects of medication with behavior, as well as awareness of the potential for chronic overuse resulting in permanent side effects for the client, such as tardive dyskinesia, motor restlessness, and others.[37]

The treatment setting may be such that pharmacological management is necessary. In those unfortunate circumstances, medications should be closely monitored because they can often lose effect. In such circumstances, the choice may be between no medication, trial periods of alternative medications, or medication dosages to the point of sedation. Once a person has progressed beyond acute hospitalization, many behavior medications can be tapered while closely observing the person's behavior within the structure of a behavior program.[38] This approach makes it much easier to reach an educated decision regarding continuation of the medication.

ETHICS

Applied behavior analysis (sometimes referred to as *behavior modification*) has always been plagued by controversy. The mere mention of behavior modification is usually enough to elicit a strong response from professionals and the public alike. For many, the use of behavior modification principles and techniques is, in some way, forcing a person to change against his or her will. Deep-rooted concepts regarding democracy, free will, and humanism are threatened by the notion of applying scientific methods to change human behavior.

What some fail to realize is that human behavior is continuously being modified by our environment. Influences from politicians and parents to television and teachers help shape and pattern our behavior. Applying behavior analysis is not meant to assume an authoritarian role over a person, but to analyze the relationship between events and behavior. The goal is to increase, not decrease, personal freedom by expanding the behavioral options available to the person, thereby enhancing opportunities for community, social, and family interaction. Such opportunities are severely restricted for people with behavior problems. Applied behavior analysis is a structured technique for reducing behaviors that limit independence and increasing actions that empower a person.

Of course, misuse of applied behavior analysis has occurred, and punishment techniques have been overused. However, the notion that applied behavior analysis should not be used, or more specifically, that punishment should be severely limited, is neither rational nor practical. The alternatives to applied behavior analysis are typically medication, physical restraint, or life in a locked institution, all of which carry their own ethical ramifications.[47] Applied behavior analysis, used within proper guidelines, is an effective and humane method for reducing maladaptive behaviors and teaching new skills.

Alberto and Troutman [48] have outlined a number of basic concepts regarding the ethical use of behavior analysis.

- **Use the least restrictive setting:** Clients should be living in the least restrictive setting and be provided a therapeutic environment that is safe, fun, and offers access to a variety of activities. Recreational activities and social/community involvement are essential elements of an effective rehabilitation environment.
- **Benefit the client:** The goal of any behavior procedure should be to benefit the client and protect his/her welfare, not to improve staff convenience. For example, pharmacological management of behavior is very often used with the latter objective in mind.
- **Provide competent and trained staff:** Clients should be treated by competent staff who are trained and supervised by experienced professionals. Behavior programs are only as sound as the staff that implements them.
- **Teach functional skills:** Clients should be taught functional skills to replace maladaptive behaviors. Behavior problems may be a result of the client's reduced ability to perform independently in his/her environment or of a decreased behavioral repertoire.
- **Evaluate programs systematically:** Behavior programs should be methodically evaluated for effectiveness. Data analysis is a crucial component of this process.

- **Choose reinforcement programs first:** Behavior programs that include punishers should be used only after other reinforcement programs have been exhausted. Long-term maintenance and generalization are only two of many reasons why reinforcement programs are the procedure of first choice.

We have added some additional guidelines to consider:

- **Use the least aversive procedure:** When two programs are deemed effective, the least aversive procedure should be used. Aversive procedures typically produce more side effects.
- **Select appropriate target behaviors:** Make certain that determinations of behaviors as maladaptive are not based on personal values of staff. The inappropriateness of many behaviors is subjective.
- **Monitor side effects:** While reducing target behaviors, closely observe for an increase in other inappropriate behavior(s). This is particularly important when implementing an aversive procedure.
- **Use reasonable intervention procedures:** All maladaptive behaviors exhibit a "degree" of inappropriateness that has implications for the type of procedure recommended. For example, verbal aggression would generally not require a physical restraint.

As the number of people with traumatic brain injury increases, rehabilitation programs will face difficult ethical questions.[49] Accountability is the key. All facilities carrying out behavior programs should have clear goals, comprehensive data collection, and the ability to provide rationale for starting, continuing, and ending a behavior program. This includes a means of closely monitoring all the previously discussed guidelines to operate ethically sound behavior programs. Applied behavior analysis is a powerful tool for changing behavior. If used correctly, clients are given the opportunity to relearn many lost skills and to become as independent as possible in the shortest amount of time.

GENERAL MANAGEMENT GUIDELINES

The environmental conditions posed by treatment and care settings for people with traumatic brain injury can have significant impact on behavior. Organizing the therapeutic setting and carefully planning your approach to the client can increase opportunities for successful learning and decrease the chances of a behavioral episode. The following are ten recommendations for structuring a positive learning environment for the person with TBI:

1. **Increase rest time.** People with TBI, especially in the initial stages of recovery, can be extremely fatigued. Monitor the person's behavior and schedule rest periods during those times related to an increased probability of problem behavior. A word of warning though — do not forget to reduce these rest periods as the person recovers and gains endurance.
2. **Keep the environment simple.** People with TBI are easily overstimulated by their surroundings. The inability to filter out external stimuli can lead to confusion and increase the chances of a behavioral episode. Interruptions and distractions should be kept to a minimum and the session format kept consistent.
3. **Keep instructions simple.** Instructions, prompts, and cues should be kept as concrete and simple as possible. This may mean writing down instructions, as well as stating them. It may also mean keeping verbal prompts to a minimum. Many people with TBI have difficulty processing auditory information. Instead, try using nonverbal instruction techniques, such as modeling or gestural cueing.
4. **Give feedback and set goals.** Self-monitoring skills can be diminished with the traumatically brain injured. They must rely on others to provide feedback until the ability is relearned. Provide frequent and consistent positive feedback for success. Most people respond well to supportive encouragement. Setting goals helps the client predict where he/she is "going" with therapy and provides him/her with some incentive for completing therapeutic tasks.[39]

5. **Be calm and redirect to task.** People who cannot control their own behavior need others to model and structure a stable, nonthreatening environment. Remaining calm, while the client is escalated, can help reduce agitation and decrease the chances of inadvertently reinforcing the client with attention for acting out. A method gaining widespread attention, "gentle teaching", uses a variation of this approach as a central technique.[40,41] It involves ignoring the exhibited behavior, redirecting the client to the task, and rewarding successful performance. However, the rather unstructured approach of gentle teaching, its lack of scientific support, and its philosophical assumptions contrast sharply with traditional behavior analysis.[42]

6. **Provide choices.** Research indicates that providing clients with choices can reduce serious behavior problems.[43] Giving them opportunities to choose tasks can be an effective technique when working with the traumatically brain injured. It allows clients an element of freedom and a measure of control over their environment. Some clients, however, require "limited" choices which decrease the range of choices so that they are not overwhelmed or left with an open-ended opportunity to say, "No".

7. **Decrease chance of failure.** Do not work above the client's level of ability. This will only lead to frustration and increase the chance of a behavioral episode. Try to keep the success rate above 80%. This ensures that the client is challenged, while at the same time feels successful. A variation of this technique is known as *behavioral momentum.* This procedure involves presenting tasks with which the client is likely to comply immediately before presenting tasks which are likely to be more problematic.[44] This establishes a high rate of performance (and, it is hoped, reinforcement) just prior to more difficult tasks, with the idea that compliance will be more likely to continue.

8. **Vary activities.** Although there is a need for consistency and repetition when working with the traumatically brain injured, there is also a need to keep the session interesting. Therapy can become boring and frustrating if the same tasks are endlessly repeated. Vary the activities to maintain interest and increase success. Also, try interspersing easy tasks (those likely to be done correctly) among more difficult tasks. Studies have shown this procedure to be effective in reducing the likelihood of aggression.[45]

9. **Over-plan.** Do not approach a session with only a few ideas or activities to complete. There will be days when the client finishes everything quickly and you are left with nothing else to do, or the client may be having a difficult time (e.g., more confused) and you need some alternate activities more suited to the functioning of the client that day. Be prepared for anything and you'll be less likely to have to confront a behavior problem.

10. **Task-analyze.** Try breaking a task down into smaller steps. Each step can then be treated as a complete task. Functional skills, such as dressing, hygiene and grooming, etc., are particularly suited to this approach; [46] however, just about any activity or task can be "dissected" into its component parts.

BASIC PRINCIPLES

The basic principles of applied behavior analysis are relatively easy to understand. Within a short time, most of the fundamental concepts of behavior analysis, and what is termed *operant conditioning,* can be grasped. Simply put, behavior analysis focuses on the behavior of people and the environmental influences that precede and follow the behavior, as opposed to their thoughts and feelings. We can refer to these factors as a person's *behavioral condition.* The components of a person's behavioral condition are the antecedent, the behavior, and the consequence. Behavior analysis attempts to explain the relationship between these components. A relationship is referred to as a *contingency.* For example, reinforcers are delivered "contingent" upon performance of a certain behavior.

Antecedent

To begin with, all target behaviors (those behaviors we wish to modify) are preceded by some event in the person's environment. This preceding event is called the *antecedent.* This event can be a broad-based condition that influences behavior (setting event) or a more specific stimulus (stimulus event). In a manner of speaking, the setting event sets the stage for the occurrence of the behavior.[50] For example, fatigue resulting from a lack of sleep may be a setting event for behavior problems the next day. Stimulus events are more discrete. For example, a phone ringing means that a behavior (answering the phone) will be reinforced (talking to someone). The antecedent may be an event occurring externally to the person (e.g., lighting, noises, instructions) or internally to the person (e.g., headache, flu, seizure, medication). One word of caution — even though one has to take into consideration internal antecedents to behavior, the focus of behavior analysis is always on those factors external to the person. Internal antecedents to behavior (e.g., vestibular sensitivity, headache) are best dealt with via medical and therapeutic disciplines within the rehabilitation regimen.

It is important for staff members to realize that external antecedents are under staff control. Tone of voice, body language, therapeutic demands, and physical setting are some of the variables that staff can adjust to decrease the likelihood of a behavioral episode.

Necessary tasks, however, should not be avoided simply because they can, at times, be antecedents to behavioral episodes. Continued progress toward independence is often reliant on the person's participation in such tasks at a very intense level of rehabilitation. Avoidance of difficult therapy tasks to reduce "problem" behaviors can be very seductive to staff, but it may simultaneously teach the client to actually exhibit more negative behavior as a means to escape the rigorous demands of therapy. Therapists and behavioral programmers need to survey all environmental antecedents and weigh the advantages and disadvantages of the therapeutic regimen before eliminating or modifying any requirements. Lowering therapeutic expectations because of potential acting-out by the person may negatively impact the person's long-term independence.

Likewise, internal antecedents should be evaluated for other potential treatments which may assist in the person's behavioral improvement. These should not be viewed as reasons to avoid implementation of a behavioral program. Let's say, for example, that a person has a vestibular lesion which causes him to be quite sensitive to motion. One day, after a motor vehicle trip, the person is not feeling well and, during therapy, is quite escalated and trying to avoid participation. He strikes a staff member. Some therapists would be inclined to believe that the individual did not feel well and that the therapist who was struck should not have persisted in treatment. While this reasoning may seem sound, it is limited by the fact that under no circumstances is it acceptable to strike another person. Thus, the behavioral program would include recognition of the contribution of the vestibular component but would also include a means for de-escalating behavioral agitation and for responding to physical aggression.

Behavior

An antecedent event is followed by the occurrence of a behavior. If the behavior has been chosen for modification, to either increase or decrease, it is referred to as the *target behavior*. People with traumatic brain injury can exhibit a wide variety of behaviors that require intervention. A target behavior must be observable and immediately recordable. The target behavior must also be very clearly defined in terms of observable actions. This is known as an *operational definition*. Two therapists, for instance, can have very different ideas about what constitutes a behavior. For example, take the behavior "physical aggression". Does it include "spitting" or "threatening"? What about "self-injurious behavior"? Should "throwing or breaking objects" be included? Clear and concise definitions of target behaviors are critical to identifying the behaviors and to implementing programs consistently.

People with traumatic brain injury can exhibit a number of maladaptive behaviors. Behavior disorders (Table 10.1) can be categorized as those of excess (occurring too often), those of deficit (not occurring often enough), and those of stimulus control (not occurring in the correct context).

TABLE 10.1 Behavior Categories and Examples

Excess	Deficit	Stimulus Control
Noncompliance	Compliance	Overfamiliarity
Angry language	Self-control	Public sexual behavior
Socially inappropriate talk	Social skills	Public grooming behavior
Disinhibition	Timeliness	Public discussion of private events
Physical aggression	Initiation	Undressing in public
Exiting	ADL's	
Hoarding		
Tardiness		
Impulsivity		
Sexually aberrant		
Perseveration		
Self-abuse		
Stealing		
Property destruction		
Overfamiliarity		

Excess behaviors tend to be the most noticeable and, thus, receive the most attention from other persons. Examples of excess behavioral disorders typically seen with the traumatically brain injured are noncompliance,[51-53] angry language,[50,51,54] hoarding, exiting,[55] physical aggression,[50,53] socially inappropriate talk,[56] impulsivity,[54] and tardiness.[52] Some other excess behaviors which may be exhibited are sexually aberrant behavior, perseveration, self-abuse, stealing, property destruction, and overfamiliarity. These behaviors can be disruptive to other clients, frighten others, and/or increase the risk of injury during treatment, thus increasing exposure to legal liability. If severe enough, they can result in a person not receiving proper therapeutic services or, worse yet, being isolated from family, friends, and community in an institutional setting.

Common deficit behaviors of people with traumatic brain injury are activities of daily living,[57] communication,[55] social skills,[58,59] and initiation.[52] Rehabilitation of these skills is of paramount importance in a client's progress toward more independent living. It is also important that excess behaviors which have been eliminated or reduced through structured behavioral programming be replaced with more appropriate behaviors occurring at a proper rate. Such behaviors will allow the client access to a wider range of naturally occurring reinforcers, thereby increasing the opportunity for successful generalization and maintenance of skills.

Stimulus control disorders can occur with any behavior which occurs in the wrong situation (e.g., brushing teeth, hugging another person, etc.). For example, the behavior may occur at the wrong time or place, or with the wrong person. The problem of stimulus control as a behavioral disorder has not been fully explored in TBI literature even though our experience indicates it to be a very common problem with this population. Most people with traumatic brain injury are adults who have already acquired many life skills. Their injury does not necessarily result in loss of the skill but, seemingly, loss of knowledge of the more abstract situation in which the behavior should occur. Antecedent or stimulus control behavior programs are tailor-made to positively impact these disorders.

Consequence

Target behaviors are followed by a consequent event that is going to affect the future rate, duration, and/or intensity of the behavior. Consequences are either *reinforcing* or *punishing*. Reinforcers will increase and punishers will decrease the future occurrence of the target behavior. Consequences do not inherently possess the quality of being either a reinforcer or a punisher. The effect of a consequent event on the frequency of a target behavior (i.e., whether it increases or decreases the target behavior) defines it as a reinforcer or a punisher. Let's use chocolate as an example. For a person who likes chocolate, its availability after the occurrence of a behavior may increase the frequency of that behavior, thereby defining it as a reinforcer. For a person who dislikes chocolate, its availability may actually decrease the frequency of target behavior, thus defining it as a punisher.

There are two types of positive reinforcers: *primary* and *secondary*. Primary reinforcers do not require any type of special training to develop their value. Food and water are two examples of primary reinforcers. Secondary reinforcers have gained their value through learning. Examples of secondary reinforcers are praise and money. Secondary reinforcers can be developed by pairing them with a primary reinforcer. For example, if praise is not a reinforcer for a person and food is, food can be paired with praise during behavioral procedures until praise serves as a reinforcer. Food can then be discontinued as a reinforcer.

There are also two types of punishment. One type involves presenting an aversive event following the behavior and the other removes a positive event following the behavior. For example, getting a ticket for speeding can be an aversive event, while having your driver's license taken away after three tickets is the removal of a positive event.

One of the most misunderstood concepts of behavior analysis is *negative reinforcement* — but it is important that those who work with people with traumatic brain injury understand this term. Negative reinforcement increases the occurrence of a behavior by eliminating the aversive event after the behavior has occurred.[60] In TBI rehabilitation, being allowed to escape and avoid therapeutic tasks is a common example of negative reinforcement.

Another basic principle of behavior analysis is *extinction*. Extinction does not involve either presenting or taking away consequences to behavior, but rather discontinues the reinforcement of a behavior. Not reinforcing the behavior eventually decreases or eliminates the occurrence of the behavior. *Ignoring* is probably the best example of an extinction procedure. Ignoring behaviors that were previously given attention (e.g., complaining, yelling, etc.) can be an effective technique when combined with reinforcement of positive behaviors.

It is recommended that reinforcement programs be attempted before implementing a punishment program. Reinforcement programs teach people what to do, are generally more effective for long-term maintenance of the desired behavior, and do not elicit many of the negative side effects inherent in punishment programs.

Prompting and Fading

Teaching behaviors involves *prompting* to help initiate the behavior. Instructions, gestures, and modeling are all examples of prompting. They are antecedents to the target behavior. The way in which prompting is utilized can have significant impact on how easily a client learns. A person with language deficits will have difficulty following verbal prompts. In this case, using physical gestures and cues can be more effective. Different types of prompts can be combined to facilitate the desired behavior. Shaping and chaining procedures rely on competent use of various prompting techniques (e.g., backward and forward chaining) to teach new skills.

The goal is for the behavior to occur independently without prompting. The method for accomplishing this is called *fading*. Fading is the systematic and gradual removal of prompting. If prompting is ended too quickly, the behavior may not continue. A more gradual reduction in prompting is recommended until the behavior is performed independently, or with as little prompting as possible. For example, teaching a person with traumatic brain injury a showering sequence may start with actual physical guidance through many of the steps. Next, some of the physical cues could be reduced to gestures (e.g., pointing) and then to verbal cues. Later, a written checklist could be placed in the shower, listing each step of the showering sequence. The checklist could then be removed and the client allowed to perform the task independently.

Generalization

Like fading, *generalization* is an important procedure in developing the independence of a person with traumatic brain injury. There are two types of generalization — *stimulus generalization* and *response generalization*. Whereas fading involves decreasing a behavior's dependence on prompts, stimulus generalization reduces a behavior's dependence on the conditions under which it was learned. All of us would agree that rehabilitation takes place in a restricted environment. It is the goal of stimulus generalization that behaviors learned under these conditions be transferred to other settings. For instance, the goal of learning to read in a clinic setting is that it will generalize to reading the newspaper at home or the grocery list at the supermarket. Learning to control physical aggression in the clinic, to give another example, is not as important as the ability to control aggression in the community.

Response generalization involves behaviors rather than the conditions under which they occur. In other words, if you reinforce or punish a behavior, other similar behaviors will also be affected. We have seen this occur with clients. A behavior treatment plan that focuses on reducing the most problematic behavior decreases other less severe behaviors at the same time. This experience lends support to the saying, "Worry about the big things and the little things will take care of themselves". Target the most severe behaviors first and you may never have to treat the small ones.

BEHAVIORAL DIAGNOSTICS

Prior to writing a behavioral treatment plan, it is essential that a comprehensive assessment of the client's history, current status, and future goals be performed. The success of a behavior program depends as much on an accurate evaluation of the client's behavior as on the intervention plan itself. The evaluation must analyze all the potential factors contributing to a client's behavior. The three basic behavioral diagnostic tools are 1) a historical survey, 2) a current status evaluation, and 3) a functional analysis.

Historical Survey

Collecting historical information helps the behavior programmer understand how the client may respond to the rehabilitation process, and what he or she expects to gain from treatment.[61] The first half of a historical survey covers a range of demographic data. This includes information on age, sex, marital status, children, parents, friends, religious preference, his or her living conditions prior to the injury, education, work history, and recreational interests. Information we have found to be particularly important is that concerning eating preferences, sleeping patterns, personal likes and dislikes, daily routines, and lifestyle characteristics. Many behavior problems can be averted with an understanding and appreciation of a client's lifestyle prior to the injury. Requiring the client to conform to unfamiliar schedules, foods, people, and situations that can be reasonably modified creates a potential setting event.[62] As we explained in the previous section, a setting event increases the likelihood of a problem behavior occurring. This can happen when facilities develop schedules that are easier or less expensive to manage. This inflexibility can contribute to unnecessary behavior problems which are actually more difficult and expensive to manage.

The second half of the historical survey concerns medical and rehabilitation history. It can be helpful for the behavior programmer to know the location and etiology of injury, the elapsed time since injury, and the course of treatment that has been provided. This furnishes the programmer with an idea of the client's rate of recovery. Additionally, knowledge of a client's medical history can be beneficial. For example, any diseases, major illnesses, or substance abuse problems which may have affected him or her before the injury may contribute to the client's current behavioral sequelae and future prognosis.

Most of the above information can be gathered from medical records, discussions with the previous treating staff, and an interview with the client and/or significant others, such as family and friends. Contact with prior treatment facilities provides insight into behaviors exhibited by the client since the injury, under what circumstances the behavior occurred, and staff response. Interviews with the client and/or significant others help to determine the client's premorbid behavior pattern which, in part, determines his or her response to the demands of rehabilitation and life after a traumatic brain injury.

Current Status

Traumatic brain injury usually involves more than just damage to the brain. Many medical and psychological complications can result from the TBI. These complications can also be setting events for behavior problems. For example, if a person is in pain or constantly dizzy, his or her behavioral control will likely be diminished. This is why a comprehensive evaluation of a client's current status is important.

A current status evaluation reviews a client's medical and psychological status and therapeutic testing results and examines the relationship of these to behavioral issues. A comprehensive review of the medical status involves looking at the cardiac, vascular, and respiratory systems, orthopedic and muscular capability, the sensory system, bowel and bladder functioning, and other areas of physiological functioning. Of all possible medical problems, medication usually has the most direct relationship to behavior. Medications can profoundly affect behavior, thus programmers need to be educated and informed on the subject.

A traumatic brain injury has an impact not only on the client but family and friends as well. It is important that programmers understand the dynamics between the client and significant others. After discharge from rehabilitation, family or friends may be required to carry out behavioral procedures with their loved one or, at the very least, maintain an environment which is conducive to continued learning and development.

One of the most important assessments of current status is a functional skills evaluation. How well is the client able to perform activities of daily living such as hygiene, grooming, dressing, and toileting? Is the client able to cook meals and clean the house? What about community mobility, driving, and shopping? Is the client able to manage his money? All of these issues are fundamental to some level of independent functioning. They will prescribe the type of living arrangement and level of assistance the client will require. Also, relearning functional skills can help to replace maladaptive behaviors while reducing the need for aversive procedures.

A review of therapeutic testing results completes the current status evaluation. Standard therapeutic testing includes cognitive, physical, and psychological evaluations, as well as a neuropsychological examination. A client's cognitive level can dictate the type of behavioral procedure that is implemented. Clients with severe cognitive impairment, for instance, will probably not participate in a contracting program because it requires more abstract thinking. Physical issues can also directly affect the treatment plan. For example, overcorrection or contingent restraint procedures can be especially ill-suited for clients with orthopedic concerns. The neuropsychological examination brings all of the client's skills and deficits into focus, helping the behavior programmer to design an appropriate treatment plan.

Functional Analysis

A functional analysis is central to the design of the treatment plan. Its purpose is to identify the function that each target behavior serves.[63] A functional analysis is composed of three parts: 1) describing the behavior and its surrounding events, 2) predicting the factors that control the behavior, and 3) testing the predictions by manipulating the identified factors.

A functional analysis begins by describing the behavior. This is accomplished by interview and/or direct observation. Direct observations should constitute the primary source of information because anecdotal reports from interviews can be clouded by subjective perceptions. Nevertheless,

FUNCTIONAL ANALYSIS	Time					
Behaviors						
Antecedent/Setting Events						
Demand/Request						
Difficult Task						
Perceived Functions						
Get/Obtain						
Attention						
Desired item/activity						
Escape/Avoid						
Demand/Request						
Activity						
Person						
Consequences						

FIGURE 10.1 Functional analysis form.

in cases where direct observations are not possible, interviews may be the only method for gathering the information needed to start a treatment plan. Interviews are conducted with those who have direct contact with the client, such as family members, caregivers, therapists, or paraprofessionals. The interview consists of identifying the target behavior, the conditions under which it normally takes place (antecedent or setting events), what events occur following the behavior (consequence), and what function the behavior serves (e.g., communicating needs). Some behavior problems can be reduced by simply improving the function that the behavior is attempting to perform.[64] For example, if behavior problems are being caused by an inability to effectively communicate one's needs, then improving a client's communication skills may decrease the problem behaviors. Although interviews are important to functional analysis, if possible they should be a secondary source of information.

Functional analysis is usually based on direct observations. The most precise method for collecting observational data is by recording the events surrounding behavioral episodes. An excellent form for organizing this information was designed by O'Neill et al.[65] Figure 10.1 is a modified version of this form. It includes a place to write in the time of each behavioral event, possible setting events (e.g., difficult task, demands, etc.), the perceived function of the behavior (e.g., attention, avoiding activity, etc.), and the consequence to the behavior. The completed form can then be analyzed for patterns of behavior and the conditions in which they most frequently occur. From this analysis, hypotheses can be formulated regarding conditions maintaining the behavior.

The last step in a functional analysis is to test the conclusions drawn from the interviews and direct observations. This involves manipulating specific conditions and observing whether the behavior changes. The idea is that, by changing the conditions surrounding the behavior (antecedents, setting events, and consequences), the behavior will change. Once the conditions for changing the behavior in the desired direction (higher or lower) have been identified, then a treatment plan can be implemented. For example, if physical aggression occurs with a client during 25% of the intervals while in therapy, but only during 5% of the time before starting therapy, one may try allowing the client "alone time" after completing a specified amount of therapy.

Of course, the time and financial constraints of rehabilitation may make it difficult to always complete this last step of a functional analysis before implementing a treatment plan. However, identifying the conditions that maintain behavior and monitoring the effects of changing these conditions can, at the very least, be utilized during the treatment plan.

BEHAVIOR PLAN FORMAT

A behavior treatment program includes four major components: 1) short- and long-term goals, 2) operational definitions of target behaviors, 3) data collection system and materials needed, and 4) staff procedures (Figure 10.2). The behavior programmer must synthesize diagnostic data (historical information, current status, and functional analysis) with goals of the client, family, treaters, and payer to create an individualized treatment program. The treatment plan should be written as clearly as possible and in an easy-to-follow structure. The programmer has to strike a balance between including all the necessary information and, at the same time, presenting it in a way that is concise and readable. The degree of staff behavioral training will dictate the level of sophistication with which the program can be written and followed with consistency. However, the reality of most rehabilitation environments, be it acute, postacute, or in the home, is that there is a wide range of behavioral competence. It is our experience that, even after extensive training, there are significant differences in the degree of natural ability among staff to carry out effective behavioral treatment. This being the case, a step-by-step procedural outline, combined with close monitoring of staff performance, is the most practical format with which to run behavior treatment plans.

Goals

Behavior treatment goals are separated into short- and long-term goals. Short-term goals are objectives that define the desired measurable change in the target behavior. A specific time frame for accomplishing the objective should be clearly stated. For example, physical aggression (the target behavior) will be reduced to 5% of the total recorded intervals within 30 days. Short-term goals help the client and staff focus on tangible achievements while continuing to strive toward long-term goals.

Long-term goals, on the other hand, describe the projected functional outcome of the treatment plan. For example, the client will increase independent living to a minimal supervision level (group home) or will be able to work in a part-time volunteer employment position. Long-term goals are defined by the client, family, caretakers, funding source, and other responsible parties.

All goals and objectives should include three parts: 1) how they will be assessed, 2) how often they will be reviewed, and 3) what type of report will be generated. Many regulating agencies, such as the Commission on the Accreditation of Rehabilitation Facilities (CARF), require these guidelines for accreditation. The assessment of goals can be accomplished by many available or in-house rating scales. For example, long-term goals of disability level can be gauged by the Disability Rating Scale.[66] Short-term goals can be evaluated by a standard data collection system (e.g., frequency count, time-sampling, etc.). Short- and long-term goals should include a statement concerning the frequency of review (e.g., weekly, biweekly, monthly) and what type of report will be produced.

Target Behavior

Target behaviors are the focus of the treatment plan. They are the behaviors that are interrupting therapy, impeding progress, endangering others, disrupting activities, or otherwise interfering with a person's ability to live independently in the community. They can be behaviors of excess (e.g., physical aggression), deficit (e.g., hygiene and grooming), or stimulus control (e.g., public sexual behavior).

Each target behavior must be defined operationally. The operational definition describes what the behavior looks like in objective, observable terms. For example, labeling a target behavior "physical aggression" without an operational definition leaves it wide open to interpretation. The more interpretation allowed in a behavior program, the less consistent it will be. Not only does an operational definition describe what a behavior is, but it also describes what it is not. For example, "physical aggression" could be defined as any attempted or actual hit, strike, kick, pinch, or grab by the client, not including spitting.

Operational definitions sometimes require that the context in which the target behavior will occur be identified. For example, "hand waving" is only a problem when it interferes with writing activities. The definition may also need to include the duration or rate at which the behavior must occur before it is considered a target behavior. For example, "refusing to participate in therapy for more than 30 seconds" may be the minimum criterion for "noncompliance".

Materials and Data Collection

The third section of a behavior treatment plan outlines all the materials required to carry out the prescribed procedures and the data collection system for tracking the rate and/or duration of the target behavior. Many behavior treatment plans require specific materials for implementing procedures. For example, a stopwatch may be needed for a "differential reinforcement of other behavior" program that calls for reinforcing the client after a specified period of time in which the target behavior does not occur. Any supplies or items that are used to implement the treatment plan (e.g., timer, tokens, tape recorder, etc.) need to be described in this section.

The second half of this section describes the data collection system. All behavior programs should have a procedure for gathering information which will be used to determine the effect of the treatment plan. The Data Collection and Graphing section of this chapter details methods for systematically recording and analyzing behavioral data. Without consistent data collection, it is difficult to ascertain whether the program is working. Anecdotal reports (i.e., verbal feedback from staff) are usually not reliable enough, due to their subjectivity, to make important decisions concerning the effectiveness of behavior programming. Frequency, interval, duration, or time-sampled data of operationally defined target behaviors gives the behavior programmer ample information, which, together with staff feedback, will allow for better treatment decisions.

BEHAVIOR TREATMENT PLAN

Client Name: C. G.
Program Start Date: 11-30-91
Implemented By: Clinical therapists and staff aides.

GOALS:

Short-Term Goal: To decrease physical aggression by 5% of total intervals from last month.

Long-Term Goal: To increase independent living scale (ILS) score to more than 80/100 pts. (min-mod. supervision).

Evaluation of Goals: Weekly summary of interval data.

TARGET BEHAVIORS:

Primary:

Physical Aggression (PA) - attempting to and/or striking out with an object or body part; may include hitting, kicking, pinching, grabbing without permission, scratching, throwing items at someone etc.; includes attempted or actual contact; does not include verbal threats or invasion of personal space.

Property Destruction (PD) - ramming, throwing, tearing, striking or breaking property (even if accidental; or attempts to do so), property does not have to be damaged.

No Cooperation (None) - did not participate in therapy at all and exhibited at least one target behavior. May be in therapy area, yet did not attempt any activities.

Secondary:

Angry Language (AL) - cursing, yelling, threats, hostile language, demands delivered with increased volume (above conversational level) lasting more than two seconds.

Refusal to Work (R) - active or passive statements or actions meant to evade start, interrupt or stop therapy tasks or directives; must be more than one minute; does not include slow processing time or lack of ability.

Exiting (E) - attempted to and/or left place of required activity.

Partial Cooperation (Part) - attempted and/or completed some therapy tasks as directed. Displayed one or more target behavior, but was able to be redirected to task or attempted the task prior to any behavior episode.

Full Cooperation (Full) - attempted and/or completed all therapy tasks as directed. No target behaviors displayed.

FIGURE 10.2 Example of a behavior treatment plan.

Treatment Procedures

The fourth, and main, section of the treatment plan describes the procedures of the behavior program. It outlines the staff's response to the target behavior (consequence) and arranging of environmental conditions prior to the behavior (antecedent). The section on behavior plan procedures details a variety of behavior treatment plans.

The treatment plan describes each step a staff member is to take before and after the occurrence of the target behavior. Every step needs to be described in concrete, understandable terms in a language that can be understood by a wide range of people, including the client,

MATERIALS AND DATA COLLECTION:

1.　　15-minute interval data sheet.
2.　　Two-minute Therapy Chart.
3.　　Two-minute board with countdown timer.

TREATMENT PROCEDURES:

Outline - This program will consist of several key components including: 1) a two-minute fixed interval DRO, 2) primary target behaviors of PA and PD, 3) a reward contingent upon completion of the 5 two-minute blocks of therapy with no occurrence of the target behaviors, 4) a graduated guidance program contingent on the occurrence of non-compliance, and 4) relaxation practice each hour.

Relaxation - Begin each hour with two minutes of timed relaxation practice. Tell C. G. to "take a couple of minutes to relax". Ask him to close his eyes, take a deep breath, and let his mind and muscles relax. Make every effort to keep the surrounding therapy area quiet during his relaxation time.

DRO - Following the relaxation period, post the two-minute board on a straight back chair near the task area where C. G. can see it clearly. Inform him that when each of the boxes has an "X" in it, then he can go outside. Set the timer for two minutes and begin therapy. Each time the timer sounds and C. G. has not exhibited a primary target behavior, "X" out a box on the board, quickly reset the timer, and continue therapy. Try and keep therapy tasks flowing comfortably while maintaining awareness of the timer. Immediately after the final (fifth) box has been "X'd", state to C. G. "Great, you stayed calm, we can go now" and take him for a short walk outside. Have C. G. walk himself during the walk unless he asks for assistance. Reflect to him that this is his time and he has earned it. After about 3-5 minutes, redirect C. G. back to therapy. Do not allow him to manipulate or slow his return to therapy. Assist as needed. Immediately reset the timer and repeat the above sequence.

Graduated Guidance - If a C. G. displays noncompliance (i.e., refusing to start a task), **immediately** provide hand-over-hand guidance. Have tasks available that C. G. can be physically guided through. For example, tasks requiring pointing, reaching, touching etc. As soon as noncompliance begins, start prompting the current task or immediately switch to an activity requiring motor involvement. Provide guidance until C. G. begins complying, then fade physical prompting. Once guidance has been discontinued, return to the task and/or approach used before the behavior occurred.

FIGURE 10.2 (continued).

staff, and family. More often than not, the success of a program rests on the ease with which the procedures can be followed. Figure 10.2 is an example of a completed treatment plan.

BEHAVIOR PLAN PROCEDURES

The staff member responsible for writing behavior programs has many designs from which to choose (Table 10.2). The types of behaviors exhibited by the client, the setting for implementing the program, and the level of staff skills and experience are all factors to be considered in choosing the most suitable behavior program. Once these factors have been identified and weighed, one can then choose a treatment procedure which is either *accelerative* (designed to increase the frequency or duration of a target behavior), *decelerative* (designed to decrease the frequency or duration of a target behavior), or *complex* (having characteristics of both accelerative and decelerative programs). Combinations of these procedures, in a multicomponent approach, can also be used simultaneously to increase the speed and stabilization of behavioral change.[67]

We will outline procedures for the most common behavior programs and provide illustrations (for most procedures) of actual cases encountered in behavioral treatment. Some of

TABLE 10.2   Behavior Program Treatment Procedure Designs

Accelerative	Decelerative	Complex
Positive programming	DRI	Contracting
Shaping and chaining	DRO	Stimulus control
	DRL	Token economy
	Overcorrection	
	Stimulus change	
	Stimulus satiation	
	Time-out	

the techniques we will not be covering in this chapter are group-based programs, peer-administered contingencies, biofeedback, and cognitively based treatment (e.g., stress reduction, problem-solving skills, self-statements, etc.). These methods are either not often used, not practical for people with traumatic brain injury (e.g., group-based programs, peer-administered contingencies), or fall more into the realm of counseling (e.g., cognitively based treatment).

Accelerative Programs

Positive Programming

Positive programming is nothing more than teaching an individual new skills through the use of reinforcing consequences.[68] Activities of daily living, functional communication, and social skills training are all examples of positive programming. This technique is familiar to most of us since we have been exposed to learning new skills (e.g., reading) and being rewarded for our performance (e.g., grade).

An advantage of positive programming is that it is constructive in nature. It teaches people how to do something. Positive programming helps to reduce undesirable behaviors that are incompatible with the new skill (e.g., the social skill of shaking hands is incongruous with hitting). Generalization and maintenance of skills taught through positive programming are also often supported by naturally occurring contingencies (e.g., learning to verbalize allows one to express and receive one's needs).

A disadvantage of positive programming can be its lack of quick results — positive programming takes time. Because of the tremendous costs involved in rehabilitation of people with traumatic brain injury, pressures are exerted on rehabilitation programs to bring about behavioral change as quickly as possible. This does not infer that positive programming should be excluded, rather that efficient programming must be developed to meet the needs of payers. To help accomplish this, positive programming can be integrated with other behavior programs that focus on decreasing undesirable behaviors. The result should be increased efficiency and rate of behavioral change.

Case Illustration

H. H. was a 32-year-old male injured in a motor vehicle accident. H. H.'s physical and cognitive skills were severely impaired. Expressive language, in particular, was extremely difficult. Most of his severe behavior, which included physical aggression and self-injurious behavior, occurred when his wife would leave for home at the end of his day at the clinic. When she would inform him she was leaving, he would start yelling, attempt to attack her or anyone intervening, and throw himself out of his chair. On one occasion, he even stabbed himself with a pencil that was lying nearby.

The program for reducing his aggressive behavior was to replace it with more appropriate social and communication skills. H. H. was taught to wave good-bye to his wife before she departed for the evening. This was accomplished by having the client, during counseling sessions, practice saying good-bye to a videotaped presentation of his wife. If he completed the sequence correctly, and without any negative behavior, then he was allowed to color in one section of a black-and-white drawing of his house. The drawing was divided into seven sections. When he completed coloring in the seven sections, he earned a supervised weekend home visit. Once he succeeded at the videotape presentation and earned a visit home, the client practiced saying good night to his wife in person. The same reinforcement procedure was used again. Seven successful trial sessions resulted in a weekend home. H. H. successfully completed both training procedures within approximately 30 days and never presented the problem again during the rest of his stay in rehabilitation. The more appropriate social skills of saying good night and waving good-bye had replaced the maladaptive behaviors of physical aggression and self-injurious behavior.

Shaping

Shaping refers to the reinforcement of gradual approximations to a target behavior and is generally used with behaviors which do not require urgent change. For example, if a therapist wants a client to remain seated during the therapy session, she may start by reinforcing the client for remaining seated for five continuous minutes at a time. Once the client is able to accomplish this consistently, the time can be increased to ten minutes, and so on, until the client remains seated the entire session. Although shaping is used primarily for skill building (e.g., learning a single step of a dressing procedure — pulling one's shirt all the way down), it can also be used to modify maladaptive behaviors. For example, if a client is constantly late for therapy, he or she could be reinforced for approximating closer correct arrival times to therapy.

Chaining

Chaining, often confused with shaping, involves teaching a sequence of steps to a task. The basic sequences in which such a task may be taught are termed *forward chaining, backward chaining,* and *whole task method.*[69] For example, putting on a pullover shirt would involve teaching a person the steps of 1) putting his arms through the sleeves, 2) pulling the shirt over his head, and 3) pulling the shirt down over his body. In forward chaining, one would begin teaching with the first step (putting arms through the sleeves), then combine steps 1 and 2, and finally connect the sequence of Steps 1 through 3. In backward chaining, one actually begins teaching the last step first (e.g., pulling shirt down), then combines Steps 3 and 2, and finally Steps 3 through 1. In whole-task method, the most common teaching technique, the entire sequence (Steps 1–3) is taught each time. Evidence is not clear as to which of these methods is most effective; however, backward and forward chaining are usually used if one is trying to reduce the number of errors produced by the client during learning.

Case Illustration

K. T. was a 38-year-old female who was injured in a motor vehicle accident. The injury left K. T. with severe cognitive and behavioral problems. Her most difficult behavior was an intense motor restlessness and inability to sustain attention. She was constantly moving her legs and arms and would exit from therapy every few minutes. A shaping program was introduced to try to increase her ability to sit in a chair and participate in therapy. The procedure started with having K. T. sit on the floor for 30 seconds. If she completed this successfully, she was allowed up and a poker chip token was placed in a circle on a board with ten total circles. When all ten circles were filled with a token, K. T. was taken for a walk around the clinic or outside. After she mastered floor sitting for 30 seconds with minimal failures, she was instructed to sit in a chair for 30 seconds. The same procedure was repeated. The 30-second time period was systematically increased over several weeks, with the structured introduction of tabletop activities, until she could sit at a therapy table for 45 minutes and work on therapeutic tasks without exiting. K. T.'s ability to sit quietly and work on cognitive activities had been shaped to a length commensurate with that of most clients participating in rehabilitation. The same program was used with K. T. in her living environment to help her sit at the dining table and finish eating a meal.

Decelerative Programs

Differential Reinforcement of Incompatible Behaviors (DRI)

Differential reinforcement of incompatible behaviors (DRI) involves reinforcing behaviors which are topographically different from, or incompatible with, the target behavior.[70] For example, the behavior of keeping one's hands in the lap, or to the side, is topographically different from hitting oneself. The production of the topographically different behavior actually competes with, or disallows, the production of the target behavior. Thus, reinforcing the client for keeping his hands in his lap, or to his side, is said to differentially reinforce an incompatible behavior.

Careful monitoring of behaviors during a DRI program is required to make certain that the target behavior is actually decreasing and not only that the incompatible behaviors are increasing. Using the above example, one could imagine that the client's time with hands in his lap or to his side (incompatible behaviors) could increase and self-hitting (target behavior) could remain unchanged. If this occurs, use of a DRO *(Differential Reinforcement of Other Behaviors)* program may be more effective.

Case Illustration

E. N. was a 43-year-old male who was injured in a motor vehicle accident. E. N. exhibited a variety of ticklike behaviors. He would touch or pick at his nose and face and grab his crotch area constantly throughout the day. As you can probably guess, social interaction with others was severely limited by this behavior. A DRI program was implemented to help reduce these socially unacceptable behaviors. During therapy sessions, E. N. was reinforced with tokens for keeping his hands either on the table or engaged in hand-involved therapeutic tasks. The tokens were exchangeable for certain privileges in his living environment. Over a period of several months, E. N.'s ticklike behaviors decreased to a socially acceptable level. His inappropriate behavior (i.e., touching nose, face, or crotch) had been replaced by incompatible behaviors (i.e., hands on table or engaged in a task). It was not possible for E. N. to exhibit both behaviors at the same time.

Differential Reinforcement of Other Behaviors (DRO)

Differential Reinforcement of Other Behaviors (DRO) is defined as reinforcing any behavior other than the target behavior for a specific interval of time.[71] For example, if the target behavior is "physical aggression", the therapist would reinforce the client at the end of every designated time interval in which the physical aggression was not exhibited. One can keep the time intervals absolute (e.g., every 15 minutes) or relative (e.g., resetting the clock after every occurrence of the target behavior). If the client exhibits physical aggression, the clock is reset for another 15 minutes. Once there is an increase in the number of intervals in which aggression does not occur, or when it is occurring at a predetermined lower rate, the interval size can be systematically lengthened and eventually eliminated.

There are, however, a few precautions to take when implementing a DRO program. DRO programs are not designed to reduce high-rate behaviors. High-rate behaviors do not allow enough time to reinforce the client between episodes of the targeted inappropriate behavior. Also, by their nature, DRO programs reinforce any other occurring behaviors. Therapists need to be aware that they may inadvertently reinforce another undesirable behavior.[72] As with many decelerative programs, DRO procedures do not teach people new skills and, thus, are more effective if implemented in concert with positive programming.

Case Illustration

C. I. was a 27-year-old male who was injured in an industrial explosion. As a result of the accident, C. I. had severe cognitive deficits and could not ambulate independently. He also had severe aggressive behavior problems that were significantly interfering with all rehabilitative therapy. C. I. exhibited hitting, kicking, biting, yelling, exiting, and noncompliance in therapy.

A DRO program was started to reduce the above-mentioned behaviors. C. I. was required to participate in the therapy task for a total of two minutes without any of the target behaviors. If he was successful, an "X" was marked over one of five squares on an erasable dry ink board. A picture of an outdoor scene was attached to the board at the end of the five-square sequence. Any time C. I. displayed one of the target behaviors, the clock was reset to zero and a new two-minute interval would begin. As soon as five squares were marked, C. I. was taken for a walk outside of the clinic (the identified reinforcer). When he was able to complete two-minute intervals approximately 80% of the time without resetting, the time was increased to five minutes and then to ten minutes. Eventually, C. I. was able to participate in therapy for a full 45 minutes before taking a break. He was being reinforced for any behaviors "other" than the target behaviors.

Differential Reinforcement of Low Rates of Behavior (DRL)

Differential Reinforcement of Low Rates of Behavior (DRL) programs provide reinforcement if a specified interval of time has elapsed since a target behavior last occurred or if a specified number of occurrences of the target behavior have occurred during the interval.[73] For example, if the target behavior is "yelling", a DRL program may state that a client is to be reinforced for each 15-minute interval of time that passes since yelling last occurred or for each time interval in which the target behavior occurs below a certain rate (e.g., five occurrences or less of yelling every 15 minutes). The time intervals can then be lengthened (e.g., from 15 minutes to 30 minutes) or the number of occurrences allowed can be decreased (e.g., five occurrences to two occurrences every 15 minutes) until the target behavior is eliminated or reduced to an acceptable level. Baseline data must be collected to determine either the initial time interval length or the initial number of occurrences to be allowed for the client to receive a reinforcer. For example, if a behavior is occurring four times per hour, an appropriate interval length may be 15 minutes, or reinforcement for every 15 minutes that the behavior occurs only once. This interval length will assure initial success by the client and help develop reinforcer strength.

Some of the advantages of DRL programs are that interval times can be adapted to fit therapy sessions (e.g., 45-minute sessions can be divided into 15-minute intervals) and high-rate behaviors, for which DRO programs are not designed, can be systematically reduced. Like DRO programs, however, DRL programs do not teach new skills. Instead, the focus is on reduction of maladaptive behaviors. DRL programs, therefore, should be supplemented with positive programming of some type.

Case Illustration

K. C. was a 36-year-old male who was injured when the bicycle he was riding was hit by a car. K. C. presented several behavior problems, including verbal and physical aggression. If he displayed any target behavior, the DRL program stated he must go to his kitchen and remove one of four keys hanging on a cork board. If, at the end of three days, he still had one key remaining, he could unlock a box and choose one of several available reinforcers (e.g., ten dollars). When K. C. was able to earn his three-day reinforcer three consecutive times, the reinforcer period was increased to four days, and so on, until it reached a one-week reinforcer time period. The number of keys was then reduced until only two keys were available. This meant he could only exhibit one target behavior per week and still earn a reinforcer. K. C.'s target behaviors had been systematically reduced to lower rates.

Overcorrection

There are two types of *overcorrection* procedures.[74] One is known as *restitutional overcorrection* and the other as *positive-practice overcorrection*. Restitutional overcorrection requires that a person returns the environment (e.g., therapy room) to a state better than before the behavioral episode. For example, if an agitated client knocks over a chair, he or she is required to pick up not only that chair, but to straighten all other chairs in the room as well.

Positive-practice overcorrection requires repeated practice of an appropriate behavior. For example, if a client walks with poor posture, he or she may be asked to practice walking with upright posture for specified periods of time.

Overcorrection can be an alternative to other, more punitive punishment procedures. The disadvantages are that overcorrection can be time-consuming and can elicit aggression in circumstances where overcorrection requires physical guidance to obtain compliance.

Case Illustration 1

O. H. was a 42-year-old female who was injured in a motor vehicle accident. She had spent approximately one year in a locked psychiatric institute on multiple psychoactive medications prior to admission for rehabilitation. She exhibited behaviors of yelling, hitting, stripping, exiting, and noncompliance with therapy. Although continent of bowel and bladder, O. H. would periodically urinate small amounts on furniture during therapy. A restitutional overcorrection program was implemented to reduce this behavior. If O. H. urinated on a chair, she was required to change her clothing, put the dirty clothes in the wash, clean the chair that was soiled, and wipe off all other chairs in the room. O. H.'s inappropriate urination ended within a few weeks.

Case Illustration 2

S. D. was a 29-year-old female who fell into a diabetic coma and lost oxygen (anoxia) to her brain. S. D. displayed yelling and noncompliance to therapy and was also incontinent of bladder. A positive-practice overcorrection program was started to reduce her incontinence. If S. D. was incontinent between her scheduled bathroom visits, she was required to go to the bathroom and practice a series of five "correct" toileting sequences (i.e., adjust clothing, sit on toilet, get up, clean self, adjust clothing, wash hands). After several months, S. D. was continent of bladder and able to live in a supervised group home.

Stimulus Change

Stimulus change is the sudden introduction of an unrelated (nonfunctional) stimulus, or change in stimulus conditions, that results in a temporary reduction of the target behavior.[75] For example, clapping loudly once while a client is engaged in yelling, or suddenly shouting the client's name if he is engaged in aggressive behavior, may cause a lapse in the behavior.

An advantage of stimulus change programs is that their effectiveness can be determined very quickly. There is no need for any long-term assessment of the program. The disadvantage of a stimulus change program is that its effect may be temporary (startle effect) and/or the client may quickly adapt to the stimulus event and return to the maladaptive behavior. Stimulus change programs are almost exclusively used as emergency programs to quickly stop destructive behavior.

Stimulus Satiation

Stimulus satiation programming allows unrestricted access to the reinforcer of an undesirable behavior.[76] The unconditional availability of the reinforcer will eventually weaken its relationship to the target behavior. Stimulus satiation weakens the reinforcer through the process of satiation (complete satisfaction) and deprivation of other reinforcers.[77]

Case Illustration

C. F. was a 32-year-old male who, while working on a rooftop, was electrocuted and fell. C. F. exhibited a number of severe behavior problems; however, one unusual behavior was his obsession with staying on the toilet. When cued to leave the bathroom, C. F. would become extremely agitated and start yelling. If anyone tried to help him out, he would become physically aggressive. His time in the bathroom was becoming increasingly longer and his behavior more severe. A stimulus satiation program was implemented to reduce his time in the bathroom. The program allowed the client to stay in the bathroom, and on the toilet, for as long as he desired. Over a period of two weeks, C. F.'s time on the toilet increased to over 19 consecutive hours in one day. The following two weeks saw his time in the bathroom decrease gradually to what would be considered normal lengths of time. Unlimited access to toilet-time eventually weakened its reinforcement quality (i.e., satiation).

Time-Out

Time-out procedures (also known as *contingent withdrawal*) can be either *nonseclusionary* or *exclusionary*. Nonseclusionary time-out involves withdrawing attention from a person while remaining in their presence. Exclusionary time-out consists of removing the person from a reinforcing environment following the occurrence of a target behavior. For example, when a client exhibits verbal threats, one can either ignore the statements (nonseclusionary) or remove the client from the area (exclusionary). Time-out procedures are more effective if the reinforcer sustaining the behavior is attention from others. A third type of time-out procedure, *seclusionary,* involves the use of a time-out room when the client exhibits a specific target behavior. Strict guidelines need to be followed to operate seclusionary time-out procedures safely:[78]

1. The duration of seclusionary time-out should be as brief as possible (e.g., one–five minutes).
2. The room should be well lit, ventilated, and free of dangerous objects (e.g., light fixtures).
3. The room should have provisions for visually monitoring the person.
4. The room should not be locked, only latched.
5. Records should be kept for each use of the time-out room. At a minimum, records should include the client's name, description of the behavioral episode, and start/end time of the procedure.

An advantage of time-out procedures is that they are easy for staff to understand. The disadvantage is that, in reality, time-out procedures can be very difficult for staff to implement. It is extremely difficult for staff to completely ignore a client's target behavior (e.g., threats, cursing) 100% of the time. If the target behavior is not ignored, it can be inadvertently intermittently reinforced. Intermittently reinforced behavior is actually strengthened. Also, a client should not be removed from the therapy area as part of an exclusionary time-out procedure if the behavior is to escape and avoid therapy. Time-out procedures should always be combined with positive, skill-building procedures (e.g., positive programming, shaping) to develop functional skills to replace the behavior being extinguished.

Case Illustration

L. I. was a 24-year-old male who was injured in a motor vehicle accident. L. I. exhibited behaviors of verbal aggression, threatening behavior, and noncompliance. He was a mild traumatic brain injury case. If L. I. did not want to participate in a therapeutic activity, he began by arguing, then escalated to yelling and threatening physical aggression. A nonseclusionary time-out procedure was started to reduce his aggressive behavior and increase his compliance with therapy. "Attention from staff" was the identified reinforcer. Any time that L. I. began arguing and refusing to follow instructions, therapists were instructed to inform L. I. that they were going to their office and would return when he was ready to stop yelling and cooperate. Other staff were also instructed to ignore L. I. if he was not with his therapist during therapy time. Cooperation increased to an acceptable level over a two-week period.

Complex Programs

Contracting

Contracting is a technique which involves a written agreement between the client and another person.[79] A key to behavioral contracting is that the elements of the contract are agreeable and understandable to both parties. Contracting can shift the focus of therapy away from the demands of a therapist to one of cooperative problem-solving. Clients may be more likely to follow therapeutic guidelines when they feel part of the decision-making process and can see behavioral steps and reinforcers outlined in a written format. Contracting should include a definition of the target behavior or goal, how the behavior or goal will be measured or monitored, rewards for following the contract, and the signatures of both parties. Contracting can work well for behaviors such as tardiness, cooperation, and quality of performance, which are typically thought of as involving "higher" levels of self-control.

Case Illustration

> T. K. was a 36-year-old female who, while working as a junior high teacher, was injured when hit in the head by a student. T. K. was diagnosed as having "mild" head injury. Most of her symptoms were related to psychological functioning and high-level abstract thinking. One specific symptom that caused her difficulty was a sensitivity to light. Following the injury, she could not tolerate bright light, including indoor fluorescent lighting. She developed a habit of wearing dark glasses, both outdoors and indoors. As therapy progressed, she still felt the need to wear dark glasses indoors. T. K. stated that she wanted to stop wearing dark glasses inside; however, she could never fully cooperate. Various procedures were attempted to reduce her dependence on dark glasses, but none worked. Contracting was finally adopted. T. K. signed a contract stating she would cooperate with systematically reducing her time wearing glasses based on gradually increasing periods without "dark glasses on". Once the goals were outlined and the contract signed, full cooperation from T. K. was achieved. She completed her rehabilitation and was discharged without the need to wear dark glasses indoors.

Stimulus Control

Stimulus control programming involves bringing the target behavior under the control of a specific stimulus or set of conditions.[80] Many behaviors are deemed acceptable, or unacceptable, based on the circumstances under which they occur. Sexual intimacy, for example, is considered an acceptable behavior if it occurs between consenting adults in the privacy of their home. If it occurs at the supermarket or on a public bus, however, it would not be considered acceptable. The goal of stimulus control programs, then, is to bring behaviors which may be occurring at the wrong time, place, or frequency into more appropriate, or more easily controlled, stimulus conditions. Behaviors are brought under stimulus control by reinforcing the target behavior at the time and/or location where the behavior should naturally or acceptably occur (e.g., masturbating in the bedroom rather than in public). Behaviors can also be brought under a specific stimulus control which is then progressively reduced, decreasing the frequency of the behavior as access to the stimulus decreases. Stimulus control programs are considered positive in nature because the behavior is being reinforced, in most cases, for occurring in a more appropriate environment or time.

It is not recommended that stimulus control programs be used with more violent or destructive behaviors (e.g., physical aggression, self-injurious behavior). Severe behaviors are potentially dangerous to the client and others and, thus, are not acceptable even at low rates of occurrence or in selected settings.

Case Illustration

> D. K. was a 37-year-old male who was injured in a motor vehicle accident. As a result of severe brain injury, D. K. displayed physical and verbal aggression, exiting, and noncompliance with therapy. His verbal behavior (i.e., threats, cursing, and yelling) was his predominant problem. A stimulus control program was implemented to reduce verbal agitation. A therapy room was set aside as the stimulus control environment. A lamp, with a blue incandescent light bulb, was placed on the table to increase the uniqueness of the room. To begin with, all therapy sessions were done in this room. If D. K. exhibited any verbal target behaviors, he was reinforced with a variety of

edibles and verbal praise. To insure a high reinforcer rate, if D. K. did not exhibit a target behavior within 60 seconds, he was cued by staff to "please yell". In contrast, when D. K. was outside of the room (for walks, bathroom breaks, etc.), all target behaviors were ignored. After three weeks of using the stimulus control room exclusively for therapy, D. K. was systematically moved to conventional rooms at a rate of one per week. Again, he was reinforced for exhibiting target behaviors only in the stimulus control room, whereas target behaviors were ignored in all other conditions.

Token Economies

Token economies require the use of secondary reinforcers (tokens) that a person has earned and which can be traded later for something of value to the person.[81] For example, plastic poker chips are commonly used as tokens that are earned for positive behaviors such as compliance with therapy. Clients can then trade in the chips daily, weekly, etc. (depending on the reinforcement interval length required) for any activity, privilege, or item identified as a reinforcer (e.g., dining out, movies, money). One can also include a response-cost aspect to a token program. This involves losing tokens for exhibition of specific behaviors. For example, a client may earn tokens for compliance with therapy and lose tokens for exhibiting any physical aggression.

The most difficult aspect of a token program is deciding the value of each token and how often the client can earn it. Baseline data on the frequency of the target behavior is necessary to determine the potential earning power of the client. Token programs should be neither too easy nor too difficult for a client. An earning rate of about 70 to 80% is probably a good rule of thumb. Advantages of token programs are that they provide for structured, concrete feedback, delay of gratification, and ease of use across many settings (e.g., therapy room, community, home).

Case Illustration

S. X. was a 28-year-old male who was injured while working as a motorcycle highway patrolman when he was hit by a motorist. S. X. suffered a severe brain injury which left him with significant cognitive and physical deficits. With the exception of physical therapy, S. X. was limited to using a wheelchair for mobility. While sitting, S. X. would let his head fall forward and begin drooling. He would also let his left hand pull up to his chest, instead of keeping it in a more neutral position on his lap. A token program was started to decrease the above-mentioned behaviors. He could also earn bonus tokens for each 15-minute interval in which he added inflection to his monotone voice. A response-cost element was added to decrease his habit of transferring out of the wheelchair without supervision. He was given a "transfer ticket", which cost him tokens, if anyone witnessed him transferring without another person present. Tokens were earned on a 15-minute interval basis (determined by baseline data on the rate of target behaviors) and could be cashed in for food outings and extra walking time. By time of discharge, S. X.'s drooling and hand position had been resolved and he was placed in a semi-independent living environment and a part-time position with the police force as an office clerk.

Summary

The design of an effective behavioral program may require combining a number of the procedures just described. No single design can be used universally. Consequently, it is often necessary to begin with one procedure and switch to another when the first plan fails or loses its effectiveness.

Recent studies have also stressed the importance of *contextual control* in choosing treatment plans.[82] Contextual control recognizes the role that context (stimulus setting) plays in altering the effect of behavior programs. A treatment plan designed to modify behavior in one environment may not be effective in another.[83]

DATA COLLECTION AND GRAPHING

Behavior programming requires a procedure for systematically recording and graphing behavior data. Decisions regarding the effectiveness of treatment plans should be data based and this demands comprehensive data collection. When possible, collect data throughout the entire day and evening — not just in structured settings. Behavior data from the home and community are just as important as those from a school or rehabilitation facility. Long-term maintenance is questionable if behavior changes do not generalize to other, more natural environments. This section will cover methods of data collection, graphing and analysis of data, and the use of computer technology to assist in data management. Although comprehensive data collection and graphing can be time consuming and somewhat rigorous to implement, there are a number of important reasons to do so. Collecting data on a consistent basis will provide:

- Baseline information prior to starting a behavior program. Before beginning any behavior program, it is recommended that data be collected on the person's target behaviors. Baseline data provides the behavior programmer and staff with a clear picture of the frequency of maladaptive behaviors being exhibited by the person. This information bears directly upon the design of the treatment plan. For example, if, after baseline data analysis, it is determined that the target behavior rate is extremely high, then one would not choose to implement a Differential Reinforcement of Other Behavior program which is suited for low-rate behaviors.
- A method for judging the ongoing effectiveness of the behavior program. Systematic collection and graphing of data is important in tracking the progress of a treatment plan. Trends in data can be analyzed to support any changes necessary to the initial program. Modifications to the program should be data driven and not based on anecdotal staff reports alone.
- Feedback to family, staff, payers, and client. Behavior data provide important information to those responsible for the client's well-being and/or funding. People typically respond more favorably to observationally recorded data of behavior rather than statements such as "He's behaving better." Graphs based on collected data help the client, staff, and others visualize and understand the impact of the behavioral intervention plan. Graphs can also assist the client in developing self-monitoring skills.
- Valuable information for research and program development. If the person is in a school or rehabilitation program, systematic collection of behavior data assists those responsible for clinical research, conference presentations, preparation of professional manuscripts, and program development. These activities require the support of reliably collected data.

Data Collection

There are many methods for collecting data. The three most common and practical methods are *event recording, interval recording,* and *time-sample recording.* These three data collection methods are known as *direct observational recordings* (Table 10.3).

Event Recording

Event recording (Figure 10.3) is probably the easiest direct observational recording system. The only requirement is to mark on a piece of paper each time a specific target behavior occurs. Handheld devices, such as golf counters, can be used to make counting easier for high-frequency behaviors. The drawback to event recording is that it can be difficult to judge when one occurrence of a behavior ends and another occurrence begins. In tallying angry language, for example, if a person is yelling for several minutes, it would be difficult to judge how many instances of angry language actually occurred. The person recording would have to decide whether to count the entire period as one event or try to tally each statement as a separate occurrence. In addition, high-frequency and long-duration behaviors are more difficult to count because of the amount of attention required. Event recording requires constant observation of the client so all occurrences of the target behavior are recorded, thus making it one of the most time-consuming of the data collection procedures.

TABLE 10.3 Direct Observational Data Collection Methods

Method	Definition	Considerations
Event recording	Tally *each* occurrence of target behavior.	Requires constant observation. Difficult to judge beginning and end of behavior.
Interval recording	Record each occurrence or nonoccurrence of target behavior *during* each interval.	Requires constant observation. Results in approximations of behavior duration and frequency.
Time-sample recording	Record occurrence or nonoccurrence of target behavior at the *end* of each interval.	Broad approximation of behavior duration and frequency.

Client Name: **John Doe**   Date: **4-14-92**   Time: **1-2 pm**

Therapist Name: **Mary Smith**   Therapy: **OT**

Instructions: Tally the *number of occurrences* of each target behavior.

Target Behaviors	Tallies	Total
1. Physical Aggression Definition - attempting to and/or actual striking of an individual with an object or body part.	I I	2
2. Angry Language Definition - cursing, threats, or any hostile language delivered with increased volume.	I I I I I	5
3. Property Destruction Definition - attempting to and/or actual damaging of property.	I	1
4. Refusal Definition - not starting, interrupting, or stopping therapy or instructions > 60 seconds.	I I I I I I I	7
5. Exiting Definition - attempting to and/or leaving the place of required activity.	I I I	3

FIGURE 10.3 Example of an event recording sheet.

Interval Recording

Interval recording (Figure 10.4) eliminates the task of judging the beginning and ending of behavioral episodes and tallying high-frequency or long-duration behaviors. Instead, interval recording divides the therapy session (or observation period) into equal time intervals (e.g., 15-minute periods) and requires the person recording to mark whether the target behavior occurred during each interval. It does not matter how many times the behavior occurred during the interval, only that it occurred at least once. Interval recording requires choosing an

Client: **John Doe**	Day: **Monday**	Date: **4 / 14 / 94**

Instructions: *Every 15 minutes you are to mark any **target behaviors**, and level of **cooperation**, listed below that occurred during that period by circling the letter corresponding to the behavior. The interval begins at the listed time (e.g., mark in the 2:00 period behaviors seen from 2:00 to 2:15). Note any observations and **comments** in the space provided.*

Target Behaviors: PA = Physical Aggression, AL = Angry Language, PD = Property Destruction, R = Refusal to Work, E = Exiting

Cooperation: None = No cooperation (with behavior),   Part = Partial cooperation (with behavior),   Full = Full cooperation (no behavior)

Therapy SP	9:00 a.m.	9:15 a.m.	9:30 a.m.	9:45 a.m.
Target Behaviors >	PA AL PD R E	PA AL PD R E	PA AL PD R E	PA AL PD R E
Cooperation >	None Part Full	None Part Full	None Part Full	None Part Full
Comments/Other >				
Therapy OT	10:00 a.m.	10:15 a.m.	10:30 a.m.	10:45 a.m.
Target Behaviors >	PA AL PD R E	PA AL PD R E	PA AL PD R E	PA AL PD R E
Cooperation >	None Part Full	None Part Full	None Part Full	None Part Full
Comments/Other >				
Therapy ED	11:00 a.m.	11:15 a.m.	11:30 a.m.	11:45 a.m
Target Behaviors >	PA AL PD R E	PA AL PD R E	PA AL PD R E	PA AL PD R E
Cooperation >	None Part Full	None Part Full	None Part Full	None Part Full
Comments/Other >				
Therapy PT	1:00 p.m.	1:15 p.m.	1:30 p.m.	1:45 p.m.
Target Behaviors >	PA AL PD R E	PA AL PD R E	PA AL PD R E	PA AL PD R E
Cooperation >	None Part Full	None Part Full	None Part Full	None Part Full
Comments/Other >				
Therapy RT	2:00 p.m.	2:15 p.m.	2:30 p.m.	2:45 p.m.
Target Behaviors >	PA AL PD R E	PA AL PD R E	PA AL PD R E	PA AL PD R E
Cooperation >	None Part Full	None Part Full	None Part Full	None Part Full
Comments/Other >				
Therapy SP	3:00 p.m.	3:15 p.m.	3:30 p.m.	3:45 p.m
Target Behaviors >	PA AL PD R E	PA AL PD R E	PA AL PD R E	PA AL PD R E
Cooperation >	None Part Full	None Part Full	None Part Full	None Part Full
Comments/Other >				

FIGURE 10.4 Example of an interval recording sheet.

appropriate interval size. Time intervals should approximate the frequency rate of the behavior. High-rate behaviors require short time intervals (e.g., one–five minutes), and low-rate behaviors need long time intervals (e.g., 15–60 minutes). For example, if a person uses angry language approximately once every ten minutes, an observation interval of ten or 15 minutes would capture most of the variability in the behavior. If the interval size is too long, the rate of behavior may change and not be reflected in a measurement of percent of interval change. When the intervals are extremely short (e.g., 30 seconds), every other interval should be used

Client Name: **John Doe**			Date: **4-14-92**	Time: **2-3 pm**	
Therapist Name: **Mary Smith**				Therapy: **OT**	

Instructions: At the times listed in the left column, observe the client for 30 seconds then put an X under *Yes* if the target behavior occurred, or under *No* if the target behavior did not occur.

Target Behavior			Definition		
Angry Language			Cursing, threats, yelling, or any hostile language delivered with increased volume.		

Time	Yes	No	Time	Yes	No
9:00	X		9:32		X
9:03		X	9:35	X	
9:10		X	9:40	X	
9:15	X		9:47		X
9:23		X	9:51		X
9:25		X	9:56	X	

Data Calculation:

Total Yes's **- 5**   Total Yes's/ Total Samples **- 5/12**

Total No's **- 7**

Total Samples **- 12**   **42%** of time-samples

FIGURE 10.5 Example of a time-sample recording sheet.

for marking the data sheet. This achieves greater accuracy because the observer does not miss occurrences of behavior while attending to the recording sheet. If several target behaviors are being tracked simultaneously, the use of behavioral codes is recommended to simplify the procedure. At the end of each interval, the person recording marks the behavioral code (e.g., PA = physical aggression) for those behaviors which occurred during the interval. As in event recording, interval recording requires the undivided attention of the person recording. It is necessary to track both interval time and occurrence of target behaviors.

Time-Sample Recording

The last data collection method to be covered is *time-sample recording* (Figure 10.5). Time-sample recording is similar to interval recording except that it does not require constant attention by the person recording. Behavior is only periodically sampled. A therapy session (or observation period) can be divided into equal or variable (random) periods at the end of which (during a brief time sample) the person recording marks the occurrence or nonoccurrence of the target behavior. The advantages of this method are that the person recording does not have to monitor the client's behavior continuously and it is minimally intrusive on any activities, which also makes it ideally suited for monitoring high-frequency behaviors. It does

PA = Physical Aggression, AL = Angry Language, PD = Property Destruction, R = Refusals, E = Exiting,
T = Total Intervals

John Doe

Week 1		PA	AL	PD	R	E	T
	4/10	1	5	0	2	1	24
	4/11	0	2	0	1	0	20
	4/12	3	5	1	3	1	24
	4/13	1	1	0	0	0	20
	4/14	2	4	1	2	1	24
Total		7	17	2	8	3	112
Percent		6.25	15.18	1.79	7.14	2.68	

FIGURE 10.6 Example of a computer summary data sheet.

require a device, such as a timer, to signal the end of each time period. The disadvantage is that time-sample recording results in an even broader approximation of behavior frequency than does interval recording.

Computer Management of Data

With the advent of powerful and affordable personal computers, a number of spreadsheet programs have been made available which are well suited to managing and graphing behavior data. If your facility handles a fair number of clients with behavior difficulties, we would highly recommend using one of these programs. Organizing data is a time-consuming activity that can be streamlined with the help of computer technology. Quattro Pro for Windows®* is one program we have found to be very useful for this purpose. It includes both spreadsheet functions and graphing capabilities. Figure 10.6 is an example of a computer summary sheet covering one week of interval data. It includes columns for the date, day, each target behavior (e.g., PA = physical aggression), and the total number of intervals recorded. All that is required is to write simple formulas for each of the percent calculations and design a master form which can be retrieved for each new client.

Graphing

Due to its single-case structure, behavior analysis does not lend itself to statistical procedures to judge the effectiveness of treatment interventions. Graphs are the traditional means of accomplishing this task. They provide an overall visual impression of behavior that is easy for staff, families, clients, and others to understand. As it is common for behavior problems to accelerate before decreasing after the introduction of the treatment intervention, graphs are an easy way to track learning curves. Graphs can be produced by hand or with one of the numerous commercially available computer graphics programs, such as Harvard Graphics®** or Quattro Pro® — two programs we have used extensively for graphing and data management.

There are two fundamental concepts to remember when graphing. First, what information goes with the vertical line (ordinate, or *y*-axis) of the graph and, second, what information goes

---

* Registered Trademark of Borland International, Scotts Valley, CA, 1993.
** Registered Trademark of Software Publishing Co., Santa Clara, CA, 1987.

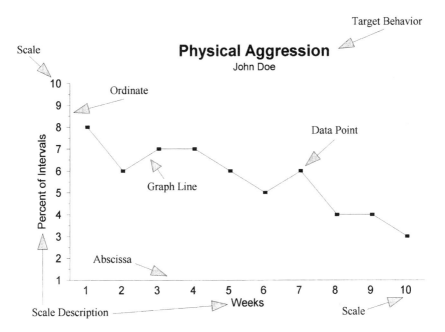

FIGURE 10.7 Components of a graph.

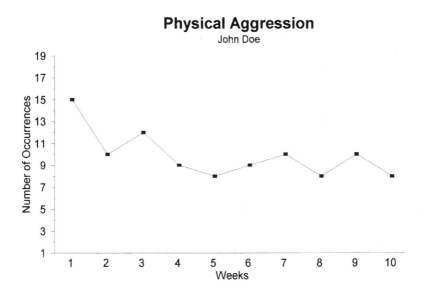

FIGURE 10.8 Example of an event graph.

with the horizontal line (abscissa, or *x*-axis) of the graph. Figure 10.7 labels all the basic components of a graph.

For event-recorded data, the ordinate indicates the number of occurrences of the target behavior (e.g., physical aggression) and the abscissa indicates the time across which the behavior was recorded (e.g., days, weeks). For example, if one were graphing the number of occurrences of physical aggression on a weekly basis, the graph would look something like Figure 10.8.

In addition, choose the maximum value for the ordinate scale based on a number that is slightly higher than the highest frequency that has occurred with the person. For example, if

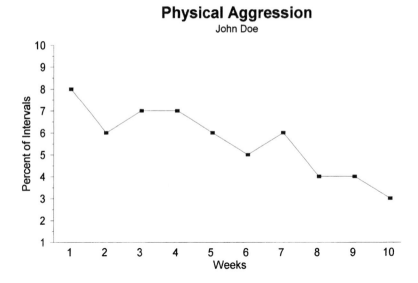

FIGURE 10.9 Example of an interval or time-sample graph.

the highest number of occurrences of physical aggression in a week was four, then choose five as your maximum value for the ordinate scale.

For interval or time-sample recording, the ordinate of the graph indicates the percentage of intervals (or time samples) in which the target behavior has occurred. The abscissa of the graph represents the time period during which the behavior was recorded. For example, if one were graphing the percentage of intervals for physical aggression on a weekly basis, the graph would look something like Figure 10.9.

Choose the maximum percentage for the ordinate scale based on a slightly higher percentage than the maximum that has occurred with the person. For example, if the highest percentage of intervals with physical aggression in a week was 20%, then choose 25% as your maximum value for the ordinate scale.

Interpreting graphs can sometimes be very difficult. Behavior that is either highly variable or changes very little can make analysis a challenging proposition. One can look for a general trend or slope, or one can begin grouping data and comparing means (averages) to help detect changes in behavior.

A graphing technique we have found to be extremely useful in situations where interpretation is difficult is called *trend graphing*. This graph is tedious to complete by hand, but both the Harvard Graphics® and Quattro Pro® computer programs we have mentioned have the ability to calculate a "line of best fit" graph. If we take a behavior (e.g., physical aggression) and create a trend graph, it will show us the future projected change of physical aggression based upon the current observed rate of change. Figure 10.10 is an example of a trend graph. It clarifies the effect of the treatment and indicates when a target behavior might be expected to reach a projected goal. Of course, there are numerous variables which can have an impact on goal attainment, so care must be taken when interpreting trend graphing.

CRISIS PREVENTION AND INTERVENTION

Assaultive behavior, such as physical aggression, is common in the field of traumatic brain injury rehabilitation. All of the planning and programming described in the previous sections cannot always prevent or predict the occurrence of assaultive behavior by a client. In some cases, behavioral programming may even elicit aggression when it exerts control over sensitive aspects of a client's environment. Assaultive situations can be a frightening experience.

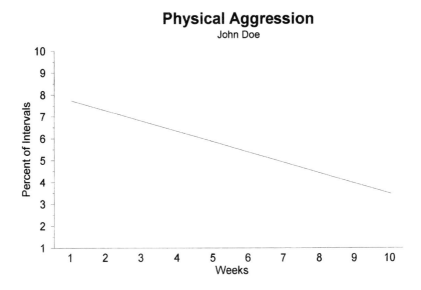

FIGURE 10.10 Example of a trend graph.

People can be combative during the acute phase of recovery as they reorient themselves to the world around them and during postacute rehabilitation (i.e., when a person has reached medical stability) as they develop awareness of functional deficits. Severe behavior is a reality of the rehabilitation process and staff can learn to take measures, when possible, to prevent its occurrence. However, if a crisis situation does occur, staff should also be equipped with techniques to de-escalate the client and decrease the likelihood of injury to the client and others.

This section will cover some basic models of the assault cycle, common reasons for assaultive episodes, techniques for preventing the development of crisis situations, and useful interventions if a crisis episode occurs. However, this chapter is not a replacement for a certified course in crisis intervention or management of assaultive behavior. There are several good quality training programs available to train staff directly or to certify staff members as instructors. We highly recommend all facilities, schools, or families that work with people with traumatic brain injury with behavior problems to incorporate this training as standard practice. The content, structure, and training methodology of these courses, including the practice of self-defense and restraint techniques, is an effective means of comprehensively equipping a person to handle assaultive situations safely.

Models of Assault

Paul Smith,[84] founder of Professional Assault Response Training (PART)®*, has proposed seven models of assaultive behavior. They are the *Common Knowledge Model, Stress Model, Communication Model, Environmental Model, Legal Model, Developmental Model,* and *Socio-Cultural Model.* We will only concern ourselves here with the first five. The developmental and socio-cultural models are not typically related to the field of TBI rehabilitation.

Common Knowledge Model

Smith[84] believes that the underlying reasons as to why people attempt to injure one another are relatively simple and that one can apply intervention techniques to respond to these events effectively. He states that assaultive incidents can be reduced to four common motives: fear, frustration, manipulation, and intimidation.

---

* Registered Trademark of Professional Assault Response Training, Citrus Heights, CA, 1983.

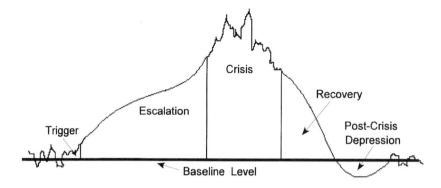

FIGURE 10.11 The assault cycle. (From Smith, P., Professional Assault Response Training® Workshop Syllabus, 1983. With permission.)

When people are afraid, or feel that their well-being is threatened, their behavior may escalate to physical aggression as a means of defending themselves. To reduce fear, staff can respond to the client with a relaxed posture, use slow and natural gestures, keep a safe distance from the client, stand off to the side, position oneself below the client's eye level, use a firm, yet reassuring voice, stay logical, and encourage calm reflection.

When a client's behavior escalates as a result of frustration, staff need to follow different guidelines than those used with a fearful client. Staff should demonstrate control with a more commanding posture, use forceful gestures such as pointing, stay directly in front of the person but just out of reach, keep the tone of voice quiet yet forceful and confident, and repeat commands.

If a client is escalating behaviorally as a means of manipulation, a role of "detachment" is the technique recommended by Smith.[84] This method involves maintaining a closed, yet relaxed posture, mild gestures of disapproval (e.g., finger tapping), positioning far enough away from the client to show noninvolvement, turning slightly away from the client, using a detached, slightly bored tone of voice, and quiet, repetitive commands.

If the client is attempting to intimidate through escalated behavior, the technique Smith[84] advises is *consequation*. The basic premise is that clear communication of the consequences of an assaultive act will reduce the probability that the episode will occur. Staff should be poised and ready to react (without giving the impression of fear), keep gestures to a minimum, position oneself for protection (e.g., behind a chair or desk), maintain a monotone, emotionless tone of voice, and give clear and direct statements of consequences.

Stress Model

The *stress model* views assaultive behavior as a reaction to extreme stress. The rehabilitation process, as we know, is an extremely stressful situation for a person. When a client perceives a threat to his well-being (e.g., daily confrontation of deficits), he can either fight or flee from the situation. In TBI rehabilitation, we see both of these responses. Some clients try to escape the stress of their condition by either escaping or avoiding therapy. Others become combative when stressed. Each client has specific responses to stress, which can be detected and recognized as predictable patterns. A common tool for visualizing these response patterns is "The Assault Cycle" graph (Figure 10.11). It is divided into five separate phases: 1) triggering event, 2) escalation, 3) crisis, 4) recovery, and 5) postcrisis depression.

The triggering event is any stimulus or event that exceeds the client's tolerance for stress (e.g., demands for compliance, being touched, etc.). This begins the assault cycle. Any prevention techniques (e.g., arranging of environment, level of demands, etc.) would have to occur before the triggering event. The escalation stage is characterized by increasing levels of agitation or changes in the normal (i.e., baseline) behavior of the client. De-escalation techniques are used during this phase to try to help the client return to a baseline level of behavioral activity. The sooner de-escalation techniques are used during this stage, the less likely more restrictive measures will have to be implemented. The crisis stage is characterized by the client physically acting out. At this point, de-escalation techniques have failed and physical intervention may be necessary. During the recovery phase, the client's level of activity is decreasing. Once the person regains self-control, decrease any external control that may have been introduced. The last stage, postcrisis depression, is characterized by activity which falls below baseline levels. The client may require a short period of rest, or less active tasks, until recovery occurs.

Communication Model

The *communication model* focuses on the balance of communication between the therapist and client. On one end of the spectrum is "withdrawal" and on the other end "assault". Smith[84] believes that the best means for achieving a balance that decreases the chances of triggering an assaultive cycle is with assertive communication. Smith[84] states that both manipulation and intimidation by the client can be accounted for by this model. When staff respond with either intimidating aggressiveness or submissive nurturing, they contribute to an imbalance of communication and increase the opportunity for an assaultive situation. Smith[84] emphasizes that "when staff respond to a potential assault with balanced and assertive communication, they automatically reduce the chances that an assault will occur."

Environmental Model

Smith[84] describes the *environmental model* from the perspective that assaultive behavior is, for the most part, a product of the circumstances in which it occurs. This is the model which most closely fits the fundamental philosophy of behavior analysis. Although Smith[84] does not discuss consequences to behavior as part of his model, he does emphasize the role of antecedents and setting events in triggering or setting the stage for assaultive behavior. Such things as weather conditions, level of sound, crowding, and scheduling of activities are given as examples of events which can "predispose people to assaultive behavior." The important point to make concerning the environmental model is that staff is in control of most environmental antecedents to behavior. Schedules, noise level, tone of voice, etc., are usually under the control of the staff. Staff can take advantage of this opportunity to prevent "trigger events" and minimize assaultive behavior.

Legal Model

Assaultive behavior can be separated into legal categories. They are: 1) simple assault, 2) assault and battery, and 3) aggravated assault. The staff can legally protect itself against these varying degrees of assault, but is limited to using only "reasonable force". As Smith[84] states, "A reasonable amount of force is just enough for effective self protection...." For example, with simple assault (i.e., threatening gestures or speech), communication techniques would be the maximum force that could be legally applied. With assault and battery (i.e., use of physical force and threats), evasive self-defense would probably be the maximum reasonable force allowed. If aggravated assault (i.e., attempt to cause serious bodily harm) occurs, a controlling self-defense (i.e., restraint) and physical intervention would be reasonable. The use of physical techniques for self-defense and other interventions requires intensive training. Unless a staff member has completed this training, he should have limited contact with clients exhibiting severe behavior disorders.

General Techniques and Methods

There are many techniques for preventing a crisis situation or intervening once it has started. We have covered many of those methods in the previous section. Smith's[84] recommendations regarding body posture, tone of voice, content of speech, and use of gestures are invaluable aids to dealing effectively with a crisis episode. There are other techniques which can be added to this list.

To help prevent a crisis situation from being "triggered," review the guidelines outlined in the section *General Management Guidelines*. These included 1) increasing rest time for the client, 2) keeping the environment simple, 3) keeping instructions simple, 4) giving feedback and setting goals, 5) staying calm and redirecting the client to task, 6) providing choices, 7) decreasing chances of task failure, 8) varying the type of activities, 9) overplanning, and 10) utilizing task-analysis procedures. If one can implement these environmental controls and combine them with a sensitivity to patterns of interaction and sharpened observational skills, most assaultive events can be prevented. For those that are unavoidable, intervention techniques for de-escalating the client must be employed.

Once the escalation phase of an assault cycle has begun, measures by staff change from one of prevention to one of intervention. The intervention techniques used during the escalation stage are an attempt to de-escalate the client before the cycle reaches the crisis stage. The earlier the intervention, the less restrictive the measures. If the client progresses to the crisis stage, de-escalation techniques will not be useful and may, in fact, prolong the crisis. Physical intervention by staff, unfortunately, becomes likely.

Some of the most effective de-escalation techniques staff can utilize are active listening, orientation, setting limits, redirection, withdrawal of attention, and contracting.

Active listening: Active listening is a technique incorporating a variety of listening skills.[85] Active listening begins on a nonverbal basis. The staff member should make eye contact with the client, maintain a relaxed posture that shows interest, and use natural gestures. Once this nonverbal basis has been established, verbal statements can be utilized. These consist of paraphrasing, clarifying, and perception checking. *Paraphrasing* is a method of restating the client's message in fewer words. Its purpose is to indicate to the client that you are trying to understand his message. *Clarifying* focuses on the more abstract messages from the client. The staff member admits confusion about a statement and tries a restatement or asks for clarification — for example, "I'm confused. Is what you are saying...?" *Perception checking* involves asking the client for verification of your perception — for example, "You seem to be very mad at me. Is that correct?"

Orientation: Memory deficits are one of the most common consequences of a TBI. People can experience periods of severe disorientation. Disorientation has been found to be a key factor in the severe behavior of people with traumatic brain injury.[31] Orienting a client to the time, to his location, and to whom he is with can sometimes help to de-escalate a client. It helps the client feel less threatened by the environment when he can understand where he is and why he is there.

Setting limits: As stated earlier, setting limits can be a useful technique. This is especially true for clients who are trying to intimidate staff by threatening severe behavior. Although these can be frightening experiences, escalation can be curtailed if the staff member remains calm and confident and outlines the consequences of the threatened behavior — for example, "If you throw that chair at me, you will be restrained by four other staff members until you are calm."

Redirection: Redirection is useful when a client is in the early stages of escalation. Staying calm and redirecting a client to another task or activity can interrupt the escalation phase and refocus the client on something else. It also decreases the opportunity for inadvertently reinforcing the client with attention which may be the behavior problem's maintaining reinforcer.

Withdrawal of attention: This technique is the opposite of active listening. Whereas *active listening* provides undivided attention to the client during escalation, *withdrawal of attention* discontinues any attention during escalated behavior. Withdrawal of attention is usually more effective with manipulative types of behavior. Clients exhibiting this type of behavior thrive on attention from others. Withdrawing attention for brief periods of time when they begin to escalate helps establish a relationship between "attention" and cooperative, calm behavior.

Contracting: Contracting, like other de-escalation techniques, is a skill which takes some practice. The reason, however, is that contracting has the potential for being misused. If used incorrectly, it becomes a method of "buying" good behavior which may lead to further behavior problems from the client. For example, if a client is escalated over completing an unpleasant task and you "contract" with him that he does not have to finish the task if he calms down, you have set yourself up for future problems when the client does not want to complete a task. You may have reinforced the escalated behavior. A more constructive response may be to tell the client he can switch to another task for the moment and finish the difficult task later in that session. This teaches the client that he can let you know when he has reached his limit of frustration with an activity and would like to work on something else for a while.

The models of assault, as outlined by Smith,[84] provide us with a structure in which to view crisis episodes. Techniques for prevention should be the first line of defense in dealing with severe behavior problems. Behavior treatment plans should always include instructions for controlling antecedents and setting events to help prevent problem behaviors from occurring. If they do occur, the treatment plan outlines the consequences to the behavior and provides procedures for staff to follow. All crisis situations, however, cannot be predicted or prevented by a behavior program. This is why it is important for staff to be trained in techniques and methods of crisis intervention. It is hoped the techniques described in this section, although not a substitute for direct training, will at least assist staff and family members with basic approaches to crisis intervention. Recommended training courses are given by:

Professional Assault Response Training (PART)
Professional Growth Facilitators
P.O. Box 5981
San Clemente, CA 92674-5981
(714) 498-3529

National Crisis Prevention Institute, Inc. (CPI)
3315-K North 124th Street
Brookfield, WI 53005
(800) 558-8976

STAFF AND FAMILY TRAINING

A fundamental component to the implementation of a sound behavioral treatment plan is staff training. To be successful in treating people with traumatic brain injury with behavioral difficulties, rehabilitation facilities must be committed to providing adequate staff training and support. This commitment is not only one of allocating the time and financial resources for training, but also providing philosophical support of behavioral principles, use of its techniques, and sufficient staffing levels to carry out behavior programs effectively. Without this foundation, it would be very difficult for a facility to realize the full benefit of behavioral programming. These issues aside, training consists of the following steps:.

Basic principles: Training must begin with an understanding of basic behavioral principles. Staff should be able to identify environmental influences (antecedents and setting events) and responses (consequences) that help to maintain target behaviors. It is especially important for staff and families to understand the importance of consistency in implementing treatment plans and in responding to the client behavior.

Data collection: Staff require training to enable them to observe client behavior accurately and record data reliably. This can include training to criteria. For example, staff can observe client behavior on videotape and fill out data sheets until they are within 90% agreement of preestablished scoring.

Behavior procedures: It is important for staff and families to understand the structure of behavior treatment design — for example, the differences between accelerative programs (e.g., positive programming), decelerative programs (e.g., DRO), and complex programs (e.g., token economy). Staff are better able to consistently follow programs that they understand.

Ethical issues: It is recommended that staff and families be informed of current ethical issues and guidelines regarding the use of behavior programs. Applied behavior analysis can be a powerful and controversial intervention for behavioral change. The procedures must be implemented with great care, understanding, and sensitivity.

Environmental validity and generalization: Staff and families need to understand the concepts of environmental validity (the teaching of skills at the proper time and natural setting) and generalization (the transfer of skills from one setting to another). Skills are not useful if they cannot be performed in the correct context or cannot be transferred from a clinical setting to the home and community. For example, being able to dress in a clinic treatment room at 11:00 A.M. is not the same as being able to dress at 7:00 A.M. in your own bedroom.

Team approach: Training should emphasize the importance of a team approach to applied behavior analysis. Assisting one another in crisis situations or helping when a client or staff member is not "having a good day" are just a couple of situations which illustrate the need for staff to act as a team. Staff members are more confident at implementing behavior programs when they know others are there to help if the circumstances warrant.

Management of assaultive behavior: Even the most effective behavior programs may not always prevent a crisis situation. Several courses provide training in management of aggressive behavior and crisis intervention. They typically include methods of observation, de-escalation, self-defense, and physical restraint. This training, in our experience, affords one of the best means for instilling confidence in staff to work with behaviorally difficult clients effectively. It provides for a systematic approach to aggression and a structure in which all behavioral interactions and interventions can be gauged. These courses tend to emphasize early intervention in the client's *assault cycle,* before it reaches a crisis stage that requires physical intervention. This training also provides a useful means for ensuring adherence to the legal requirements of balancing the restraint of clients and self-defense.

Behavior staffings: Staff require a forum to openly address and discuss current behavioral issues. Weekly behavior staffings, of at least one-hour duration, are a minimum requirement for keeping abreast of the latest behavioral concerns. They also provide an excellent venue for continuing staff education on behavior methodology.

Family training: Many clients continue to have behavior problems that persist after being discharged from a facility. Those people who will play a significant role in the client's life after rehabilitation will need training in the proper use of behavior analysis and access to behavior specialists for ongoing support. Facilities can provide families with the same training as their staff. Family members can practice behavior procedures (with the client) under the guidance of the facility. Without this training, maintaining behavior change after leaving a facility is less likely to last.

PUTTING IT ALL TOGETHER

- Perform behavioral diagnostics
- Identify potential conditions maintaining the behavior
- Collect baseline data
- Design and implement treatment procedures
- Continue data collection
- Graph and analyze behavior data
- Fine-tune treatment procedures (if needed)
- Plan for generalization and maintenance of changed behavior

This chapter has described the basic components of effective behavior program designs. However, each component does not stand alone. All of the steps are integrated and must be completed systematically in order to reach the desired behavioral outcome.

Behavioral diagnostics: First, a thorough assessment must be performed. This consists of reviewing historical information about the client which helps the behavior programmer understand how the client may respond to rehabilitation, and what he or she expects to gain from treatment.[61] It involves evaluating the client's current functional skills and analyzing clinical test results which can dictate the type of behavioral procedure that is implemented. Most important, a thorough behavioral assessment includes a functional analysis that identifies the function served by each target behavior.[63]

Identify maintaining conditions: The result of behavioral diagnostics should be the identification of conditions that might be supporting the target behavior. Is there an antecedent or setting event to the behavior? Are there responses to the behavior which are reinforcing? What function might the behavior be serving? The three parts of a functional analysis are: 1) identification of the target behavior and its surrounding events, 2) predicting the factors that control the behavior, and 3) testing of the behavioral hypothesis by manipulating those factors.

Baseline data: Once the assessment is complete, the target behavior defined, and the maintaining conditions identified, baseline data can be collected. Baseline data will provide valuable information concerning the frequency and duration of the target behavior, and a means for judging the effectiveness of the treatment procedure. The behavior programmer can choose an event, interval, or time-sample recording method based on the characteristics of the target behavior. Event recording is better suited to discrete behaviors (i.e., those with a clearly defined beginning and end). Time-sample recording is more appropriate for high-rate behaviors that are ill-suited to constant observation, and interval recording works for general-purpose data collection.

Treatment procedures: After baseline data has been collected, a treatment plan can be designed and implemented. The behavior program should include short- and long-term goals, clear operational definitions of the target behavior, a list of any materials needed, a description of the data collection system, and procedures for staff to follow. Procedures can be accelerative (designed to increase the target behavior), decelerative (designed to decrease the target behavior), or complex (having characteristics of both accelerative and decelerative programs). Effective behavioral programming may even require combining more than one of these procedures simultaneously.

Continued data collection: Once the treatment plan has started, data collection should continue as a means of monitoring the progress of the client. Data recording sheets should be completed on a daily basis in as many environments and conditions as possible. Systematic data collection allows the programmer, staff, client, family, and others to be kept abreast of the client's progress. People typically respond more favorably to observationally recorded data of behavior than to statements such as "She's behaving better."

Graph and analyze behavior: Behavior data should be routinely summarized and graphed. Graphing is one of the best means for analyzing the effect of a treatment plan. It provides an overall visual impression of behavior that is easy to understand and an effective way of tracking learning curves. The behavior programmer can then base any modifications to the treatment plan on more objective data rather than anecdotal reports.

Modify treatment procedures: Treatment procedures should be altered only when there is sufficient evidence in the data to indicate a failure in the procedure's effectiveness, or when the data indicates a need for a transition to a less structured approach. This can happen when the original behavior problem has been resolved. In this situation, the use of trend graphing can be useful. Trend graphs show the future projected change in a behavior based on the current observed rate of change.

Generalization and maintenance: Treatment plans are not successful if a behavioral change is not generalized to other environments and conditions and maintained over time. As treatment and recovery progress, procedures require modification — for example, thinning a reinforcement schedule or decreasing dependence on prompts.

If the client will be living with others after rehabilitation, training of these individuals in basic principles and treatment procedures is essential for a successful outcome. Long-term maintenance of behavior changes can hinge on the ability of family and friends to continue the treatment plan after a client has been discharged from a facility.

CONCLUDING REMARKS

As the field of traumatic brain injury rehabilitation grows beyond its infancy, behavioral treatment procedures are being recognized as an essential component of successful client outcome. Applied behavior analysis provides the structure and consistent feedback required by people with traumatic brain injury. Although many facilities understand the concepts of behavior analysis and recognize the need for its implementation, the authors have seen very few facilities actualize this ideal. Usually, this is a result of a division between a behavioral approach on the one hand and a therapeutic approach on the other. Behaviorally oriented staff focus primarily on the behavior of a client, whereas therapists' main concern is with recovering of lost cognitive and physical skills. Both need to work together, recognizing the contribution each makes to the total rehabilitation of the client. The result of any such division is that a behaviorally challenged client is undertreated, not able to progress to his or her highest level of independence, and, in many cases, placed in a long-term restrictive environment.

Reductions in the use of aversive procedures and emphasis on nonaversive techniques is forthcoming. Legal and ethical concerns related to the use of aversive procedures are making these programs increasingly more difficult to implement,[78] which, in our opinion, will be an unfortunate and impractical consequence. The full spectrum of behavior technology can be properly utilized with comprehensive ethical guidelines and monitoring.

Applied behavior analysis is an essential component to helping the person with traumatic brain injury rebuild his or her life. Helping these individuals reintegrate into the home, community, and work settings presents a great challenge to the field of rehabilitation. Behavior analysis provides an effective means for achieving this goal.

REFERENCES

1. Slifer, K. J., Cataldo, M. D., Babbitt, R. L., Kane, A. C., Harrison, K. A., and Cataldo, M. F., Behavior analysis and intervention during hospitalization for brain trauma rehabilitation, *Arch. Phys. Med. Rehabil.*, 74, 810, 1993.
2. DiCesare, A., Parente, R., and Anderson-Parente, J., Personality changes after traumatic brain injury: Problems and solutions, *Cognit. Rehabil.*, 8, 14, 1990.
3. Denny-Brown, D., Disability arising from closed head injury, *J. Am. Med. Assoc.*, 127, 429, 1945.
4. Levin, H. S. and Grossman, R. G., Behavioral sequela of closed head injury: Quantitative study, *Arch. Neurol.*, 35, 720, 1978.
5. Corrigan, J. D., Mysiw, W. J., Gribble, M. W., and Chock, S. K. L., Agitation, cognition, and attention during post-traumatic amnesia, *Brain Injury*, 6, 155, 1992.
6. Corrigan, J. D. and Mysiw, W. J., Agitation following traumatic head injury: Equivocal evidence for a discrete stage of cognitive recovery, *Arch. Phys. Med. Rehabil.*, 69, 487, 1988.
7. Brooke, M. M., Questad, K. A., Patterson, D. R., and Bashak, K. J., Agitation and restlessness after closed head injury: A prospective study of 100 consecutive admissions, *Arch. Phys. Med. Rehabil.*, 73, 320, 1992.
8. Peters, M. D., Gluck, M., and McCormick, M., Behaviour rehabilitation of the challenging client in less restrictive settings, *Brain Injury*, 6, 299, 1992.
9. Duncan, P. W., Physical therapy assessment, in *Rehabilitation of the Adult and Child with Traumatic Brain Injury*, Rosenthal, M., Griffith, E. R., Bond, M. R., and Miller, J. D., Eds.,, F. A. Davis Company, Philadelphia, 1990, 264.
10. Adamovich, B. L. B., Cognition, language, attention, and information processing following closed head injury, in *Cognitive Rehabilitation for Persons with Traumatic Brain Injury: A Functional Approach*, Kreutzer, J. S. and Wehman, P. H., Eds., Paul H. Brookes Publishing Co., Baltimore, 1991, 75.

11. McNeny, R., Deficits in activities of daily living, in *Rehabilitation of the Adult and Child with Traumatic Brain Injury*, Rosenthal, M., Griffith, E. R., Bond, M. R., and Miller, J. D., Eds., F. A. Davis Company, Philadelphia, 1990, 193.

12. Armstrong, C., Emotional changes following brain injury: Psychological and neurological components of depression, denial and anxiety, *J. Rehabilt.*, 2, 15, 1991.

13. MacNiven, E. and Finlayson, M. A. J., The interplay between emotional and cognitive recovery after closed head injury, *Brain Injury*, 7, 241, 1993.

14. Bendiksen, M. and Bendiksen, I., A multi-dimensional intervention for a toxic solvent injured population, *J. Cognit. Rehabil.*, 10, 20, 1992.

15. McMillan, T. M., Papadopoulos, H., Cornall, C., and Greenwood, R. J., Modification of severe behaviour problems following herpes simplex encephalitis, *Brain Injury*, 4, 399, 1990.

16. Mild Traumatic Brain Injury Committee, Definition of mild traumatic brain injury, *J. Head Trauma Rehabil.*, 8, 86, 1993.

17. Alexander, M. P., Neuropsychiatric correlates of persistent postconcussive syndrome, *J. Head Trauma Rehabil.*, 7, 60, 1992.

18. Harrington, D. E., Malec, J., Cicerone, K., and Katz, H., Current perceptions of rehabilitation professionals towards mild traumatic brain injury, *Arch. Phys. Med. Rehabil.*, 74, 579, 1993.

19. Boake, C., Bobetic, K. M., and Bontke, C. F., Rehabilitation of the patient with mild traumatic brain injury, *NeuroRehabilitation*, 1, 70, 1991.

20. Verduyn, W. H., Hilt, J., Roberts, M. A., and Roberts, R. J., Multiple partial-like symptoms following "minor" closed head injury, *Brain Injury*, 6, 245, 1992.

21. Swiercinsky, D. P., Price, T. L., and Leaf, L. E., *Traumatic Head Injury: Cause, Consequence, and Challenge*, The Kansas Head Injury Association, Inc., Shawnee Mission, KS, 1987.

22. Katz, D. I., Neuropathology and neurobehavioral recovery from closed head injury, *J. Head Trauma Rehabil.*, 7, 1, 1992.

23. Coutant, N. S., Rage: Implied neurological correlates, *J. Neurosurg. Nurs.*, 14, 28, 1982.

24. Crompton, M. R., Hypothalamic lesions following closed head injury, *Brain*, 94, 165, 1971.

25. Elliott, F. A., The neurology of explosive rage, *Practitioner*, 217, 51, 1976.

26. Grafman, J., Sirigu, A., Spector, L., and Hendler, J., Damage to the prefrontal cortex leads to decomposition of structured event complexes, *J. Head Trauma Rehabil.*, 8, 73, 1993.

27. Goldman-Rakic, P. S., Specifications of higher cortical functions, *J. Head Trauma Rehabil.*, 8, 13, 1993.

28. Hart, T. and Jacobs, H. E., Rehabilitation and management of behavioral disturbances following frontal lobe injury, *J. Head Trauma Rehabil.*, 8, 1, 1993.

29. Rose, M. J., The place of drugs in the management of behavior disorders after traumatic brain injury, *J. Head Trauma Rehabil.*, 3, 7, 1988.

30. Yablon, S. A., Posttraumatic seizures. *Arch. Phys. Med. Rehabil.*, 74, 983, 1993.

31. Galski, T., Palaz, J., Bruno, R. L., and Walker, J. E., Predicting physical and verbal aggression on a brain trauma unit, *Arch. Phys. Med. Rehabil.*, 75, 403, 1994.

32. Rao, N. R., Jellinek, H. M., and Woolston, D. C., Agitation in closed head injury: Haloperidol effects on rehabilitation outcome, *Arch. Phys. Med. Rehabil.*, 66, 30, 1985.

33. Chandler, M. C., Barnhill, J. L., and Gualtieri, C. T., Amantadine for the agitated head-injury patient, *Brain Injury*, 2, 309, 1988.

34. Brooke, M. M., Patterson, D. R., Questad, K. A., Cardenas, D., and Farrel-Roberts, L., The treatment of agitation during initial hospitalization after traumatic brain injury, *Arch. Phys. Med. Rehabil.*, 73, 917, 1992.

35. Mooney, G. F. and Haas, L. J., Effect of methylphenidate on brain-injury related anger, *Arch. Phys. Med. Rehabil.*, 74, 153, 1993.

36. Speech, T. J., Rao, S. M., Osmon, D. C., and Sperry, L. T., A double-blind controlled study of methylphenidate treatment in closed head injury, *Brain Injury*, 7, 333, 1993.

37. Silver, J. M. and Yudofsky, S. C., Pharmacologic treatment of neuropsychiatric disorders, *NeuroRehabilitation*, 3, 15, 1993.

38. Cantini, E., Gluck, M., and McLean, A., Jr., Psychotropic-absent behavioural improvement following severe traumatic brain injury, *Brain Injury*, 6, 193, 1992.

39. Miller, D. L. and Kelly, M. L., The use of goal setting and contingency contracting for improving children's homework performance, *J. Appl. Behav. Anal.*, 27, 73, 1994.

40. Jones, R. S. P. and McCaughey, R. E., Gentle teaching and applied behavior analysis: A critical review, *J. Appl. Behav. Anal.*, 25, 853, 1992.

41. McGee, J. J., Gentle teaching's assumptions and paradigm, *J. Appl. Behav. Anal.*, 25, 869, 1992.

42. Bailey, J. S., Gentle teaching: Trying to win friends and influence people with euphemism, metaphor, smoke, and mirrors, *J. Appl. Behav. Anal.*, 25, 87, 1992.

43. Dyer, K., Dunlap, G., and Winterling, V., Effects of choice making on the serious problem behaviors of students with severe handicaps, *J. Appl. Behav. Anal.*, 23, 515, 1990.

44. Mace, F. C. and Belfiore, P., Behavioral momentum in the treatment of escape-motivated stereotypy, *J. Appl. Behav. Anal.,* 23, 507, 1990.

45. Horner, R. H., Day, H. M., Sprague, J. R., O'Brien, M., and Heathfield, L. T., Interspersed requests: A nonaversive procedure for reducing aggression and self-injury during instruction, *J. Appl. Behav. Anal.,* 24, 265, 1991.

46. Wheeler, A. J., Miller, R. A., Duke, J., Salisbury, E. W., Merritt, V., and Horton, B., *Murdoch Center C & Y Program Library: A Collection of Step-By-Step Programs for the Developmentally Disabled,* Murdoch Center, Butner, NC, 1977.

47. Cope, D. N., Legal and ethical issues in the psychopharmacological treatment of traumatic brain injury, *J. Head Trauma Rehabil.,* 4, 13, 1989.

48. Alberto, P. A. and Troutman, A. C., *Applied Behavior Analysis for Teachers,* Macmillan Publishing Co., New York, 1990, Chap. 2.

49. Scofield, G. R., Ethical considerations in rehabilitation medicine, *Arch. Phys. Med. Rehabil.,* 74, 341, 1993.

50. Kennedy, C. H. and Itkonen, T., Effects of setting events on the problem behavior of students with severe disabilities, *J. Appl. Behav. Anal.,* 26, 321, 1993.

51. Tate, R. L., Behavior management techniques for organic psychosocial deficit incurred by severe head injury, *Scand. J. Rehabil. Med.,* 19, 19, 1987.

52. Hegel, T. M., Application of a token economy with a non-compliant closed head-injured male, *Brain Injury,* 2, 333, 1988.

53. Zencius, A., Wesolowski, M. D., and Burke, W. H., Comparing motivational systems with two non-compliant head-injured adolescents, *Brain Injury,* 3, 67, 1989.

54. Turner, J. M., Green, G., and Braunling-McMorrow, D., Differential reinforcement of low rates of responding (DRL) to reduce dysfunctional social behaviors of a head injured man, *Behav. Residential Treat.,* 5, 15, 1990.

55. Zencius, A., Wesolowski, M. D., Burke, W. H., and McQuade, P., Antecedent control in the treatment of brain-injured clients, *Brain Injury,* 3, 199, 1989.

56. Giles, G. M., Fussey, I., and Burgess, P., The behavioral treatment of verbal interaction skills following severe head injury: A single case study, *Brain Injury,* 2, 75, 1988.

57. Giles, G. M. and Clark-Wilson, J., The use of behavioral techniques in functional skills training after severe brain injury, *Am. J. Occup. Ther.,* 42, 658, 1988.

58. Braunling-McMorrow, D., Lloyd, K., and Fralish, K., Teaching social skills to head injured adults, *J. Rehabil.,* Jan.–Mar., 39, 1986.

59. Blair, D. C. and Lanyon, R. I., Retraining social and adaptive living skills in severely head injured adults, *Arch. Clin. Neuropsychol.,* 2, 33, 1987.

60. Steege, M. W., Wacker, D. P., Cigrand, K. C., Berg, W. K., Novak, C. G., Reimers, T. M., Sasso, G. M., and DeRaad, A., Use of negative reinforcement in the treatment of self-injurious behavior, *J. Appl. Behav. Anal.,* 23, 459, 1990.

61. Jacobs, H. E., *Behavior Analysis Guidelines and Brain Injury Rehabilitation: People, Principles, and Programs,* Aspen Publications, Gaithersburg, MD, 1993.

62. Wahler, R. G. and Fox, J. J., Setting events in applied behavior analysis: Toward a conceptual and methodological expansion, *J. Appl. Behav. Anal.,* 14, 327, 1981.

63. Iwata, B. A., Vollmer, T. R., and Zarcone, J. R., The experimental (functional) analysis of behavior disorders: Methodology, applications, and limitations, in *Perspectives on the Use of Nonaversive and Aversive Interventions for Persons with Developmental Disabilities,* Repp, A. C. and Singh, N. N., Eds., Sycamore, Sycamore, IL, 1990, 301.

64. Durand, M. V. and Carr, E. G., Functional communication training to reduce challenging behavior: Maintenance and application in new settings, *J. Appl. Behav. Anal.,* 24, 251, 1991.

65. O'Neill, R. E., Horner, R. H., Albin, R. W., Storey, K., and Sprague, J. R., *Functional Analysis of Problem Behaviors: A Practical Assessment Guide,* Sycamore, Sycamore, IL, 1990.

66. Rappaport, M., Hall, K., Hopkins, K., Belleza, T., and Cope, D., Disability rating scale for severe head trauma: Coma to community, *Arch. Phys. Med. Rehabil.,* 63, 118, 1982.

67. Carr, E. G. and Carlson, J. I., Reduction of severe behavior problems in the community using a multicomponent treatment approach, *J. Appl. Behav. Anal.,* 26, 157, 1993.

68. LaVigna, G. W. and Donnellan, A. M., *Alternatives to Punishment: Solving Behavior Problems with Non-Aversive Strategies,* Irvington Publishers, Inc., New York, 1986.

69. Walls, R. T., Zane, T., and Ellis, W. D., Forward and backward chaining and whole task methods, *Behav. Modification,* 5, 61, 1981.

70. Mulick, J. A., Leitenberg, H., and Rawson, R. A., Alternative response training, differential reinforcement of other behavior, and extinction in squirrel monkeys, *J. Exp. Anal. Behav.,* 25, 311, 1976.

71. Reynolds, G. S., Behavioral contrast, *J. Exp. Anal. Behav.,* 4, 57, 1961.

72. Cowdery, G. E., Iwata, B. A., and Pace, G. M., Effects and side effects of DRO as treatment for self-injurious behavior, *J. Appl. Behav. Anal.,* 23, 497, 1990.

73. Skinner, B. F., *The Behavior of Organisms*, Appleton-Century-Crofts, New York, 1938.
74. Azrin, N. H. and Foxx, R. M., A rapid method of toilet training the institutionalized retarded, *J. Appl. Behav. Anal.*, 4, 89, 1971.
75. Azrin, N. H., Some effects of noise on human behavior, *J. Exp. Anal. Behav.*, 1, 183, 1958.
76. Ayllon, T., Intensive treatment of psychotic behavior by stimulus satiation and food reinforcement, *Behav. Res. Ther.*, 1, 53, 1963.
77. Alderman, N., The treatment of avoidance behavior following severe brain injury by satiation through negative practice, *Brain Injury*, 5, 77, 1991.
78. Czyzewski, M. J., Sheldon, J., and Hannah, G. T., Legal safety in residential treatment environments, in *Behavior Analysis and Therapy in Residential Programs*, Fuoco, F. J. and Christian, W. P., Eds., Van Nostrand Reinhold Co., New York, 1986, 194.
79. DeRisi, W. J. and Butz, G., *Writing Behavioral Contracts: A Case Simulation Practice Manual*, Research Press, Champaign, IL, 1975.
80. Catania, A. C., Ed., *Contemporary Research in Operant Behavior*, Scott, Foresman & Co., Glenview, IL, 1968.
81. Ayllon, T. and Azrin, N. H., *The Token Economy: A Motivational System for Therapy and Rehabilitation*, Appleton-Century-Crofts, New York, 1968.
82. Baer, D. M., Wolf, M. M., and Risley, T. R., Some still current dimensions of applied behavior analysis, *J. Appl. Behav. Anal.*, 20, 31, 1987.
83. Haring, T. G. and Kennedy, C. H., Contextual control of problem behavior in students with severe disabilities, *J. Appl. Behav. Anal.*, 23, 235, 1990.
84. Smith, P., Professional Assault Response Training (PART) Workshop Syllabus, Citrus Heights, CA, 1983.
85. Brammer, L. M., *The Helping Relationship: Process and Skills*. Prentice-Hall, Inc., Englewood Cliffs, NJ, 1973.

11

Cognition, Language, Communication: Some Challenging Issues

John R. Muma and William E. Harn

CONTENTS

INTRODUCTION

One of the most fascinating areas of endeavor in rehabilitation of the person with traumatic brain injury (TBI) is the area of cognition. The role of cognition in achievement of functional independence and return to normalized, age-appropriate activities is the subject of much concern for rehabilitation professionals dealing with the TBI population. Assessment of cognition, however, must be undertaken in indirect ways, especially if one is to gain an understanding of cognition as a dynamic process within an individual. Assessments which are of the paper-and-pencil variety are not often available for the patient with significant cognitive impairment. Thus, assessment of cognitive function must occur via behavioral observation of the individual within an environment and/or via linguistic channels of access to cognitive processing. The interrelation of language and cognition has been studied for some time, though perhaps it is the person with brain injury that presents both the greatest clinical challenge and the greatest clinical opportunity for enhancement of our understanding of the seeming interdependence of language and cognition.

The purpose of this chapter is to provide the reader with information relating what our current understanding is about the relation of cognition to language and to discuss developments in the cognition literature that have far-reaching implications for understanding TBI and for developing appropriate clinical services. These developments raise many challenges for the traditional views, policies, and practices. Furthermore, the paradigm shifts away from behaviorism and reinforcement theory to constructionism, functionalism, and experiential realism have defined intentionality and functional contexts as crucial issues for rendering appropriate clinical services. These perspectives and challenges are placed within the perspective of speech act theory and a model for the cognitive bases of language.

This is a challenging time for the emerging field of service professionals dealing with traumatic brain injury. It is challenging because of the need to work within a shared, interacting team of health providers with diverse areas of expertise and varied service provider locations ranging from hospitals and clinics to work locations and homes. And, it is a challenging time because many relatively new developments in the literature have questioned traditional views, policies, and practices. The purpose of this chapter is to discuss the latter with particular attention given to the changes in the literature concerning cognition and language.

From a brief historical perspective concerning many traditional and pervasive views of clinical practice, several issues are raised. Indeed, several cherished issues have become questioned by virtue of developments in the literature. It is especially timely to address these issues in an effort to separate productive clinical ventures from less productive ones. It is timely simply because these issues have come to the fore in the recent literature and because clinical fields addressing services for TBI individuals are currently marshalling their expertise in a concerted effort.

There is no question that the literatures on cognition, language, and communication are crucial to an understanding of TBI and for conceptualizing appropriate perspectives, policies, and practices regarding assessment and interventions. Therefore, it is necessary to have a general appreciation of these literatures, especially as they interface with one another in a unified perspective. This can be achieved by the following topics: Historical Perspective; Paradigm Shifts; Cognitive Bases of Language: A Model; and Two Castles. In the course of discussing these topics, the central issues have been extracted and identified as particular issues to facilitate reading; thus, a series of 14 issues have been raised across these topics.

HISTORICAL PERSPECTIVE

At the turn of the century, thought and language were regarded as separate and distinguishable human abilities. With Watsonian empiricism, efforts were made to assess thought and language independently. On the one hand, the measurement of thought was invested in the notion of intelligence testing[1] whereas developmental norms were obtained for language.[2,3] These two somewhat independent perspectives became prominent in rendering clinical services. Even today, some clinical assessment and intervention views and practices reflect the notion that thought and language should be separated.

As Frank Sinatra would say, 1957 was a very good year. Two major developments occurred which were closely related to a third. First, Chomsky[4] raised some fundamental questions about the inadequacies of traditional taxonomic linguistics — normative inventories. The essential issue was that Chomsky approached the study of language from a psychological perspective — competence. Rather than viewing language as a collection of structures, Chomsky was interested in what individuals know in order to comprehend and produce language. This placed the study of language within cognitive science. Thus, language was no longer independent of thought. Furthermore, the cognitive issues raised concerning the generative nature of language were not about intelligence but about mental processes that enable one to produce or comprehend messages.[5]

Second, Grice gave the 1957 William James Lecture at Harvard University in which he formally proposed Speech Act Theory. A revised version of this theory was published a decade later.[6] And, more eloquent renditions have subsequently appeared.[5,7] The importance of speech act theory is that it broadened the study of language to a study of communication within the rubric of cognitive socialization. The four primary issues in speech act theory were intent, explicit content in relation to implicit content, the message itself (grammatical and phonological realizations), and the effects of a message on a listener. Thus, this perspective deals with cognitive-linguistic-pragmatic aspects of language in a unified way. With the functionalistic movement over the past two decades, these dimensions could be regarded as

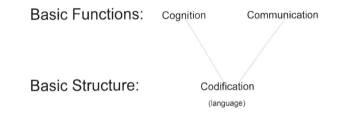

FIGURE 11.1   Cognition, codification, communication: function and form.

cognition, codification, communication; and, cognition and communication have become regarded as the basic functions of language whereas language per se, or codification, constitutes the subsumed structure for realizing cognition and communication. Figure 11.1 depicts these issues.

This model is very important because it defines language structure or form operating within cognitive and communicative functions and it distinguishes function from form. These form-function distinctions have major clinical implications. Paramount among these implications is the principle that function has priority over form. That is, form operates in the service of function.

Issue I: Function has priority over form.

This issue is very important simply because some clinical fields have traditionally operated in conflict with this principle. Specifically, many clinical services have been based on frequency counts (or percentages) of language structures rather than indicating how these structures *function* to realize actual thinking or communicative objectives. It is more appropriate to ascertain how structures function in particular communicative contexts than to merely count instances of structure. Second, it is necessary to ascertain an individual's repertoire of skills for grammatical and pragmatic systems as evidence of available options for communicating, available strategies of learning, and evidence of active loci of learning. One would be hard pressed to find clinical practices based on estimated repertoires of skills, strategies of learning, and active loci of learning.

Third, Brown[8] was instrumental in launching the study of language acquisition from the perspective of cognitive socialization; he indicated that language acquisition is "a process of cognitive socialization." This is a very important comment because it indicates that cognition and socialization (or communication) comprise the two basic functions of language and that the linguistic domains, or forms, are subsumed. This, in turn, means that the two basic communicative functions, notably intent and content, have priority over form which is the functionalistic message of the past two decades or so.

It can be safely said that developments in the past four decades in cognition, language, and communication have not only come together in a unified perspective of cognitive socialization but they have given fuller realization to what Brown and Grice had posited. Brown[9] provided another comment which underscores the centrality of the communicative function of language, "If you concentrate on communicating, everything else will follow." Bruner[10] indicated that "context is all" — and, "everything is use".[11] These all recognize that it is how language *functions* in context that is essential rather than the actual forms or frequencies of forms. And, it should be noted that Bruner was referring to both internal and external contexts in recognition of the fact that messages do not work as intended unless they are functioning in relation to implicit knowledge of the world. This perspective is amplified further below. At present, it is only necessary to indicate the importance of context. Thus, form is not meaningful as an entity by itself; rather, form is meaningful as it functions in particular contexts.

Issue II: Context is all.

Traditional clinical assessment and intervention characteristically have violated the importance of context. Notice how many tests remove contexts and how many intervention approaches have individuals perform a skill in isolation — removed from actual communicative contexts. Strange as it may sound, many studies that used behavior modification are bewildered because of a lack of generalization. Yet, these studies have not only removed behaviors from contexts, but they relied on elicited rather than intentional behaviors and relied on a stochastic (distributed practice) model of presumed rule learning when algebraic (abstract) models more accurately represent language acquisition.[12-15]

Two other closely related notions are the problems of reductionism and quantification — both of which are richly evident in the clinical fields and have a lineage extending back to the Watsonian era at the turn of the century. *Reductionism* is the view that domains such as language may be reduced to their elements to understand them. But, just as water would not be understood by reducing it to hydrogen and oxygen, language would lack an understanding by reducing it to semantics, syntax, phonology, and pragmatics, and cognition would not be understood well by reducing it to sensation, perception, discrimination, memory, concepts, and ideas. The literatures in cognition and language over the past three decades have long since dashed the view that reductionism is very productive.

Issue III: Reductionism has not been very productive.

It is not difficult to find clinical assessment tests and intervention programs that are reductionistic in dealing with cognition and language. For example, clinicians still claim to measure memory by the number of digits recalled forward and backward and the number of commands executed. Yet, these views and practices were shown to be invalid many years ago.[16,17] Similarly, reductionism in language is alive and well in the clinical fields. Bruner[11] made the following comment about reductionism in language: "I have tried to show that it is self-defeating to establish the psychological reality or relevance of syntactical, semantic, and pragmatic distinctions, each on their own and in isolation from the others."

The *quantification* issue might be summarized by the following: What is gained, or lost, by converting behavior into numbers? Again, in both cognition and language, there are large risks in attempting to convert behaviors to numbers. The risks are due to the fact that these behaviors are not reducible, they are not linear but hierarchical, and they function in context. Therefore, if quantification were used, it would be necessary to not only quantify a behavior of interest, but also how it functions in particular contexts. Needless to say, the clinical fields have not entered this arena with a full-fledged appreciation of the issues.

Indeed, notice how many clinical papers in the journals and clinical reports of clients misuse quantification, especially the misuse of percentages. It is not difficult to find instances where percentages have been used for instances of behavior that are much less than 100. For example, Washington and Craig[18] applied percentages for samples of subjects well under 100, specifically 12, 14, and 19. Such uses of percentages inflate the data. Furthermore, when such percentages are used in comparative ways (pre-post comparisons; comparisons between clients, between behaviors, or between programs), there is the added problem whereby disproportionate comparisons occur.

Issue IV: Quantification may be a disservice.

There is an irony in the clinical literature on language because it has been oriented traditionally on modalities, specifically the expressive and receptive modalities and the oral and written modalities. Yet, a person would be hard pressed to find much of the scholarly literature oriented on modalities. Rather, the scholarly literature has indicated that modality aspects of information are purged very early in information processing[5,7,19,20] with the bulk of the information processing occurring in a nonmodality way. Specifically, such information processing operates on general cognitive capacities, notably categorization, inference, and problem solving, toward the realization of intent.[11,21-24] With the clinical fields so committed to a modality perspective and the scholarly literatures focused on inherent cognitive capacities, there is the very real risk that the clinical fields have been dealing with tangential, rather than basic, issues of cognition and language.

Issue V: Modality perspectives may be tangential to basic issues of cognition and language.

PARADIGM SHIFTS

So that clinicians will not despair, it is useful to turn to philosophical views and theoretical perspectives that have received scholarly attention and support because they provide anchors for "righting the ship" in a stormy burlesque of claimed expertise and rendered services.

There have been some paradigm shifts whereby some basic cherished notions in the clinical fields have become questioned. Prominent in the shifts is the overthrow of behaviorism by constructionism, functionalism, and experiential realism. The basic tenet of *constructionism* is that an individual is an active processor of information. The implication is that it is desirable to ascertain an individual's repertoire of skills, alternative learning strategies, and active loci of learning rather than impose systems in the normative test format in an attempt to ascertain what an individual can do. As indicated above, the basic tenet of *functionalism* is that function has priority over form. The implication is that purpose or intent of a behavior has priority over its form. The basic tenet of *experiential realism* is that experience defines what is real for an individual. The implication is that objectivity is merely formalized subjectivity.[25]

Many scholars have recognized this paradigm shift. Pinker[26] referred to the failings of behavior modification in the following way: "With the virtual demise of classical learning theory as an explanation of language development." Bruner[27] indicated that the positivist views (behaviorism) merely resulted in "corrosive dogma". And, in this vein, Bruner[27] indicated that the centrality of *intent* for the above philosophical views has replaced *reinforcement* as a viable account of language acquisition.

Another major issue in the contemporary literature on language acquisition is the debate about modularity. Fodor[28] has advocated the modularity view. In essence, the modularity view is that language acquisition, use, and impairment may be modular. This means that various aspects of language may be learned, used, and disrupted with the other aspects relatively unaltered or intact. The clinical implication is that language services could be compartmentalized, i.e. semantic, syntactic, phonological, and pragmatic.

Issue VI: Modularity is not very promising.

However, the literature has provided many counterissues not only about language but also cognition.[25] The pragmatic movement has been especially prominent in dethroning the modularity view.[11,21,23,24] But, the renditions of pragmatics in the clinical fields come perilously close to impressionism.[29] Thus, putting the modularity notion aside, it may be useful to turn to a model of the cognitive bases of language devised by Muma[22] that conforms to the basic premises of speech act theory.

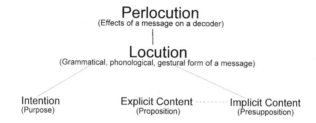

FIGURE 11.2   The structure of a message in actual social commerce in accordance with speech act theory.

Level	Domain
I	General cognitive capacities: possible worlds, categorization, inference, problem solving
II	Substantive aspects: intent, implicit content, explicit content
III	Encoding and decoding processes: planning and execution, construction, and utilization
IV	Metalinguistic skills: reflection

FIGURE 11.3   The cognitive bases of language in accordance with the centrality of communicative intent.

COGNITIVE BASES OF LANGUAGE: A MODEL

The reason that it is imperative to establish a model that is compatible with speech act theory is that this theory is one of the most, if not the most, prominent theories in the scholarly literature on cognition and language[30] over the past three decades or so and because this theory has been relatively successful in obtaining descriptive and explanatory adequacy.[5,7,31]

Speech act theory[6] posited that the central issue is the realization of communicative intent and that all of the other cognitive, linguistic, and pragmatic issues operate to realize communicative intent. The *centrality of communicative intent* has major clinical implications. Directly put, it means that clinical assessment should be predicated on what an individual actually does in natural spontaneous communication if the objective is to ascertain what he/she can do. This raises the distinction between elicited (test performance, *a priori* checklists) vs. spontaneous (intentional) behavior as providing the most viable information for what an individual can do. Similarly, language intervention should be based on how an individual actually functions when he/she intends to communicate. As it stands, much of what is done clinically in both assessment and intervention relies on elicited rather than intentional behavior.

Issue VII: Communicative intent is the central issue.

In addition to the centrality of intention, speech act theory has three other major dimensions: (a) explicit content (proposition) with respect to requisite implicit content (presupposition); (b) message form (grammatical, phonological, gestural); and (c) perlocution (effects of a message on the decoder). These are depicted in Figure 11.2.

Given speech act theory and the centrality of communicative intent, a model of the cognitive bases of language must place intent as a function in perspective with other functions and structures in a coherent way. Figure 11.3 gives the model of the cognitive bases of language derived from Muma;[22] this model is compatible with speech act theory.

From this perspective, it behooves clinicians to establish assessment and intervention views, policies, and practices for these domains. Level I deals with general cognitive capacities.

These capacities have an indirect relation to language acquisition and use. They deal with what has been variously termed as an individual's: *knowledge of the world*,[10] *theory of the world*,[32] or *possible worlds*.[11] This is what Schlesinger[33] regarded as "the interpretation problem". That is, individuals strive to learn about the world and interpret which aspect of general knowledge may be needed for learning language. Thus, language acquisition, and recovery, is predicated on basic knowledge of the world. Knowledge of the world, or possible worlds, is the product of perceptual, inferential, and problem-solving processes that categorize experience. The categories themselves are prototypic representations of experiences.

Issue VIII: Knowledge of the world, or possible worlds, is the general cognitive base for language acquisition and recovery.

The literature on event knowledge is especially relevant to Level I issues. Event knowledge is, first and foremost, a social affair. "Events are always 'socially and culturally meaningful'."[34] Young children come to know who the participants are and their roles in regular events; they come to know about social and nonsocial objects, about location, time, and order. To the extent that they are willing participants in social events, even as early as nursing, there is a nucleus of intent. Event knowledge invested in intentionality within a social arena is important for young children acquiring language and TBI adults recovering from language loss.

Issue IX: Event knowledge is an important arena for rendering clinical services because it entails intentionality within a social agenda.

Returning to the general perspective of knowledge of the world, it is needless to say that it would be useful to ascertain the extent to which an individual with brain injury may have difficulty with categorization. For example, Burger and Muma[35] showed that aphasics with word-finding difficulties had significantly more trouble with categorizing peripheral exemplars, as contrasted to focal exemplars,[36,37] than aphasics who had grammatical difficulties and age-matched normal adults. This indicates that, while prototypic knowledge of categories may have remained intact, extended or overlapping aspects may have been disrupted. All of the same subjects had significantly more trouble with categorizing pictures than objects; this is an issue of cognitive distancing which is discussed below in Level III. The implications are that categorization activities, especially those dealing with peripheral exemplars, are warranted, and objects should be used before pictorials in clinical assessment and intervention.

In addition to categorization, other general cognitive skills may be disrupted. Muma and Muma[38] have compiled a battery of tasks (MAP) from the cognitive psychology literature. These have been described elsewhere[19,22] and are listed here: Piagetian sensorimotor skills (object permanence, anticipation, causality, deferred imitation, alternative means); perceptual salience; iconic/symbolic processing; rule/nonrule-governed learning; technology of reckoning; part/whole and alternatives; cognitive tempo; and production deficiency.

Regarding the Piagetian sensorimotor skills, Uzgiris and Hunt[39] have developed contrived tasks for assessing these skills. Donaldson[40] has shown that different results can be obtained if the Piagetian tasks make "human sense" rather than being contrived in an *a priori* manner. Bronfenbrenner[41,42] has raised a similar concern which is that it is necessary to have "ecologically valid" evidence rather than mere test performance. With these and other related developments, there has been a general shift away from *a priori* psychometric tests to *a posteriori* descriptive assessment.[18,22]

And finally, it should be stressed that problem solving and inference are necessary general cognitive skills for producing and comprehending messages.[5,7] Some psycholinguists have maintained that the mental skills for language are uniquely different from those for dealing with cognition in general. However, Lakoff[25] argued that the notion that language relies on unique cognitive skills does not make much sense. It is far more likely that the same basic cognitive skills are shared with language. "It seems extremely unlikely that human beings do not make use of general cognitive capacities in language. It is bizarre to assume that language ignores general cognitive apparatus, especially when it comes to something as basic as categorization."

Level II in the cognitive bases of language model pertains to the substantive aspects of language, specifically intent, explicit content, and implicit content. *Intent* is the purpose of a message. Some messages have direct and some have indirect intentions. *Explicit content* is the proposition of a message which may, or may not, be fully coded in a sentence. It could be partially coded in other ways such as posture, facial expression, gesture, etc. *Implicit content* is that requisite information about the world that is presumably shared, implied, or presupposed in order for a message to work as intended. Thus, presupposed information is needed for utterances such as the following to work as intended: "I like apples." It is presumed that the listener knows that "like" means taste and that "apples" are edible, otherwise the sentence does not work as intended.

A speaker strives to produce messages that take into account what is informative in relation to what may be mutually known. Explicit content is the result of decisions to code new information in the context of old in order to be informative.[5,43] The result is that some messages are "messages-of-best-fit"[44] whereas others may need to be negotiated further to play the communication game. Brown[45] described the attempt to provide a message-of-best-fit in the following way: "A sentence well adapted to its function is, like a piece in a jigsaw puzzle, just the right size and shape to fit the opening left for it by local conditions and community understandings." This whole enterprise is ladened with decisions about what information is needed in a particular communicative context and what should be negotiated to achieve a message-of-best-fit. Such perspectives raise major questions about the viability of clinical assessment and intervention practices that are prepackaged. These *a priori* approaches strip away basic substantive skills of language that are needed for making messages informative.

> **Issue X:** *A priori* prepackaged assessment and intervention approaches strip away basic substantive skills of language that are needed for making messages informative.

Level III pertains to mental processes that are entailed in encoding and decoding messages. These have been detailed by Clark and Clark.[5] One point should be stressed regarding presumed auditory and visual processing. The clinical fields are very shortsighted regarding this literature. The thinking in the clinical fields is that, if one sees something, he is visually processing and, if one hears something, he is processing auditorily. This is so, but it is very naive because the literature has shown that modality (visual, auditory) information is purged very early with the bulk of the work committed to problem solving, inferencing, and categorization.[5,7,20] Thus, to devote clinical assessment and intervention to presumed modality deficits without addressing the major aspects of verbal processing is surely shortsighted, just as surely as the notion that the number of commands executed is considered a measure of memory.

The theory of cognitive distancing[22,46] pertains to mental processing. It is based on the premise that motoric processing is early, relatively easy, and more primitive than perceptual processing. Indeed, that is the crux of the Piagetian theory whereby sensorimotor skills provide the bases for subsequent skills. Similarly, Bruner[47] held that enactive processing (motoric) precedes perceptual functioning. The implication is that actions on objects should precede the use of pictures and the use of pictures should precede the use of words, for both children and adults, if ease or degree of information processing is at issue. Indeed, the findings by Burger and Muma[35] were that aphasic and elderly individuals had significantly more trouble processing pictures of objects than the objects themselves.

Issue XI: In accordance with cognitive distancing, objects are easier to process than pictures and pictures are easier than words.

Level IV pertains to metalinguistic skills.[48-51] These skills are the abilities to reflect on and possibly play with language. It is fairly common for preschool and early school aged children to engage in spontaneous play with language and to entertain themselves with various verbal jingles about language. Muma[19,22] held that such play is potentially useful for developing language and offers good potential for language intervention. vanKleeck[52] has developed a language intervention program based on metalinguistic skills. It is noteworthy that adult individuals with brain injury are usually not good at understanding humor. Of course, it is necessary to distinguish between understanding humor and a happy facade that is sometimes used as a deception by the brain injured.

TWO CASTLES

Perhaps the model just discussed should be placed in a larger perspective. Bruner[11] has discussed two modes of thought which have become institutionalized as two professional castles: the castle of science and the castle of human affairs. The two modes of thought are paradigmatic (logico-scientific) and narrative.[11] These two castles, or modes of thought, have major ramifications for the conceptualization and implementation of clinical services. But first, a brief discussion of them is needed.

These are discussed in detail elsewhere.[53] Briefly, the castle of science is predicated on categorization and logical relations between categories to eventually address the irreducible nucleus of science, which is causality. In contrast, the castle of human affairs is predicated on the irreducible nucleus of *intentionality functioning* in context. Variance is intolerable for science simply because causality is presumably accountable even for the smallest element. However, variance is intrinsic to human affairs simply because intent varies from person to person in varying contexts. "'Intention and its vicissitudes' constitute a primitive category system in terms of which experience is organized, at least as primitive as the category system of causality."[11]

Science is context independent whereas human affairs, or narrative, is context sensitive; the former is oriented outward to an external world whereas the other is oriented inward concerning what one feels or imagines is "right". "Both of them surely trade on presupposition."[11] And, both are illusionary.

The reason that the distinctions between science and human affairs should be raised in the consideration of cognition and language for the TBI individual is that there has been a traditional reliance on a scientific view even when this view has been imposed on human affairs. For example, the reliance on psychometric normative testing to deal with cognition and language constitutes an imposition of science on human affairs. More specifically, performances on intelligence and achievement tests are compared to norms in an effort to claim that an individual evidences a particular psychometric level, but no effort is made to ascertain how the individual actually performs (intentionality) within his ecology. Ironically enough, the psychometric indices are used to draw inferences about how the individual may function; yet, direct evidence of how he actually functions is not only dismissed but actually viewed with disdain because it is presumably subjective. Yet, it is such evidence that deals with intent and human affairs. The same circumstance occurs in language assessment in the clinical fields. There is a tendency to rely on psychometric test results while ignoring what an individual actually does. And again, the irony is evident when test results are used to draw inferences about what an individual may do while evidence about what he actually does is dismissed. This irony is often rationalized by claiming that test performance provides objective evidence whereas observations of actual performance are subjective. However, this argument has been shown to be false.[24] Nevertheless, the clinical fields have held tenaciously to this perspective. In a word, the clinical fields have bought into the view that science should rule human affairs.

Issue XII: The irreducible nucleus of science is causality whereas it is *intentionality* for human affairs or narrative.

The clinical implications of the distinction between science and human affairs are considerable. For example, the use of "diagnostic" categories in medicine makes sense in dealing with medical conditions where causal relations are known but may actually be a hindrance when they are unknown. And, in the human affairs arena, the use of "diagnostic" procedures may not be only a hindrance but truly detrimental by virtue of the fact that individuals may be forced into preconceived categories with virtually no heed given to their particular status and functioning in their particular ecology.[41,42] This is what has come to be known as *the lethal label* problem.[54] Moreover, the issue of causality is often a moot issue clinically; rather, it is more useful to ascertain motivations (intentions) for participation in intervention.

The psychometric perspective, as an instance of the imposition of science on human affairs, is not just a problem of *a priori* categorization, but some other cherished issues have been scrutinized. Specifically, it was traditionally believed that psychometric normative tests (a) are objective, (b) provide relevant information, and (c) provide necessary and sufficient information. However, the recent literature has raised some major questions about the validity of these claims. Yet, this has been the empirical mentality, especially in the United States, since the turn of the century.

Issue XIII: Psychometric tests have been questioned in regard to objectivity, relevance, and necessary and sufficient information.

Perhaps it would be appropriate to make a few brief comments about some cherished notions or beliefs concerning psychometric tests. Some developments in the literature on the theory of science, notably Bruner[11] and Lakoff,[25] have raised some fundamental threats to the basic premises of psychometric normative testing. One threat is the *objectivity myth*; essentially, it is that objectivity is inaccessible, resulting in the undeniable recognition that everything is subjective, the normative solution notwithstanding. Indeed, it should be acknowledged that subjectivity is richly evident, both going in (test development) and coming out (test use).

Another threat is whether psychometric tests provide *relevant information*. Where is the evidence, either rational or empirical, that the information on a particular test is relevant to the existing scholarly literature?

For example, the Peabody Picture Vocabulary Test (PPVT-R)[55] is undoubtedly the most widely used clinical test even though it has some fundamental violations of the literature on word or vocabulary acquisition. Muma[56] showed that the PPVT-R misses intentionality because it relies on elicited responses for named pictures, misses referential meaning of words,[57] and misses relational meaning of words.[57] These are the most basic issues of vocabulary; yet, clinicians remain undaunted in the claim that the PPVT-R provides relevant information about an individual's vocabulary. Perhaps a summary of the literature on vocabulary learning[58] would be useful to appreciate the nakedness of this test and the claims of expertise for individuals who use it in this way. Said differently, this test, and many others in the clinical fields, lacks the most important issue of assessment — construct validity.[59]

Issue XIV: Many clinical tests lack the central issue of assessment — construct validity.

Still another fundamental threat to psychometric tests is whether they provide *necessary and sufficient information* to warrant assessing abilities. This is an issue that is regularly ignored in the clinical fields. In a sense, this issue is the other side of the relevance issue, because the relevance issue pertains to what the scholarly literature has to offer and the issue of necessary and sufficient information pertains to the relevance of information to warrant a conclusion about an individual's presumed abilities. Returning to the PPVT-R, it is noteworthy that claims are made about an individual's presumed vocabulary skills from performance on this test while no attempt is made to ascertain the individual's repertoire of available vocabulary. A typical retort is that this test provides a shorthand estimate of these abilities. This is valid if the test actually provides necessary and sufficient information — a claim that is woefully in need of substantiation. As for shorthand estimates of presumed skills, Muma et al.[60] have shown that the traditional clinical practices of using 50- or 100-utterance language samples have excessive error rates — on the order of 60% to 40%, respectively.

The descriptive approach to clinical assessment offers some solutions to the problems facing psychometric normative testing. Rather than test scores, it may be more efficacious to estimate actual repertories of skills from representative samples with attendant attribution criteria, available acquisition strategies, and active loci of learning.[21,61] For example, an estimate of an individual's repertoire of skills for subject nominals would provide evidence of the available alternatives for coding communicative intents. This is very important because, when a particular code does not work as intended, a speaker has recourse to other available codes. To this end, such information could provide necessary and sufficient information for ascertaining what an individual can do.

This chapter has delineated several major issues in the contemporary scholarly literature that have the potential of changing some basic clinical practices for the TBI. Furthermore, the clinical implications of these issues were made explicit. In so doing, it is hoped that the emerging field of clinical services providers for TBI will respond favorably to these challenges.

REFERENCES

1. Wechsler, D., Intelligence defined and undefined: a relativistic appraisal, *Am. Psychol.,* 30, 135, 1975.
2. McCarthy, D., The language development of the preschool child, *Institute of Child Welfare, Monograph Series, No. 4*, University of Minnesota Press, Minneapolis, 1930.
3. Templin, M., *Certain Language Skills in Children: Their Development and Interrelationships*, University of Minnesota Press, Minneapolis, 1957.
4. Chomsky, N., *Syntactic Structures*, Mouton, The Hague, 1957.
5. Clark, H. and Clark, E., *Psychology and Language*, Harcourt, Brace, and Jovanovich, New York, 1977.
6. Grice, H., 1957 William James Lectures, Harvard University, (Published in part as "Logic and conversation"), in *Syntax and Semantics: 3. Speech Acts*, Cole, P. and Morgan, J., Eds., Seminar Press, New York, 1967, 41.
7. Sperber, D. and Wilson, D., *Relevance: Communication and Cognition*, Harvard University Press, Cambridge, MA, 1986.
8. Brown, R., Language and categories, in *A Study of Thinking*, Bruner, J., Goodnow, L., and Austin, G., Eds., Wiley, New York, 1956, 247.
9. Brown, R., Introduction, in *Talking to Children,* Snow, C. and Ferguson, C., Eds., Cambridge University Press, New York, 1977, 1.
10. Bruner, J., The social context of language acquisition, *Language Commun.,* 1, 155, 1981.
11. Bruner, J., *Actual Minds, Possible Worlds*, Harvard University Press, Cambridge, MA, 1986, 87.
12. Bowerman, M., Commentary, in *Mechanisms of Language Acquisition*, MacWhinney, B., Ed., Erlbaum, Hillsdale, NJ, 1987, 443.
13. Fodor, J. and Crain, S., Simplicity and generality of rules in language acquisition, in *Mechanisms of Language Acquisition*, MacWhinney, B., Ed., Erlbaum, Hillsdale, NJ, 1987, 35.
14. Macken, M., Representation, rules and overgeneralization in phonology, in *Mechanisms of Language Acquisition*, MacWhinney, B., Ed., Erlbaum, Hillsdale, NJ, 1987, 367.
15. Ninio, A., On formal grammatical categories in early child language, in *Categories and Processes in Language Acquisition*, Levy, Y., Schlesinger, I., and Braine, M., Eds., Erlbaum, Hillsdale, NJ, 1988, 99.
16. Blankenship, A., Memory span: A review of the literature, *Psychol. Bull.,* 35, 1, 1938.
17. Jenkins, J., Remember that old theory of memory? Well, forget it! *Am. Psychol.,* 29, 785, 1974.

18. Washington, J. and Craig, H., Dialectal forms during discourse of poor, urban, African-American preschoolers, *J. Speech Hear. Res.,* 37, 816, 1994.

19. Muma, J., *Language Handbook: Concepts, Assessment, and Intervention*, Prentice-Hall, Englewood Cliffs, NJ, 1978.

20. Tallal, P., Fine-grained discrimination deficits in language-impaired children are specific neither to the auditory modality nor to speech perception, *J. Speech Hear. Res.,* 33, 616, 1990.

21. Bloom L., Beckwith, R., Capatides, J., and Hafitz, J., Expression through affect and words in the transition from infancy to language, in *Life-Span Development and Behavior*, Volume 8, Baltes, P., Featherman, D., and Lerner, R., Eds., Erlbaum, Hillsdale, NJ, 1988, 99.

22. Muma, J., *Language Acquisition: A Functionalistic Perspective*, PRO-ED, Austin, TX, 1986.

23. Nelson, K., *Making Sense: The Acquisition of Shared Meaning*, Academic, New York, 1985.

24. Nelson, K., *Event Knowledge: Structure and Function in Development*, Erlbaum, Hillsdale, NJ, 1986.

25. Lakoff, G., *Women, Fire, and Dangerous Things: What Categories Reveal About the Mind*, University of Chicago Press, Chicago, 1987.

26. Pinker, S., Learnability theory and the acquisition of a first language, in *The Development of Language and Language Researchers*, Kessel, F., Ed., Erlbaum, Hillsdale, NJ, 1988, 97.

27. Bruner, J., Foreword, in *Action, Gesture and Symbol*, Lock, A., Ed., Academic Press, New York, 1978, vii.

28. Fodor, J., *The Modularity of Mind*, MIT Press, Cambridge, MA, 1983.

29. Muma, J., Impressions: Clinical Views of Pragmatics in *Cognition, Codification, Communication, Expression,* Muma, J., Erlbaum, Hillsdale, NJ, forthcoming Appendix D..

30. Perera, K., Editorial: Child language research: Building on the past, looking to the future, *J. Child Language,* 21, 1, 1994.

31. Ingram, D., *First Language Acquisition*, Cambridge University Press, Cambridge, England, 1989.

32. Palermo, D., Theoretical issues in semantic development, in *Language Development*, Volume 1, Kuczaj, S., Ed., Erlbaum, Hillsdale, NJ, 1982.

33. Schlesinger, I., The role of cognitive development and linguistic input in language acquisition, *J. Child Language,* 4, 153, 1977.

34. Nelson, K., Event knowledge and the development of language functions, in *Research on Child Language Disorders,* Miller, J., Ed., PRO-ED, Austin, TX, 1991, 125.

35. Burger, R. and Muma, J., Cognitive distancing in mediated categorization in aphasia, *J. Psycholinguist. Res.,* 9, 355, 1980.

36. Anglin, J., *Word, Object, and Concept Development*, Norton, New York, 1977.

37. Rosch, E., Natural categories, *Cognit. Psychol.,* 4, 328, 1973.

38. Muma, J. and Muma, D., *MAP (Muma Assessment Program)*, Natural Child, Lubbock, TX, 1981.

39. Uzgiris, I. and Hunt, J., *Assessment in Infancy: Ordinal Scales of Psychological Development*, University of Illinois Press, Urbana, IL, 1975.

40. Donaldson, M., *Children's Minds*, Norton, New York, 1978.

41. Bronfenbrenner, U., Developmental research, public policy, and the ecology of childhood, *Child Dev.,* 45, 1, 1974.

42. Bronfenbrenner, U., *The Ecology of Human Development*, Harvard University Press, Cambridge, MA, 1979.

43. Greenfield, P., Going beyond information theory to explain early word choice: A reply to Roy Pea, *J. Child Language,* 7, 217, 1980.

44. Muma, J., The communication game: Dump and play, *J. Speech Hear. Disord.,* 40, 296, 1975.

45. Brown, R., *A First Language: The Early Stages*, Harvard University Press, Cambridge, MA, 1973.

46. Sigel, I. and Cocking, R., Cognition and communication: A dialectic paradigm for development, in *Interaction, Conversation, and the Development of Language*, Lewis, M. and Rosenblum, L., Eds., Wiley, New York, 1977, 207.

47. Bruner, J., The course of cognitive growth, *Am. Psychol.,* 19, 1, 1964.

48. Cazden, C., Play with language and metalinguistic awareness: One dimension of language experience, in *Dimensions of Language Experience,* Winsor, C., Ed., Agathon Press, New York, 1975.

49. Hakes, D., *The Development of Metalinguistic Abilities in Children*, Springer-Verlag, Berlin, 1980.

50. Menyuk, P., Metalinguistic abilities and language disorders, in *Research on Child Language Disorders,* Miller, J. Ed., PRO-ED, Austin, TX, 1991, 387.

51. Winner, E., New names for old things: The emergence of metaphoric language, *J. Child Language,* 6, 469, 1979.

52. vanKleek, A., Metalinguatic skills: Cutting across spoken and written language and problem-solving abilities, in *Language Learning Disabilities in School-Age Children*, Wallach, G. and Butler, K., Eds., Williams & Wilkins, Baltimore, 1984, 128.

53. Muma, J., Science and Human Affairs: Clinical Implications in *Cognition, Codification, Communication, Expression,* Muma, J., Erlbaum, Hillsdale, NJ, forthcoming Appendix B.

54. Mercer, J., The lethal label, *Psychol. Today,* 44, 1972.

55. Dunn, L. and Dunn, L., *Peabody Picture Vocabulary Test-revised*, American Guidance Service, Circle Pines, MN, 1981.

56. Muma, J., *Language Primer for the Clinical Fields*, PRO-ED, Austin, TX, 1981.

57. Brown, R., How shall a thing be called? *Psychological Review*, 65, 18, 1958.

58. Kuczaj, S. and Barrett, M., *The Development of Word Meaning*, Springer-Verlag, Berlin, 1986.

59. Messick, S., Test validity and the ethics of assessment, *Am. Psychol.*, 35, 1012, 1980.

60. Muma, J., Morales, A., Day, K., Tackett, A., Smith, S., Daniel, B., Logue, B., and Morriss, D., *Language Sampling: Repertoire and Sample Size* in *Cognition, Codification, Communication, Expression,* Muma, J., Erlbaum, Hillsdale, NJ, forthcoming Appendix E.

61. Muma, J., Experiential realism: Clinical implications, in *Pragmatics of Language: Clinical Practice Issues,* Gallagher, T., Ed., Singular Publishing Group, San Diego, CA, 1991, 229.

12

Cognitive Disorders: Diagnosis and Treatment in the TBI Patient

Mark J. Ashley and David K. Krych

CONTENTS

HISTORICAL PERSPECTIVES

Human cognition has been contemplated, in one form or another, even in the times of ancient philosophers. Great thinkers pondered man's condition and the manner in which he dealt with his situation via his mental, emotional, and spiritual faculties. Development of the field of psychology and subsequently development of subspecialty areas would later bring some refinement to the way man would reflect upon his circumstance and abilities.

In the clinical dealing with brain injury, cognition has become a focal issue. Cognitive rehabilitation, essentially nonexistent in the early 1970's, was born in the late 1970's as medical and therapeutic personnel came to recognize the sequelae of traumatic brain injury. These sequelae were unparalleled in their complexity and pervasiveness. Furthermore, traditional medical diagnoses were simply inadequate for understanding and addressing traumatic brain injury. While various brain injury diagnoses preexisted the traumatic brain injury diagnosis, they were not very useful.

As a consequence, professionals in many disciplines began to focus upon the complexities of the brain and its function. Service providers soon realized that physical restoration of motor and sensory functions often preceded restoration of "mental function". As the field developed through the 1980's and emerged into the 1990's, there also developed considerable confusion over just what cognition is and what efforts are most efficacious to enhance cognitive functioning following traumatic brain injury. Part of the confusion dealt with the meaning of cognitive terms, for example, *executive function, higher intellectual skills,* etc.

Webster's New World Dictionary of the American Language[1] classifies "cognition" as a noun and defines it as "1) the process of knowing, perceiving, etc., 2) an idea, perception, etc." The field of cognitive rehabilitation has long viewed cognition as an *entity,* though it may be better understood if seen as a *process.* Specific skill subsets of cognitive function have likewise been viewed as independent entities rather than as interrelational and componential to the process of perceiving, learning, and knowing. As a result, efforts undertaken in this field have been largely fragmented and have rarely been based upon sound theoretical constructs.

According to Tulving,[2] "Memory is made up of a number of interrelated systems, organized structures of operating components consisting of neural substrates and their behavioral and cognitive correlates". In Tulving's view, memory systems exist as organized structures of elementary operating components. He cited evolutionary influences in the development of the individual organism and the implication for ordering these developments from "lower" to "higher" systems or from less advanced to more advanced. Tulving's concept of a "memory system" required that intervention at any level in the system would necessarily affect all learning and memory functions that depend upon the system as a whole. Interventions, therefore, should respect the premises of evolutionary order and usefulness as well as the premise that impairments observed constituted elements of a process rather than individual entity impairments, which cannot be dealt with independently of one another.

Neuroscientist Vernon Mountcastle[3] said, "I frequently use the word 'minding' as a verb rather than 'the mind' as a separate entity." Similarly, memory is often viewed as an entity with qualifiers placed to segregate short-term from long-term, visual from auditory, etc. Historically, *memory* has often been placed structurally within the brain in the region of the hippocampus. The immediate question which comes to mind, however, is, "Which memory?". We do not tend to view motor function as a memory, or sensory function as a memory, yet the neural structures controlling motor or sensory function probably operate quite similarly to the neural structures responsible for auditory or any other type of memory. That is to say, the basic parameters regulating neuronal firing and communication from one neuron to another can be presumed to be much the same though different neurotransmitter, neuropeptide, and amino acid substances may be involved in actual synaptic transmission. Perhaps *memory,* like Mountcastle's *mind,* should be viewed as *remembering.*

Memory is perhaps the most recognizable cognitive construct and, at the same time, the most elusive rehabilitation goal. This chapter will attempt to explain the comparative elusiveness of *memory* by demonstrating the componential cognitive processes involved in not only *remembering* but other cognitive processes as well. We will attempt to deal with cognition as it relates to the ability to mentally represent, organize, and manipulate one's environment. Consistent with this broad definition, one must recognize the impact of all neural systems on cognition. In order to achieve a mental representation of one's environment and one's experience with that environment, neural structures which deal with all sensory and motor modalities must input, albeit differentially, to the representational process.

Literature in related disciplines of psychology, cognitive psychology, child language development, psycholinguistics, and anatomical/physiological research contains a great deal of information from which one can derive a sound theoretical basis to approach cognition. The literature review contained herein is taken from these disciplines, and an attempt is made first to develop a theoretical construct supportive of cognition as a process vs. cognition as an entity. Therapeutic applications based upon the theoretical construct for cognition are then explored.

FUNCTION FOLLOWS FORM

Just as there appears to be merit in the field of physical therapy to respect developmental concepts in neurodevelopmental therapy (NDT),[4-6] it is also important to understand and respect the impact of these principles on cognitive development and rehabilitative efforts to be undertaken following traumatic brain injury. The basic developmental sequences provide a guide as to which skills should be present and when. These developmental guidelines also help the service provider to understand which skills, when absent, should be reestablished and in what order. Tulving[2] states, "Different systems have emerged at different stages in the evolution of the species, and they emerge at different stages in the development of the individual organism."

While the purpose of this chapter is not to review neurologic ontogeny or phylogeny in detail, it is useful, nonetheless, to understand some basics regarding evolution of the nervous system. The idea that ontogeny or natal development is the recapitulation of phylogeny or evolutionary development is not a new concept. While the concept was initially taken quite literally and considerable controversy arose, the concept is more widely accepted today as a general principle by which ontogenic milestones can be predicted. Likewise, postnatal development can frequently be seen to mirror ontogenetic development. Meader and Muyskens[7] indicated that newly arising and more complex structures and functions incorporated earlier structures and their functions and retained their characteristics. Meader and Muyskens's comments bear considerable similarity to those of Tulving[2] pertaining to the ordering of developments in memory from lower to higher systems. It is generally accepted that the brainstem, cerebellum, and structures composing the limbic system are the oldest structures of the brain, phylogenetically. The telencephalon, by contrast, is a relatively new addition. As the human central nervous system (CNS) has evolved, new structures have been developed and new functions or skills have been overlaid on older ones.

Embryologic development is such that the telencephalon is among the last structures to develop and mature. The pallium or forebrain is derived from a rostral continuation of the ventral thalamus and subthalamic matrix, as suggested by embryologic development of the cerebral vesicles.[8] "Throughout phylogeny, the thalamus has few descending fibers; its efferent discharge is almost entirely projected into the forebrain; neither structure functions completely independently of the other, particularly in higher mammals."[9] These matters will bear greater significance as we examine known information about anatomical substrates of attentional processes.

Myelination of the neural structures can be seen to follow a specific pattern which roughly parallels embryological development of neural structures. Figure 12.1 shows the myelogenetic fields of Flechsig.[10] It is interesting to note the parallels between myelination progression (Figure 12.1) and the organization of the cortical structures as proposed by Luria (Figure 12.2).[11] As can be seen in Figure 12.1, considerable similarity exists between the earliest maturing myelin fields and the "primary" areas proposed by Luria. Likewise, there is a fair degree of overlap between the intermediate myelin fields and the secondary Lurian areas. Of course, both the primordial myelin fields and Luria's primary areas correlate with the known primary areas of the brain, those responsible for vision, audition, tactile sensation, and motor movement.

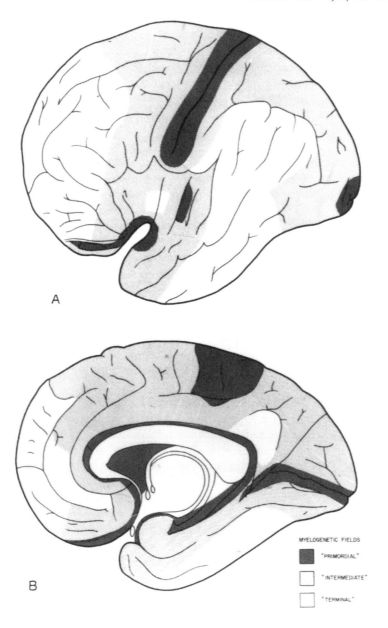

MYELOGENETIC FIELDS

■ "PRIMORDIAL"

□ "INTERMEDIATE"

□ "TERMINAL"

FIGURE 12.1 The myelogenetic fields of Flechsig, modified from Yakovlev (1962) to demonstrate "primordial", "intermediate", and "terminal" fields. Primordial fields show stainable myelin before or at term. Intermediate fields myelinate at 6–12 weeks. Terminal fields myelinate after the fourth postnatal month. (A) Lateral surface, (B) medial surface. (Reprinted with permission from *An Introduction to the Neurosciences* (p. 461) by B. A. Curtis, S. Jacobson, and E. M. Marcus. Copyright 1972 by W. B. Saunders Company.)

It is not possible, nor desirable, to fully enumerate the phylogenesis or ontogenesis of the human central nervous system in these pages. It is enough to understand that function must logically follow form and that the form has been achieved in a progressive manner. Consequently, a specific function must be viewed in concert with its developmental acquisition. We know it is pointless to attempt to teach a four-month-old infant to ambulate bipedally because prerequisite motor skills to be acquired through crawling, tall-kneeling, etc., have not been fully mastered at that age. A similar case might be made for cognitive processes.

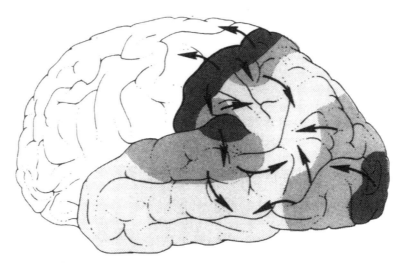

A The sensory unit

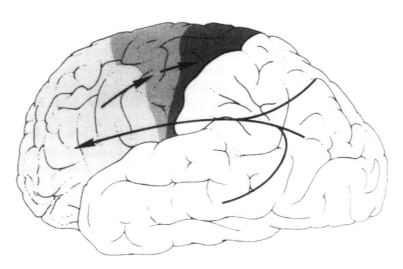

B The motor unit

FIGURE 12.2 (A) The first functional unit of the cortex — the sensory unit. (Dark-shaded areas are primary zones; medium shaded, secondary zones; light shaded, tertiary zones.) Sensory input travels from primary to secondary to tertiary and is thereby elaborated from sensation into symbolic processes. (B) The second functional unit of the cortex — the motor unit. Symbolic processes from the sensory unit are translated into intentions in the tertiary motor zones and then into patterns of action in the secondary and primary motor zones. (Reprinted with permission from *The Working Brain* by A. R. Luria. Copyright 1973 by Penguin Publishers.)

Neuroanatomical Review

We will next focus on sensory processes and their neural substrates to review these systems and their interconnections. Tactile sensory experience with the environment is registered primarily through three pathways. The three pathways (Table 12.1) are described as they relate

TABLE 12.1   Tactile Pathways

Pathway	Termination	Sensation
Lateral spinothalamic tract	Post-central gyrus	Pain and temperature
Dorsal column-medial lemniscal pathway	Post-central gyrus	Conscious proprioception and discriminative touch
Anterior spinothalamic tract	Post-central gyrus	Simple touch
Ventral and dorsal spinocerebellar tracts	Cerebellum	Unconscious proprioception

to the various types of stimuli for which they are responsible. The spinal cord organization of these pathways is of lesser interest to us in this discussion, while the confluence of these pathways upon various nuclei of the thalamus is of primary importance. The *lateral spinothalamic tract* (responsible for pain and temperature) projects to the ventral posterior nucleus of the thalamus, prior to continuation via thalamocortical fibers in the posterior limb of the internal capsule to the postcentral gyrus of the frontal lobe. Collateral fibers from the spinothalamic tract are given off at several levels within the neuraxis and, of particular interest, collaterals in the brain stem synapse with neurons contained in the reticular formation. The *dorsal column-medial lemniscal pathway* (responsible for conscious proprioception and discriminative touch) also projects to the ventral posterior nucleus of the thalamus, continuing via the thalamocortical fibers in the posterior limb of the internal capsule to the postcentral gyrus of the frontal lobe. The dorsal column also includes fibers composing the *anterior spinothalamic tract* (responsible for perception of simple touch). The fibers of the anterior spinothalamic tract follow essentially the same course as the medial lemniscal fibers above the level of the brainstem. The third pathway responsible for tactile sensation of the environment is composed of the *ventral and dorsal spinocerebellar tracts* (responsible for unconscious proprioception). These tracts, however, terminate at the level of the cerebellum.

Sensory pathways for visual stimuli travel from the retina through the optic canal as the optic nerve. The optic nerves join in the optic chiasm and continue through the optic tracts to the lateral geniculate nuclei of the thalamus. The visual pathway continues from the lateral geniculate nuclei through the optic radiations known as the *geniculocalcarine tract* and terminate in the calcarine fissure of the occipital lobe.

Sensory pathways for auditory stimuli leave the dorsal and ventral cochlear nuclei of the pons and project to the medial geniculate bodies of the thalamus. They continue to the auditory cortex of the temporal lobes bilaterally. Vestibular pathways of the eighth cranial nerve synapse on the superior, medial, lateral, and inferior vestibular nuclei in the upper medulla and lower pons. Information is then projected to the spinal cord, cerebellum, reticular formation, and nuclei of cranial nerves III, IV, and VI via the medial longitudinal fasciculus.

Olfactory stimuli enter the CNS at a supratentorial level, as do visual stimuli. Fibers project to the rhinencephalon, an area at the base of the brain. Projections course to the piriform area of the medial temporal lobe, the anterior perforated substance and terminal gyri of the medial basal frontal lobe, and the anterior uncus on the medial surface of the temporal lobe. There are also connections with the amygdala and the hippocampal gyrus.

Reticular Formation

The ascending projectional system consists of fibers arising from the reticular formation. Pathways which provide afferent input to the reticular formation include collateral branches from the spinothalamic and lemniscal pathways, and fibers from the cortex descending via the corticoreticular fibers. These fibers arise from widespread cortical areas as well as from collateral branches of the corticospinal and corticobulbar tracts. Afferents are also received from the cerebellum, basal ganglia, hypothalamus, cranial nerve nuclei, and the colliculi.

The projections from the reticular formation project directly to the hypothalamus and the nonspecific nuclei of the thalamus. There are no specific tracts which carry these projection fibers to the hypothalamus and thalamus. Instead, the fibers are found through the brainstem and diencephalon. Additional projections from the reticular formation form the descending reticulospinal fibers.[12]

The hippocampus is widely regarded as critical for memory encoding. As structures of the limbic system, the hippocampal gyri are critical for encoding recent memory. The hippocampus has been shown in primates to receive afferent inputs from the association areas of the cerebral cortex. These include the parietal cortex which processes spatial information, the temporal lobe visual and auditory areas, and the frontal cortex.[13] An interesting loop is formed as fibers project to the anterior nuclei of the hippocampus from the entorhinal cortex, project from there to the cingulate gyrus, and then return to the entorhinal cortex.[14]

The hippocampal projections have been shown in the squirrel monkey to project to the amygdala, the septum, the fornix, the thalamus, the mammillary bodies, the medial preoptic area, and the perifornical nucleus of the hypothalamus. Willis and Grossman[14] state, "Activity in the hippocampus can reach widely distributed regions of the brain rather directly." The hippocampus has been demonstrated to be largely excitatory to other structures in primates.[15] The anterior hippocampus exerts a direct effect on most of the nuclei of the amygdala and is thought, therefore, to modulate functions associated with the amygdala.[16] Its effect is excitatory via the amygdala, inhibitory via the fornix, and both excitatory and inhibitory on the ventromedial nucleus of the hypothalamus. The amygdala is involved in feeling and expressive states associated with self-preservation, such as the search for food, feeding, fighting, and self-protection.[17] The anterior hippocampus projects, via the amygdala, to the hypothalamus and the basal forebrain. Anterior hippocampal projections via the fornix connect to the preoptic area. The posterior hippocampus projects, via the fornix, to the basal forebrain, preoptic area, and the hypothalamus. Lastly, the hippocampal gyri project to each other via the hippocampal commissure.

There appear to be two different types of cells within the hippocampus, at least on the basis of electrophysiological studies. Complex spike cells appear to be activated by voluntary movement, whereas theta cells are activated by novel stimuli.[18] The hippocampus is repeatedly implicated for its impact on attentional processes. Anterograde amnesia results from damage to the hippocampus or to the ventromedial nucleus of the thalamus in humans.[19,20]

Hypothalamus, Thalamus, and Basal Ganglia

The hypothalamus acts as the major integrator of visceral afferents. It receives projections from the cerebral cortex, thalamus, rhinencephalon, and reticular formation and is responsible for regulation of reflex responses of the visceral and endocrine systems.

Having reviewed the major sensory system afferent pathways, we can now move to subcortical structures to review their relative roles in sensory information management and relay. The pathways reviewed, thus far, are systems which relay to specific thalamic nuclei and act more directly upon the sensory cortex via thalamic nuclei. The reticular formation, however, acts indirectly to provide sensory input to the cortex via the nonspecific thalamic nuclei. The nonspecific thalamic nuclei project to all areas of the cortex, as opposed to sensory cortex, as in the case of projections arising from specific thalamic nuclei. This system is known as the *ascending projectional system.*

Diffuse thalamocortical projections are present from the nonspecific nuclei of the thalamus to widespread cortical areas. The thalamocortical pathways of the thalamic-specific nuclei project primarily to sensory cortex.

The basal ganglia (caudate nucleus, putamen, and globus pallidus) provide for anatomic loops which act chiefly as control circuits for information related to organization and execution of movement,[21] though there is speculation that the basal ganglia may organize information from the limbic system as well.

Commissural and Association Tract Fibers

Next, the means by which information is moved from one cerebral area to another must be examined. This is accomplished by projectional fibers which link subcortical to cortical areas. These fibers constitute the *internal capsule*. Fibers of the internal capsule carry information both toward and away from the cortex. Axons of the internal capsule spreading out to all areas of the cortex are known as the *corona radiata*. Fibers from the thalamus projecting to the cortex travel in the internal capsule. Projections from the anterior and medial thalamic nuclei carry visceral and other information and project to the frontal lobe via the anterior limb of the internal capsule. Projections from the ventral anterior and ventral lateral nuclei of the thalamus travel in the genu and posterior limb of the internal capsule and reach the motor and premotor areas of the frontal lobes. Fibers from the ventral posterior and medial thalamic nuclei travel via the posterior limb of the internal capsule and reach sensory cortex in the parietal lobes. Optic radiations and auditory information project via the posterior limb of the internal capsule.

Commissural fibers allow connections between the two hemispheres. The corpus callosum carries a great deal of information; however, two smaller commissural bundles exist. The anterior commissure connects anterior temporal areas, and the hippocampal commissure interconnects the hippocampal areas of both hemispheres.

Finally, association fibers allow intrahemispheric interconnection. The uncinate fasciculus joins the temporal and frontal lobes. The cingulum interconnects medial surfaces of the frontal, temporal, and parietal lobes. The cingulum connects the cingulate gyrus to the orbitofrontal cortex and the hippocampal cortex. It also carries projectional fibers from the thalamus.[12] Shorter association fibers which connect adjacent gyri are known as *arcuate fibers*.

Neurophysiological Principles

We shall see in later sections of this chapter how this brief review of neural structures will become important to the study of cognition. However, prior to moving into discussions of cognitive function, some basic neurophysiological information should be reviewed. This order of presentation is quite different from the order of our acquisition of information. Psychologists and others have been studying cognition, or components thereof, via psychological experimentation for some time. Tremendous insight into the probable cellular mechanisms underlying information processing through these methods has been gained. But only recently have we begun to be able to uncover some of the actual cellular and synaptical phenomena which serve information processing. This is all very interesting when one stops to consider the hypotheses of early scientists who theorized that learning and memory involved reverberating circuits.[22] In fact, psychological experimentation for memory for verbal material continues to focus on the concept of a neural trace.

Neurotransmission

At a cellular level, it has been demonstrated that different types of memory formation place different demands on the cellular mechanisms for protein synthesis. Protein synthesis occurs within the nucleus of the neuron in direct response to learning. Protein synthesis does not occur, though, for all types of memory. Short-term memory does not require protein synthesis. "All of the proteins, including receptors, ion channels, enzymes, and transporters, required for short-term memory formation and temporary storage are already present in sufficient abundance. In sharp contrast, however, long-term memory absolutely depends on the synthesis of new proteins or the increased synthesis of already existing proteins."[23]

When neuronal activation occurs, it leads to synaptic activation and transmission. Neuroscientists have long suspected that synaptic transmission caused changes to occur within the nucleus, axon, dendrite, and/or synapse itself to either encourage or discourage subsequent synaptic transmissions. The evolution of understanding of long-term potentiation (LTP) has allowed for an improved understanding of this phenomenon.[24] LTP is triggered when a neuron receives several simultaneous signals, and that LTP "strengthens" a synapse. In addition to LTP, two other forms of potentiation have been identified. Posttetanic potentiation (PTP) has been observed to last for a minute or less. Short-term potentiation (STP) lasts somewhat longer than PTP, and both PTP and STP can involve increases in the number of quanta released or the strength of their postsynaptic effect, or both.[25]

It appears as though LTP has an inhibitory counterpart, known as long-term depression (LTD). LTD, a decrease in synaptic responsivity which is activity dependent, has been recently demonstrated to be induced postsynaptically, and it is possible that LTD may require the production of a retrograde messenger as well.[26] Both LTP and LTD are viewed as cellular mechanisms involved in learning and memory.

The findings of Schubert[27] relating to the release of glycoproteins into the synaptic cleft, reduction of the synaptic cleft, and broadening of the axonal and dendritic end-plates allow for an understanding of some physiological changes underlying learning. Glycoproteins serve to bind the synaptic end-plates together. As the size of the synaptic cleft is reduced, neurotransmitters have less distance to travel. Likewise, the broadening and flattening of the end-plates expose the synaptic vesicles, allowing more rapid release and uptake of neurotransmitters from the synapse.

Neurons are organized within the CNS in a manner such that adjacent columns of cells tend to serve similar functions. In fact, activation of a single neuron can be observed to increase electrical activity in adjacent cells and actually cause a focal neuronal LTP response. Most recently, this widespread effect of LTP on adjacent cells[28] was brought into clearer view when the role of nitric oxide and carbon dioxide were hypothesized to act as retrograde messengers in neurotransmission.[29]

The effects of nitric oxide release are not restricted to a single synapse. Nitric oxide release can be experienced by closely adjacent, activated synapses as well,[28] thus the realization that neurons do not necessarily function as a single unit; rather, that aggregate groups of neurons probably function together.[30] Nitric oxide is understood to be relatively short-acting, thereby limiting its geographic sphere of influence and duration of activation.

Nitric oxide has been demonstrated to exert an effect on working vs. reference memory only in rat hippocampal studies.[31,32] Similar findings were reported by these authors for changes occurring following cerebral ischemia. In these studies, working memory is roughly the equivalent of short-term memory, whereas reference memory is an approximate equivalent to long-term memory.

Neurotransmission and Learning

A difference exists, from a neurophysiological perspective, between simple neural activation and neural activity associated with learning. Underlying neural activation associated with learning is a process known as *reactive synaptogenesis*. Synaptogenesis, which refers to new dendritic spine formation at synapses following repeated neurotransmission, appears to be a significant neurophysiological underpinning for learning. The process of synaptogenesis is fairly rapid. In fact, the discovery of at least one retrograde messenger, nitric oxide, that can operate rapidly to mediate both pre- and postsynaptic changes, aids considerably in a formulation of synaptogenesis as a neural substrate to learning. It is now known that reactive synaptogenesis occurs very rapidly in the CNS.[33] Studies in this area have shown that reactive synaptogenesis occurs within 10–15 minutes. The changes may have occurred earlier; however, the researchers only evaluated for the changes within the 10–15 minute time frame. Synaptogenesis has been found to occur only during learning and not during neural activity where no learning was evident.[34,35]

In order for synaptogenesis to occur, not only must learning occur, but there must be appropriate support available from glial cells, specifically astrocytes,[36] and blood supply[34] in the affected region.

Anatomical Substrates of Attentional Function

Experimentation that has been reviewed thus far indicates that synaptogenesis is a dynamic event and, together with LTP, one that occurs on a focal neuronal basis as opposed to a single-cell basis. Neural activity alone, without learning, does not result in synaptogenesis. Sensory input pathways have been reviewed as well as extensive interconnections which exist at multiple levels on the neuraxes. Constant sensory input occurs, and access to higher cortical structures is regulated by the thalamic nuclei acting in concert with cortical neurons. Thus, the focus can be turned to cognitive psychology and psycholinguistic literatures as an attempt to translate this information into experientially based terms.

Specific structures and their relative contributions to certain cognitive functions can now be examined. Included in these structures are the reticular formation, the thalamus and its cortical projections, and cortical structures (Figure 12.3).

The basic premise which has been presented is that the subcortical and cortical organization of the brain predisposes the system to its function. The sensory end-organs, brainstem, thalamus, thalamic projections, and intercerebral and intracerebral commissural and association tracts constitute the anatomical basis of attentional processes. Trexler and Zappala[37] provide a review of three neuroanatomical systems which regulate attentional processes. They indicate that the systems are hierarchically integrated and highly interdependent.

Attentional functions associated with the brainstem are tonic arousal of the telencephalon. Posner[38] pointed to the superior colliculus as responsible for covert orientation of attention to visual space in humans. Denny-Brown and Fischer[39] and Goldberg and Wurtz[40] also provided insight into the role of the midbrain in orientation of attention. Gummow et al.[41] cited the role of both the diffusely organized thalamic nuclei and the mesencephalic reticular formation in the maintenance of arousal level, and Brown[42] demonstrated that lesions of nonspecifically organized thalamic nuclei produced attentional losses. These nuclei were shown earlier to receive projections from the mesencephalic reticular formation by Scheibel and Scheibel[43] and, as was earlier noted, to send projections to widespread cortical areas. Disorders associated with the brainstem may result in loss of consciousness or coma.

Controlled or selective attentional processes are thought to be controlled by thalamic projections, specifically, the thalamofrontal gating system. Phasic activation of the cerebral cortex, in particular the associative cortex, is brought about through the diffuse thalamic projection system. Disturbances of the diffuse thalamic projection system may result in "distractibility", while impairments of the thalamofrontal gating system may produce increased difficulty with interference and problems with integrational behaviors such as judgment, planning, and social-communicative appropriateness.[37]

"By facilitating or inhibiting transmission of neural impulses through sensory pathways, the consciousness system enhances or attenuates responses to incoming stimuli, directing attention to a specific input while other incoming signals are suppressed. Electrical activity reaching the cortex via specific sensory pathways is not perceived unless it is followed by activity via the diffuse projection paths".[12] The stimuli to receive attention are selected and other, competing stimuli are attenuated until such time as their characteristics are changed in some fashion so as to cause a shift in directed attention.

Goodglass and Kaplan[44] indicated that the neocortex was involved in response selection based upon cognitive or semantic dimensions. Eidelberg and Schwartz,[45] Näätänen,[46] Watson

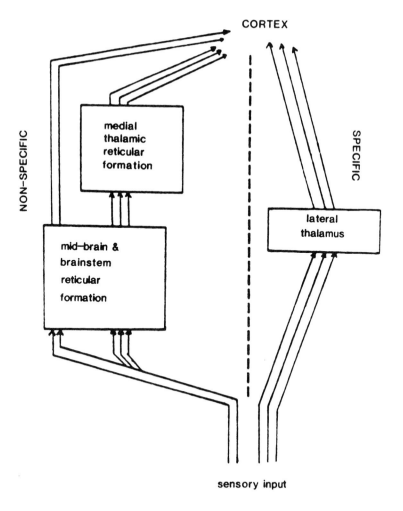

FIGURE 12.3 Specific and nonspecific activation systems. (Reprinted with permission from "Neuropathological determinants of acquired attention disorders in traumatic brain injury" by L. E. Trexler and G. Zappala, *Brain Cognit.*, 8, 293. Copyright 1988 by Academic Press, Inc.)

et al.,[47] and Heilman and Valenstein[48] have demonstrated the role of the frontal, posterior parietal, and cingular cortices in attentional processing. Goff[49] and Vaughan and Ritter[50] suggested that vertex responses of EEG were heavily dependent upon activity in the association cortex. Mesulam and Geschwind[51] held that the most advanced portions of association cortex were involved in attention. They demonstrated that these same regions have direct projections to limbic structures responsible for modulation of emotional and motivational behavior, making an interesting neural connection between attention, emotion, and motivation. The authors contend that many disorders of attention and emotion, perhaps even schizophrenia, may be conceptualized in terms of disruption of fibers connecting the neocortex and limbic structures. Clearly, from a clinical perspective, emotionally charged experience seems to be more readily retained in some form as compared to nonemotionally charged experience. The circuitous connections which link the cerebral cortex, the limbic system, and the corpus striatum as well[21] may allow for the overall fluidity of attentional processes.

Thompson and Bettinger[52] proposed a hypothesis relating cellular activity in the association areas of the cortex to attention. They suggested that, since there is increased cell activity in the association cortex during novel stimulation, the number of cells of the nonspecific association system available to be activated by another stimulus was decreased in proportion to the increase in ongoing cellular activity resulting from the first novel stimulus. Posner and

Snyder[53] showed that subjects who begin to attend to a signal by use of the limited-capacity conscious mechanism showed facilitation of specific pathways but also evidenced inhibited processing of other signals. These data support the concept that deliberate or conscious processing could be accompanied by widespread inhibitory consequences for other stimuli. In fact, Kahneman[54] noted a decrement in the detectability of new stimuli during conscious processing.

Conscious direction of attention occurs in conjunction with specific changes in the autonomic nervous system. Kahneman[55] noted substantial autonomic nervous system changes, including changes in heart rate, vascular dilation, pupil size, and galvanic skin response during directed orientation of attention. Initially, the system seems to be a reflexive one which allows for the input of specific stimuli by the organism in a selective fashion. Attentional processes may later become inhibited and used selectively or incorporated as a part of a more complex attentional function. Such a sequence would mirror the sequence of motor reflexes and their subsequent inhibition and incorporation into more sophisticated motor movements. Clearly, there exists, in the developmental literature, information about perceptual fixation, which is thought to be used by a child to limit attentional focus to a specific perceptual attribute. This matter will be more fully expanded upon later in this chapter. Once again, however, the influence of lower brain systems can be seen in the autonomic nervous system responses during initial orientation. The thalamic structures and cortical association areas differ in regional responsivity during various attentional processes.

ATTENTION

Anderson[56] states: "Attention is a very limited mental resource that can only be allocated, at most, to a few cognitive processes at a time. The more frequently that processes have been practiced, the less attention they require; eventually, they can be performed without interfering with other cognitive processes. …Processes that are highly practiced and require little or no attention are referred to as *automatic*. Processes that require attention are called *deliberate*." Anderson indicated, after review of visual and auditory report task studies, that automatic processes seemed to be completed without subject control. These studies indicated that registration of sensory stimuli appeared to be an automatic process. Likewise, comprehension of language and even many aspects of operating an automobile appear to be automatic. By contrast, deliberate processing seemed to require conscious control of the subject. Tasks requiring such deliberate conscious control would include many higher cognitive processes, such as performing mental arithmetic.

Anderson[56] provides a useful schema for reviewing the initial phases of attention. He states: "When information first enters the human system, it is registered in sensory memories. These sensory memories include an *iconic* memory for visual information and an *echoic* memory for auditory information." Recognition of brief visual memory store as an icon was done initially by Neisser.[57] Moray et al.[58] and Darwin et al.[59] provided evidence for a brief auditory sensory store mechanism which Neisser later called echoic memory.

Sensory memories can store a great deal of information but only for brief periods of time. This visual store was first demonstrated by Spurling.[60] Information is initially stored for very brief periods of time (less than 60 seconds) in iconic and echoic store mechanisms. Information which is retained beyond this time period is thought to have been processed and integrated into other memory structures or other cognitive processes. Note the similarity between these concepts and those of PTP, STP, and LTP.

Apparently, the role of a sensory store mechanism is to store information briefly so it can be processed by a higher level mental routine. It is interesting to note that the sensory store mechanism is particularly vulnerable to "wash out". That is to say, incoming information can rapidly override previously stored information. This would suggest that this brief sensory store is of sufficiently limited capacity as to disallow retention of much information.

Treisman,[61] following dichotic listening studies, held that it was apparent that large amounts of information were screened in dichotic listening tasks. Information was retained seemingly on the basis of specific features which were selected by the listener. Thus, while large amounts of information enter sensory stores, only selected information is actually retained. We will examine next the nature of these specific features used for selection.

FEATURE IDENTIFICATION

Sokovlov[62] studied autonomic nervous system and EEG changes observed following novel stimulus presentation and subsequent habituation to stimuli. In this work, Sokovlov found that the slightest change in the perceptual characteristics of the stimulus following habituation would be made manifest in changes in autonomic nervous system and EEG reactions. This phenomenon is behaviorally observable in infants, toddlers, and young children.

Olson[63] proposed that the human system was inherently designed to give priority to certain types of perceptual cues over others. Olson attributed this, presumably, to evolutionary usefulness. Rosch[64] provided some evidence of the impact of perceptual cues and found that certain classification schema ("natural categories") were basically universal to persons of different languages and cultures, thereby supporting the concept of physiological predisposition.

Certainly, that sensory systems should respond to environmental information is not a new concept. Environmental information must be experienced in a manner that is compatible with the physiology of the attending organism; otherwise, the information cannot be processed at all. The visual system provides for specific variables to be attended to, while different sensory systems, i.e., touch, hearing, or smell, allow yet other variables to be dealt with. These variables have been referred to as *perceptual attributes,* and they are both physiologically and, to a lesser degree, experientially dependent.

Cortical representation during the initial stages of information processing will now be considered. Voss[65] refers to encoding for memory as the "process by which certain aspects or features of the stimulus event are employed in establishing the internal representation of the event." These features are termed by Voss as *attributes*. The attributes are used, together with information contained in the external and internal context of the event, for encoding purposes. *External context* refers to the contextual events which may be encoded with or as a part of a stimulus, while the *internal context* refers to other encodings which occur with or as part of the encoding of the stimulus. Virtually every object and concept that is encountered has features associated with it.[64,66] These features or characteristics can be simply defined by many common terms such as color, size, weight, shape, construction, texture, or function. The actual complexity of available characteristics, however, cannot be understood with such a simplistic representation. In fact, every adjective and adverb of a language represents a potential feature. Additionally, nouns, verbs, and prepositions can represent features. Each decision made in a day is made on the basis of pertinent featural attributes. How these important characteristics enter into decision making will be reviewed, but, first, more discussion of features is necessary.

Features fall into essentially two classifications. *Iconic* features are those attributes which are descriptive of a physical characteristic. These would include color, size, weight, shape, etc. *Symbolic* features relate to functional characteristics. The iconic features of a chair might be "made of wood, 42 inches high, a rectangular seat and back, four legs, and brown." The most obvious symbolic feature of a chair is that it is used to sit upon.

Attributes are more or less readily described from terms common to us in discussion of perceptual domains. A simplified representation might be iconic attributes such as color or size in a visual domain or intensity and pitch in an auditory domain. More complex representation may be obtained by combinations of simpler attributes. To make the obvious extension, our language is replete with opportunities for simple and complex representation. Experiential representation of a classroom lecture might be undertaken by utilization of the available, though probably the most salient, attributes assignable to the lecture. The lecture may be described by or associated with the following attributes: boring, interesting, difficult to understand, new information, old information, cold room, uncomfortable seating, unusual dress of the lecturer, etc. — in addition to subject matter.

The most salient attributes are utilized individually and in relation with one another to compose a representation of the experience. Each attribute, and only those attributes used for input, can then function as an attribute by which the information can be recalled, since research has demonstrated that information to be used in retrieval must already be stored at the time of output.[67,68] This information, however, is converted into mental representation; thus, input attributes become purged.

Long-term retention and recall appear to be impacted by the attributes which are encoded at the time of stimulus presentation. Long-term retention is also viewed as dependent upon the integrity of the organizational structure developed at the time of acquisition.[69,70]

Manipulation of iconic features may alter the symbolic status of an object. Continuing with the example of the chair above, the function of the chair can be changed from an object which is used to sit upon to one of an object which is used to attain height (a ladder). The iconic feature pertaining to the height of the seat of the chair is what allows the transformation from *chair* to *ladder*. Other characteristics which would enter into a featural assay allowing transformation from *chair* to *ladder* might include the construction of the seat (solid vs. webbed vs. cushion), the stability of the chair (solid vs. rickety), and the number of legs on the chair (four legs vs. three).

An individual may engage in problem solving to the extent to which he/she accurately and completely reviews features encompassing a given circumstance and uses those features to find a solution to a particular problem. In the example above, in order to obtain a *ladder*, one must be able to call upon a memory of a chair being used as a ladder, or one must be able to intentionally and discriminately direct attention to the appropriate set of features which allows the transformation of function from *chair* to *ladder*.

The potential influence of attentional deficits during this process may be considerable. Any interruption of the assay process might well interfere with a successful solution for a particular problem. A creative solution to a problem might well be dependent upon the individual's ability to move freely amongst available features or their representations.

A phenomenon in feature identification called *perceptual salience* has been observed by such authors as Odom and Corbin,[71] Odom,[72] Odom and Guzman,[73,74] and Caron.[75] Perceptual salience has been described as an inordinate focus on a perceptual domain such as color, shape, position, size, etc., to the exclusion of information in other available perceptual domains. This phenomenon is observed regularly, for example, with preschool and early school-age children who show a strong orientation to a specific perceptual attribute (iconic feature). This orientation can be so strong as to interfere with other cognitive processing. It is thought that perceptual salience provides a means by which the developing child can acquire knowledge about the environment and develop conceptual awareness. Perceptual salience seems to act as a natural means of limiting attention until concept development is attained.

There is evidence for the existence of a developmental process in perceptual salience such that, in time, the individual gains selective control over perceptual processes. Odom and Guzman[73] studied variability and constancy in preschool and older children and found that preschool-age children were more perceptually salient for variability than for constancy. They also found that older children showed no differential sensitivity between variability and constancy. Saltz and Sigel[76] found that six-year-olds made more overdiscrimination errors than older subjects. The feature differences which were irrelevant and led to judgment errors were found to be more salient for the younger children than were the task-relevant invariants. In other studies, Kagan[77,78] found that reflectivity increased and impulsivity decreased with age.

The phenomenon of perceptual salience and the natural changes which can be observed therein correlate with changes in age and with neural pathway changes occurring in the maturing central nervous system. Thus, following the motor skills analogy, a reflexive tendency toward variability may be inhibited to gain mastery of the ability as a directable skill.

An individual's perseveration on a particular piece of clothing or failure to complete a task properly may well be explained by perceptual salience. Wayland and Taplin[79] argue that performance of brain-injured subjects on recognition memory tasks evidenced difficulty in processing featural information. The pattern of results observed suggested major difficulties in responding to complex, multidimensional stimuli. The most common response was to base decisions about category membership according to one salient feature. The relation of perceptual features to categorization will now be examined.

CATEGORIZATION

Features, then, have much to do with the likelihood that information will be processed and with the manner in which information is stored. These attributes readily become categorical descripters and, as such, heavily influence the long-term storage of information. From the very earliest developmental stages, learning is guided by the ability to recognize similarities and differences. Learning is affected by experiential sophistication and the ability to recognize subtle vs. gross differences. In order to adequately handle large amounts of information from the environment, information is grouped or clustered so that it can be handled efficiently. Tyler[80] indicates that classification allows for infinite variabilities to be shrunk to manipulable size. Bruner et al.[81] felt that nearly all cognitive ability involved, and was dependent upon, the process of categorization. The integration of iconic or symbolic similarities among objects and the development and importance of categorization is emphasized by Bowerman.[82] These are crucial to the transfer of information from attentional stores to subsequent longer term storage and use of that information.

Clark and Clark[83] state: "In dealing with the world, people have a system for classifying objects into categories. The system makes these classifications on the basis of salient attributes like shape, size, function, and activity. ...The systems for classifying and for naming are not really distinct."

A featural approach to category naming was developed by Rosch,[64,66] as well as by Rosch and Mervis,[84] Rosch et al.,[85] Smith et al.,[86] Rips,[87] and Shoben.[88] These individuals studied categorical internal structures that were not captured in hierarchical analysis that had preceded their work, as put forth by Collins and Quillian.[89,90]

The featural approach introduced the idea of *typicality* of category membership. The concept of typicality suggested that, for many common categories, there was a prototype which was highly typical of a category. Additionally, there were category members which were less typical, or actually atypical, of the category though they belonged in that category. Clark and Clark[83] stated that "typicality is critical in the process of comprehending category names." Of course, typicality is dependent upon the features defining categorical inclusion/ exclusion. An object which is typical of a particular category can be viewed as having a group of features which are characteristic of the category and represent the category. These features may or may not be critical to actual inclusion in the category, however.

Typicality was studied further by Rips et al.[91] and Rosch,[64] who showed that the more typical the member was of a category, the more quickly it was judged to be a member of that category. Thus, verification time was introduced to the concept of category inclusion or exclusion. According to Smith et al.[92] categories have both defining features and characteristic features which probably impact verification time. *Defining features* were those features required of an item to be included in the category. *Characteristic features* were those most commonly seen but not necessarily properties of all members of the category. They are instead so common that they are felt to be characteristic of the category.

The effects of categorization complexity have been explored through reaction-time studies. Differing times for determination of categorical inclusion have been evidenced, reflecting differences in access to categorical information and differences in categorical complexity.[88] Thus, processing time and word finding may well be affected by deficits in attentional, perceptual feature, and/or categorizational skills.

Bowleska[93] argues that naming is an act of categorization and, as such, is not a speech mechanism disturbance. She believes that word finding problems among aphasic patients should be viewed as concept formation disturbances.

It is quite apparent, then, that categorization is both impacted by and impacts upon the perception of the world. In a study conducted by Glucksberg and Wiseberg,[94] the impact of labeling on problem-solving capabilities was shown. Their findings indicated that, when persons attempted problem solving with objects which were labeled, speed of problem solving was improved over the same problem-solving task with unlabeled objects. It was felt that the labeling of the objects encouraged the problem solver to view the objects as separate and distinct entities, allowing more rapid manipulation of the objects for the problem-solving task. It can be seen that the role of labeling or categorization is substantial and may impact performance in problem solving, word retrieval, and processing speed.

Much work has been done in defining categorizational processes. It may be useful to review the manner in which categorization skills emerge. Developmentally, the acquisition sequence for categorization skills is as follows: 1) piling, 2) keychaining, 3) iconic categorization, 4) symbolic categorization.[95]

Piling is characterized by simple grouping of all items into one large, nondescript group. There is no specific common attribute which defines inclusion in the group at this level. As *keychaining* emerges, items are serially ordered rather than grouped, with one feature shared between adjacent items. Item 1 may share color with Item 2. Item 2 may share shape with Item 3. However, Items 1 and 3 may be totally unrelated. This has also been referred to by Vygotsky[95] as *edge matching*. Vygotsky refers to keychaining as the use of one central object by which others are associated via one iconic feature and then another. Piling and keychaining emerge about the same time and, for the purposes of this chapter, are considered in tandem.*

Hartley and Jensen[96] reviewed narrative and procedural discourse comparing closed head injury patients to normals. They concluded that the brain-injured group evidenced impairment of productivity, content, and cohesion. These findings appear to lend credence to the difficulty of respecting cognitively distant categorical boundaries such as those utilized during language usage.

Iconic categorization occurs next, using physical attributes as requisites for category inclusion, such as color, size, shape, etc. Multiple items are grouped at this level because of a single attribute which is shared by all items in the group. *Symbolic categorization* occurs based upon a common functional characteristic of items in the group. Categorization can become as complicated as needed for a given scenario, categorizing on the basis of more than one iconic or symbolic attribute or categorizing on some combination of iconic and symbolic features.

Clearly, the complexities of categorizational processes cannot be readily depicted by a simplistic model. The available complexities can be best reflected, perhaps, by the complexities of language itself. Each noun in a language can be viewed as a category. Using the noun *car*, it can be easily established that an item is either included in or excluded from the category "car". This is a binary process. The category can be further defined or restricted by adding one or more adjectives, for example, *red*. Now the original category has changed. Addition of the adjective *large* restricts the category further, as does addition of the adverb *fast*. Now the category is "fast, large, red car". One can see the use of iconic features in categorical definition.

---

* Tangential speech evidenced by many individuals with traumatic brain injury may occur due to an inability to respect categorical boundaries in conversation. These boundaries are quite cognitively distant, as is all language, and so difficulties with categorization are compounded by problems with cognitive distance.

While the example above depicts the construction of more and more restrictions on a category, the process can be reversed as well. Imagine that you see a car. You might notice its color, make, shape, speed, and/or size. This information is readily available. As you record information about the perception of the car, its descripters or attributes are logged also. The individual who shows a perceptual salience for a particular attribute may not make an adequate log of the remaining perceptual attributes, thereby losing information and reducing the number of associations or cross references that the perceptual experience can be logged under.

Likewise, the individual who has difficulty directing attention may treat all perceptual attributes with equal importance, being unable to adequately classify the perceptual experience into a useful category. The filing of the perceptual experience becomes dependent upon whatever information can be processed from iconic or echoic store mechanisms, with no predictability or consistency observed in how information is selected for long-term storage. Thus, in selective reminding tasks, the individual may have stored information in long-term storage; however, the selective reminding process must progress until the attributes which were used for storage are happened upon.

The neural substrates of categorization are not clear, yet clues to categorizational topography may be obtained via review of literature pertaining to individuals' performance where more discrete and focal neurological lesions are involved. Grossman and Wilson[97] noted that individuals with left hemisphere lesions evidenced problems in categorizing fruit and vegetable items, but not items categorized on the basis of perceptual features alone. The reverse was the case for right hemisphere lesioned individuals. Individuals with left posterior hemisphere lesions had weak categorical boundaries and even reclassified items, while those with left anterior hemisphere lesions evidenced highly categorical responses and less differentiation of items within a category. Left posterior lesion individuals had problems imposing functional categorical boundaries on the continuum of items, but individuals with a left anterior lesion respected categorical boundaries and judged items somewhat rigidly.

Others[98,99] found that individuals with left posterior disease had problems sorting words or pictures of objects into appropriate piles representing categories. Such performance may constitute evidence of problems not only with categorization but also with cognitive distance. Grober et al.[100] and Grossman[101,102] found fluent aphasics had more or less difficulty, depending upon "representativeness" or typicality of the stimulus along the category's continuum.

Caramazza et al.[103] found that fluent aphasics had difficulty utilizing perceptual or contextual information in recognition naming (categorization) tasks. Broca's aphasics and normals, however, were able to use this information. Broca's aphasics and individuals with right hemisphere lesions have been observed to be more competent than fluent aphasics but have difficulty with categorization on occasion.[102,104,105] Nestor et al.[106] studied the relation between memory, abstraction, and categorization skills with temporal lobe volume as measured by MRI in schizophrenic patients. Significant correlations were evidenced between poor skills in verbal memory, abstraction, and categorization and reduced temporal lobe volume, including the parahippocampal gyrus and both the right and left posterior superior temporal gyri. Visual memory skills were not correlated with temporal lobe abnormalities.

A number of studies point to the influence of categorization on various skills. These studies also show deficits of performance for individuals having sustained damage to cortical structures. In a study conducted by Channon et al.,[107] verbal memory involving recall of categorized and noncategorized word lists was evaluated in epileptic patients with left or right temporal lobectomies compared to normals. Recognition and recall performance was poorer for the left temporal group as compared to normals. The right temporal group did not differ significantly from normals for recognition, but neared significance for recall. Performance for both groups was better for the categorized word lists. Hirst and Volpe[108] studied verbal learning among amnesiacs and frontal lobe patients. They found that the frontal lobe patients failed to spontaneously categorize a "categorizable" word list, whereas the amnesiacs did categorize the lists. Frontal lobe patients performed better when categorization was forced. Hough[109] evaluated fluent and nonfluent aphasics' ability to verify category membership and generate exemplars. Both groups required extended verification time and evidenced difficulty with generating atypical categorical exemplars. Both groups were better at generating typical category exemplars. Hough concluded that these findings pointed to diminished representations of the boundaries around a category's referential field.

Electrophysiological correlates of categorizational access of long-term memory were investigated by Rosler et al..[110] Potential amplitudes in the bilateral parietal areas were larger for general concepts (category labels) and smaller for specific concepts (category exemplars). The amplitudes of bilaterally distributed frontal potentials increased when more diversified associative structures were searched. There is, then, supportive electrophysiological evidence to suggest that categorization occurs in a multifaceted manner neurophysiologically and involves the temporal, parietal, and frontal lobes.

Certainly, the individual with traumatic brain injury cannot be characterized as readily as the populations described above in that far more diffuse neurological damage occurs in such cases. However, the information above lends substantial support to the presence of difficulties with feature recognition and manipulation as well as categorizational and cognitive distance issues.

COGNITIVE DISTANCE

It has been noted that the nature of encoding of features is dependent upon the integrity of the sensory end-organs, attentional processing mechanisms, perceptual feature skills, and categorical skills. While one does not need, necessarily, to have proximity with an object to be able to have information about that object's features, it is far easier to have more complete and reliable information if the object is within physical proximity. It is far more difficult, of course, to have a concept in physical proximity. These comments bear upon the issue of *cognitive distance* which was first discussed by Piaget.[111]

Piaget noted that, as an individual became better able to represent experience cognitively, he was better able to do so while being physically removed from the experience itself. Sigel[112] proposed a three-level system of cognitive distance — dealing with objects, then pictorials, and, lastly, words. This system can be broken down further on the basis of a progression of fewer and fewer features available for direct observation. For example, the features of an object are readily available to the individual. The object is available for manipulation, viewing, feeling, and so on. A color photograph of that object allows less opportunity for features to be discerned through direct experience. Instead, in order to have a complete featural assay of the pictured object, the individual must rely upon memory of that object or of a similar object. The object's weight cannot be discerned from the photograph, as an example. Likewise, a black-and-white photograph of the same object will render less information, and a line drawing less information still.

Linguistically, there is more information available about an object in a paragraph written about the object than in a sentence, and in a sentence than the word alone. Thus, an order exists in cognitive distance, moving from the object, to a color photograph, to a black-and-white photograph, to a line drawing, to a word in a paragraph, to a word in a sentence, to a word alone.

Burger and Muma[113] showed that cognitive distance was a factor in aphasic and elderly nonaphasic individuals, whose performance was enhanced with manipulation of objects in contrast to performance with pictorials of the same objects. Muma[114] noted similar discrepancies in performance with learning-disabled, mentally retarded, and autistic children.

It is important to understand the role of cognitive distance in our therapeutic interventions. Muma[114] reported improved performance in an autistic child when play with items in a real house with a real kitchen was compared to play with items in a toy house. The influence of cognitive distance can be seen throughout attentional, perceptual feature assay, and categorizational processes.

INTERVENTION TECHNIQUES AND STRATEGIES

Intervention strategies which attempt to encompass the theoretical and scientific constructs presented thus far can now be considered. Of course, cognitive rehabilitation is required for systems which have undergone serious physiological damage. Consequently, discussion of specific interventions and strategies necessitates review of a few prerequisites to therapy, together with a few philosophical statements pertaining to the therapeutic milieu.

Conditions for Cognitive Rehabilitation

In order to work most effectively in cognitive rehabilitation, it is of extreme importance that the metabolic milieu of the CNS be at least normalized, though evidence may be evolving that will suggest enhancement of specific metabolic conditions to effect maximal neuronal function recovery (specifically, investigations into nerve growth factor and its impact on neuroregeneration). When traumatic brain injury occurs, neuronal death ensues as well as neuronal compromise. Becker[115] refers to "metabolic paralysis", which occurs to cells which have been compromised following injury, though not seriously enough to have succumbed. These cells are able to generate action potentials of amplitudes only one seventh of that of a normal action potential. Becker indicates that, when the metabolic milieu is normalized for the impaired neurons, they become able, once again, to generate normal action potentials. Becker also points out that the metabolically paralyzed cells are unable to survive subsequent ischemic events as would normal cells.

The effects of traumatic brain injury are complicated by the nearly ever-present effects of shearing forces.[116] These forces impact not only cell bodies, but axonal and dendritic processes, glial cells, and blood supply at arterial, venous, and capillary levels. Damage sustained to axonal and dendritic processes, depending upon the distance from the cell body, may undergo some measure of repair via processes known as *axonal regeneration* and *collateral sprouting*.[117] Collateral sprouting does not appear to require damage to the neuron to be elicited. It is not clear whether glial cell and capillary damage, however, can undergo similar repair.

Glial cells and capillary structures are critical to the metabolic processing undertaken by neurons; thus, the availability and viability of these structures is of great importance. Studies have shown that there is a clear increase in the number and availability of these structures in cortices of animals raised in stimuli-enriched environments,[36,118] pointing to the importance of the environment upon the postnatal development of cortical structures. Dendritic tree density is also highest in these animals. Since it is known that reactive synaptogenesis is an active neurophysiological component of normal learning, this process will, of course, also be impacted by glial cell activity and capillary support.

These points are raised to bring to light the importance of the metabolic milieu of the CNS following traumatic brain injury and/or ischemic events of the brain. For example, repetitive seizure activity may, in fact, cause additional neuronal damage. Pulmonary compromise or medications may impact the CNS metabolic milieu and should, therefore, receive greater attention for potential impact on cognitive recovery.

Additionally, the impact of thyroid and steroid hormones on neural structures must be considered. Cytoskeletal proteins necessary in neuronal growth are regulated by thyroid hormone.[119] Thyroid deficiency can result in memory problems, deafness, and cerebellar ataxia. The highest concentration of thyroid hormone receptors has been found in the adult rat hippocampus, amygdala, and cerebral cortex.[120] Removal of the thyroid in adult rats results in a significant reduction in the number of dendritic spines of cerebral cortex neurons in adult rats.[121-123] Thus, information processing capacity of neurons can be impacted by thyroid hormone's impact on dendritic spine density.

Estrogen has been implicated as well in cognitive function. Estrogen has been shown to impact dendritic spine density as well as acetylcholine synthesis,[124,125] and estrogen therapy has been shown to be an effective therapy for female Alzheimer's patients.[126]

Glucocorticoid (a steroid produced by the adrenal glands) insufficiency can likewise result in central nervous system complications. McEwen et al.[127] reported a limbic system representation for glucocorticoid receptors, particularly in the hippocampus. Symptoms associated with glucocorticoid insufficiency include apathy, depression, irritability, and psychosis.

Taken as a whole, cognitive rehabilitation should not be undertaken in a void of adequate evaluation and address of matters which will impact the overall metabolic milieu of the CNS. The therapeutic approaches which will follow in this chapter assume that all that needs to be done to normalize the neurological metabolic milieu has been done and/or is ongoing.

Finally, the information contained in this chapter points to the highly interconnected nature of the CNS and its inherent ability to act as a powerful information processing system. A single neuron can interconnect with up to 10,000 other neurons, creating a richly networked system, one which seems to have some system redundancy. The role of the environment as a source of constant, complex stimuli in rehabilitation cannot be overemphasized.

The rich stimuli of the environment can be both helpful and harmful to the recovering brain-injured patient, as perceptual mechanisms for proper information gating and processing may be such that overload occurs easily. The key is found in balancing the stimuli availability while facilitating improvement in the actual functioning of the perceptual mechanisms involved in information processing. The nature of multiple attribute encoding may be such that the concept of generalization may be as much dependent upon where therapy is performed as upon what the therapy is.

Neurobehavioral programs, for example, conducted in isolated settings may not allow for adequate acquisition of generalizable skills to environments of greater stimuli availability. Likewise, cognitive rehabilitation programs which focus on individual skill sets such as number repetition or rely upon devices such as memory notebooks may not be effective in overall cognitive rehabilitation. In fact, when one considers the impact of reinforcement upon learning and memory formation, a memory notebook actually would seem to be contraindicated for development of neural substrates which serve normal cognitive function. Neural traces would not be required to store information once that information is "dumped" to a paper form of memory storage.

It is clear that, overall, the system appears to revert to the level of least effort as it attempts to process massive amounts of incoming stimuli on a continuing basis. Anecdotal clinical reports are available of patients' recent memory worsening following implementation of memory notebooks, with subsequent return to baseline and further improvement noted following cessation of utilization of the notebook system. The CNS is really not different than other portions of the body in that structures which are utilized are enhanced and structures which are not utilized are likely to be diminished in some fashion.

Having established a common base from which to view cognitive skills and processes, it is now possible to discuss intervention techniques and strategies. A common theme which must be reflected throughout any intervention process is recognition of and respect for the importance of developmental acquisition sequences. The developmental and anatomical influences on cognitive skill acquisition have been illustrated together with the interrelated nature of cognitive skills and processes.

The intervention techniques and strategies to be discussed are designed in consideration of these matters. It is important to realize that an intervention strategy designed in the traditional manner of deficit definition through testing and targeted remediation of skills found to be in deficit cannot be expected to be very successful. This type of approach will result in changes to targeted skills as well as to skills which were untargeted by the therapeutic approach. These unanticipated changes may not always be beneficial, and our clinical experience suggests that this type of approach is less effective and efficient than treatment which is sequenced developmentally.

As has been previously discussed, Tulving[2] stated that memory systems are interrelated and hierarchically arranged. He indicated that higher level systems acted on lower level systems in an interrelated manner. It is through this mechanism that both anticipated and unanticipated changes in targeted and untargeted skills, respectively, can occur when therapeutic endeavors are directed by deficit identification and not by developmental issues. Consequently, it logically follows that intervention strategies must respect both the hierarchical and interrelated nature of cognitive systems.

A more appropriate and prudent approach to cognitive skill development is one which mirrors the postnatal progression of skill acquisition in infancy and childhood. Skills which are acquired at developmentally later periods act on those skills previously acquired, in some cases causing a refinement, inhibition, maturation, or some other change in the skill set. This process is not unlike that seen with motor development, where the infant gradually learns to inhibit and utilize reflexive motor acts. Motoric patterns reflect maturation of gross movement patterns prior to fine movement patterns, with the latter being superimposed upon the stable base of the prior.

The therapeutic hierarchy suggested herein is one which places attention as the most basic cognitive skill set, followed by feature identification skills, and then categorizational skills. Cognitive distance is a process which is superimposed on a number of other cognitive skill sets and, thus, is dealt with at nearly all levels of cognitive rehabilitation. It should be understood that these cognitive skill sets are basic to and serve as the foundation for other cognitive processes such as episodic memory, problem solving, reasoning, creativity, judgment, etc.

While there may exist a variety of ways to deal with delivery of cognitive rehabilitative services which respect the aforementioned matters, it is helpful to create modules which allow for a consistent and systematic application of these principles. Since the intent of this chapter is to discuss therapeutic techniques specifically derived on the basis of theoretical and scientific constructs presented herein, cognitive remediation programs and practices in general will not be reviewed. The approaches to be outlined are remediative in nature, rather than compensatory, and are illustrative, in general, of the various modules which are currently used in our clinical practice. The general approach is to undertake formal and informal testing procedures to document pretreatment cognitive functioning. The "bias for action" assumption to treatment is to treat every individual with each level of each module in a prescribed order, progressing from attention through categorization as outlined above. Those individuals who are competent at various levels move through those levels rapidly, however, but benefit from the overall, developmentally oriented presentation of therapeutic activities.

Attention

Attentional deficits are thought to be highly characteristic of cognitive dysfunction following traumatic brain injury. Jennett and Teasdale[128] state that the vast majority of persons sustaining traumatic brain injury will manifest with attentional deficits. These deficits take several forms, the most common of which will be dealt with here.

Terminology used in the rehabilitation world does not always do justice to the therapist attempting to undertake remediative efforts for a particular diagnosis. Therapists, for example, who are attempting to treat an individual who is distractible, are often readily able to recognize the need to modify the treatment environment to compensate for the individual's distractibility. The term *distractibility*, however, does little to describe the actual nature of the individual's problem. Therefore, remediative efforts can remain elusive for the struggling therapist. The same is the case for the individual who exhibits perseverative behaviors. Again, the term *perseveration* does little to convey the actual nature of the problem.

A descriptive approach to deficit definition is far more helpful in both assessing and treating. The individual who is distractible actually has difficulty directing and/or maintaining a focus of attention. The therapist must improve the individual's ability to direct and/or maintain a focus of attention. Therapeutic activities can be designed to do so. Systematic manipulation of three basic therapeutic concepts can be accomplished in order to develop a successful approach to attentional skill building. These include manipulation of environmental stimulus, task complexing, and cognitive distance.

First, the nature of the disorder itself requires some compensatory adjustments in the treatment environment in order for treatment to be undertaken. Thus, treatment should be done in an environment where as many sensory stimuli as possible can be controlled. The treatment room should be designed such that lighting, temperature, and furnishings can be manipulated. Some individuals may require a treatment environment initially without furniture, with low lighting, with temperature adjusted to their liking, with the therapist and patient in an unfurnished room, on the floor (or mat), and with sound levels controlled. The therapist may need to wear a smock to reduce color stimuli from clothing and remove jewelry, etc., as potential visual stimuli distractors.

The treatment environment can then be stimulus-enhanced as the individual's performance on quantified, therapeutic activities warrants. Distractors can be introduced on a controlled basis, moving from least salient to most salient and moving in one sensory modality at a time. That is to say, a young man who enjoys country/western music by a particular group and is neutral about other types of music might have low-level, calm, symphonic music as a background introduced first, progressing to more "active" music at louder levels, ending with the type of music the young man enjoys most and knows well.

A similar hierarchy can be created for visual stimuli. The entire environment must be considered, including the therapist's attire, furniture, treatment materials, and patient equipment. It is not unusual for all treatments by all disciplines to be done in such a sensory-controlled environment. Specific activity to enhance the ability to maintain attentional focus can also be performed in this environment, both separate from and in tandem with other therapeutic activities. It is sometimes necessary, with the most severely impaired individual, to be prepared to undertake a single therapeutic activity for extended periods of time in an effort to build rudimentary attention skills which will allow interaction with a therapist beyond a few seconds.

Next, therapeutic attention activities should take into account the principles of cognitive distance. Objects should be utilized first, and any tasks to be performed should be done on a physical basis. That is, the task should comprise physical activity alone or in combination with actions on an object such as moving the object to relative positions between the patient and treater. Once the individual is able to handle the stimulus of a single object, the activity can be expanded to include the same action on a small group of objects. Other examples might include the therapist asking for a motorically simple act such as, "Please sit down on the mat until I count to ten." After criteria is met (say, the individual sits down for ten seconds, eight out of ten times), the time frame can be lengthened progressively until sitting time is long enough (one to two minutes) to allow engagement in other tasks.

It is often useful, with an individual at this basic level, to utilize the *Premack principle*[129] to identify potential positive reinforcers for use in a predetermined reinforcement schedule. The Premack principle allows us the assumption that any behaviors which are spontaneously produced may be viewed as reinforcing to the organism. This subject is discussed further in Chapter 10 of this volume.

When therapy has progressed to the point at which other activities can be overlaid on the progressive sitting schedule, those activities should consist of other actions on, or interactions with, a single object, progressing to multiple objects. The therapist needs to continually monitor performance accuracy and time-to-complete for signals indicating when progression to a more complex level is warranted.

TABLE 12.2   Order of Distractor Presentation

	No distractor	Simple auditory or visual distractor	Multisensory distractor
Physical task	1	2	3
Physical/Mental task	4	5	6
Mental task	7	8	9

The treatment scenario outlined above is necessary only for the most severe attentional deficits. Many individuals can begin at a higher level but should always begin in a stimulus-controlled environment and with a physical task. In this way, persistence can be improved and the individual readied for more cognitively distant concentration activities. The environment can be complicated at the therapist's discretion and in accordance with accuracy and time-to-complete data collected from ongoing therapy tasks. Ultimately, the progression should occur to the point that the therapy takes place outside the environmentally controlled area, preferably, in the most challenging environment(s) available. Again, it is important to recognize that quantifiable data should be collected continually throughout the therapeutic activity.

It may be necessary and advisable to reduce the task complexity and the cognitive distance of the required task as more environmental stimuli are introduced. A good rule of thumb is 90–95% accuracy as a criterion for progression to a higher level of task complexity, cognitive distance, or environmental stimulus. Baseline measures of time-to-complete allow variations due to physical impairments, and subsequent simultaneous determinations of at least a 20% improvement over baseline for time-to-complete scores are required before progression to the next therapeutic level.

As can be seen, there are numerous ways in which the creative therapist can systematically manipulate the activities in respect to the three primary variables of environmental stimulus, task complexity, and cognitive distance. One example might be utilizing the sorting of hardware, such as nuts and bolts, by size and color under varying and controlled degrees of auditory and/or visual stimuli. Tasks such as sorting or ordering index cards alphabetically or serially by number can be used. The task should be one which requires physical action upon an object or group of objects.

Therapy should progress to tasks which are increasingly cognitively distant or abstract, reducing physical cues available and increasing reliance upon mental representation and manipulation of the object(s). Abstract tasks might consist of performance of mental arithmetic problems or description of named objects, requiring a specified number and nature of perceptual attributes in the description. Table 12.2 depicts the multivariate nature of therapeutic design which must be considered and controlled for, the nature of distractors to be used, and the order of therapeutic task presentation.

Another form of attentional deficit is seen in many perseverative behaviors. It is important to realize that the term *perseveration* does not truly convey the nature of the problem. A perseverative response may be based wholly upon perceptual salience and, as such, may actually represent a deficit in the individual's ability to freely shift attention among perceptual feature. Perseveration can be thought of as an inability to shift a focus of attention. Therapeutic activities which reduce perceptual salience and build featural assay skills tend to bring about reductions in perseverative responses. It should also be recognized, however, that some perseverative behaviors may occur for reasons of perceptual salience in other sensory domains, e.g., "rocking" as a vestibular stimulus. Remediation of perceptual salience will be expanded upon later in this chapter.

Discussions of attentional deficits often include problems with what is termed *vigilance*. Vigilance refers to an individual's ability to maintain a focus of attention and monitor incoming stimuli for a specific set of features. In order to be successful, the individual must be able to rapidly take into sensory stores (such as iconic and/or echoic) large amounts of information and screen that information for the desired feature(s). The individual must be able to resist loss of focus of attention for the incoming stimuli, either in favor of other stimuli or other perceptual attributes within the attended stimulus field. As can be seen, this is both a complicated and cognitively distant process. Vigilance represents one of the more complicated attentional skills and, therefore, therapy should concentrate on remediation of the componential skills involved in vigilance, i.e., maintaining a focus of attention in a stimulus-rich environment, as well as building cognitive distance skills.

The ability to shift between activities with the least amount of disruption to information stores, task sequencing, and task accuracy is referred to as *cognitive shift*. This cognitive skill is frequently impaired in the traumatically brain-injured individual. It is hierarchically more complicated than any of the attentional skills discussed thus far and, as such, should be reserved for treatment until the other arenas have been improved.

Cognitive shift activities must be designed respecting cognitive distance and environmental stimuli presentation and complexity. The therapist can create activities which begin with two simple physical tasks, requiring a change from one activity to the other and back. Data is collected on time-to-complete a specified number of changes and on the accuracy of task completion. As competence warrants, the tasks are varied to become more complicated and numbered. Finally, the tasks should progress from physical only, to physical and mental, then to mental only. The tasks can be complicated further by the addition of environmental stimuli intended to serve as potential distractors. The order of presentation of such distractors can be the same as that used in activities designed to enhance more basic attentional skills.

Feature Identification

At the first level of remediation of feature identification skills, the individual learns to attend to and identify iconic features of real objects. The seven iconic features utilized in this exercise can include color, shape, construction, size, weight, texture, and detail. This is not an all-inclusive list. These perceptual attributes are suggested due to the nature of the attributes themselves and the comparative degree with which they reflect some of the "linguistic universals" referred to by Rosch.[66] Furthermore, an object can be described by its main function (a symbolic feature), bringing the total number of features used to eight. Identification of a symbolic feature is also required at the first level.

Remediation of cognitive distance is introduced at Level I. The individual begins by describing the iconic features and symbolic features of an object. Successful completion for this step comprises description of at least six of the eight potential features (iconic and symbolic) of ten consecutive objects. Next, the task progresses through a hierarchy consisting of objects, color photographs of objects, black-and-white photographs of objects, line drawings of objects, written words, and spoken words. This progression requires increasingly greater reliance upon mental representation of features that are no longer represented physically.

Initially, the individual may be provided a checklist of the eight features. The checklist is faded as success in identifying the features emerges, until an individual is capable of providing spontaneous description of the items without the checklist. After successful completion of feature identification of real objects, an individual progresses to the next step in the hierarchy, which is color photographs of objects. Throughout Level I, an individual is required to identify the eight previously described features of items presented in increasingly more abstract representations.

Criterion for successful completion at this level is dependent upon the individual with whom the task is being performed. Generally, the criterion for movement to the next level in the module is 75% accuracy in description of features for ten items at each level. Completion must occur within a time frame deemed reasonable to the task and should not be extensive. This criterion may be modified for an individual functioning at a lower level, with the individual perhaps repeating the module at a later date with a more stringent criterion applied.

At the next level, the tasks focus on broadening the feature identification skills. The purpose of this activity is to further develop and refine feature identification skills by identifying each of the eight features and identifying another object which exhibits one of the eight features. The individual is required to identify all the features of an object, one by one, and to provide an example of an item that shares the same feature. The alternate object provided as an example by the individual must be different for each attribute. In this way, maximum benefit toward improvement of the individual's word finding and memory skills is realized. Also, the example must be an object not visible in the immediate environment. Once again, the hierarchy of cognitive distance — real objects through spoken words — is followed.

The next level focuses on abstract negation. The purposes of this section are to continue the development and refinement of feature identification skills and to begin a focus on categorization skills. This section requires the individual to identify and describe items in terms of what they are not, utilizing the eight salient features. For example, when presented with a baseball, the individual identifies the object and a feature that it does not have, i.e., "the baseball is not green". At this point, the individual is then required to give an example of another object that does not share this feature, i.e., "a car tire is not green". Real objects are utilized first, and the cognitive distance hierarchy is followed, through description by spoken words.

Categorization

Now that the individual is able to readily identify and deal with features, the next goal is to develop the ability to define iconic categories and then maintain categorical boundaries. The goal of this activity is to have the individual categorize objects according to the seven iconic features. Real objects are utilized first and the individual is required to name the iconic feature shared by different items grouped together. Upon successful completion at this level, the individual is required to come up with three objects which can be grouped on the basis of a given iconic feature. For example, given the inclusive feature "yellow", the individual indicates that a pencil, a banana, and a lemon all share the same yellow color. With successful completion at this level, color photographs are introduced and categorized according to iconic features. Black-and-white photos, line drawings, and written words are next used in this activity.

Finally, symbolic categorization skills are developed and expanded. The process of symbolic categorization may seemingly be less difficult for some individuals than the more basic step of iconic categorization. While symbolic categorization may be more easily stored,[130] it does not provide evidence for an intact feature processing system. Therefore, what may seem to be a good understanding of symbolic features may only be a superficial understanding of common functional attributes of objects and not representative of competence in feature identification and categorization processes. In addition, symbolic representation may, in fact, be evidence of old learning. Old information is most likely to return following traumatic brain injury, while new information processing is most impaired. It is possible that the presence of skills at a symbolic level may cause a false assumption of competence.

The purpose of this section is to develop the ability to define symbolic or functional categories and maintain and manipulate these categorical delineations. First, the individual is required to identify the symbolic features, or functional properties, of objects. Upon successful completion of this step, the individual is next required to modify or "extend" the functional use of an object. The goal is to identify an abstract, atypical function. For example, a fork can be used as a small crowbar due to its size, shape, and strength. Next, the individual is asked to identify two or more objects that can be used for the same abstract, atypical function. For example, a pen and a screwdriver can also be used as small crowbars.

Finally, the individual is to manipulate an entire object array into categories of self-defined, atypical use. He is required to provide reasons for the groupings he chooses. These explanations should be reasonable in the therapist's judgment, and only one rule is allowed per group. That is to say, a group of objects must all share the same symbolic feature. Care should be taken to discourage repetitive responses, encouraging, instead, a broad array of patient-defined atypical uses. After successful completion of these four steps with real objects, the process is repeated using color photographs.

Following successful completion of symbolic categorization, the individual then moves to extended negative categorization. The individual is required to describe an object, including its function, and then describe a function that the object cannot be used for. For example, a fork is used for eating but cannot be used for toasting bread. This procedure is repeated using color photographs, line drawings, and written and spoken words.

As can be seen, the cognition module demands cognitive shift abilities. Cognitive skills, including attention, feature identification, categorization, and cognitive distance are de-manded simultaneously. Through the use of seven iconic features, perceptual salience (an inordinate focus on a particular perceptual feature) is avoided. Categorization abilities are maximized throughout the module, beginning first with iconic features and progressing to symbolic features. Also, each step addresses the issue of cognitive distance, increasingly requiring the individual to rely on mental representation of objects by reducing the number of physical cues present.

The intervention strategies discussed herein are designed to rebuild basic-level cognitive skills. These skills are thought to be the foundation upon which higher level thought processes and memory are based. It should be stressed that the cognition module is not a single entity but, instead, an integral part of the overall rehabilitation program. Separate modules exist for development of attentional and cognitive shift skills. As each area is substantially complex, they have been separated to provide concentrated remediative intervention.

SUMMARY

This chapter presented information derived from cognitive psychology, experimental psychol-ogy, child language development, psycholinguistics, embryology, neuroembryology, neu-roanatomy, neurophysiology, and aphasiology to develop a theoretical and scientific construct upon which a treatment rationale for cognitive rehabilitation can be built. Such a treatment rationale has been presented with very specific treatment approaches outlined and examples provided. In many cases, compensatory strategies are used as the sole intervention process in cognitive therapy. Cognitive rehabilitation which is undertaken respecting the remediative principles outlined herein can be highly effective in the treatment of cognitive disorders following traumatic brain injury.

REFERENCES

1. Guralnik, D. B., *Webster's New World Dictionary of the American Language*, 2nd college edition, World Publishing Company, New York, 1970, 276.
2. Tulving, E., How many memory systems are there? *Am. Psychol.*, 40, 385, 1985.
3. Mountcastle, V., Interview, *Omni*, 13, 62, 1991.
4. Bobath, B., *Adult Hemiplegia: Evaluation and Treatment*, 2nd edition, William Heineman Medical Books, Ltd., London, 1978.
5. Bobath, K. and Bobath, B., Cerebral palsy. Part 1. The neurological approach to treatment, in *Physical Therapy Services in the Developmental Disabilities*, Pearson, P. H and Williams, C. E., Eds., Charles C. Thomas, Springfield, IL, 1980, 114.
6. Farber, S. D., *Neurorehabilitation: A Multisensory Approach*, W. B. Saunders Company, Philadelphia, 1982.
7. Meader, C. L. and Muyskens, J. H., *Handbook of Biolinguistics. Part 1: The Structures and Processes of Expression with Introduction to Biolinguistics*, Revised edition, Waverly Press, Baltimore, 1962.
8. Yokoh, Y., Early development of the cerebral vesicle in man, *Acta Anat.*, 91, 455, 1975.

9. Sarnat, H. B. and Netsky, M. G., *Evolution of the Nervous System*, 2nd edition, Oxford University Press, New York, 1981.
10. Marcus, E. M., Cerebral cortex: Cytoarchitecture and electrophysiology, in *An Introduction to the Neurosciences*, Curtis, B. A., Jacobson, S., and Marcus, E. M., Eds., W. B. Saunders Company, Philadelphia, 1972, 447.
11. Luria, A. R., *The Working Brain*, Penguin Publishers, Harmondsworth, England, 1973.
12. Daube, J. R., Sandok, B. A., Reagon, T. J., and Westmoreland, B. F., *Medical Neurosciences: An Approach to Anatomy, Pathology, and Physiology by Systems and Levels*, Little, Brown and Company, Boston, 1978.
13. Rolls, E. T., Neurophysiological and neuronal network analysis of how the primate hippocampus functions in memory, in *The Memory System of the Brain*, Delacour, J., Ed., World Scientific, Singapore, 1994.
14. Willis, W. D., Jr. and Grossman, R. G., *Medical Neurobiology: Neuroanatomical and Neurophysiological Principles Basic to Clinical Neuroscience*, C. V. Mosby Company, St. Louis, MO, 1977.
15. Poletti, C. E., Kinnard, M. A., and MacLean, P. D., Hippocampal influence on unit activity of hypothalamic, preoptic, and basal forebrain structures in awake, sitting squirrel monkeys, *J. Neurophysiol.*, 36, 308, 1973.
16. Poletti, C. E., Is the limbic system a limbic system? Studies of hippocampal efferents: Their functional and clinical implications, in *The Limbic System: Functional Organizational and Clinical Disorders*, Doane, B. K. and Livingston, K. E., Eds., Raven Press, New York, 1986.
17. MacLean, P. D., Culminating developments in the evolution of the limbic system: The thalomocingulate division, in *The Limbic System: Functional Organization and Clinical Disorders*, Doane, B. K. and Livingston, K. E., Eds., Raven Press, New York, 1986.
18. Ranck, J. B., Jr., Studies on single neurons in dorsal hippocampal formation and septum in unrestrained rats, *Exp. Neurol.*, 41, 461, 1973.
19. Milner, B., Amnesia following operation on the temporal lobes, in *Amnesia*, Whitty, C. W. M. and Zangwill, O. L., Eds., Butterworths, London, 1966.
20. Squire, L. R. and Moore, R. Y., Dorsal thalamic lesions in a noted case of chronic memory dysfunction, *Ann. Neurol.*, 6, 503, 1979.
21. Nauta, W. J. H., Circuitous connections linking cerebral cortex, limbic system, and corpus striatum, in *The Limbic System: Functional Organization and Clinical Disorders*, Doane, B. K. and Livingston, K. F., Eds., Raven Press, New York, 1986, 43.
22. Hebb, D. O., *The Organization of Behavior*, John Wiley & Sons, New York, 1949.
23. Brinton, R. E., Biochemical correlates of learning and memory, in *Learning and Memory: A Biological View*, Martinez, J. L. and Kesner, R. P., Eds., Academic Press, San Diego, CA, 1991.
24. Kandel, E. R., Cellular mechanisms of learning and the biological basis of individuality, in *Principles of Neuroscience*, Kandel, E. R., Schwartz, J. H., and Jessell, T. M., Eds., Elsevier, New York, 1991.
25. Hannay, T., Larkman, A., Stratford, K., and Kack. J., A common rule governs the synaptic locus of both short-term and long-term potentiation, *Curr. Biol.*, 3, 832, 1993.
26. Bolshakov, V. Y. and Siegelbaum, S. A., Postsynaptic induction and presynaptic expression of hippocampal long-term depression, *Science*, 264, 1148, 1994.
27. Schubert, D., The possible role of adhesion in synaptic modification, *Trends Neurosci.*, 14, 127, 1991.
28. Schumann, E. M. and Madison, D. V., Locally distributed synaptic potentiation in the hippocampus, *Science*, 263, 532, 1994.
29. Hawkins, R. D., Zhuo, M., and Arancio, O., Nitric-oxide and carbon-monoxide as possible retrograde messengers in hippocampal long-term depression, *J. Neurobiol.*, 25, 652, 1994.
30. Baringa, M., Learning by diffusion: Nitric oxide may spread memories, *Science*, 263, 466, 1994.
31. Ohno, N., Yamamoto, T., and Watanabe, S., Intrahippocampal administration of the NO synthase inhibitor L-name prevents working-memory deficits in rats exposed to transient cerebral ischemia, *Brain Res.*, 634, 173, 1994.
32. Ohno, N., Yamamoto, T., and Watanabe, S., Deficits in working-memory following inhibition of hippocampal nitric-oxide synthesis in the rat, *Brain Res.*, 632, 36, 1993.
33. Chang, F.-L. F. and Greenough, W. T., Transient and enduring morphological correlates of synaptic activity and efficacy changes in the rat hippocampal slice, *Brain Res.*, 309, 35, 1984.
34. Black, J. E., Sirevaag, A. M., and Greenough, W. T., Complex experience promotes capillary formation in young visual cortex, *Neurosci. Lett.*, 83, 351, 1987.
35. Anderson, B. J., Isaacs, K. R., Black, J. E., Vinci, L. M., Alcantara, A. A., and Greenough, W. T., Synaptogensis in cerebellar cortex of adult rats after less than 15 hours of visuomotor training over 10 days, *Soc. Neurosci. Abstr.*, 14, 1239, 1988.
36. Sirevaag, A. M., Smith, S., and Greenough, W. T., Rats reared in a complex environment have larger astrocytes with more processes than rats raised socially or individually, *Soc. Neurosci. Abstr.*, 14, 1135, 1988.
37. Trexler, L. E. and Zappala, G., Neuropathological determinants of acquired attention disorders in traumatic brain injury, *Brain Cognit.*, 8, 291, 1988.

38. Posner, M. I., Psychobiology of attention, in *Handbook of Psychobiology*, Gazzinaga, M. S. and Blakemore, C., Eds., Academic Press, New York, 1975, 441.

39. Denny-Brown, D. and Fischer, E. C., Physiological aspects of visual perception. II. The subcortical visual direction of behavior, *Arch. Neurol.,* 33, 228, 1976.

40. Goldberg, M. E. and Wurtz, R. H., Activity of superior colliculus in behaving monkeys. II. Effect of attention on neuronal responses, *J. Neurophysiol.,* 35, 560, 1972.

41. Gummow, L., Miller, P., and Dustman, R. E., Attention and brain injury: A case for cognitive rehabilitation of attentional deficits, *Clin. Psychol. Rev.,* 3, 255, 1983.

42. Brown, J. W., Thalamic mechanisms in language, in *Handbook of Behavioral Neuropsychology: Vol. 2: Neuropsychology*, Gazzinaga, M. F., Ed., Plenum, New York, 1979.

43. Scheibel, M. E. and Scheibel, R. M., Structural organization of nonspecific thalamic nuclei and their projection toward cortex, *Brain Res.,* 6, 60, 1967.

44. Goodglass, H. and Kaplan, E., Assessment of cognitive deficit in the brain-injured patient, *Handb. Behav. Neurobiol.,* 2, 3, 1979.

45. Eidelberg, E. and Schwartz, A. S., Experimental analysis of the extinction phenomenon in monkeys, *Brain*, 94, 91, 1971.

46. Näätänen, R., Orienting and evoked potentials, in *The Orienting Reflex in Humans*, Kimmed, H. D., Van Olst, E. H., and Orlebeke, J. F., Eds., Wiley, New York, 1979.

47. Watson, R. L., Heilman, K. M., Cauthen, J. C., and King, F. A., Neglect after cingulectomy, *Neurology*, 23, 1003, 1973.

48. Heilman, K. M. and Valenstein, E., Frontal lobe neglect in man, *Neurology*, 22, 660, 1972.

49. Goff, W. R., Evoked potential correlates of perceptual organization in man, in *Attention in Neurophysiology*, Evans, C. R. and Mulholland, T. B., Eds., Appleton, New York, 1969.

50. Vaughan, H. G. and Ritter, W., The sources of auditory evoked responses recorded from the human scalp, *Electroencephalogr. Clin. Neurophysiol.,* 28, 360, 1970.

51. Mesulam, M. and Geschwind, N., On the possible role of neocortex and its limbic connections in the process of attention and schizophrenia: Clinical cases of inattention in man and experimental anatomy in monkey, *J. Psychiatr. Res.,* 14, 249, 1978.

52. Thompson, R. F. and Bettinger, L. A., Neural substrates of attention, in *Attention: Contemporary Theory and Analysis*, Mostofsky, D. L., Ed., Appleton, New York, 1970.

53. Posner, M. I. and Snyder, C. R. R., Facilitation and inhibition in the processing of signals, in *Attention and Performance V*, Rabbitt, P. M. A., Ed., Academic Press, New York, 1975.

54. Kahneman, D., Remarks on attention control, *Acta Psycholog.,* 33, 118, 1970.

55. Kahneman, D., *Attention and Effort*, Prentice-Hall, Inc., Englewood Cliffs, NJ, 1973.

56. Anderson, J. R., *Cognitive Psychology and Its Implications*, W. H. Freeman & Company, San Francisco, 1980.

57. Neisser, U., *Cognitive Psychology*, Appleton, New York, 1967.

58. Moray, N., Bates, A., and Barnett, T., Experiments on the four-eared man, *J. Acoust. Soc. Am.,* 38, 196, 1965.

59. Darwin, C. J., Turvy, M. T., and Crowder, R. G., The auditory analog of the Spurling partial report procedure: Evidence for brief auditory storage, *Cognit. Psychol.,* 3, 255, 1972.

60. Spurling, G. A., The information available in brief presentation, *Psychol. Monogr.,* 74, 498, 1960.

61. Treisman, A. M., Verbal cues, language, and meaning in selective attention, *Q. J. Exp. Psychol.,* 12, 242, 1960.

62. Sokovlov, E. N., *Perception and the Conditioned Reflex*, Macmillan, New York, 1963.

63. Olson, D., Language and thought: Aspects of a cognitive theory of semantics, *Psychol. Rev.,* 77, 257, 1970.

64. Rosch, E., On the internal structure of perceptual and semantic categories, in *Cognitive Development and the Acquisition of Language*, Moor, T., Ed., Academic Press, New York, 1973.

65. Voss, J. F., On the relationship of associative and organizational processes, in *Organization of Memory*, Tulving, E. and Donaldson, W., Eds., Academic Press, New York, 1972, 174.

66. Rosch, E., Universals and cultural specifics in human categorization, in *Cross-cultural Perspectives on Learning*, Brislin, R. W., Bochner, S., and Lonner, W. J., Eds., Wiley, New York, 1975.

67. Freund, J. S. and Underwood, B. J., Restricted associates as cues in free recall, *J. Verbal Learn. Verbal Behav.,* 9, 136, 1970.

68. Tulving, E. and Osler, S., Effectiveness of retrieval cues in memory for words, *J. Exp. Psychol.,* 77, 239, 1968.

69. Mandler, G., Organization and memory, in *The Psychology of Learning and Motivation*, Volume 1, Spence, K. W. and Spence, J. T., Eds., Academic Press, New York, 1967.

70. Mandler, G., Pearlstone, Z., and Koopmans, H. S., Effects of organization and semantic similarity on recall and recognition, *J. Verbal Learn. Verbal Behav.,* 8, 410, 1969.

71. Odom, R. and Corbin, D., Perceptual salience and children's multidimensional problem solving, *Child Dev.,* 44, 425, 1973.

72. Odom, R., Effects of perceptual salience on the recall of relevant and incidental dimensional values: A developmental study, *J. Exp. Psychol.,* 92, 285, 1972.

73. Odom, R. D. and Guzman, R. D., Problem solving and the perceptual salience of variability and constancy: A developmental study, *J. Exp. Child Psychol.,* 9, 156, 1970.

74. Odom, R. and Guzman, R. D., Development of hierarchies of dimensional salience, *Dev. Psychol.,* 6, 271, 1972.

75. Caron, A., Discrimination shifts in three year olds as a function of dimensional salience, *Dev. Psychol.,* 1, 333, 1969.

76. Saltz, E. and Sigel, I. E., Concept over-discrimination in children, *J. Exp. Psychol.,* 73, 1, 1967.

77. Kagan, J., Reflectivity-impulsivity and reading ability in primary grade children, *Child Dev.,* 36, 609, 1965.

78. Kagan, J., Developmental studies in reflectional analysis, in *Perceptual Developments in Children,* Kidd, A. and Rivoire, J., Eds., International University Press, New York, 1966, 487.

79. Wayland, S. and Taplin, J. E., Feature-processing deficits following brain injury. 1. Overselectivity in recognition memory for compound stimuli, *Brain Cognit.,* 4, 338, 1985.

80. Tyler, S., *Cognitive Anthropology,* Holt, Rinehart and Winston, New York, 1969.

81. Bruner, J., Goodnow, J., and Austin, G., *A Study of Thinking,* Science Editions, Inc., New York, 1956.

82. Bowerman, M., Semantic factors in the acquisition of rules for word use and sentence construction, in *Normal and Deficient Child Language,* Morehead, D. and Morehead, R., Eds., University Park Press, Baltimore, 1976.

83. Clark, H. and Clark, E., *Psychology and Language,* Harcourt, Brace & Jovanovich, New York, 1977.

84. Rosch, E. and Mervis, C. B., Family resemblances: Studies in the internal structure of categories, *Cognit. Psychol.,* 7, 573, 1975.

85. Rosch, E., Simpson, C., and Miller, R. S., Structural bases of typicality effects, *J. Exp. Psychol.,* 2, 491, 1976.

86. Smith, E. E., Shoben, E. J., and Rips, L. J., Structure and process in semantic memory: A featural model for semantic decisions, *Psychol. Rev.,* 81, 214, 1974.

87. Rips, L. J., Inductive judgements about natural categories, *J. Verbal Learn. Verbal Behav.,* 14, 665, 1975.

88. Shoben, E. J., The verification of semantic relations in a same-different paradigm: An asymmetry in semantic memory, *J. Verbal Learn. Verbal Behav.,* 15, 365, 1976.

89. Collins, A. M. and Quillian, M. R., Retrieval time from semantic memory, *J. Verbal Learn. Verbal Behav.,* 8, 240, 1969.

90. Collins, A. M. and Quillian, M. R., Experiments on semantic memory and language comprehension, in *Cognition in Learning and Memory,* Gregg, L. W., Ed., Wiley, New York, 1972.

91. Rips, L. J., Shoben, E. J., and Smith, E. E., Semantic distance and the verification of semantic relations, *J. Verbal Learn. Verbal Behav.,* 12, 1, 1973.

92. Smith, E. E., Rips, L. J., and Shoben, E. J., Semantic memory and psychological semantics, in *The Psychology of Learning and Motivation,* Volume 8, Bower, G. H., Ed., Academic Press, New York, 1974.

93. Bowleska, A., Some aspects of conceptual organization in aphasics with naming disturbances, *Z. Psychol. Z. Angew. Psychol.,* 189, 67, 1981.

94. Glucksberg, S. and Wiseberg, R. W., Verbal behavior and problem solving: Some effects of labeling in a functional fixedness problem, *J. Exp. Psychol.,* 71, 659, 1966.

95. Vygotsky, L., *Thought and Language,* Revised edition by Kozulin, A., MIT Press, Cambridge, MA, 1986.

96. Hartley, L. L. and Jensen, P. J., Narrative discourse after closed head injury, *Brain Injury,* 5, 267, 1991.

97. Grossman, M. and Wilson, M., Stimulus categorization by brain-damaged patients, *Brain Cognit.,* 6, 55, 1987.

98. Lhermitte, F., Derouesne, J., and Lecours, A. R., Contribution a l'etude des troubles semantiques dans l'aphasie, *Rev. Neurol.,* 125, 81, 1971.

99. Goldstein, K., *Language and Language Disorders,* Grune & Stratton, New York, 1948.

100. Grober, E., Perecman, E., Kellar, L., and Brown, J., The status of semantic categories in aphasia, *Brain Lang.,* 10, 318, 1980.

101. Grossman, M., The game of the name: An examination of linguistic reference after brain damage, *Brain Lang.,* 6, 112, 1978.

102. Grossman, M., The figurative representation of a superordinate's referents after brain damage, paper presented at the meeting of the International Neuropsychological Society, San Francisco, 1980, February.

103. Caramazza, A., Berndt, R. S., and Brownell, H. H., The semantic deficit hypothesis: Perceptual parsing and object classification by aphasic patients, *Brain Lang.,* 15, 161, 1982.

104. Cavalli, M., de Renzi, E., Faglioni, P., and Vitale, A., Impairment of right brain-damaged patients on a linguistic cognitive task, *Cortex,* 17, 545, 1981.

105. Gainotti, G., Caltagirone, C., Miceli, G., and Masullo, G., Selective semantic-lexical impairment of language comprehension in right brain-damaged patients, *Brain Lang.,* 13, 201, 1981.

106. Nestor, P. G., Shenton, M. E., and McCarley, R. W., Neuropsychological correlates of MRI temporal lobe abnormalities in schizophrenia, *Am. J. Psychiatry,* 150, 1849, 1993.

107. Channon, S., Daum, I., and Polkey, C. E., The effect of categorization on verbal memory after temporal lobectomy, *Neuropsychologia*, 27, 777, 1989.

108. Hirst, W. and Volpe, B. T., Memory strategies with brain damage, *Brain Cognit.*, 8, 379, 1988.

109. Hough, M. S., Categorization in aphasia — Access and organization of goal-derived and common categories, *Aphasiology*, 7, 335, 1993.

110. Rosler, F., Heil, M., and Glowalla, U., Monitoring retrieval from long-term memory by slow event-related brain potentials, *Psychophysiology*, 30, 170, 1993.

111. Piaget, J., *Play, Dreams, and Imitation in Childhood*, Norton, New York, 1962.

112. Sigel, I., Language of the disadvantaged: The distancing hypothesis, in *Language Training in Early Childhood Education*, Lavatelli, C., Ed., University of Illinois, Urbana, IL, 1971.

113. Burger, R. and Muma, J., Mediated Categorization Behavior in Two Representational Modes: Fluent Aphasics, Afluent Aphasics, and Normals, unpublished manuscript, 1977.

114. Muma, J. R., *Language Handbook: Concepts, Assessment, Intervention*, Prentice-Hall, Inc., Englewood Cliffs, NJ, 1978.

115. Becker, D. P., Brain cellular injury and recovery — Horizons for improving medical therapies in stroke and trauma, *West. J. Med.*, 148, 670, 1988.

116. Gennarelli, T. A., Thibault, L. E., Adams, J. H., Graham, D. I., Thompson, C. J., and Marcincin, R. P., Diffuse axonal injury and traumatic coma in the primate, *Ann. Neurol.*, 12, 564, 1982.

117. Crutcher, K. A., Anatomical correlates of neuronal plasticity, in *Learning and Memory: A Biological View*, Martinez, J. L. and Kesner, R. P., Eds., Academic Press, San Diego, CA, 1991.

118. Black, J. E., Jones, A. L., Anderson, B. J., Isaacs, K. R., Alcantra, A. A., and Greenough, W. T., Cerebellar plasticity: Preliminary evidence that learning, rather than repetitive motor exercise, alters cerebellar cortex thickness in middle-aged rats, *Soc. Neurosci. Abstr.*, 13, 1596, 1987.

119. Nunez, J., Effects of thyroid hormones during brain differentiation, *Mol. Cell. Endocrinol.*, 37, 125, 1984.

120. Dussault, J. H. and Ruel, J., Thyroid hormones and brain development, *Ann. Rev. Physiol.*, 49, 321, 1987.

121. Ruiz-Marcos, A., Abella, P. C., Garcia, A. G., del Rey, F. E., and de Escobar, G. M., Rapid effects of adult-onset hypothyroidism on dendritic spines of pyramidal cells of the rat cerebral cortex, *Exp. Brain Res.*, 73, 583, 1980.

122. Ruiz-Marcos, A., Sanchez-Toscano, F., Obregon, M. J., Escobar del Rey, F., and Morreale de Escobar, G., Thyroxine treatment and recovery of hypothyroidism-induced pyramidal cell damage, *Brain Res.* (Netherlands), 239, 559, 1982.

123. Ruiz-Marcos, A., Cartagena, A. P., Garcia, G. A., Escobar del Rey, F., and Morreale de Escobar, G., Rapid effects of adult-onset hypothyroidism on dendritic spines of pyramidal cells of the rat cerebral cortex, *Exp. Brain Res.* (West Germany), 73, 583, 1988.

124. Wooley, C. S. and McEwen, B. S., Estradiol regulates synapse density in the CA1 region of the hippocampus in the adult female rat, *Soc. Neurosci. Abstr.*, 16, 144, 1990.

125. Luine, V. N., Estradiol increases choline acetyltransferase activity in specific basal forebrain nuclei and projection areas of female rats, *Exp. Neurol.*, 89, 484, 1985.

126. Fillit, H., Weinreb, H., Cholst, I., Luine, V., McEwen, B., Amador, R., and Zabriski, J., Observations in a preliminary open trial of estradiol therapy for senile dementia-Alzheimer's type, *Psychoneuroendocrinology*, 11, 337, 1986.

127. McEwen, B. S., Weiss, J. M., and Schwartz, L. S., Selective retention of corticosteroid by limbic structures in rat brain, *Nature*, 220, 911, 1968.

128. Jennett, B. and Teasdale, G., *Management of Head Injuries*, F. A. Davis Company, Philadelphia, 1982.

129. Premack, D., Toward empirical behavior laws: I. Positive reinforcement, *Psychol. Rev.*, 66, 219, 1959.

130. Bruner, J., The course of cognitive growth, *Am. Psychol.*, 19, 1, 1964.

13

Management of Residual Physical Deficits

Velda L. Bryan

CONTENTS

0-8493-9463-5/95/$0.00+$.50
© 1995 by CRC Press Inc.

AN HISTORICAL PERSPECTIVE

Since World War II, an internationally scattered group of occupational therapists (OT) and physical therapists (PT) have developed and advocated theories and treatment procedures to address sensorimotor deficits in the neurologically impaired patient.[1-7] However, until the early 1980's, training and practice of these techniques were usually found only in specialty clinics and in advanced professional workshops. The majority of general practice therapists were neither trained in nor practiced a therapeutic approach based on neurophysiological or developmental principles. Among those with training, some therapists were strong advocates of only one approach while others were applying bits and pieces of all the then-known treatment approaches. Their patients were usually of cerebral palsy, stroke, multiple sclerosis, and other neurological etiologies.

Survivors of traumatic brain injury (TBI) prior to the 1970's were encouraged to use functional extremities, were put into wheelchairs and braces, and were eventually sent home or to an institution. Treatment was usually dictated by medical personnel who were not rehabilitation oriented. An early entry into the "therapy department" was rare and usually awaited the TBI patient's ability to "respond" or "cooperate".

Most ICU's were not familiar territory for therapists until the mid-1980's, when it was realized that early, consistent range of motion and positioning would later enhance general care and rehabilitation outcome. As early as the 1960's, Bobath[1] advocated that nurses and therapists should develop cooperative relations at the ICU and acute floor levels. Building a bridge of understanding and cooperation between nurses and therapists required careful diplomacy and patience. Despite graphic instructions on the walls over patients' beds, continuity of positioning care was poor. Abnormal postures became habitual, and the limitations of contractures hindered mobility long down the rehabilitation road. Today, it is not uncommon to see multisensory stimulation programs undertaken by the rehabilitation staff in the ICU. In fact, it is generally accepted that this practice is beneficial overall, though there may be some question whether physiological or biochemical benefit is derived for persons with severe diffuse traumatic brain injury.[8]

The "brain injury unit", as an important, separate, and distinct unit, was not prevalent in general or acute rehabilitation hospitals prior to the 1980's. A focused, comprehensive team approach was absent, and vital supportive components were missing. The various therapy departments represented distinct territories, each treating a designated anatomical portion of the patient. Speech and occupational therapists often bickered over the territory of oral feeding programs. Physical and occupational therapists did battle over the upper extremity, and some were concerned when a speech therapist would attempt to ambulate or transfer a patient during a session.

Physical rehabilitation essentially focused on strengthening the "good" side and rarely challenged the impaired or "bad" side. We neglected the potential of the patient as a "whole".

Bobath[1] warned of the inherent failure of this "compensatory rehabilitation" approach. Many therapists made assumptions about a patient's skills from the narrow view of the clinical setting rather than from a broader "real world" perspective.

Severe cognitive and perceptual deficits and inappropriate behaviors often overwhelmed the physical rehabilitation effort, and these patients were usually discharged due to "lack of progress", "lack of motivation", or as "uncooperative". Behavior modification training to support the treating staff was nonexistent. Therapies were frequently further hindered by use of psychoactive medications. TBI patients were often discharged to nursing homes or to locked psychiatric hospitals or, without other options, many were discharged to frightened families. The TBI patient was puzzling, and many wrong assumptions were made about the sequelae of brain injury. In the process, the notion that the person with acquired brain injury could not appreciably benefit from rehabilitation was perpetuated.

Meanwhile, emergency neurotrauma and neurosurgical technology dramatically improved as a result of the Korean conflict and the Vietnam experience. By the mid-1970's, the TBI survivor population was increasing, and the institutionalization of these patients became more and more unacceptable. Although early, aggressive involvement of therapists in the acute facility had not yet captured great enthusiasm, therapists began to question the old points of view and began to be truly challenged by TBI patients. By the late 1970's, a handful of therapists dedicated themselves to organizing a postacute TBI rehabilitation environment. These people knew inherently that they could expand the horizon for this special population and, soon, their vision became a reality. A chance for "life" after head injury was coming into view.

In the early 1980's, professional attendance at the first TBI conferences and response to initial publications revealed an intensified international interest. Jennett and Teasdale[9] and Rosenthal et al.[10] brought the broad scope of TBI into clearer view and the idea of continuity of care to our attention. During this time, many postacute admissions presented with unnecessary contractures, unattended heterotopic ossification, misdiagnosed or ignored vestibular and oculomotor deficits, poorly defined cognitive deficits, and polypharmacy for aggressive behaviors. Until the mid-1980's, many postacute TBI clients lost valuable time, at tremendous expense, due to the fact that they required "reconstructive therapy." This loss ultimately reflected a less-than-optimal outcome. Although it was a frustrating time for clients and therapists, many knew that more could be accomplished.

During this time, the expansion of a continuity of rehabilitation care from the acute through the postacute directed many therapists to reflect on the seemingly obscure lessons of the past. New enthusiasm for Bobath's[1] teachings and Ayres'[7] concept of sensory integration emerged. The notion of hierarchical development in the human being was revisited. Therapeutic intervention was noted to be more successful when directed in the appropriate developmental order. The complex nature of TBI residuals requires, and was recognized to benefit from, an organized, integrated, progressive approach which utilizes theories and treatments from all rehabilitation disciplines.[11] Alternative views regarding posture and movement control emerged and gave therapists fresh avenues through which to evaluate and treat balance and movement deficits.[7,12-14]

By 1990, increasing involvement of therapists during the acute stage was evidenced. Recent authors point out that *good preventative care must begin at the acute level* for the severely brain-injured patient.[15-17] As a result, early and consistent positioning, use of inhibitory and facilitatory techniques, and orienting activation of the TBI patient are provided.[18,19] Greater focus is now placed on treatment team communication and cooperation. The "brain injury unit" offers a more structured and less distracting rehabilitation environment within the acute setting. Supportive systems to address aggressive and other inappropriate behaviors now assist staff in the acute rehabilitation facility. The results of all these efforts are reflected in the patient's subsequent improved status when discharged from the acute phase and admitted to postacute rehabilitation.

Sazbon and Groswasser[20] reviewed TBI sequelae in relation to the length of postcomatose unawareness (PCU) relative to physical rehabilitation. The review of 72 patients with postcomatose unawareness periods of greater than one month showed that approximately one third of all patients achieved full ambulation, 38.9% achieved aided ambulation, and 27.8% required wheelchairs for mobility. The patients were classified into four groups according to length of postcomatose unawareness. Of those patients in PCU for 31–60 days, 55.2% progressed to full ambulation, 34.2% to aided ambulation, and 10.5% to wheelchair mobility. Conversely, of those patients who fell into the PCU group of 91–180 days, only 10% progressed to full ambulation, 20% to aided ambulation, and 70% to wheelchair mobility. Since PCU is, essentially, a manifestation of severity of injury, it can be seen that the more severely injured individuals were, not surprisingly, the individuals most likely to present in physical and occupational therapies with long-term rehabilitation needs. These patients were also the most likely to have significant problems with aphasia, speech disorders, behavior disturbances, and cognitive disturbances.

It is becoming common practice for physical and occupational therapists to consult with pharmacists and physicians about medications administered to their patients. With feedback from therapists about the positive or negative impact of medications on therapeutic efforts, physicians have been able to make better choices. For example, they have found that, in many situations, antispasticity or psychoactive medications can be avoided with appropriate treatment approaches by well-trained and supported therapists[18,21] (see Chapter 10 in this volume for information on behavior management) except in cases of severe spasticity, flaccidity, or behavioral disturbance. Severe spasticity which is not amenable to therapeutic or conventional pharmacological management has been demonstrated to respond well to intrathecal baclofen (Lioresal®*) management.[22] Flaccidity has been treated successfully with conventional techniques, EMG/biofeedback,[23] and, in some cases, administration of dopaminergic medications such as Sinemet®**.[24-26] Cooperative effort between physicians, nurses, psychologists, and therapists has greatly enhanced patient progress.

As TBI patients are provided excellent early acute rehabilitative care, they move into the postacute phase as "clients" with greater potential for progress. Now, the level of expectation of both the postacute therapist and the TBI client has been raised. The therapeutic approach (how) and the environment (where) become influential factors to successful outcomes. In this process, the ultimate exchange occurs as the client learns and teaches as much as the therapist teaches and learns.

The postacute rehabilitation experience is at its best when provided in environmentally valid settings with teams experienced in comprehensive neurorehabilitation working with the client and family toward a common goal. With a broader and more realistic scope of treatment settings, therapists are allowed to more fully challenge their clients. Intensified treatment, with graded structure and proper generalization of skills, translates into shorter lengths of stay, reduced costs, and more favorable outcomes.

Purpose and Focus

A truly comprehensive postacute TBI rehabilitation program is qualified to admit a broad range of clients, and therapists must treat clients with severe, moderate, or mild levels of disability. A severely impaired client may have significant sensorimotor, perceptual, language/communication, and cognitive deficits and may be wheelchair-bound, have a gastrostomy, and be incontinent. A severe level of disability can also include the ambulatory, physically functioning client who is significantly confused and behaviorally difficult. The moderately impaired individual may have some perceptual and cognitive deficits while being capable of independent ambulation and performance of simple ADL's with supervision.

---

* Medtronic, Inc., Minneapolis, MN.
** DuPont Pharmaceuticals, Wilmington, DE.

The person suffering sequelae from mild traumatic brain injury (MTBI), also known as *postconcussion syndrome,* may not routinely appear as an early referral to the TBI rehabilitation program. It is more likely that this client will be first referred to and treated by an orthopedic therapist for commonly associated musculoskeletal complaints. It is important to question subtle or occasionally bizarre complaints from these clients and make appropriate referral for assessment and treatment. This cooperative effort will prevent a comparatively minor injury from becoming a catastrophic one.

Brain-injured persons may be two weeks or two years, or more, postinjury upon admission to postacute rehabilitation programming. They may be directly admitted from the acute hospital or may come from home, a psychiatric hospital, a nursing home, or another postacute program. TBI may be combined with various levels of spinal cord injuries, unresolved orthopedic/neurosurgical injuries, and diseases or dysfunctions of various systems. Consequently, the evaluative process and the management of the residual physical deficits need to be thorough and capable of addressing neurological, musculoskeletal, psychological, cognitive, and behavioral influences to physical functioning.

The purpose of this chapter is to offer some practical information to physical and occupational therapists treating TBI clients at the postacute rehabilitation level. The focus of this chapter is to address the continuum of evaluation and management of residual physical deficits which complicate the postacute phase of recovery. Although it may appear that specific areas of evaluation and treatment have been designated to the PT or the OT, there is no intent to imply that these designations are, necessarily, as described. The important point is that every area must be appropriately evaluated and aggressively treated by the best therapist for the task.

THE EVALUATIVE PROCESS

The purpose of a complete evaluation is to identify both obvious and subtle deficits in order to set the stage for an effective continuum of treatment and achievement of realistic goals. It is important to not only evaluate problem areas, but to evaluate all systems for proper identification and treatment of specific deficits within those systems.[11] The therapist is a teacher, but the teacher must be able to identify the "component(s) of a skill that is missing or that is preventing the client from accomplishing the task".[18] It is not uncommon in the TBI population to encounter persons with seemingly more advanced skills than are actually present. A good example can be found in the person who is able to ambulate reasonably well but testing of protective reactions demonstrates these reactions to be delayed. Such a person is in greater jeopardy for reinjury following a loss of balance or a fall.

In an efficient admission to the postacute TBI rehab program, the therapeutic team will be informed in advance about the client's injury, medical and early rehabilitation histories, and will be given a glimpse into the preinjury history and lifestyle prior to the commencement of the individual's therapy. Recommendations, pertinent factors to explore, and discussion of possible discharge options should be reviewed prior to admission. The collection and presentation of this information should be provided by experienced field evaluators (see Chapter 1 in this volume).

All therapists should be able to recognize the influence of various cognitive deficits which impact the client's ability to problem solve, organize, and sequence motor acts. The rehabilitation team needs to understand impairments in perception and integration of the senses influencing movement, balance, and position in space.

Agitation or otherwise inappropriate behaviors can seriously hinder progress. Therefore, proper staff training and effective approaches to behavior management should be expected in a comprehensive TBI program (see Chapter 10 in this volume). Behavioral deficits are fairly common sequelae in TBI. Many persons are tactilely defensive and/or easily overstimulated by even modest amounts of stimuli. Disorientation adds to the likelihood that verbal or physical aggression or withdrawal from treatment will occur. The proximity of physical and occupational therapy treatments, together with the factors above, makes it quite likely that therapists in physical rehabilitation will require substantial behavioral intervention.

Behavioral programming should be superimposed on treatment in either physical or occupational therapy. Application of defined behavioral strategies and programs can be best achieved in tandem with physical rehabilitation programming. Occasionally, it will be necessary for behavioral programming to supplant other programming; however, careful monitoring should be conducted to ensure that rehabilitation programming is undertaken as soon as possible. It is not realistic, nor necessary, for behavioral issues to be completely resolved prior to initiation or continuation of rehabilitation programming. In fact, there are very few instances where rehabilitation programming should be deemed "nonfeasible" due to behavioral deficits.

Emotional problems may manifest in problems with cooperation or motivation. It is hoped a team member is available to assist in the address of such problems; however, the physical or occupational therapist may become the de facto counselor to the brain-injured person. Often, the intimacy of the physical rehabilitation treatment setting allows for the breakdown of psychological defense mechanisms or allows the development of a level of trust and understanding which will allow access to the person's emotional status. Overall, discussion amongst team members will allow for all aspects of the clinical presentation to be shared and treatment approaches to be developed by the appropriate discipline.

As the client enters the initial PT and OT evaluation sessions, the therapist should explore him as a whole. There should be no assumptions made about functional skills despite the report of previous diagnoses, treatment records, or initial appearances. Such premature assumptions can lead to inappropriate or absent treatment.[27]

Evaluation should be performed in a variety of clinical, residential, and community settings. Although personal, lifestyle, and medical histories were introduced in the preadmission information, the initial session should still allow time for getting acquainted. During this interaction, trust and understanding should be nurtured. To signify respect, the therapist should attempt to explain the purpose of each test or exercise and relate it to tasks in daily life. Most clients will respond to this type of interaction and will probably attempt to rise to a realistic level of expectation. A vital aspect of the therapist's role is that of motivator.

The evaluation should be thorough and well-documented in quantitative and qualitative terms. Utilization of videotape is an excellent tool to assist in recording the client's performance progress from evaluation throughout treatment to discharge. If the client is unable to follow directions or is uncooperative, document observations of how the client functions. For example, in an evaluation of a client who was heavily medicated, depressed, and unable to respond to usual evaluative techniques, the client was asked to tie his shoe. After a significant delay, presumably for processing, the client sat down in a chair, slowly brought his left leg to his right knee, and tied the shoe. Observation allowed for comment about probable range of motion impairments, at least, for the observed joints in movement, dexterity, truncal flexibility, strength of the left hip and knee flexors, and antigravity muscle groups during standing. There were no obvious impairments of gait, other than speed. Flexibility of the trunk was demonstrated by reaching to tie the shoe during sitting. Obvious impairments of dexterity, possibly related to medication, were observed as well. It was also obvious that the client was able to respond to a verbal command, was able to follow through, did not demonstrate evidence of apraxia, and was cooperative within his capabilities. When the ability to respond becomes more appropriate, more conventional testing can be performed and documented.[28-31]

The neurological rehabilitation field is currently responding to an increasing demand for assessment tools to provide better documentation of functional skills and outcomes.[29,32,33] Such assessments as the Barthel Index,[34] the Disability Rating Scale,[35] the Tuft's Assessment of Motor Performance (TAMP),[36] the Tinetti Performance-Oriented Assessments of Mobility,[37] and the Functional Independence Measurement (FIM)[38] have been utilized. More recently, "functional status measurements" are being developed to measure performance during daily activity which includes cognitive, social, and psychological functioning.[27] Therapists should be acquainted with these measures and should choose the most appropriate tool for the level of client and the information desired. Rating systems provide ongoing comparative data to review the flow of progress.

Additional information can be obtained from pertinent family members.[39,40] Their insights about the client's previous lifestyle and their perception of changes since the injury can reveal information which may help the therapist to understand and, perhaps, enhance motivation. Also, in appropriate situations, the family can be included in treatment sessions so as to educate and prepare them as potential participants in the client's future discharge environment.

During the initial interview, the therapist may wish to expand upon preadmission information by exploring the client's perception of the accident. Indications of retrograde or anterograde amnesia may be detected. If available, the family may provide their perceptions or additional insights for a confused or otherwise noncommunicative client. Documentation should include review of preinjury and postinjury history of fractures, surgeries, medications, and visual and/or auditory dysfunctions.

The subjective review should also include the client's perception of current symptoms and any changes in activity levels which may be related to endurance, musculoskeletal complaints, sensorimotor deficits, pain, or vestibular dysfunction as they impact the person's quality of life. The person should also be asked to provide the therapist with an understanding of both short- and long-term goals for treatment. As the client relates problems in a given area, it may be helpful to provide a checklist (Figure 13.1) to further elicit information about the nature of the problem prior to evaluation.

Range of Motion and Dexterity

A thorough evaluation and documentation of active and passive hip, knee, ankle, and cervical/lumbar spine ranges of motion must be conducted. Evaluation should also review upper extremity ranges of motion, including the shoulders, elbows, wrists, and fingers. Documentation (Figure 13.2) of flexibility should include an assessment of the hamstrings, the gastrocnemius (with the knee extended), Thomas test, long sitting, trunk extension in the prone position, and trunk flexion from a seated position.

When evaluating upper extremity and hand function, hand dominance should be documented. Observe the client's ability to control gross grasp and release and perform lateral pinch, tripod pinch, and palmar prehension. Upper extremity and hand function are further observed for the ability to hold, stabilize, and carry a variety of both light and heavy objects. Gross motor coordination of the upper extremity can be documented during timed performance testing via the Box and Block Test of manual dexterity.[41]

Fine motor coordination and selective movements are assessed during timed performance tests (e.g. the Nine Hole Peg Test[42] or a Twenty Hole Peg expanded version) and through functional task observation. The Jebson Hand Function Test[43] measures prehension and nonprehension tasks of both hands. The Purdue Pegboard[44] and the Minnesota Rate of Manipulation[45] are useful tests for the moderately or mildly impaired client. If desired, additional prevocational assessments of dexterity, cognitive, and perceptual functions can be attained with such tests as the Crawford Small Parts Dexterity Test[46] and the Bennett Hand Tool Dexterity Test.[47] Objects which are pertinent to the client's lifestyle should be used in the functional task evaluation, e.g. razors, toothbrushes, combs, buttons, zippers, eating utensils, pencils/pens, kitchen tools, cards, and work tools. Any complaints of pain, or observations of edema, tremors, or changes in muscle tone, should be documented.

The Neurological Examination

While the comprehensive neurological examination takes place in the initial field evaluation and, subsequently, by other treatment professionals (see Chapter 2 by Gelber in this volume),

A. **VESTIBULAR SYMPTOMS CHECKLIST**

 1.   Current symptoms:_____

 2.   Activity level change:_____

 3.   Rate baseline dizziness on a scale of 0-10:_____

 4.   Do any of the following activities make you dizzy?

     Yes   No

     _____   _____   riding on escalators

     _____   _____   riding in elevators

     _____   _____   walking up/down stairs

     _____   _____   walking in the dark

     _____   _____   walking on a busy street

     _____   _____   walking on grass or thick carpet

     _____   _____   driving in a car

     _____   _____   bending over

     _____   _____   grocery shopping

     _____   _____   making the bed

     _____   _____   getting into or out of bed

     _____   _____   rolling over in bed

     _____   _____   reaching up

 5.   Do you have a history of becoming motion sick prior to your injury?

         Y   N

B. **SELF-PERCEPTION:**

 1.   Self-Reported Deficits:_____
     _____
     _____

 2.   Self-Reported Goals:_____
     _____
     _____

C. **OTHER PERTINENT INFORMATION:**_____
     _____
     _____

FIGURE 13.1   Vestibular symptoms checklist: Used to collect initial evaluative information about the nature of problems from the client's perspective.

this does not relieve the need for further assessment by the OT and the PT. A focused neurological examination is necessary to look at those components that will be eventually addressed by the OT and the PT.

Sensation and Proprioception

Although the structure of documentation varies in each clinical setting, a complete sensory evaluation should be performed (Figure 13.3). Tactile sensation is tested for light/firm and sharp/dull discrimination and hot/cold temperature discrimination. Responses should be recorded

```
┌─────────────────────────────────────────────────────────────────────┐
│                         FLEXIBILITY EVALUATION                        │
├─────────────────────────────────────────────────────────────────────┤
│                                                                       │
│                                          LEFT              RIGHT       │
│                                                                       │
│   A.  HAMSTRING                       _____        _____     │
│   B.  THOMAS TEST                     _____        _____     │
│   C.  GASTROCNEMIUS (knee extended)   _____        _____     │
│   D.  LONG SIT TEST                         _____                  │
│   E.  PRONE TRUNK EXTENSION                 _____                  │
│   F.  SEATED FLEXION                        _____                  │
│                                                                       │
└─────────────────────────────────────────────────────────────────────┘
```

FIGURE 13.2   Flexibility evaluation form: Used to document information about the lower extremities and trunk.

as intact, hypersensitive, or impaired. Proprioception testing includes the ability to name movements, mirror movements, and detect vibration. Graphesthesia (the ability to identify numbers written on the skin by the examiner's finger) and stereognosis (the ability to identify objects by touch) should be tested and documented. Record responses to proprioceptive testing as intact or impaired.

Deep Tendon Reflexes and Pathological Reflexes

These reflexes influence responses to movement. Record responses to the Patellar and Achilles reflex tests as hyper (3+), normal (2+), hypo (1+), and absent (0) (Figure 13.4). The Babinski reflex should also be tested and recorded as present or absent.

Cerebellar Tests

Cerebellar reflexes have significant influence on the performance of smooth movements. Tests should include performances of 1) finger-to-finger, 2) finger-to-nose, and 3) heel-to-shin. Record findings as normal, hypermetric, ataxic, or with intention tremor (Figure 13.5). Diadokokinesis is tested symmetrically and asymmetrically and is recorded as normal, ataxic, or unable.

Urbscheit[14] discussed the frustration encountered by many therapists in the evaluation and treatment of cerebellar deficits. Many therapists are unable to adequately diagnose and treat cerebellar dysfunction. Swaine and Sullivan[48] reviewed interrater reliability for measurement of clinical features of finger-to-nose testing and reported fairly poor interrater reliability for determination of the presence of dysmetria. The therapist working with this population must become proficient in cerebellar evaluation and treatment.

The client must be observed for hypotonicity, dysmetria, difficulty with rapid alternating movements, and movement decomposition. These deficits may be observed in gait, pace of gait, and activities of daily living (ADL's), e.g. brushing teeth, stirring food, eating, or trying to walk at a fast pace. Complaints of difficulties with vision while the client is in motion may be related to cerebellar dysfunction as well as vestibular dysfunction.

The Manual Muscle Test, Tone, and Muscle Endurance

Muscle testing is performed not only to evaluate a muscle group's ability to produce force against gravity, but also the person's ability to isolate a muscle's movement and force. Manual

---

NEUROLOGICAL EVALUATION

I. SENSATION

		UPPER EXTREMITY		LOWER EXTREMITY	
		LEFT	RIGHT	LEFT	RIGHT
A.	Light/Firm	Intact Hyper Impaired	Intact Hyper Impaired	Intact Hyper Impaired	Intact Hyper Impaired
B.	Sharp/Dull	Intact Hyper Impaired	Intact Hyper Impaired	Intact Hyper Impaired	Intact Hyper Impaired
C.	Hot/Cold	Intact Hyper Impaired	Intact Hyper Impaired	Intact Hyper Impaired	Intact Hyper Impaired

II. PROPRIOCEPTION

		UPPER EXTREMITY		LOWER EXTREMITY	
		LEFT	RIGHT	LEFT	RIGHT
A.	Naming Movements	Intact Impaired	Intact Impaired	Intact Impaired	Intact Impaired
B.	Mirroring Movements	Intact Impaired	Intact Impaired	Intact Impaired	Intact Impaired
C.	Vibration	Intact Impaired	Intact Impaired	Intact Impaired	Intact Impaired
D.	Graphesthesia	Intact Impaired	Intact Impaired	Intact Impaired	Intact Impaired
E.	Stereognosis	Intact Impaired	Intact Impaired	Intact Impaired	Intact Impaired

FIGURE 13.3   Neurological evaluation form: Used to document sensory and proprioceptive functions.

muscle tests document strengths in musculature of the neck, shoulders, arms, hands, hips, knees, ankles, abdominals, and trunk extensors.

Muscle tone may remain a factor significantly influencing movement. In initial observations, many clients seem to have minimal to nil abnormal tone. However, the client should be closely observed during active functional movements. This is another reason for evaluating the client while performing functions in various environments. The evaluation should begin with an analysis of the motor control present in each extremity. Keenan and Perry[49] provide a useful schema for classifying motor control based upon description of the type of control observed. Hypotonicity with no active motion is classified as "Flaccid" and is Grade 1. A spastic, rigid extremity without any volitional or reflexive movement is classified as "Rigid" and Grade 2. Patterned or synergistic motor control which occurs as a mass flexion or

REFLEX TESTING

I. DEEP TENDON REFLEXES

A. Patellar

Left	Hyper (3 +)	Normal (2 +)	Hypo (1 +)	Absent (0)
Right	Hyper (3 +)	Normal (2 +)	Hypo (1 +)	Absent (0)

B. Achilles

Left	Hyper (3 +)	Normal (2 +)	Hypo (1 +)	Absent (0)
Right	Hyper (3 +)	Normal (2 +)	Hypo (1 +)	Absent (0)

II. PATHOLOGICAL REFLEXES

A. Babinski Reflex

Left	Absent	Present
Right	Absent	Present

FIGURE 13.4   Reflex testing form: Used to document reflex testing information.

CEREBELLAR TESTS

A. Finger - Finger

Left	Normal	Hypermetric	Ataxic	Int. Tremor
Right	Normal	Hypermetric	Ataxic	Int. Tremor

B. Finger - Nose

Left	Normal	Hypermetric	Ataxic	Int. Tremor
Right	Normal	Hypermetric	Ataxic	Int. Tremor

C. Heel - Shin

Left	Normal	Hypermetric	Ataxic	Int. Tremor
Right	Normal	Hypermetric	Ataxic	Int. Tremor

D. Diadokokinesis

Symmetrical	Normal	Ataxic	Unable
Asymmetrical	Normal	Ataxic	Unable

FIGURE 13.5   Cerebellar tests form: Used to document cerebellar functions.

extension and only in response to a noxious stimulus is classified "Reflexive mass pattern" and Grade 3. Patterned or synergistic movement which can be at least volitionally initiated is classified as "Volitional mass pattern" and Grade 4. Grades 1 through 4 are quite primitive and of no functional use in the upper extremity. When motor control is classified as "Selective with pattern overlay", movement can be initiated in specific joints with minimal overflow to

---

MUSCLE ENDURANCE

1. TRUNK ENDURANCE

   Sit-Ups   _____ repetitions   (1 minute)

   Push-Ups   _____ repetitions   (maximum)

   Bridging   _____ seconds   (norm: 1 minute)

   Hyperextension   _____ seconds   (norm: 1 minute)

---

2. LOWER EXTREMITY ENDURANCE

   Wall Slide (90⁰/90⁰)   _____ seconds   (norm: 1 minute)

   Airdyne bike
   (Goal: 1.5 kps, 12 minutes) _____ kps   _____ minutes

   RPE   @ 1 minute   _____
                               @ 6 minutes   _____
                               @ 12 minutes   _____

	Heart Rate	Blood Pressure
Pre-exercise	_____ bpm	_____/_____ mm/Hg
Post-exercise	_____ bpm	_____/_____ mm/Hg
Post-exercise: 1 minute	_____ bpm	_____/_____ mm/Hg

   If exercise is stopped before 12 minute mark:
       What caused you to stop exercise?
       1. Fatigue   (location: _____)
       2. Pain   (location: _____)
       3. Other   (describe: _____)

FIGURE 13.6   Muscle endurance form: Used to document trunk, lower extremity, and cardiovascular endurance.

adjacent joints and is Grade 5. Volitional control of individual joints independently of adjacent joints is classified as "Selective" and is Grade 6.

Observations pertaining to lack of movement or minimal movement, in particular in cases where the dopaminergic system may have been impacted by the injury, may suggest the application of dopaminergic medication to enhance motor function. Conversely, persons who present with significant spasticity will generally not benefit from such an approach. The response of spasticity to stretching, relaxation, positioning, and medication will need to be explored together with an appraisal of the likelihood of response to chemical neurolysis and casting. Spasticity should be differentiated from rigidity in the hypertonic patient. Rigidity may respond to dopaminergic drugs, whereas spasticity may be worsened. The PT and OT can provide quite valuable information to the physician in these arenas. The influence of emotion, pain, fatigue, and varying demands of motion and posture should be considered in evaluation of movement.

Muscle endurance of the trunk and lower extremities is also assessed by the PT. Trunk endurance (Figure 13.6) testing documents the maximum number of sit-ups performed in one minute and the maximum number of push-ups the client is able to produce. Bridging and hyperextension are each sustained as long as possible (Figure 13.6). Acceptable performance is

---

* Schwinn Bicycle Co.

considered to be one minute for each. Lower extremity endurance can be tested with the Wall Slide Test, and cardiovascular endurance with the stationary Airdyne®* bike test (Figure 13.6).

Differential diagnosis of cardiorespiratory endurance problems and vestibular dysfunction cannot be undertaken completely at this point in the evaluation; however, findings of nystagmus during testing may point to vestibular dysfunction and should be noted for consideration during subsequent vestibular testing.

Mobility Evaluation

Although the majority of severely disabled TBI persons may have become quite mobile during the acute rehabilitation stay, there will be an occasional need for full evaluation of bed mobility, transfers, tub/shower, and wheelchair skills. In the residential setting, most people will be able to sleep in standard double size (or larger) beds. Bathrooms should be an appropriate size and equipped for wheelchair, walker, or cane mobility.

Beyond the expected physical components for bed mobilization and bed/tub/toilet transfers, other areas which impact mobility, such as cognitive abilities, safety judgment, and systems impacting postural control, should be observed and documented. The evaluation should document the client's ability to perform the tasks independently or with assistance and include notation of the quality of performance.

Bed mobility (Figure 13.7) explores scooting up and down as well as to the right or left sides. Is the client able to turn him/herself to either side and attain sitting and supine positions? Wheelchair mobility (Figure 13.7) assessments include the client's ability to mobilize on even and uneven surfaces, inclines and declines, through doorways, and over curbs. Note the approximate height of the curb and time to cover specific distances.

Document the client's preparation for transfer (Figure 13.7). Record any need for verbal and/or physical cues as well as the need for physical assistance. Note performance in transferring from the wheelchair to a level surface, an elevated surface, the floor, and floor to wheelchair.

Observations of the client's general ability to ambulate should be documented (Figure 13.7) whether the individual has detectable mobility problems or appears quite normal. The evaluation should include observations from clinical, residential, and community settings. Observe and document ambulation indoors, outdoors, on uneven terrain, on inclines and declines, and negotiating curbs and stairs. Document the client's ability to rise from sitting to standing. Note the need for assistance and the use of any supportive devices.

When evaluating ambulatory skills, an initial impression of minimal or no obvious abnormalities may change when the situation moves from a well-lit, even-surfaced, clinical setting to a less ideal environment with low light and uneven terrain, i.e., darkened room with plush carpeting or evening time on grassy/rocky terrains. Impairments in sensorimotor and/or vestibular system-related performances may be revealed under more realistic and demanding circumstances. The evaluation may even be extended to include movement onto or off of escalators and into or out of elevators. Watch for a tendency to avoid or complain about tasks in noisy or busy environments. Subtle changes in fluidity of body movement during ambulation can point to vestibular, cerebullar, or oculomotor problems.

During ambulation evaluations, document reduced or absent reciprocal arm swing, slowed pace of walking, reduced head turning or visual scanning, drifting or "wall walking", and slight or obvious hesitancy when changing directions.

Posture and Gait Evaluation

Notations should be made regarding the client's posture during sitting and standing activities as well as any gait deviations.[50] Observations should also note apparent influences from muscle weakness, leg length discrepancies, pain, vestibular, cerebellar, or ocular dysfunctions,

---

MOBILITY EVALUATION

I. BED MOBILITY   <u>Assist</u>   <u>Quality</u>

    A.   Scooting
          1. Up   _____   _____
          2. Down   _____   _____
          3. Left   _____   _____
          4. Right   _____   _____
    B.   1/2 Rolls
          1. Left   _____   _____
          2. Right   _____   _____
    C.   Attain Sitting   _____   _____
    D.   Attain Supine   _____   _____

II. WHEELCHAIR MOBILITY   <u>Assist</u>   <u>Quality</u>

    A.   Even Surfaces   _____   _____
    B.   Uneven Surfaces   _____   _____
    C.   Inclines   _____   _____
    D.   Declines   _____   _____
    E.   Doorways   _____   _____
    F.   Curbs   _____ inches   _____   _____

III. TRANSFERS   <u>Assist</u>   <u>Quality</u>

    A.   Preparation   _____   _____
    B.   Wheelchair to level surface   _____   _____
    C.   Wheelchair to elevated surface   _____   _____
    D.   Wheelchair to floor   _____   _____
    E.   Floor to wheelchair   _____   _____

IV. AMBULATION   <u>Assist</u>   <u>Quality</u>

    A.   Sit to stand   _____   _____
    B.   Assistive device   _____   _____
    C.   Indoors   _____   _____
    D.   Outdoors   _____   _____
    E.   Uneven terrain   _____   _____
    F.   Inclines/declines   _____   _____
    G.   Curbs   _____   _____
    H.   Stairs   _____   _____

FIGURE 13.7 Mobility evaluation form: Used to collect information on bed, wheelchair, transfer, and ambulation activities.

cognitive/perceptual deficits, poor endurance, loss of flexibility, and impairments in somatosensory functions.[13,14,18,51,52]

Neurodevelopmental Sequence Evaluation

To gather a baseline on a variety of movement patterns, the neurodevelopmental sequence is a good place to start. Assessment of the motorically intact client is just as important as assessing the motorically impaired client. Omission of this evaluation for high level clients may prevent observations of subtle deficits in sensorimotor integration. Observe closely for inefficient movement patterns.

NEURODEVELOPMENTAL SEQUENCE EVALUATION

		Assist	Quality
I.	**LOG ROLLING** A. Left B. Right	_____ _____	_____ _____
II.	**PRONE ON ELBOWS** A. Assume B. Maintain	_____ _____	_____ _____
III.	**QUADRUPED** A. Assume B. Maintain	_____ _____	_____ _____
IV.	**CONTRALATERAL BALANCE** A. Left Knee B. Right Knee	_____ _____	_____ sec. _____ sec.
V.	**IPSILATERAL BALANCE** A. Left Knee B. Right Knee	_____ _____	_____ sec. _____ sec.
VI.	**RECIPROCAL CRAWLING** A. Forward B. Backward	_____ _____	_____ _____
VII.	**TALL KNEEL** A. Assume B. Maintain C. Weight Shift	_____ _____ _____	_____ _____ _____
VIII.	**KNEE WALK** A. Forward B. Backward	_____ _____	_____ _____

IX.	**HALF KNEEL**
	 A. Assume Left Knee
	               Right Knee
	 B. Maintain Left Knee
	               Right Knee
		_____
		 _____
		 _____
		 _____
			_____
			 _____
			 _____
			 _____

X.	**HALF KNEEL TO STAND** A. Left Foot B. Right Foot	_____ _____	_____ _____

FIGURE 13.8 Neurodevelopmental sequence evaluation form: Used to document information on various movements through the sequence.

The ability to perform independently or with assistance is recorded as well as the quality of performance. Video recording of this initial evaluation further documents quality of performance. Of course, recording is repeated at various intervals throughout the treatment process.

The evaluation follows a very basic sequence of movement patterns (Figure 13.8). It begins with log rolling to both sides. Next, observe the client's ability to assume and maintain a prone-on-elbows position followed by the quadruped or all-fours position. Contralateral (Figure 13.9-A) and ipsilateral (Figure 13.9-B) positions are assumed next and the maintained positions are timed. Reciprocal crawling is observed forward and backward. Tall-kneel position is observed for the ability to assume and maintain the position as well as the ability to weight shift. Knee walking is also observed in forward and backward. The half-kneel position is assumed and maintained for both sides. The half-kneel-to-stand position is also observed from both sides.

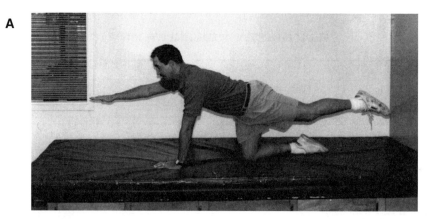

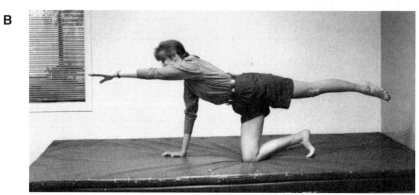

FIGURE 13.9   (A) Illustration of contralateral position in the neurodevelopmental sequence. (Photo courtesy James
E. Eaton.) (B) Illustration of ipsilateral position in the neurodevelopmental sequence. (Photo
courtesy Lynda R. Eaton.)

Vestibular Evaluation

It has already been pointed out that an important aspect of the evaluation is to identify subtle
deficits impacting upon oculomotor, gross motor, and ADL performance. Proper identification of the problem leads to a better choice of treatment avenues. Assessment should include
walking tests, postrotary nystagmus, and provoked vertigo testing. The walking tests begin
with evaluation for Romberg's sign, wherein balance is assessed in standing with the eyes
closed, head in neutral, feet together, and arms outstretched and together in front of the patient
at shoulder level. Be sure to spot the patient during all these evaluations to prevent injury from
falling. The Unterberger's sign is evaluated by asking the person to march in place with eyes
closed. The person should not rotate or drift in either direction. Rotation or drift generally
occurs toward the side of lesion. The Walking Test is performed with eyes closed. The person
is asked to walk forward ten to twelve feet and reverses direction, when the therapist touches
the chest, for the same distance. The forward/backward motion is repeated at least five times
and observation is made of deviation from the straight line. Deviation occurs generally toward
the side of lesion. Care should be taken to disallow the influence of light or sound sources
which may facilitate spatial orientation despite the eyes being closed.

Postrotary nystagmus can be clinically evaluated in a motorized or nonmotorized rotary
chair. The person is placed in the chair and rotated, with eyes open, for ten rotations at a
moderate pace (30–45 rpm). The eyes are viewed for nystagmus, and the duration and
direction of nystagmus are noted. The procedure is performed in both directions. The norm
for duration of nystagmus is 20 to 30 seconds. Provoked vertigo testing rates dizziness

---

VESTIBULAR EVALUATION

I. WALKING TESTS
    A. Romberg's Sign: Positive   Negative
    B. Unterberger's Sign (stepping):   Positive   Negative
                                              R / L _____ °
    C. Walking Test (stars):   Positive   Negative
                                              R / L _____ °

II. POSTROTARY NYSTAGMUS
    A. Clockwise: _____   Norms: 20 to 30 seconds
    B. Counterclockwise: _____

III. PROVOKED VERTIGO (Vestibular Sensitivity Scale)
     Score: Intensity: 0-10
             Duration: 0 = 0 sec., 1 = 1-10 sec.,   2 = 10-30 sec., 3 = 30-60 sec., 4 = 60 sec. +

	Intensity	Duration
1. Baseline (seated)	0 1 2 3 4 5 6 7 8 9 10	0 1 2 3 4
2. Head - Look Right	0 1 2 3 4 5 6 7 8 9 10	0 1 2 3 4
3. Head - Look Left	0 1 2 3 4 5 6 7 8 9 10	0 1 2 3 4
4. Head - Look Up	0 1 2 3 4 5 6 7 8 9 10	0 1 2 3 4
5. Head - Look Down	0 1 2 3 4 5 6 7 8 9 10	0 1 2 3 4
6. Head - Look to Side	0 1 2 3 4 5 6 7 8 9 10	0 1 2 3 4
7. Head - Up & Down	0 1 2 3 4 5 6 7 8 9 10	0 1 2 3 4
8. Sit to Supine	0 1 2 3 4 5 6 7 8 9 10	0 1 2 3 4
9. Roll to Right	0 1 2 3 4 5 6 7 8 9 10	0 1 2 3 4
10. Roll to Left	0 1 2 3 4 5 6 7 8 9 10	0 1 2 3 4
11. Supine to Sit	0 1 2 3 4 5 6 7 8 9 10	0 1 2 3 4
12. Bend to Floor - Left -Head Down	0 1 2 3 4 5 6 7 8 9 10	0 1 2 3 4
13. Return to Vertical	0 1 2 3 4 5 6 7 8 9 10	0 1 2 3 4
14. Bend to Floor - Right - Head Down	0 1 2 3 4 5 6 7 8 9 10	0 1 2 3 4
15. Return to Vertical	0 1 2 3 4 5 6 7 8 9 10	0 1 2 3 4
16. Sit to Stand	0 1 2 3 4 5 6 7 8 9 10	0 1 2 3 4

Total Points: V.S.S.
          Intensity _____ + 150 = _____
                                                    + _____ = _____ + 2 = _____
          Duration   _____ + 60 = _____

FIGURE 13.10 Vestibular evaluation form: Used to score the vestibular sensitivity scale.

intensity and duration as reported by the patient following each of the listed maneuvers. The total points for intensity is divided by 150 and added to the total points for duration divided by 60. The resulting number is divided by two to reach a Vestibular Sensitivity Scale score.[53] Figure 13.10 illustrates a convenient form for information collection during this phase of evaluation.

The therapist should be trained in the assessment and treatment of various vestibular dysfunctions,[13,54-56] though much of the training in this subject matter is available largely through postgraduate coursework. Lingering problems related to balance, postural control, and spatial orientation can disable any TBI client. The reader is directed to Chapter 6 of this volume. Assessment and treatment approaches are excellently reviewed and clearly demonstrated and, therefore, will not be discussed herein.

Sensorimotor Integration and Dynamic Balance Evaluations

In a normal central nervous system, purposeful activity of the extremities depends upon the stabilization of the trunk. When postural control is maintained, significant influence is exerted on limb tone, range of motion, and control.[50] However, the client with moderate to severe sensorimotor impairment may find that extremity movement is less than functional when selective movement is reduced to gross movement patterns influenced by primitive reflexes.

The ability to maintain standing balance in static or dynamic conditions requires the complex interaction of several systems — vision, vestibular, and somatosensory systems. However, these systems must be coupled with appropriate motor programs, muscle contractions, body alignment, and ranges of motion to allow for smooth and well-coordinated, purposeful movements.

The sensorimotor integration evaluation considers the manner in which postural control, reflexes, and feedback from vision, vestibular, and proprioceptive systems impact upon motor control and programming. The evaluation should, therefore, document postural control in sitting and standing (Figure 13.11). In the sitting position, observe the client's body alignment. While the client is sitting, note responses to weight shifting in lateral and anterior/posterior directions. While the client orients the head, rights the trunk, or resumes the vertical position, note the direction of shift. Notice responses to dizziness, dysequilibrium, and protective responses.

The Tinetti Performance-Oriented Assessment of Mobility[37] includes an assessment of balance deficits in more impaired clients during movement in functional tasks. The assessment calls for observation of the client during sitting, arising, standing, and walking. Balance reactions are also observed while the client turns around (360 degrees), sits down, and attempts single-foot support. The test provides a scoring system for comparative data. As the client reaches scoring criteria, they can be advanced to more appropriate tests.

Persons without severe impairments to postural control and balance/coordination may also benefit from evaluation of sensorimotor integration (Figure 13.11).[57,58] In the standing position, balance skills can be evaluated through observation of postural control strategies used during both active and induced weight shifts as well as standing one-foot balance evaluation. Observation of active weight shifts (initiated by the client) to anterior/posterior and lateral positions assesses the client's use of ankle, hip, stepping, or other types of postural control strategies. Presence or absence of dizziness is noted. Induced weight shifts (imposed by the examiner) measure the same positions.

Standing one-foot balance is measured by the length of time maintained and the postural control strategy utilized (i.e., ankle, hip, stepping, or other) should be noted. Give the client two to three trials and average the times. Sensory organization, that is, the integration of proprioceptive and vestibular input, is measured by timing and the amount of sway with eyes open and eyes closed on a firm surface and on a foam surface. Care should be taken to disallow any potential for orientation which might be available from a continuous light or sound source during balance and sensorimotor testing (Figure 13.11).

The dynamic balance evaluation (Figure 13.12) again documents the type of postural control strategy (ankle, hip, stepping, falls) used in dynamic gait activities, heel-toe ambulation, balance beam ambulation, winding strip ambulation, and step-ups. The dynamic gait activity task involves walking forward for twelve feet to an abrupt stop. Note the postural control strategy utilized and complaints of dizziness. Next, have the client walk forward for twelve feet and, then, sharply pivot to the right. Repeat to the left. Note the strategy utilized and any complaint of dizziness. The final dynamic gait activity task involves walking with the head moving first horizontally and then repeated with the head moving vertically. Note the strategy utilized and any complaint of dizziness.

```
┌─────────────────────────────────────────────────────────────────────────┐
│                  SENSORIMOTOR INTEGRATION EVALUATION                      │
```

I. POSTURAL CONTROL

  A. Sitting:

    1. Alignment:

    2. Weight shifts:

		Eyes Open			Eyes Closed		
		Lateral	Ant/Post		Lateral	Ant/Post	
a.	Shifts Weight:	+	·	+	·	+	·	+	·
b.	Head Oriented:	+	·	+	·	+	·	+	·
c.	Trunk Righted:	+	·	+	·	+	·	+	·
d.	Resume Vertical:	+	·	+	·	+	·	+	·
e.	Dizziness:	+	·	+	·	+	·	+	·
f.	Dysequilibrium:	+	·	+	·	+	·	+	·
g.	Protective Response:	+	·	+	·	+	·	+	·

  B. Standing:

    1. Active weight shifts:

a.	Anterior/posterior:	ANKLE	HIP	STEPPING	OTHER
b.	Lateral:	ANKLE	HIP	STEPPING	OTHER
c.	Dizziness	YES	NO		
d.	Comments:				

    2. Induced weight shifts:

a.	Anterior/posterior:	ANKLE	HIP	STEPPING	OTHER
b.	Lateral:	ANKLE	HIP	STEPPING	OTHER
c.	Dizziness:	YES	NO		
d.	Comments:				

    3. Standing One-Foot Balance: A = Ankle   H = Hip   S = Stepping   O = Other

	Left		Right	
	Time	Strategy	Time	Strategy
Trial 1	___	___	___	___
Trial 2	___	___	___	___

    4. Sensory Organization: Time   Sway

a.	Eyes Open, Firm Surface	___	___
b.	Eyes Open, Foam Surface	___	___
c.	Eyes Closed, Firm Surface	___	___
d.	Eyes Closed, Foam Surface	___	___

FIGURE 13.11 Sensorimotor integration evaluation form: Used to document postural control in sitting and standing positions.

Heel-toe and balance beam ambulation evaluation should document required assistance levels and the quality of performance for going forward, backward, sideways, and during Carioca or braiding step maneuvers. The winding strip ambulation test (heel-toe walking following a piece of string or fabric laid out in a curvilinear fashion on the floor) (Figure 13.13) is conducted for forward, backward, and sideways walking. Step-ups are repeated 20 times, first leading with the left and then with the right. Note the time needed to perform this task. The careful notation of the times will provide a window on the progress of the improvement as it occurs.

DYNAMIC BALANCE EVALUATION

I.   DYNAMIC GAIT ACTIVITIES:

Strategy: A = Ankle   H = Hip   S = Stepping   F = Falls

		Strategy	Dizziness
A.	Walk 12 ft., stop abruptly	_____	_____
B.	Walk 12 ft., pivot sharply		
1.	Left	_____	_____
2.	Right	_____	_____
C.	Walk with head motion		
1.	Horizontal	_____	_____
2.	Vertical	_____	_____

II. HEEL-TOE AMBULATION:

		Assist	Quality
A.	Forward	_____	_____
B.	Backward	_____	_____
C.	Sideways	_____	_____
D.	Carioca	_____	_____

III. BALANCE BEAM AMBULATION:

		Assist	Quality
A.	Forward	_____	_____
B.	Backward	_____	_____
C.	Sideways	_____	_____
D.	Carioca	_____	_____

IV. WINDING STRIP AMBULATION:

		Assist	Quality
A.	Forward	_____	_____
B.	Backward	_____	_____
C.	Sideways	_____	_____

V.   STEP-UPS (20 repetitions)

		Assist	Time
A.	Left	_____	_____
B.	Right	_____	_____

FIGURE 13.12   Dynamic balance evaluation form: Used to document performances during dynamic activities.

Quick Reciprocal Movement Evaluation

For evaluation of higher level balance and coordination disorders, movements to be assessed include straddle jumps, straddle crosses, reciprocal jumping, pendulum, slalom (forward and backward), four-point, shuffling (left/right), running Carioca (left/right), skipping, and reciprocal marching (forward/backward) (Figure 13.14).

Straddle Jump

The *straddle jump* is performed beginning in a standing position with the feet together. The individual jumps from the feet-together position and lands with the feet separated via hip abduction as in a jumping jack exercise (Figure 13.15).

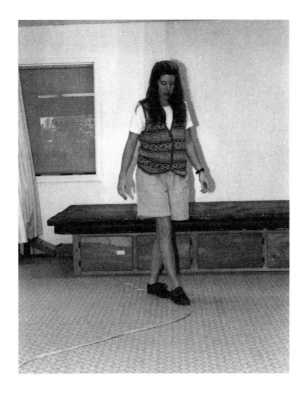

FIGURE 13.13   An illustration of the winding strip ambulation test. (Photo courtesy Caryn Murphy.)

Straddle Cross

The *straddle cross* is performed beginning in the same position as the straddle jump; however, rather than separating the feet while in the air, the individual crosses the feet and lands in a legs-scissored position. The second straddle cross reverses the front leg position with the back leg position (Figure 13.16).

Reciprocal Jumping

Reciprocal jumping is accomplished by beginning in a standing position with the feet together. The individual jumps and lands with one foot outstretched in a forward, hip-flexed position while the other foot is in a backward, hip-extended position. The arm swing should be reciprocal as in normal walking. The second reciprocal jump reverses the leg and arm positions (Figures 13.17-A and 13.17-B).

Pendulum

The *pendulum* maneuver is accomplished by beginning in the standing, feet-together position. The individual jumps kicking one leg into hip abduction, keeping the foot in the air and landing on the opposite foot. The second pendulum "swing" is accomplished by jumping and reversing leg/foot positions (Figure 13.18).

Slalom

The *slalom* exercise begins with standing in the feet-together position. The feet are kept together as the individual jumps and lands. The first jump places the feet off to the left and the second places the feet off to the right while maintaining an upright torso. The knees should

---

QUICK RECIPROCAL MOVEMENT EVALUATION

		Assist	Quality
I.	STRADDLE JUMPS:	_____	_____
II.	STRADDLE CROSSES:	_____	_____
III.	RECIPROCAL JUMPING:	_____	_____
IV.	PENDULUM:	_____	_____
V.	SLALOM:		
	A. Forward	_____	_____
	B. Backward	_____	_____
VI.	4-POINT:	_____	_____
VII.	SHUFFLING:		
	A. Left	_____	_____
	B. Right	_____	_____
VIII.	RUNNING CARIOCA:		
	A. Left	_____	_____
	B. Right	_____	_____
IX.	SKIPPING:	_____	_____
X.	RECIPROCAL MARCHING:		
	A. Forward	_____	_____
	B. Backward	_____	_____

FIGURE 13.14 Quick reciprocal movement evaluation form: Used to document performance of quick reciprocal movements.

be flexed and pointed forward. The feet positions are similar to those used in parallel turns while downhill skiing (Figures 13.19-A, 13.19-B, and 13.19-C).

Four-Point

The *four-point* jump is initiated in the standing, feet-together position. The individual jumps using both feet, but moves one foot forward, via hip flexion, to toe-touch the floor in front of the individual in harmony with the other foot returning to the floor. On the next jump, the foot which was moved to the forward toe-touch position is moved to the side toe-touch position via rotation of the hip to a hip-abducted position. On the third jump, the foot is moved to the rear toe-touch position, via hip rotation to a hip-extended position. The final jump brings the feet back together. The exercise is performed to each side (Figures 13.20-A, 13.20-B, 13.20-C, and 13.20-D).

Shuffling

The *shuffling* maneuver is initiated with feet together in standing. Separations of the feet are accomplished via hip abduction followed by quick return to the feet-together position via hip adduction to produce a rapid sideways shuffle. The maneuver should produce sideways movement and should be conducted in both directions (Figures 13.21-A and 13.21-B).

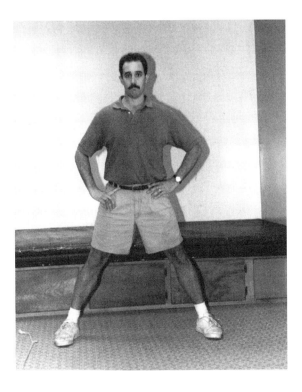

FIGURE 13.15   Illustrates the ending position of the straddle jump. (Photo courtesy James E. Eaton.)

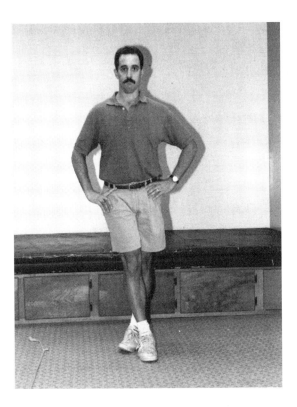

FIGURE 13.16   Illustrates the cross position of the straddle cross. (Photo courtesy James E. Eaton.)

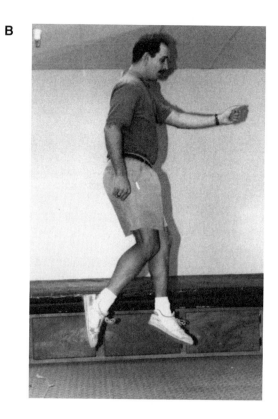

FIGURE 13.17 (A) Illustrates the ending position of the first reciprocal jump. (B) Illustrates the change of leg positions during the midjump phase of the second reciprocal jump. (Photos courtesy James E. Eaton.)

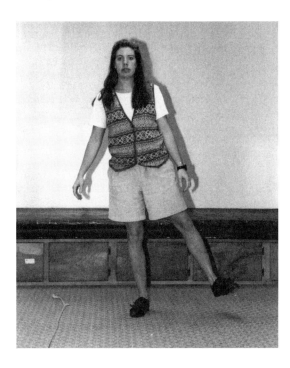

FIGURE 13.18   Illustration of the pendulum position. (Photo courtesy Caryn Murphy.)

Running Carioca

Running Carioca is a rapid production of the grapevine step or cross step.

Skipping

Skipping should be self-explanatory.

Reciprocal Marching

The *reciprocal march* is an exaggerated march step with large arm swing and exaggerated hip and knee flexion during the march.

Each of the above exercises is repeated until the evaluator has a good understanding of the person's abilities. Measure assistance required and quality of performance.

Rapid Alternating Movement Evaluation

While seated, alternate floor touching with the heel and toe and seated side steps are observed for the number of repetitions performed in ten seconds. The number of repeated standing side steps are also recorded for a ten second period. Note quality of performance (Figure 13.22).

Assessment of Smell and Taste

It is imperative that chemosensory or gustatory and olfactory senses are tested, in that they can be impaired or absent in both the MTBI client as well as the severely impaired client. Yet, these functions are often ignored in the evaluation process.

Dysfunction in olfactory and gustatory senses may have gone undetected until the client reaches the postacute phase. Anosmia is thought to occur in approximately 5.5% of the TBI population, while over one third of TBI patients have dysosmia.[59,60] As many as one third of TBI patients may have difficulty with olfactory naming and recognition. Questions should be raised

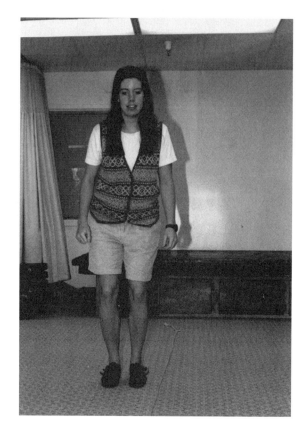

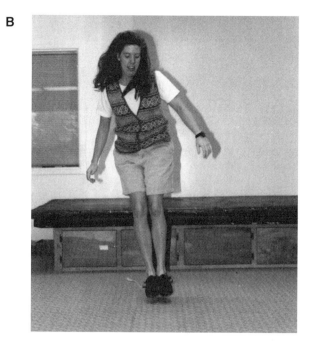

FIGURE 13.19 (A) Illustrates position No. 1 of the slalom activity; (B) position No. 2; (C) position No. 3. The sequence of FIGURE 13.19 is then repeated a specified number of times. (Photo courtesy Caryn Murphy.)

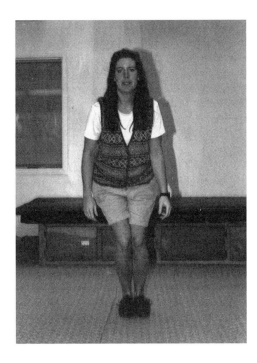

FIGURE 13.19   (continued).

by complaints of smelling foul odors, poor appetite, or unawareness of body odor or various household smells including burning or spoiled foods. Following a chemosensory screening by OT or PT, alterations in function should be examined in light of the original injury. The client will require awareness and education in ways to detect smoke, gas, other toxic fumes, and spoiled foods.[61,62] A chemosensory screening may also indicate the necessity to refer the client for additional clinical examinations by an otorhinolaryngologist or neurosurgeon.

Evaluation of Vision

The incidence of visual dysfunction following traumatic brain injury is fairly high. Schlageter et al.[63] reviewed 51 inpatients within days of admission. They found that 30 (59%) were impaired in one or more of the following: pursuits, saccades, ocular posturing, stereopsis, extraocular movements, and near/far eso-exotropia. Since the acute rehabilitation experience has become increasingly shorter in duration for this population, relatively little attention is paid to visual-motor and visual-perceptual remediative efforts. As a consequence, these deficits are frequently evidenced in postacute rehabilitation settings.

A thorough OT evaluation should include a complete vision screening test.[64] Prior to the vision screening, preliminary information is collected via the Visual Symptoms Checklist (Figure 13.23). This questionnaire not only collects subjective responses but provides an opportunity for objective documentation. For example, the client may not acknowledge symptoms. The therapist's observations, however, reveal head tilting, squinting or closing an eye, difficulty reading, or bumping into walls or furniture on one side.

The purpose of the screening is not to diagnose but to detect potentially unrecognized visual deficits which may be impacting daily life. The screening should include visual attentiveness, near and distance acuities, ocular pursuits, saccades, nearpoint convergence, strabismus, eye alignment, stereopsis, and peripheral fields. Changes in acuities may be reflected in difficulty performing tasks requiring near vision, e.g., shaving or putting on makeup, or difficulty recognizing environmental cues, e.g., facial expressions.

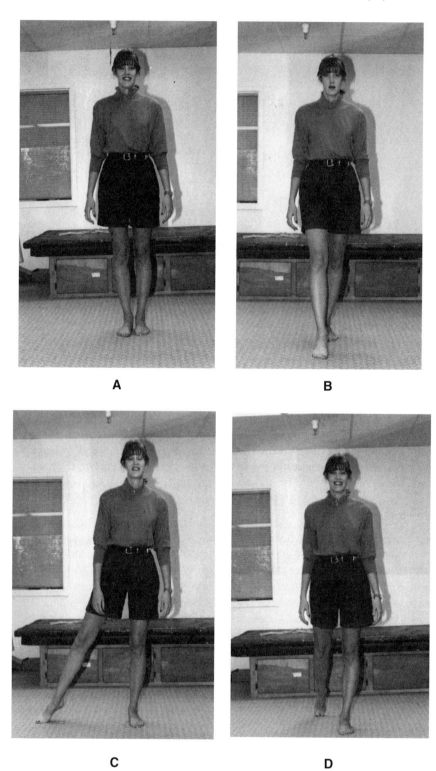

FIGURE 13.20 (A) Illustrates the starting position of the four-point which is followed by a jump to the next position. (B) Illustrates the second position of the four-point with a foot forward. (C) Illustrates the third position of the four-point with the foot to the side. (D) Illustrates the fourth position of the four-point with the foot posterior to midline. The next jump returns to the starting position in FIGURE 13.20-A, and the sequence is repeated a specified number of times. (Photos courtesy Lynda R. Eaton.)

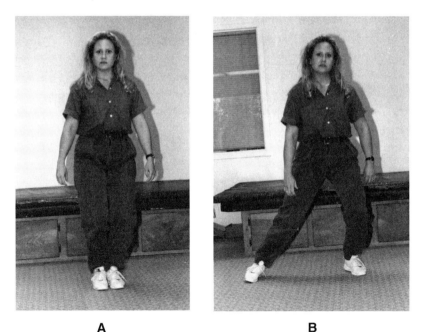

A   **B**

FIGURE 13.21 (A) Illustrates the starting position of the shuffling maneuver. (B) Illustrates the landing position during the rapidly repeated shuffle. (Photos courtesy Shannon M. Parrish.)

RAPID ALTERNATING MOVEMENT EVALUATION
(# repetitions in 10 seconds)

		Left	Right
I.	HEEL-TOE:	_____	_____
II.	SEATED SIDE STEPS:	_____	_____
III.	STANDING SIDE STEPS:	_____	_____

FIGURE 13.22 Rapid alternating movements form: a simple format for documenting rapid alternating movements.

Smooth ocular pursuits are required for such tasks as reading a line of print or a column of words or numbers. Saccades provide a rapid but accurate shift of the eye in such visual tasks as reading to the end of a line of print and rapidly shifting leftward to the beginning of the next line. Impairment in nearpoint convergence is another tracking deficit which may be manifested in double or blurred vision and decreased depth perception.

Strabismus may result in double or blurred vision as the eyes move through the visual sphere. The ability to visually scan may be impaired in such tasks as reading, writing, or reviewing a map. Eye alignment measures horizontal and vertical alignments to detect possible deviations.

VISUAL SYMPTOMS CHECKLIST

Prescription glasses: Yes _____ No _____

If yes: Were glasses worn prior to injury? _____

Since the injury only? _____

Last vision examination? _____

New prescription? _____ Date: _____

Answer **yes** or **no** to the following questions: Yes   No

1.   Do you have blurred or double vision?   _____   _____

2.   Do you tilt your head to see more clearly?   _____   _____

3.   Do you squint or close an eye to see?   _____   _____

4.   Do you get a headache while reading, watching television, riding in or driving a car? Other? _____   _____   _____

5.   Do your eyes feel "tired"?   _____   _____

6.   Do you lose your place while reading?   _____   _____

7.   Do you hold objects or reading material close to see?   _____   _____

8.   Do you avoid reading or not read as often as you did before the injury?   _____   _____

9.   Do you miss words, letters, or numbers while reading?   _____   _____

10.   Do you have difficulty distinguishing colors?   _____   _____

11.   Do you avoid dark areas or avoid driving after dark?   _____   _____

12.   Do you sometimes confuse which direction is right or left?   _____   _____

13.   Do you reverse letters, numbers, or words?   _____   _____

14.   Do you have difficulty recognizing road or street signs before it is too late to turn?   _____   _____

15.   While you are standing still, do objects seem to jump or move?   _____   _____

16.   While you are walking, do objects seem to jump around?   _____   _____

17.   Do you bump into objects on one side or the other?   _____   _____

FIGURE 13.23   Visual symptoms checklist: Used to collect information on vision from the client.

Deficits in stereopsis impact many functions requiring depth perception. The ability to judge spatial relationships in such eye-hand tasks as threading a needle, targeting food on a plate, or negotiating stairs is affected by this deficit.

Peripheral and central vision are required for a full field of vision. A loss of the peripheral field(s) will impact safe driving and will require the client's awareness and ability to compensate with appropriate head-turning.

The Perceptual Motor Evaluation for Head Injured and Other Neurologically Impaired Adults[65] is a frequently utilized assessment tool which provides various subtests to evaluate visual attention, scanning, fields, neglect, and saccades. The King-Devick Test[66] measures scanning required to read detailed and structured formats, e.g., reading a bus or train schedule. Evaluation of visual system integrity may raise suspicion of vestibular or cerebellar dysfunction.

Following the vision screening, appropriate referrals to the neuro-ophthalmologist or behavioral optometrist may be required for further in-depth assessments. See Chapters 7 and 8 in this volume for an in-depth discussion of evaluative and treatment options.

TBI clients may or may not complain of visual disturbances. Behavioral evidence of oculomotor deficits may be seen in problems with reading, writing, driving, playing video games, or watching television. Persons may report that words "jump" around on the page, or that they frequently lose their place while reading. They may relate that images move in strange ways while they are watching television or driving. They may experience dizziness or nausea during these activities. Head position adjustments can foretell oculomotor problems, as can observation of dysfluencies of gait, especially in uneven terrain such as curbs, uneven sidewalks, stairs, or multilevel surfaces.

The field of vision therapy represents a valuable evaluation and treatment process which has been practiced by too few over the years. It is now being more routinely incorporated into the clinical practice of neurological rehabilitation.[64,67,68]

Visual Perception and Perceptual Motor Evaluation

Following the vision evaluation, perceptual motor assessments should proceed. Deficits may impact upon the client's ability to adequately perform normal daily living tasks. Observations and documentation should be taken from clinical and other environments.[69-71] Clinical assessments may include information from tests performed by both the OT and the neuropsychologist.

Visual perception examines visual figure-ground, form constancy, spatial awareness or position in space, depth perception, visual memory, and spatial relationships. *Visual figure-ground* is the ability to distinguish foreground from background, and *form constancy* explores the ability to perceive subtle variations in form. *Position in space* is the ability to manage such spatial concepts as in/out, up/down, and front/behind. *Spatial relationship* examines the client's ability to perceive positioning of two or more objects in relation to themselves or other objects. It is easy to understand how frequently the client requires these functions in everyday living.

Clinical evaluations of visual perception should include such tests as the Baylor Adult Visual Perception Evaluation[72] and the Motor-Free Visual Perception Test (MVPT).[73,74] The MVPT measures the time it takes the client to process visual information and react to that information. This applies to such tasks as driving.

The Southern California Figure-Ground Test[75] is composed of two parts: Part I consists of superimposed common objects, and Part II, which is more abstract, uses superimposed geometric forms. These skills apply to such visual tasks as finding a sleeve on an all-white shirt or finding the coin or credit card slot on a machine.

The Hooper Visual Organization Test[76] examines the client's ability to organize visual stimuli by showing pieces of an object. These skills are needed to locate items in a grocery store, refrigerator, or in a cupboard. The Hooper Visual Organization Test is useful in detecting deficits in the right hemisphere and will determine actual perceptual deficits aside from performance.

An evaluation of the client's ability to perform purposeful movements on command or praxis is important for all TBI clients. Apraxia or dyspraxia may be obvious or subtle and may influence physical performances. Even in the MTBI client, initiation and sequencing of functional motor acts need close observation for potential disorganization.[77] The Solet Test for Apraxia[78] is a useful and comprehensive assessment tool for apraxia.

Skills required to produce a design in two and three dimensions (e.g. assemble various items from written or illustrated instructions) relate to constructional praxis and block design. This can be assessed via the Benton 3-D Constructional Praxis Test[79] and the Bender-Gestalt Test for 2-D.[80] Form perception is assessed via the Form Board and examines the client's ability to differentiate variations in form.

Difficulties in identifying body parts, or in right/left discrimination, impact the client's perception of body self or scheme. The OT can assess these abilities with the Draw a Person, Body Part Identification, and Body Puzzle tests.[65]

Lezak[81] warned that observations must distinguish between perceptual failures, apraxias, spatial confusions, motivation, or attention problems. Therapists have more recently responded to this need for clearer definition of deficits and better direction for treatments. In this regard, Bowler[70] noted that two assessments are beginning to be utilized to define perceptual skills and other neurological skills which contribute to overall function. The Rivermead Perceptual Assessment Battery[82] assesses deficits in visual perception and was developed for adults with brain injury. The Lowenstein Occupational Therapy Cognition Assessment[83] examines orientation, perception, visuomotor organization, and cognition and provides baseline information for treatment. Although some areas of assessment overlap, the combined tests view each function from a variety of perspectives to more distinctly define deficits.

Assessment of Activities of Daily Living

The OT is able to gather quite meaningful information from observations of the client during actual daily tasks in the residential setting or the client's home. The structure of some postacute programs allows a trained rehabilitation assistant to gather appropriately documented data of several specific tasks over several days during the initial assessment. This documentation continues throughout the program for the purpose of reassessment or as feedback data. For example, observations of the manner in which the client organizes and sequences tasks and manages time can be documented while the client plans the meal, shops for items, and prepares the meal. This continually collected data directs the OT along a progression of therapeutic focus, clinically and residentially (Figure 13.24).

Take careful note of potential dependency behaviors. The family or others may fail to recognize that tasks are innocently assisted or completely performed by them for the client. If possible, assess the client's ADL skills in a normal living environment, independent of family interaction. This approach should help to identify true problem areas and can be a good time to educate the client and the family about observed deficits and needed intervention for same.

Concomitant Injuries

Orthopedic and Spinal Cord

Therapists will encounter TBI clients with accompanying orthopedic and/or spinal cord injuries. Special orthopedic issues such as heterotopic ossification must be appropriately addressed (See Chapter 5 in this volume). Regardless of the possibility that surgical intervention may be involved, the PT and the OT will play a vital role. In a postoperative situation, therapeutic follow-up will be necessary to prevent loss of flexibility and function. Botte and Moore[84] describe, in detail, the methods for acute orthopedic management of extremity injuries. They point out the importance of anticipation of uncontrolled limb movement, avoidance of joint immobilization, and avoidance of prolonged traction methods. In the majority of cases, the acute orthopedic issues will have received adequate attention from medical staff.

At the acute level, musculoskeletal injuries are missed diagnoses in approximately 10% of patients arriving at head trauma units.[85] As patients are moved at an increasing pace through the acute phases of treatment, therapists are faced with greater demands for orthopedic management. Monitoring of casting and infections, sensory integrity in the extremity, mobility, and pain management is necessary. The therapists will need to educate the client, family, and other therapeutic staff in the possible adjustments required to allow an optimum of function.

Review of frequency of musculoskeletal injury[84] shows that the shoulder girdle, radius, and ulna are among the most common upper extremity injuries. The elbow must be watched because of frequent spasticity around the joint, development of heterotopic ossification, and possible ulnar neuropathy. Fractures of the humerus are relatively rare. In the lower extremities, fracture of the femur is most common, followed by fracture of the tibia. Pedestrian accidents will often involve the pelvis. Injuries to the acetabulum and hip are comparatively rare.

Another frequent concomitant injury is that of the temporomandibular joint (TMJ). TMJ dysfunction may arise from an associated facial injury or cervical myofascial injury.[86] Mechanisms of injury associated with MTBI can produce minor to severe TMJ dysfunction. TMJ problems may be manifested by headaches (described as fan-shaped in radiation in proximity to the joint); jaw, neck, or back pain; eating problems; or subtle postural disorders. As a matter of awareness and thoroughness in the evaluation process, the PT evaluation should include a TMJ screening assessment. If the neurological therapist is not trained in treatment of TMJ dysfunction, appropriate referrals can be made for in-depth examinations and potential treatment. Many PT's are trained and work with dentists in assessment and treatment of TMJ-related problems. Although pain behavior related to this dysfunction can represent a hindering factor to an efficiently addressed TBI rehabilitation program, TMJ dysfunction is often ignored.

Pain

Many neurological therapists have noted that pain behaviors, in general, are more frequently seen in the MTBI client than the more severely impaired client. In fact, the existence of brain injury can actually be hidden by pain behaviors.[87] Headaches are a common focus of the MTBI client.[88] Pain, whether real, exaggerated, or imagined, is pain and, along with companion emotional issues, can become a large obstacle to progress.

Perhaps the most frequent complaint of pain arises from headache.[88] Headache, though, can arise from a number of etiologies.[89] It is important to differentiate headaches arising from TMJ dysfunction from those arising from sinusitis. Injuries to the head often include injury to the sinuses. These headaches typically localize around the eyes and maxillary region in a "mask" distribution. Headaches which are occipital may represent tension headaches arising from tension in the neck and shoulder musculature. Sometimes, these headaches have a frontal regionalization as well. The patient who complains of daily headache may benefit from review of medications or substances which are known to cause rebound headache. Vascular etiology must be considered.

Headaches which arise from muscular tension or TMJ dysfunction may be improved by physical therapy for those problems. Of course, it must be determined if the etiology for the muscular tension is musculoligamentous strain, orthopedic injury, or compensatory reaction to vestibular hypersensitivity.

In management of pain, it is very important to utilize a system which allows for the patient to rate the pain experience throughout the day. Additionally, it is important for concomitant recording of the degree to which pain impacts the person's ability to function. These reference points can be utilized by the treating physician and team to determine appropriate medication and therapeutic approaches. Therapeutic approaches available include thermal treatments, ultrasound, massage, flexibility exercises, strengthening exercises, and relaxation. In some cases, pain management may be enhanced by involvement of psychological services for the individual to explore relaxation or hypnosis as potential avenues of treatment. Fortunately, the vast majority of pain management programs for TBI respond well to conservative modalities of treatment, either in isolation or in combination.

It should be understood that the brain-injured person may tend to perseverate on a painful extremity, cast, etc. The therapist must be sympathetic and pursue appropriate investigations into potential causes and treatments; however, the therapist should also be aware that the problem may appear to be larger than it truly is. It is for this reason that behavioral observation of activity restriction caused by pain can be useful in addition to the person's report.

Driving

The TBI client may appear physically and cognitively able to drive a vehicle and, yet, there may be problems. The ability to drive can be dramatically impacted by impairments in or damaged

---

ACTIVITIES OF DAILY LIVING CHECKLIST

ASSISTANCE LEVELS

0 = No assistance required to initiate, continue, or complete task
1 = Minimal verbal cues or gestural prompts
2 = Intermittent verbal cues or gestural prompts
3 = Minimal physical prompts
4 = Intermittent physical prompts
5 = Guided performance
6 = Unable

DRESSING   Date:_____

                                    Level   Comments

1.   Don shirt/blouse/dress   ____   _____
2.   Doff shirt/blouse/dress   ____   _____
3.   Don underwear   ____   _____
4.   Doff underwear   ____   _____
5.   Don pants   ____   _____
6.   Doff pants   ____   _____
7.   Buttoning (small, large)   ____   _____
8.   Zipping (tops, pants)   ____   _____
9.   Buckle/unbuckle belt   ____   _____
10. Don/doff socks/hose   ____   _____
11. Don/doff brace/splint   ____   _____
12. Accessories on/off   ____   _____
13. Shoes on/off   ____   _____

GROOMING/HYGIENE   Date:_____

                                    Level   Comments

1.   Use faucets   ____   _____
2.   Wash face/hands   ____   _____
3.   Use handkerchief/tissue   ____   _____
4.   Apply/remove glasses   ____   _____
5.   Brush teeth/clean dentures ____   _____
6.   Brush/comb hair   ____   _____
7.   Shampoo hair   ____   _____
8.   Style hair   ____   _____
9.   Shave face/legs   ____   _____
10. Apply deodorant   ____   _____
11. Apply make-up   ____   _____
12. Care for nails   ____   _____
13. Manage clothes at toilet   ____   _____
14. Cleans self at toilet   ____   _____
15. Manages feminine hygiene   ____   _____
16. Bathe/towel dry entire body ____   _____
17. Skin inspection   ____   _____

FIGURE 13.24 Activities of daily living checklist: Used to document daily performance of ADL's. This information is used by staff to produce weekly and monthly reports of the client's progress.

interconnections between the vestibular system, oculomotor and cerebellar functions, and the somatosensory system. The therapist must carefully listen to the client during discussions about driving and, when appropriate, driving should be observed. There may be denial of any problems. Ask a significant other about the client's driving habits or behavior as a passenger. Have any changes occurred? Has driving at night been significantly reduced or avoided? Does the client drive only at specific times to avoid busy traffic? Does he/she frequently become lost or drive only in certain areas of familiarity? Does the client drive more impulsively, become easily irritated, or make unsafe judgments? Has driving been abandoned altogether? Many clients cannot explain why they have experienced changes and may provide general comments such as, "I just feel weird when driving. It scares me." They may complain of motion sickness or headaches while driving. They may be very anxious passengers and complain that other vehicles are too close or moving too fast. Confusing visual perceptions, movement imperceptions, and spatial disorientation can produce frightening and disabling effects.[64,90-92]

```
HOUSEHOLD CLEANING                              Date:_____
                                        Level                    Comments
    1.   Change sheets/make bed         ____    _____
    2.   Pick up objects from floor     ____    _____
    3.   Dust                           ____    _____
    4.   Sweep/mop/vacuum               ____    _____
    5.   Transport pail of water        ____    _____
    6.   Wring out mop                  ____    _____
    7.   Clean windows                  ____    _____
    8.   Clean refrigerator/stove       ____    _____
    9.   Put out garbage                ____    _____


LAUNDRY                                         Date:_____
                                        Level                    Comments
    1.   Sort clothes                   ____    _____
    2.   Use washer/dryer               ____    _____
    3.   Use detergent                  ____    _____
    4.   Hand launder                   ____    _____
    5.   Put clothes on hangers         ____    _____
    6.   Fold clothes                   ____    _____
    7.   Put clothes away               ____    _____
    8.   Iron clothes                   ____    _____


MEAL PLANNING                                   Date:_____
                                        Level                    Comments
    1.   Plan balanced meals            ____    _____
    2.   Scan kitchen for necessary items ____  _____
    3.   Compile grocery list           ____    _____
    4.   Estimate amount of money needed ____   _____
    5.   Get to/from store              ____    _____
    6.   Locate items in store          ____    _____
    7.   Retrieve items from shelves    ____    _____


MEAL PREPARATION/CLEANUP                        Date:_____
                                        Level                    Comments
    1.   Read recipe/directions         ____    _____
    2.   Follow recipe/directions       ____    _____
    3.   Remove food from refrigerator  ____    _____
    4.   Remove items from cupboard     ____    _____
    5.   Organize and transfer items to work area ____ _____
    6.   Open packages/cans/bottles     ____    _____
    7.   Handle pots/pans/utensils      ____    _____
    8.   Use faucets                    ____    _____
    9.   Pour liquids (hot/cold)        ____    _____
    10.  Use microwave                  ____    _____
    11.  Use stove                      ____    _____
    12.  Use oven                       ____    _____
    13.  Peel/cut vegetables            ____    _____
    14.  Break eggs                     ____    _____
    15.  Stir                           ____    _____
    16.  Measure                        ____    _____
    17.  Use timer/clock                ____    _____
    18.  Set table/clear table          ____    _____
    19.  Transfer food/liquids to table ____    _____
    20.  Wash/dry dishes                ____    _____
    21.  Load/unload/use dishwasher     ____    _____
    22.  Wipe stove/microwave/table     ____    _____
    23.  Put dishes away                ____    _____
```

FIGURE 13.24 (continued).

Functioning at Heights

Some TBI clients may have the potential to return to a vocation which requires working on ladders or on roofs or other areas of height. Following stabilization of balance, postural control, visual perception, physical fitness, and some psychological issues, the client should undergo a height evaluation. Safety measures are taken by utilizing climber's gear and helmets. Various work stations should be set up with equipment commonly needed, e.g., ladders, scaffolds, etc. It is appropriate to incorporate hierarchically any items which would be typically carried by the client during a work assignment, e.g., paint bucket or lumber.

MANAGEMENT OF RESIDUAL PHYSICAL DEFICITS

Once the evaluative process has been completed and the treatment team has shared its findings, the individual rehabilitation program begins to take shape. The purpose of treatment is to facilitate the client's relearning and continue the momentum of improvement in skills and, thus, reduce dependence. The development of a management plan begins with understanding the factors which limit adequate performance. As is evidenced by the complexity of the evaluative process, the management program can be expected to be equally complicated.

Neurological rehabilitation differs from other types of rehabilitation in that patients who have sustained neurological damage frequently evidence multiple areas of impairment in addition to those areas which require physical restoration of function. These individuals often cannot be left alone to undertake therapy exercises. They require attention for safety, follow-through, motivation, documentation, and ongoing evaluation. The TBI population is best treated in one-to-one treatment settings. The therapy may be conducted with the help of a physical therapy assistant; however, the physical therapist must remain very active in the treatment of the TBI patient. Therapists must possess adequate knowledge of evaluative and treatment techniques and must also possess a repertoire of interpersonal skills which will enable them to motivate the unmotivated, calm the agitated, or educate the person in denial. There will be times when a therapy session is nearly entirely taken up by education or counseling and others where the session focuses exclusively on prescribed exercises.

The treatment environment should be such that the treatment can be segregated from high-stimulus environments that distract the client. Attentional deficits which accompany brain injury can make it quite difficult for the individual to focus on the treatment session. Overstimulation can lead to behavioral problems.

Rehabilitation of physical function requires maximal repetition. As such, the therapist should attempt to treat in blocks of time which allow for ample repetition of a wide array of therapeutic tasks that will be required in most treatment plans. Newly emerging positive responses should be focused upon until they are reliably reproducible, even if this means continuing a treatment session beyond scheduled times.

The therapist should develop the ability to approach treatment exercises hierarchically, utilizing task analysis, where necessary, to break larger tasks into smaller ones to accentuate the learning experience. TBI results in changes in the manner in which a person acquires new information, so physically restorative therapies may be expected to take longer in the neurologically impaired population as compared to other populations. To that end, quantitative measurement of treatment exercises that have been broken into smaller, more readily learned components can give a clearer picture of slowly progressing improvement.

Therapeutic Measurement

It is now more widely accepted that continued postacute rehabilitation with the traumatically brain-injured person can bring about substantial reduction in disability, improvement in living status, and improvement in occupational status.[93-98] This was not always the case, however. In the time when rehabilitation for this population was largely restricted to the acute rehabilitation experience, it was necessary to develop methods of measurement that would allow both the therapist and the consumer access to critical review of the therapeutic process. Progress could no longer be viewed through the subjectivity of the therapists' eyes; rather, a new period of accountability was emerging. Qualitative summaries of patient performance were no longer acceptable. Many therapists found the expectation for quantitative analysis to be difficult, but once accomplished, the improved objectivity about therapist/patient performance over time allowed for some major therapeutic advances. In fact, quantitative measurement allowed therapists to acquire new perspectives about breaking therapeutic tasks into hierarchical components so as to better teach skills to a learning-impaired patient. Therapy became easier to implement and monitor, and patients were better able to benefit from treatment.[11,14]

In order to most accurately understand whether a patient is benefiting from treatment, the therapist must reduce the therapeutic task to its hierarchical components, which can be operationally defined and objectively measured. For example, in evaluating ambulatory skills and progression therein, the therapist should refrain from characterization of skills as follows: "Mr. Smith is able to ambulate short distances with a hemi-cane." Rather, the therapist should characterize Mr. Smith's performance by a statement such as, "Mr. Smith is able to walk 100 feet, with a hemi-cane, in a mean of two minutes. This is an improvement from a mean of three point five minutes for the same distance last week."

Quantification can generally be achieved fairly readily. The therapist can count repetitions of a task, document specific amounts of weight or resistance being used, time performances, and/or count accurate vs. inaccurate performances to obtain a percentage correctly performed. Of course, there remains room for subjective observations as well, but therapy which is quantitatively approached is far easier for all parties to participate in, enhancing cooperation, motivation, consistency of treatment, and ultimately, progress.

The therapist should keep in mind that the brain-injured person has a number of special needs. In today's environment of managed care, it is important to keep the therapeutic focus on tasks which will translate, quickly and efficaciously, to good functional improvement. At the same time, the very measurement which is advocated herein may become the data utilized to justify continued treatment toward a longer term goal of improved functional capability. Outcomes are being viewed, increasingly, from the perspective of financial risks and benefits. Ashley et al.[93] address the idea that rehabilitation outcome translates to dollar savings for long-term care costs. These savings have their beginnings with the daily therapeutic sessions undertaken by the PT, the OT, and their allied health associates. Another study by Spivack et al.[99] demonstrated a clear relation between treatment intensity and rehabilitative outcome. Thus, in order to advocate best for the TBI person, quantification of treatment will be of critical importance.

In the process of treating the client, the therapist must teach all other pertinent staff, clinical and residential, methods that they can use to maximize the client's learning throughout the entire day. Management of physical injury residuals cannot be performed in a vacuum separated from other therapeutic disciplines or from environments which the person will be expected to function in. Therefore, an important daily goal is to generalize skills into actual activities in residential and community environments.[29,31] This is where environmentally valid learning takes place. Maximized repetition, performed in sequence and in realistic situations, maximizes the derived rehabilitation benefit.

Another factor to take into consideration is that the TBI client is not a passenger passively traveling through the rehabilitation process. In physical and psychological terms, therapy is difficult work for the TBI client. Confronting one's weaknesses is never easy. The earlier review of the client's personal history and lifestyle now provides key information to fuel motivation. Perception of purpose and realization of goal achievement are enhanced by the therapist's ability to present concrete, appropriately sequenced tasks within the scope of the client's interests. Progress requires a constant series of challenges. The therapist must be a creative motivator.

Mobility

Normal movement cannot be built on abnormal tone, and normal behaviors do not sequence from abnormal ones.[1,11,100] Functional mobilization may be influenced by such injury residuals as fractures, peripheral nerve injuries, general weakness, pain, sensory impairments, visual impairments, balance and coordination deficits as well as cognitive and behavioral factors.

Each must be addressed to allow the client to progress to more advanced performance levels. The goal is to facilitate and normalize movement, which will gradually advance into daily mobilization. Ranges of motion and adequate strengths to move are among the fundamental requirements which can usually be conventionally addressed.

The client with significant motor impairments may require immediate treatment for ongoing hypertonicity or a movement disorder, i.e., ataxia, which will be discussed later. Hypertonicity may refer to spasticity or rigidity. Although these problems are often addressed and resolved during the acute rehabilitation phase, the postacute therapist will have occasion to treat these impairments. These issues may be addressed via both a medical consultant and the therapist. Approaches can range from stretching and positioning to serial casting and chemical neurolysis. Orthopedic management of spasticity can be efficacious in obtaining temporary relief from spasticity.[101] Diagnostic blocks can be utilized to temporarily eliminate pain and muscle tone to ascertain the degree of motor control present and the amount of fixed contracture. Therapy is frequently enhanced by application of chemical neurolysis in that the patient and therapist can focus on nontreated muscle groups, obtain isolated contractions in those groups, enhance awareness of control of those groups, and allow for strengthening of those groups.

Mobility can be impacted by reductions in range of motion. Range of motion can be reduced due to neuromuscular deficits or due to restriction of the joint due to contractures or heterotopic ossification. Decerebrate or decorticate posturing during coma, or neuromuscular deficits seen most commonly after cortical or brainstem injury which result in spasticity, will frequently result in the development of joint limitations. Restrictions arising from musculoligamentous contracture should be treated through a multimodal program. Lehmkuhl et al.[16] advocate early use of such a program to include passive and active ROM, positioning, serial inhibitive casting, bivalved casts, motor point blocks, and antispasticity medication. Elbows and knees were noted by these authors to respond most quickly to therapeutic intervention, with elbows benefiting most. Increases in joint ROM can be expected to endure for at least six to nine months. Of course, it should be expected that joint limitation improvements will be maximized by long-term use of the full ROM achieved through daily functional activity.[102]

It is imperative that mobility be taught in an appropriate progression from bed mobility to transfers to ambulation. Mobility skills will improve through intense repetition appropriate to the developmental sequence of movement. The neurodevelopmental sequence (previously described in this chapter) can become an exercise routine which can be practiced at any level required. For example, the therapist may begin with segmental rolling to improve body awareness and enhance movement. Rolling should progress to assuming prone-on-elbows and, eventually, the quadruped position until each is performed independently. The sequence continues to be practiced, component to component, through tall-kneel, half-kneel, and standing. Treatment of any difficulty within each component of the sequence may come from the therapist's choice of a variety of treatment approaches, e.g., proprioceptive neuromuscular facilitation (PNF).[4] The client continues to practice, component to component, as the motor tasks are gradually progressed from the simple to the complex. Besides movement, strength, and flexibility, very basic balance skills are practiced within the sequenced exercises. The exercises may appear simple though they can be quite challenging. Do not skip over sequential components. Do not assume competence at any level until performance is demonstrated to the therapist.

Treatment of mobility skills is greatly enhanced by daily practice of these skills in the residential setting. Bed mobility can be practiced every day in the environmentally valid routines of getting up and going to bed. A trained staff member should be present to assist the client in additional home exercises, which should be designed by the clinical staff to ensure the use of proper techniques. The same is applied to all transfers, toileting, bathing, and early ambulatory routines. The client advances through these daily routines from the clinic to the residence to the community until greater independence is accomplished.

Pain

In management of pain, it is very important to utilize a system which allows for the patient to rate the pain experience throughout the day. A pain diary provides a way to document and rate pain. A rating scale of 0–10 (0 = none, and 10 = most severe) is a simple scale for the client to use. Headaches or neck and back pain in the brain-injured person can become a distracting somatic focus, and perseveration on pain may hinder progress in several aspects of the TBI program. An assumption that pain is exaggerated should not be made until complaints of pain are explored to rule out potential causes which may respond to treatment.

It is important to keep a concomitant recording of the degree to which pain impacts the person's ability to function. These reference points can be utilized by the treating physician and team to determine appropriate medication and therapeutic approaches. The physician must review all medications taken by the client and determine what modifications, if any, should be made. Dosage and frequency of medication taken should be included in a diary. The physician may elect to utilize a controlled reduction of dosages with combined pain medications via the "pain cocktail".

The therapist will have a major impact upon the client's understanding of the various causes of pain. The client who anticipates pain from movement develops increased anxiety and muscle tension and, therefore, the potential for chronic pain and stiffness. A kinesiological orientation in the initial exercise program may be an effective tool to reduce this anxiety-produced pain and allow the client to begin to move through and beyond pain. This approach teaches normalizing posture and improving body mechanics with more efficient movements to reduce pain.

Conventional therapeutic modalities include thermal treatment, ultrasound, TENS, massage, flexibility exercises, and strengthening exercises. In some cases, pain management may be enhanced by involvement of psychological services for the individual to explore relaxation or hypnosis as potential avenues of treatment. Fortunately, the vast majority of pain management programs for TBI result in a good response to these conservative modalities of treatment, either in isolation or in combination.

Postural Control and Balance

Fisher[50] describes postural deficits commonly seen in TBI patients and contrasts their postural abilities to normals. In general, the TBI patient can be observed to tend toward the relaxed sitting posture of normals, however, on an habitual basis. Trunk movements tend not to be incorporated into arm movements and, even when attempting to assume an erect sitting posture, truncal musculature strength and coordination may make achieving the erect position quite difficult. Not only do truncal weaknesses impact upper extremity function but transfers can also be impacted. In preparation for arising from sitting to standing, postural deficits frequently will maintain weight so far posteriorly as to make the attempt to arise ineffective.

Effective treatment of postural deficits focuses on strengthening of the truncal musculature. In cases where there is concomitant cerebellar dysfunction, strengthening may not be indicated so much as learning selective utilization of muscle groups with slow, controlled muscle activation. In cases, however, where a cerebellar component is not present, strengthening exercises such as bridging, sit-ups or crunches, or resistive lateral bending can be helpful. It is important to achieve stabilization at the hips, back, neck, and shoulders.

For detail regarding treatment of balance impairments related to vestibular dysfunction, the reader is referred to Chapter 6 in this volume.

Cerebellar Dysfunction

Many therapists struggle with movement disorders related to cerebellar dysfunction. Frustrations with ataxia or tremors in the extremities and/or trunk are compounded by the short period allowed for treatment and often lead a therapist to teach compensatory techniques, i.e., using the more functional limb or mobilizing from a wheelchair. Minimal to no time is then spent in therapeutic confrontation of the issue.

When undertaking cerebellar rehabilitation, it is important to keep several important factors in mind. The first is that muscle strengthening activities can result in exacerbation of tremor, causing the degree of tremor excursions to increase. The second point is that the individual must learn to relax selective muscle groups on command to reduce the excursion of tremor. Tremor results from agonist/antagonist muscle groups firing rhythmically. The client must learn to selectively turn on one muscle, while maintaining relative electrical silence in the antagonistic muscle. EMG/biofeedback training can be quite effective in teaching patients to control muscles and even specific motor units.[23,103] The third point has to do with the importance of a progression of stabilization of the trunk, to the neck and head, to the proximal extremities, to the distal extremities. In severe cerebellar dysfunction, postural tremors may be so severe as to necessitate treatment commencing in a supine position. It is useful to not only retrain truncal control in this position, but also to approach proximal extremity muscu-lature control as well. The utilization of selective muscular relaxation and activation can be particularly helpful at this stage, with positioning helpful in teaching the ability of selective relaxation and activation.

Diminished ability with rapid alternating movements, dysmetria, hypotonicity, and/or movement decomposition are manifestations of cerebellar damage which influence the client's performance in ADL's, i.e., feeding, brushing teeth, dressing, or gait functions. Reading, or other skills which require accuracy in visual scanning ability, can be impacted by oculomotor deficits related to cerebellar injury. A spastic hemiparesis may further complicate an ipsilat-eral or bilateral ataxia in one or more limbs. Acquiring a degree of movement control and normalizing functions can be frustrating to the therapist and, most certainly, to the client. However, the therapist should pursue proper identification of the dysfunction and aggressively pursue appropriate treatment.[14,104]

Establishment of a stable base of support is the initial focus of treatment. For example, the performance of any task requiring an ataxic extremity to extend away from the body requires trunk stabilization. Therefore, goals of treatment are postural stability and accuracy in extrem-ity movement during functional activities. Treatment must be pursued in a sequential manner until the client is independent in each component. That is to say, head and trunk control must be addressed and established prior to sitting or ambulatory activities.

If poor head control is evident, initiate treatment with prone-on-elbows positioning or seated at a table, feet firmly planted on the floor, with weight on the forearms. If there is poor trunk control, bolsters, wedges, or pillows will assist with support in the prone position. The neck extensors can be briefly brushed with ice, no more than five seconds, followed by a stretch and then heavy resistance to the extensors. This is followed by downward compression on the shoulders. The goal is to maintain the head in a steady, upright position.

Progression to management of trunk control will require a graduated removal of the pillow supports, and an increased demand will be placed on the elbows and shoulders. Approxima-tion through the shoulders should be provided. Weight shifting should be practiced until the client is able to sustain support on one elbow. Additional mat activities can include the quadruped position combined with joint approximation through the shoulders and hips and weight shifting. During this phase, trunk rolling and supine/prone-to-sit exercises can be practiced with graduated mild resistance given by the therapist. The client should progress to crawling activity to challenge balance, strength, and weight shifts in reciprocal patterns.

As head and trunk control improve, sitting can then be addressed. Sitting on surfaces without benefit of structural supports, i.e., the edge of a mat or chairs without arms or backs, should be used. Stabilization is promoted by joint approximation at the hips and shoulders. Weight shifting should be practiced. Another mat activity can include the tall-kneel position. The therapist should provide approximation through the shoulders and hips, and weight shifting can be practiced. Contact support can be initially provided by the therapist. As stabilization and balance improve, support is gradually reduced.

During progress in sitting and tall-kneel activities, the upper extremities should be extended from the body to challenge trunk stability. Head and trunk rotations and bending from the hips can be practiced with one or both arms extended overhead, laterally, or forward. Realistic movements should be practiced, i.e., reaching for objects overhead, to the side, or from the floor. Functional upper extremity activities may be practiced while sitting or tall-kneeling at a table. To progress stabilization, weight may be shifted from one forearm to the other while the opposing extremity is active. This support is gradually reduced until two-handed activities can be practiced. Mild resistance to the trunk and extremities for feedback is initially helpful to the client during movements. This can be provided manually by the therapist or by light wrist weights.

As head and trunk stabilization improves in sitting, supine/prone-to-sit, and tall-kneeling, the client should practice transfers. Initiate transfers from the most stable position, i.e., sliding surface to surface, and graduate in degrees of difficulty until the client is safely independent.

Much of the above activity prepares the client for standing and ambulation. Rolling, assuming and maintaining the quadruped position, crawling, and tall-kneeling are the basic neurodevelopmental sequence positions necessary preliminary to standing. Overall strengths, endurance, and balance must be adequate to launch into the demands of the upright position. The client should repeatedly practice moving through foot placement, sliding forward, flexing from the hips, and pushing upward with a sense of center of gravity and balance. Manual guidance from the therapist and visual feedback from a mirror can initially assist the client as extension of the hips and knees move the individual to the upright position.

Once stability in standing is accomplished, the ambulatory phase can be initiated. A front-wheeled walker may be the first support device required for ambulation practice. On occasion, weighted walker legs may be necessary to assist stabilization. If the client is appropriate, tall poles can be quite effective in developing a sense of rhythm, pace, and reciprocal movement.

The client with past-pointing or dysmetria will benefit from various techniques such as biofeedback,[103] PNF,[4] and Frenkel's exercises.[105] EMG biofeedback can be useful for the client during practical activities, i.e., combing hair, brushing teeth. Aquatic/pool exercises are also beneficial for the ataxic client.

Sensory Function

There is a therapeutic opportunity to address the sensory impairment of an extremity as the client is exposed to treatment in clinical, residential, and community activities. Yekutiel and Guttman[106] documented that somatosensory deficits in the plegic hand can significantly improve with intensive sensory retraining which incorporates functional tasks. The performance of basic self-care skills requires an integration of perceptual, cognitive, sensory, and motor functions. The client's ability to perform a motor task will depend upon the interactions of the residual components which are functioning throughout these systems.

An intensive effort should be made to stimulate sensory functions to normalize tactile sensitivity.[71,100] Keenan and Perry[49] noted that the sensory functions necessary for hand function included awareness of pain, light touch, temperature, proprioception, and two-point discrimination of less than 10 mm. Assessments will determine the specific deficits to be addressed. Treatment requires adequate time and opportunities to maximize repetition of stimuli. Also, incorporate visual input into treatment sessions to increase awareness.

If a significant motor impairment accompanies the sensory deficit, improvement of the motor function is usually addressed first. Tactile stimulation, however, can and should be incorporated into the initial treatment sessions. Weight-bearing on the impaired extremity, through the palmar surface, on a variety of textured surfaces (i.e., carpet, sand, or smooth metal) will facilitate motor function, proprioception, and touch. As improvement occurs in motor and sensory functions, progress the client to functional two-handed tasks. These tasks may include weight-bearing on dirt or sand while gardening, holding down paper while writing, or weight-bearing on the extremity while eating with the functional extremity.

Deficits in touch are addressed by providing a strong stimulus to the extremity. Initial sessions open with stimulus via rubbing various textures over the extremity. If possible, have the client actively move the textured material over his/her own extremity with the unimpaired hand. Make the client aware of any abnormal positions in the extremity or hand during activities. This should be immediately corrected to stimulate a sense of normal touch during movements. Functional tasks in repetitive daily routines can include washing, rinsing, and drying the hands, dusting, cleaning windows, making the bed, or folding laundry.

It is important to encourage the use of both hands in as many tasks or activities throughout the day as possible. A goal of treatment is to increase spontaneous use of the impaired side. Any therapist knows that the impaired extremity is not spontaneously used and that overuse of the unimpaired side occurs. Eggers[100] suggests a remedy by having the client wear a glove on the unimpaired hand, which should reduce overuse of the unimpaired extremity and facilitate increased use of the impaired extremity.

Proprioceptive deficits should be addressed while motor functions are performed. The impaired extremity is initially guided by the therapist. This is progressed to the client moving the impaired extremity through tasks with his/her own unimpaired extremity. If grip and strength are available, two-handed activities should then be incorporated to include lifting and movement of various objects, i.e., cans, plastic bottles, brush, etc. Engage activities which will include resistance, i.e., sanding or pushing objects. ADL tasks offer numerous opportunities to maximize therapeutic input for proprioceptive impairments. For example, dressing with a proprioceptively impaired upper extremity should begin with the practice of moving the extremity through sleeves or tubular materials. Have the client guide the extremity with the unimpaired hand and emphasize visual input as a reference. Progress to functional activities such as dressing. Practice should initiate with tasks in front of the body and overhead with visual input. As sensory function improves, progress to tasks without visual reference, i.e., tucking in a shirt or reaching for a wallet behind the back or reaching for objects under a table.

Smell and Taste

In cases where impairment of smell or taste is irreversible, the client and family need to be made aware of social, dietary, and safety implications of impaired smell and taste. The TBI client who will be living and/or working independently in the community will require training in management of perishable foods and toxic materials. Food preparation training must include visual monitoring of food while cooking and identification of altered seasoning practices which may not be healthy. Structure should be established to assist the client by labeling and dating perishable foods. Pet care, if applicable, should be undertaken systematically. Toxic materials should be moved to a safe place and labeled. Smoke and gas detection within the home should be considered and can be assisted by current electronic detection technology.[62]

The workplace must, likewise, be considered when treating for olfactory/gustatory deficits. Education of the employer and co-workers may allow the candidate for vocational placement a chance for return to work with reduced risk. The vocational rehabilitation counselor should take these types of deficits into consideration while looking or planning for vocational placement.[62]

Visual Perception and Perceptual Motor Functions

Areas frequently requiring therapeutic intervention are visual inattention, scanning, figure-ground, visuospatial perception, and visuopractic skills. In more severely impaired TBI clients, additional deficits may include color perception.

Appropriately trained rehabilitation assistants can augment the clinical program via the residential programs with home exercises as well as through functional application. Visual perception deficits, such as figure-ground, can be practiced via homework with worksheets and home exercises such as looking for specific objects in a cluttered drawer. It may be helpful, though, to teach the client to organize drawers in a less confusing manner. Puzzles, form boards, parquetry blocks, and other appropriate games can keep the client's interest while being therapeutic. Visual scanning while reading or working word puzzles may be useful. Data should be collected and reviewed over time for progress.

Neistadt[107,108] has indicated that there is an association between functional and constructional skills. The presence of constructional apraxia and visuoconstructive disorders has been shown to impact independent living by difficulties with meal preparation, dressing, changing a tire, or assembling an object. Bouska et al.[64] discuss the importance of teaching the client to approach a visuoconstructive task via sequential planning. For example, the task should begin first by visually and physically organizing the parts followed by construction of the object. The apraxic client benefits from physical guidance to initiate and carry out a simple task. With intense repetition, the ability to wash, groom, and feed should normalize. On higher levels, the dyspraxic client requires the same touch and guidance to accomplish more complex activities requiring the ability to plan, arrange, and build. The neurodevelopmental approach to improving perceptual motor skills has been found to be effective and provides a guideline to the progression of treatment as the client advances. Intensive practice is vital and should be pursued with functionally meaningful tasks in normal living environments.

For additional therapeutic approaches to visual impairments, the reader is referred to Chapters 7 and 8 in this volume.

Driving

Independence, in terms of driving skills, can be enhanced for the TBI client through perceptual training.[91] Exercises to address visual attention and scanning, visuospatial relationships, oculomotor skills, eye-hand-foot coordination, and response times are some of the components required to safely drive a vehicle. Driving evaluation and retraining should include behind-the-wheel time with a professionally trained driving instructor, in a dual-equipped vehicle.

Computer programs to address perceptual skills have become quite popular over the past decade. Many rehabilitation programs have depended heavily upon this tool as a therapeutic base. While computer-assisted therapy is a useful and motivating approach, it does not provide stimulus to or require responses from other systems, e.g., vestibular, motor, or other perceptual responses.[64] Any dysfunction in the perceptual realm may be impacted by concomitant vestibular and/or cerebellar deficits.[52] Again, the importance of hands-on therapy to reintegrate multiple systems into efficiently coordinated responses requires more than one evaluative or therapeutic approach. If driving skills are not adequate at evaluation, it may well be possible to enhance skills via training. It may be necessary to undertake driver's retraining with both classroom and behind-the-wheel instruction in order to improve driving skills. All therapeutic disciplines should be polled as to potential limitations which may be experienced prior to the driving evaluation. This information should be reviewed by the treating physician and a determination made about the propriety of the driving evaluation. This information will be invaluable to the driving evaluator as the assessment is undertaken.

Cardiovascular Fitness

As major sensorimotor deficits are improved and general mobility advances to higher levels, the client may become appropriate for an aerobic and conditioning program. These programs can be developed to fit into the client's lifestyle by gradually transferring the exercise routine from the clinical setting to a community gym. The initial exercises must be performed with the therapist's close supervision.

An aerobic and conditioning program can be created for the higher level client as well as one with significant motor impairments. Stretching should also be taught to start any exercise routine. An exercise program can be developed with stationary bicycles (standard or recumbent), treadmills, and weights. Muscle conditioning may utilize isometric exercise or full range exercise with weights, elastic exercise bands, free weights, or exercise machines. Low-impact aerobic exercise routines can be developed with walking, swimming, bicycling, and aerobic classes.

As the client becomes more independent and community reentry is developed, the therapist may assist the client in the choice of and transfer to a community-type exercise routine, i.e., a local gym or fitness center. Independent aerobic and exercise routines can be established in walking, swimming, or bicycling as well as a maintenance stretching and muscle toning exercise program, i.e., sit-ups, push-ups, etc. In some instances, even short-form Tai Chi has been utilized.

As the benefits of conditioning renew the client's sense of well-being and enhance the overall functional status, the continuation of exercise as an enjoyable routine may allow a gradual reduction of supervision.

The motorically and cognitively impaired clients also gain great benefit from a fitness program. Aside from endurance and stamina, it has been demonstrated that thinking ability and emotional status improve with physical fitness.[109,110] As a result, there are enhanced levels of energy, feelings of well-being, and independence for most TBI clients.

Pool/Aquatic Therapy

Although the healing elements of water have been used for centuries, organized therapeutic protocols for the neurologically impaired have emerged only during the past decade. Current programs for musculoskeletal injuries, e.g., neck and back, are widely accepted by therapists and well received by clients. In this regard, the use of a pool program is a positive aspect to the physical rehabilitation for the MTBI client. Aquatic therapy can address difficulties with balance and coordination, muscle weakness, poor endurance, and sensory dysfunctions. The buoyancy and warmth of the water, together with use of appliances to introduce resistive exercises, make a good combination for therapeutic application. Subtle vestibular impairments may manifest in aquatic activities as water reduces proprioceptive feedback making balance functions more dependent upon visual and vestibular feedback. Precautions for cardiac or other medical considerations should be taken prior to introduction of an aquatic program.

The more motorically impaired client can have quite positive responses to a pool program. Abnormal muscle tone, motor control, gait patterns, and range of motion deficits can be addressed by utilizing the characteristics of water. This approach can add an element of fun and should be relaxing for the client. As usual, normal precautions must be taken for cardiac, incontinence, and swallowing issues.[111,112]

SUMMARY

This chapter presents an historical review of the integration of physical rehabilitation services into the developing field of head trauma rehabilitation. The chapter provides a comprehensive review of evaluative and management protocols in areas which are most commonly observed to be problematic on a long-term basis for the person with TBI. The reader has been encouraged to adopt an expectation for continued improvement associated with continued treatment beyond acute hospitalization. Physical and occupational therapists should understand the tremendously complicated clinical presentation often associated with TBI and become familiar with treatment strategies which can be used either individually or in tandem to treat the physical residuals associated with TBI.

REFERENCES

1. Bobath, B., *Adult Hemiplegia: Evaluation and Treatment*, Revised edition 2, William Heinemann Medical Books, Ltd., London, 1978.
2. Bobath, K. and Bobath, B., Cerebral palsy. Part 1. The neurological approach to treatment, in *Physical Therapy Services in the Developmental Disabilities*, Pearson, P. H. and Williams, C. E., Eds., Charles C. Thomas, Springfield, IL, 1980, 114.
3. Stockmeyer, S. A., An interpretation of the approach of Rood to the treatment of neuromuscular dysfunction, *Am. J. Phys. Med.,* 46, 900, 1967.
4. Knott, M. and Voss, D. E., *Proprioceptive Neuromuscular Facilitation: Patterns and Techniques*, Harper & Row, New York, 1956.
5. Brunnstrom, S., *Movement Therapy in Hemiplegia: A Neurophysiological Approach*, Harper & Row, New York, 1970.
6. Brunnstrom, S., *Mechanical Principles: Application to the Human Body in Clinical Kinesiology*, F. A. Davis, Philadelphia, 1972.
7. Ayres, A. J., *Sensory Integration and Learning Disorders*, Western Psychological Services, Los Angeles, 1972.
8. Johnson, D. A., Roethig-Johnston, K., and Richards, D., Biochemical and physiological parameters of recovery in acute severe head injury: Responses to multisensory stimulation, *Brain Injury*, 7, 491, 1993.
9. Jennett, B. and Teasdale, G., *Management of Head Injuries*, F. A. Davis, Philadelphia, 1981.
10. Rosenthal, M., Griffith, E. R., Bond, M. B., and Miller, J. D., *Rehabilitation of the Head Injured Adult*, F. A. Davis, Philadelphia, 1983.
11. Umphred, D. A., Conceptual model: A framework for clinical problem solving, in *Neurological Rehabilitation*, 2nd edition, Umphred, D. A., Ed., C. V. Mosby Company, St. Louis, MO, 1990.
12. Horak, F. B. and Shumway-Cook, A., Clinical implications of posture control research, in *Balance, Proceedings of the APTA Forum*, Duncan, P. W., Ed., American Physical Therapy Assoc., Alexandria, VA, 1990.
13. Shumway-Cook, A. and Olmscheid, R., A systems analysis of postural dyscontrol in traumatically brain-injured patients, *J. Head Trauma Rehabil.,* 5, 51, 1990.
14. Urbscheit, N. L., Cerebellar dysfunction, in *Neurological Rehabilitation*, 2nd edition, Umphred, D. A., Ed., C. V. Mosby Company, St. Louis, MO, 1990.
15. Boughton, A. and Ciesla, N., Physical therapy management of the head injured patient in the intensive care unit, *Top. Acute Care Trauma Rehabil.,* 1, 1, 1986.
16. Lehmkuhl, L., Thoi, L., Baize, C., Kelley, C., Krawczyk, L., and Bontke, C., Multimodality treatment of joint contractures in patients with severe brain injury: Cost effectiveness and integration of therapies in the application of serial/inhibitive casts, *J. Head Trauma Rehabil.,* 5, 23, 1990.
17. Murdock, K., Physical therapy in the neurologic intensive care unit, *Neurol. Report,* 16, 17, 1992.
18. Smith, S. S. and Winkler, P. A., Traumatic head injuries, in *Neurological Rehabilitation*, 2nd edition, Umphred, D. A., Ed., C. V. Mosby Company, St. Louis, MO, 1990, 347.
19. Umphred, D. A. and McCormack, G. L., Classification of common facilitatory and inhibitory treatment techniques, in *Neurological Rehabilitation*, 2nd edition, Umphred, D. A., Ed., C. V. Mosby Company, St. Louis, MO, 1990.
20. Sazbon, L. and Groswasser, Z., Time-related sequelae of TBI in patients with prolonged post-comatose unawareness (PC-U) state, *Brain Injury*, 5, 1, 1991.
21. Glenn, M. B. and Wroblewski, B., Update of pharmacology: Antispasticity medications in the patient with traumatic brain injury, *J. Head Trauma Rehabil.,* 1, 71, 1986.
22. Abel, N. A. and Smith, R. A., Intrathecal baclofen for treatment of intractable spinal spasticity, *Arch. Phys. Med. Rehabil.,* 75, 54, 1994.
23. Schleenbaker, R. E. and Mainous, A. G., Electromyographic biofeedback for neuromuscular reeducation in the hemiplegic stroke patient: A meta-analysis, *Arch. Phys. Med. Rehabil.,* 74, 1301, 1993.
24. Rao, N. and Costa, J. L., Recovery in non-vascular locked-in syndrome during treatment with Sinemet, *Brain Injury*, 3, 207, 1989.
25. Lal, S., Merbitz, C. T., and Grip, J. C., Reply to Eames, *Brain Injury*, 3, 321, 1989.
26. Haig, A. J. and Ruess, J. M., Recovery from vegetative state of six month's duration associated with Sinemet (levodopa/carbidopa), *Arch. Phys. Med. Rehabil.,* 71, 1081, 1990.

27. Wilkerson, D. L., Batavia, A. I., and DeJong, G., Use of functional status measures for payment of medical rehabilitation devices, *Arch. Phys. Med. Rehabil.,* 73, 111, 1992.

28. Lewis, A. M., Documentation of movement patterns used in the performance of functional tasks, *Neurol. Report,* 16, 13, 1992.

29. McCulloch, K. L. and Novack, T. A., Upper extremity functional assessment in traumatic brain-injured patients, *J. Head Trauma Rehabil.,* 5, 1, 1990.

30. Kloos, A. D., Measurement of muscle tone and strength, *Neurol. Report,* 16, 9, 1992.

31. Cardenas, D. D. and Clawson, D. R., Management of lower extremity strength and function in traumatically brain-injured patients, *J. Head Trauma Rehabil.,* 5, 43, 1990.

32. Keith, R. A., Functional assessment measures in medical rehabilitation: Current status, *Arch. Phys. Med. Rehabil.,* 8, 74, 1984.

33. McCulloch, K., Functional assessment for adults with neurologic impairment, *Neurol. Report,* 16, 4, 1992.

34. Mahoney, F. I. and Barthel, D. W., Functional evaluation: Barthel index, *M. State Med. J.,* 14, 61, 1965.

35. Rappaport, M., Hall, K. M., Hopkins, K., Belleza, T., and Cope, D. N., Disability rating scale for severe head trauma: Coma to community, *Arch. Phys. Med. Rehabil.,* 63, 118, 1982.

36. Gans, B. M., Haley, S. M., Hallenberg, S. C., Mann, N. et al., Description and interobserver reliability of Tuft's Assessment of Motor Performance, *Am. J. Phys. Med. Rehabil.,* 67, 202, 1988.

37. Tinetti, M. E., Performance oriented assessments of mobility problems in elderly patients, *J. Am. Geriatr. Soc.,* 34, 119, 1986.

38. Hamilton, B. B., Granger, C. V., Sherwin, F. S. et al., A uniform national data system for medical rehabilitation, in *Analysis and Measurement,* Fuhrer, M. J., Ed., Brookes Publishing Co., Baltimore, MD, 1987.

39. Gronwall, D., Cumulative and persisting effects of concussion on attention and cognition, in *Mild Head Injury,* Levin, H. S., Eisenberg, H. M., and Benton, A. L., Eds., Oxford University Press, New York, 1989.

40. Rutherford, W. H., Postconcussion symptoms: Relationship to acute neurological indices, individual differences, and circumstances of injury, in *Mild Head Injury,* Levin, H. S., Eisenberg, H. M., and Benton, A. L., Eds., Oxford University Press, New York, 1989.

41. Mathiowetz, V., Volland, G., Kashman, N., and Weber, K., Adult norms for the Box and Block Test of manual dexterity, *Am. J. Occup. Ther.,* 39, 386, 1985.

42. Sharpless, J. W., The nine hole peg test of finger-hand coordination for the hemiplegic patient, in Mossman's *A Problem Oriented Approach to Stroke Rehabilitation,* Sharpless, J. W., Ed., Charles C. Thomas, Springfield, IL, 1982, 470.

43. Jebson, R. H., Taylor, N., Trieschmann, R. B., Trotter, M. J., and Howard, L. A., An objective and standardized test of hand function, *Arch. Phys. Med. Rehabil.,* 50, 311, 1969.

44. Tiffin, J., *Purdue Pegboard Test,* Lafayette Instrument Co., Lafayette, IN, 1968.

45. *Minnesota Rate of Manipulation Tests,* American Guidance Service, Circle Pines, MN, 1969.

46. *Crawford Small Parts Dexterity Test,* The Psychological Corporation, New York, 1956.

47. Bennett, G. K., *Bennett Hand Tool Dexterity Test,* Revised edition, The Psychological Corporation, New York, 1981.

48. Swaine, B. R. and Sullivan, S. J., Relation between clinical and instrumented measures of motor coordination in traumatically brain injured persons, *Arch. Phys. Med. Rehabil.,* 73, 55, 1992.

49. Keenan, M. E. and Perry, J., Evaluation of upper extremity motor control in spastic brain-injured patients using dynamic electromyography, *J. Head Trauma Rehabil.,* 5, 13, 1990.

50. Fisher, B., Effect of trunk control and alignment on limb function, *J. Head Trauma Rehabil.,* 2, 72, 1987.

51. Nutt, J. G., Marsden, C. D., and Thompson, P. D., Human walking and higher-level gait disorders, particularly in the elderly, *Neurology,* 43, 268, 1993.

52. Farber, S. D. and Zoltan, B., Visual-vestibular systems interaction: Therapeutic implications, *J. Head Trauma Rehabil.,* 4, 9, 1989.

53. Shepard, N., Telian, A., and Smith-Wheelock, M., Habituation and balance retraining therapy: A retrospective review, *Neurol. Clin.,* 8, 459, 1990.

54. Herdman, S. J., Treatment of vestibular disorders in traumatically brain-injured patients, *J. Head Trauma Rehabil.,* 5, 63, 1990.

55. Shumway-Cook, A. and Horak, F. B., Assessing the influence of sensory interaction on balance: Suggestions from the field, *Phys. Ther.,* 66, 1548, 1986.

56. Weber, C. M. and Verbanets, J., Assessing balance performance in moderate head injury, *Top. Acute Care Trauma Rehabil.,* 1, 84, 1986.

57. Shumway-Cook, A. and Horak, F. B., Rehabilitation strategies for patients with vestibular deficits, *Neurol. Clin.,* 8, 441, 1990.

58. Flores, A. M., Objective measurement of standing balance, *Neurol. Report,* 6, 26, 1992.

59. Levin H. S., High, W. M., and Eisenberg, H. M., Impairment of olfactory recognition after closed head injury, *Brain,* 108, 579, 1985.

60. Costanzo, R. M. and Becker, D. P., Smell and taste disorders in head injury and neurosurgery patients, in *Clinical Measurements of Taste and Smell*, Meiselman, H. L. and Rivlin, R. S., Eds., Macmillan, New York, 1986.
61. Doty, R. L., Diagnostic tests and assessments, *J. Head Trauma Rehabil.,* 7, 47, 1992.
62. Zasler, N. D., McNeny, R., and Heywood, P. G., Rehabilitative management of olfactory and gustatory dysfunction following brain injury, *J. Head Trauma Rehabil.,* 7, 66, 1992.
63. Schlageter, K., Gray, B., Hall, K., Shaw, R., and Sammet, R., Incidence and treatment of visual dysfunction in traumatic brain injury, *Brain Injury*, 7, 439, 1993.
64. Bouska, M. J., Kauffman, N. A., and Marcus, S. E., Disorders of the visual perceptual system, in *Neurological Rehabilitation*, Umphred, D. A., Ed., C. V. Mosby Company, St. Louis, MO, 1990, 705.
65. Zoltan, B., Jabri, J., Panikoff, L., and Ryckman, D., *Perceptual Motor Evaluation for Head Injured and Other Neurologically Impaired Adults*, Revised edition, Santa Clara Valley Medical Center, Occupational Therapy Department, San Jose, CA, 1987.
66. Leiberman, S., Cohen, A., and Rubin, J., NYSOA-K-D test, *J. Am. Optom. Assoc.,* 54, 631, 1983.
67. Gianutsos, R. and Ramsey, G., Enabling the survivors of brain injury to receive rehabilitative optometric services, *J. Vision Rehabil.,* 2, 37, 1988.
68. Strano, C. M., Effects of visual deficits on ability to drive in traumatically brain-injured population, *J. Head Trauma Rehabil.,* 4, 35, 1989.
69. Baum, B. and Hall, K., Relationship between constructional praxis and dressing in the head injured adult, *Am. J. Occup. Ther.,* 35, 438, 1981.
70. Bowler, D. F., Perceptual assessment, *Neurol. Report,* 16, 26, 1992.
71. Titus, M. N. D., Gall, N. G., Verra, E. J., Roberson, T. A., and Mack, W., Correlation of perceptual performance with activities of daily living in stroke patients, *Am. J. Occup. Ther.,* 45, 410, 1991.
72. *Baylor Adult Visual Perception Evaluation*, Occupational Therapy Department, Baylor University, Houston, TX.
73. Bouska, M. J. and Kwatny, E., *Manual for Application of the Motor-Free Visual Perception Test to the Adult Population*, Temple University, Rehabilitation Research & Training Center No. 8, Philadelphia, 1980.
74. Colarusso, R. and Hammill, D., *The Motor-Free Visual Perception Test*, Academic Therapy Publications, Novato, CA, 1972.
75. Ayers, A. J., *Southern California Figure-Ground Test*, Western Psychological Services, Los Angeles, 1966.
76. Hooper, H. E., *The Hooper Visual Organization Test Manual*, Western Psychological Services, Los Angeles, 1958.
77. Miller, N., *Dyspraxia and Its Management*, Aspen Publishers, Rockville, MD, 1986.
78. Solet, J. M., Solet Test for Apraxia, Thesis, Boston University, Boston, MA, 1974.
79. Benton, A. L. and Fogel, M. D., Three dimensional constructional praxis, a client test, *Arch. Neurol.,* 7, 347, 1962.
80. Pascal, G. K. and Suttell, B., *The Bender-Gestalt Test: Its Quantification and Validity for Adults*, Grune & Stratton, Inc., New York, 1951.
81. Lezak, M. D., *Neuropsychological Assessment*, Oxford Press, New York, 1976.
82. Whiting, S., Lincoln, N., Bhavnani, G., and Cockbun, J., *RPAB-Rivermead Perceptual Assessment Battery Manual*, Nfer-Nelson Publishing Co., Ltd., Windsor Berks, England, 1985.
83. Itzkovich, M., Elazar, B., and Averbuch, S., LOTCA Lowenstein Occupational Therapy Cognition Assessment Manual, Maddak, Inc., Pequahnock, NJ, 1990.
84. Botte, M. J. and Moore, T. J., The orthopedic management of extremity injuries in head trauma, *J. Head Trauma Rehabil.,* 2, 13, 1987.
85. Garland, D. E., Bailey, S., Undetected injuries in head-injured adults, *Clin. Orthop.,* 146, 317, 1980.
86. Grummons, D., Stabilizing the occlusion: Finishing procedures, in *TMJ Disorders: Management of the Craniomandibular Complex*, Kraus, S. L., Ed., Churchill Livingstone, New York, 1988.
87. Anderson, J. M., Kaplan, M. S., and Felsenthal, G., Brain injury obscured by chronic pain: A preliminary report, *Arch. Phys. Med. Rehabil.,* 71, 703, 1990.
88. Zasler, N., Mild traumatic brain injury: Medical assessment and intervention, *J. Head Trauma Rehabil.,* 8, 13, 1993.
89. Pearce, J. M. S., Headache, *J. Neurol. Neurosurg. Psychiatry,* 57, 134, 1994.
90. Page, N. G. R. and Gresty, M. A., Motorist's vestibular disorientation syndrome, *J. Neurol. Neurosurg. Psychiatry,* 48, 729, 1985.
91. Sivak, M., Hill, C. S., Henson, D. L., Butler, B. P., Silber, S. M., and Olson, P. L., Improved driving performance following perceptual training in persons with brain damage, *Arch. Phys. Med. Rehabil.,* 65, 163, 1984.
92. Katz, R. T., Golden, R. S., Butler, J., Tepper, D., Rothke, S., Holmes, J., and Sahgal, V., Driving safely after brain damage: Follow-up of twenty-two patients with matched controls, *Arch. Phys. Med. Rehabil.,* 71, 133, 1990.

93. Ashley, M. J., Krych, D. K., and Lehr, R. P., Jr., Cost/benefit analysis for post-acute rehabilitation of the traumatically brain-injured patient, *J. Insurance Med.*, 22, 156, 1990.
94. Ashley, M. J., Persel, C. S., and Krych, D. K., Changes in reimbursement climate: Relationship between outcome, cost, and payer type in the post-acute rehabilitation environment, *J. Head Trauma Rehabil.*, 8, 30, 1993.
95. Haffey, W. J. and Abrams, D. L., Employment outcomes for participants in a brain injury work reentry program: Preliminary findings, *J. Head Trauma Rehabil.*, 6, 24, 1991.
96. Ben-Yishay, Y., Silver, S. M., Piasetsky, E., and Rattok, J., Relationship between employability and vocational outcome after intensive holistic cognitive rehabilitation, *J. Head Trauma Rehabil.*, 2, 35, 1987.
97. Cope, D. N., Cole, J. R., Hall, K. M., and Barkan, H., Brain injury: Analysis of outcome in a post-acute rehabilitation system. Part 1: General analysis, *Brain Injury*, 5, 111, 1991.
98. Cope, D. N., Cole, J. R., Hall, K. M., and Barkan, H., Brain injury: Analysis of outcome in a post-acute rehabilitation system. Part 2: Subanalysis, *Brain Injury*, 5, 127, 1991.
99. Spivack, G., Spettell, C. M., Ellis, D. W., and Ross, S. E., Effects of intensity of treatment and length of stay on rehabilitation outcomes, *Brain Injury*, 6, 419, 1992.
100. Eggers, O., *Occupational Therapy in the Treatment of Adult Hemiplegia*, Aspen Publishers, Rockville, MD, 1987.
101. Keenan, M. E., The orthopedic management of spasticity, *J. Head Trauma Rehabil.*, 2, 62, 1987.
102. Griffith, E. R. and Mayer, N. H., Hypertonicity and movement disorders, in *Rehabilitation of the Adult and Child with Traumatic Brain Injury*, Rosenthal, M. R., Griffith, E. R., Bond, M. R., and Miller, J. D., Eds., F. A. Davis, Philadelphia, 1990.
103. Duckett, S. and Kramer, T., Managing myoclonus secondary to anoxic encephalopathy through EMG biofeedback, *Brain Injury*, 8, 185, 1994.
104. Roller, P. and Leahy, P., Cerebellar ataxia, *Neurol. Report*, 15, 25, 1991.
105. Kottke, F. J., Stillwell, G. K., and Lehmann, J. F., Eds., Krusen's *Handbook of Physical Medicine and Rehabilitation*, Edition 3, W. B. Saunders Co., Philadelphia, 1982, 423.
106. Yekutiel, M. and Guttman, E., A controlled trial of the retraining of the sensory function of the hand in stroke patients, *J. Neurol. Neurosurg. Psychiatry*, 56, 241, 1993.
107. Neistadt, M. E., Normal adult performance on constructional praxis training tasks, *Am. J. Occup. Ther.*, 43, 448, 1989.
108. Neistadt, M. E., The relationship between constructional and meal preparation skills, *Arch. Phys. Med. Rehabil.*, 74, 144, 1993.
109. Hayden, R. M. and Allen, G. J., Relationship between aerobic exercise, anxiety, and depression: Convergent validation by knowledgeable informants, *J. Sports Med.*, 24, 69, 1984.
110. Tomporowski, P. D. and Ellis, N. R., Effects of exercise on cognitive processes: A review, *Psychol. Bull.*, 99, 338, 1986.
111. Hurley, R. and Turner, C., Neurology and aquatic therapy, *Clin. Manage.*, 26, 1991.
112. Morris, D. M., The use of pool therapy to improve the functional activities of adult hemiplegic patients, *Forum Proceedings: Forum on Physical Therapy Issues Related to Cerebrovascular Accident*, Neurology Section of the American Physical Therapy Association, Alexandria, VA, 1992, 45.

14

Vocational Rehabilitation

Joe Ninomiya, Jr., Mark J. Ashley, Michael L. Raney,
and David K. Krych

CONTENTS

0-8493-9463-5/95/$0.00+$.50
© 1995 by CRC Press Inc.

INTRODUCTION

Vocational rehabilitation came into focus in the 1970's as a field that faced the challenge of returning injured persons to productive employment.[1] As medical and scientific technologies progressed, vocational rehabilitation benefited, taking advantage of advances in rehabilitation engineering, electronic and computing sciences, and improvement of medical treatment technologies overall.

As an increasing number of persons began to survive traumatic brain injury (TBI), it was only a matter of time until vocational rehabilitation would be challenged as it never had been before. Not only would vocational counselors need to consider physical limitations in job development and placement but they would also be called upon to deal with behavioral, cognitive, psychological, and social limitations.

There would be many attempts at traditional vocational rehabilitation with the traumatically brain-injured individual, only to end in frustration and failure. Over these trials, however, would emerge information that eventually led to the idea that vocational rehabilitation needed to become vocational "therapy". This transition in thinking allowed for more flexibility and the development of processes designed to meet the needs of this special population more effectively. In fact, the traditional approach of requiring completion of medical treatment prior to initiation of vocational rehabilitation efforts would, likewise, fall by the wayside, to be supplanted by more adaptable options such as job coaching and supported employment. Successful vocational rehabilitation would need to begin far earlier in the overall rehabilitation process and become integral to the establishment of treatment goals in the medical rehabilitation process.

With this historical reference point, we can consider vocational rehabilitation of the traumatically brain-injured individual in the pages that follow, remembering that much change has occurred to meet the needs of this interesting and demanding population.

This chapter will deal specifically with the problem of unemployment following TBI, issues of return to work, preparation for return to work, and the roles and responsibilities of the vocational rehabilitation counselor in bringing together a vocational rehabilitation plan which has the greatest likelihood of success.

THE PROBLEM

The TBI patient presents a challenging array of short- and long-term deficits to the rehabilitation team. As early problems resolve, more persistent deficits become apparent. Many of these deficits are the focus of other chapters in this volume and serve as focal points for intensive rehabilitative efforts on the acute and postacute level. Certain of these deficits will persist over long periods of time and appear to be either difficult or nearly impossible to impact with therapeutic activities. Dikmen et al.[2] report difficulties in psychosocial functioning to be dominant in the period of time two years postinjury and beyond. These problems related, in particular, to the fact that many moderately to severely head-injured individuals remained unable to work and unable to support themselves financially.

Brooks[3] also reported that psychosocial impairments following brain injury were evidenced in terms of changes in family life and recreational and vocational activities. These functional consequences were described as "great and prolonged". He noted, though, improvements in treatment of psychosocial matters through alterations in rehabilitation focus of late.

Outcomes following TBI can be discussed from a number of perspectives, including medical recovery, functional capabilities, supervision requirements, and occupational skills. While it is beyond the scope of this chapter to address outcomes in general, a number of studies have reviewed employment trends following TBI. These studies range from reviews of severely injured persons to those involving mild traumatic brain injury (MTBI). Jacobs[4] surveyed 142 persons with TBI and found that 40% of them had a postinjury employment experience. A total of 27% were actually working, however, at the time the survey was conducted. Rao et al.[5] followed 79 consecutively admitted patients during a two-year period. Follow-up conducted at a median of 16.5 months postdischarge found that 66% or 52 of the patients had returned to work or school, while 34% ($n = 27$) had not. They found factors of younger age, shorter length of coma, minimal CT scan neurological findings, and shorter length of stay to be significant contributors to educational/vocational outcome. McMordie et al.[6] reviewed 177 cases, and reported that 45% of the sample was engaged in some work-related activity at follow-up; however, only 19% were competitively employed. Age when injured, sex, length of loss of consciousness, and learning, motor, and ambulation impairments were related to return to work. Many of those who returned to competitive employment were noted to have done so in less demanding positions than held preinjury.

Gonser[7] studied 122 patients with severe head injury with respect to global social and vocational reintegration two to four years following injury. The finding was that less than half of the patients (43%) were found to be without "employment handicap", while the remainder showed various degrees of occupational difficulty. Gonser indicated that cognitive disorder, physical handicap, age, and duration of unconsciousness were important prognostic factors for vocational reintegration, with neuropsychological impairment being the single most important factor.

Englander et al.[8] reviewed mild TBI admissions with Glasgow coma scores of 13–15 and posttraumatic amnesia (PTA) of less than 48 hours, totaling 77 individuals. Telephone follow-up conducted between one and three months postinjury showed only 88% had returned to work or school, with 16% of those returning having done so with some continuing symptoms.

As can be seen, difficulties with employment following TBI are a common finding in both short-term and long-term studies. There is question whether these findings are due to the nature of the neurological injuries sustained, inadequacies of vocational rehabilitation programming, or shortcomings of medical rehabilitation programming resulting in failure to provide adequate assistance in recovery from TBI. It is safe to assume that the neurological injuries sustained clearly impact the degree to which recovery can be expected. The literature is replete with studies which have identified factors pointing to severity of injury and poorer prognosis for long-term outcome. Comparatively less research has focused on the latter two questions, however, though a few authors have provided some interesting insights into these areas.

Johnson[9] reviewed employment after severe head injury and its relationship to the utilization of Manpower Services Commission programs. It was indicated that these programs failed to meet the needs of the head injured because the programs were too short or use was made of them at too long an interval postinjury. The programs were depicted to deal poorly with the special training needs and flexible treatment approach necessary for successful employment following brain injury.

Hallauer et al.[10] reviewed the experience levels of vocational rehabilitation counselors (VRC's) working with the TBI population. The authors reported a surprising lack of experience with the population, wherein only two of 46 VRC's had experience with more than 100 TBI clients. In fact, the majority of VRC's had experience with fewer than ten TBI clients. These authors reviewed the perceptions of VRC's compared to actual findings via neuropsychological evaluation. The VRC's were more likely to cite memory as problematic despite an absence of actual test findings which would support such a conclusion.

In a survey of 38 VRC's, 167 service providers, and 47 individuals with TBI, 8.5% of persons with TBI who received services from the New York State Office of Vocational Rehabilitation were ultimately placed in jobs as a result of those services.[11] Sixty-nine percent of the counselors reported that they felt only "minimally" or "somewhat" prepared to deal with the residuals of TBI. Over 91% reported that they "occasionally", "almost never", or "never" referred a client with TBI for cognitive remedial services. In fact, 53% of the respondents reported that they classified persons with TBI with other disabilities. Finally, 91% of the service providers responding reported that they did not have programs which were specifically developed for the TBI population.

Michaels and Risucci[12] contrasted VRC perceptions to employer perceptions of problems encountered by the TBI client in returning to work. The VRC's were more likely to focus on workplace accommodation, believing that accommodation would be too cumbersome for the employers. Employers were less concerned with accommodation and more concerned with whether the person could actually fulfill both the main job responsibilities as well as ancillary ones.

Prognostic Variables in Return to Work

It should come as no surprise that vocational rehabilitation counseling, like other rehabilitation disciplines, would require some time to acquire requisite knowledge, skills, and perspective to address the needs of a comparatively new vocational rehabilitation population. As rehabilitation professionals have gained in experience with the TBI population, studies have begun to focus on prognostic variables impacting return to work.

In a follow-up study of severely head-injured individuals seven years following injury, Oddy et al.[13] showed that, while there were no observed changes at follow-up in physical or cognitive status, personality problems continued to be frequently reported. Not surprisingly, less disabled individuals were seen to make further progress in returning to former levels of vocational or social activity. The findings of Vogenthaler et al.[14] were largely supportive of this perspective. These authors reported on long-term productivity and independent living outcomes as related to severity of injury. They found that, in general, more severe impairment at 24 hours postinjury was associated with greater dependence and less productivity at follow-up. They also found, however, that this was not always the case. In some circumstances, individuals who were severely impaired at 24 hours postinjury had good outcomes, while several mildly impaired subjects had poorer outcomes.

van Zomeren and van den Burg[15] conducted a follow-up study of 58 patients with severe closed head injury. A correlation between posttraumatic amnesia and return to work of 0.52 was demonstrated, indicating that longer PTA duration was associated with return to work at a lower level or not at all.

Rao and Kilgore[16] also looked at prediction of return to work following traumatic brain injury using two brain injury assessment measures — the Patient Evaluation and Conference System (PECS) and the Levels of Cognitive Functioning Scale. These scales allowed prediction of return to work with 73.5 to 84.4% accuracy. Analysis of incorrect predictions showed that social factors such as substance abuse, family and community supports, and financial need to return to work also seemed to impact return to work or school.

Wehman et al.[17] reported that individuals who were more difficult to secure vocational placement for tended to be younger and had greater functional limitations. As might be expected, it was indicated that these functional limitations impacted many work-related skills.

In a study conducted by Ruff et al.,[18] age, length of coma, speed for both attending and motor movements, spatial integration, and intact vocabulary were found to be significantly related to likelihood of returning to work or school. These authors indicated that the best predictors of return to work or school were the relative strengths of the individual's verbal intellectual power, speed of information processing, and age.

Ezrachi et al.[19] noted substantial contribution to return to work relative to an individual's ability to be aware of and accept deficits associated with traumatic brain injury.

In summary, severity of injury as measured by both coma and posttraumatic amnesia duration, degree of cognitive and physical impairment, age, learning ability, intellectual power, speed of processing, awareness and acceptance of deficits, and interpersonal relationship skills have all been observed to impact return to work.

Important information about return to work has also been gained from reviews of individuals who have returned to work and subsequent study of the reasons for separations from work.

Sale et al.[20] reported on a review of reasons for separation for 38 individual job separations involving 29 persons with TBI. They reported a mean length of employment of 5.8 months before separation. The range of time observed was 0.2 to 27.6 months. It is particularly instructive to note that over 66% of the separations came within the first six months of employment. Interpersonal relationship problems were cited as the most frequent reason for separation. These problems took the form of overfamiliarity, anger displays, or inappropriate social interaction such as violation of personal space, poor conversational turn-taking, etc. Problems associated with the employment setting, problems associated with mental health/criminal activity/substance abuse, and true economic layoffs followed as reasons for separation. In many cases, more than one reason was cited.

Information reported by Sale et al.[20] pertaining to substance abuse is supported by Kreutzer et al.[21] These authors cite difficulties associated with substance abuse and the importance of familiarity with substance abuse recognition and treatment requirements for vocational rehabilitation counselors working with the TBI population.

Return to Work Models

At the same time that information was being gathered relating to identification of problems encountered in return to work and variables which would impact the likelihood of a successful return to work, VRC's were, of course, attempting to return TBI clients to work. A number of models for return to work have been developed as a consequence. The basic approach of vocational rehabilitation — wherein limitations were identified, job modification pursued, or a determination made for pursuit of alternative employment, job search, and job placement — was found to be inadequate for the TBI client. It became readily apparent that return to work would require more time than other populations and that the role of the vocational rehabilitation counselor might need to take on a therapeutic flavor. It also became more widely accepted that the most efficacious vocational rehabilitation effort was likely to come from an integration of vocational rehabilitation services with medical rehabilitation services.

Pampus[22] suggested that more comprehensive and long-term therapy was necessary in rehabilitation of the brain-injured individual and that overall improvement could be achieved by close cooperation between the hospital, rehabilitation center, attending physician, rehabilitation agencies, and employers. Hackspacher et al.[23] also pointed to the role of interdisciplinary cooperation in rehabilitation problem solving.

Additionally, in a study by Jellinek and Harvey,[24] the ability to increase the likelihood of vocational/educational success by bringing vocational rehabilitation staff on to the treatment team of a rehabilitation facility was discussed. It was found that vocational/educational placement rates for spinal cord and brain-injured clients increased from 19% to as high as 78%.

As medical rehabilitation teams began to realize the importance of incorporation of vocational rehabilitation earlier in the overall process, several models of vocational rehabilitation emerged. These models included a *cognitive remediation model*,[25] a *work hardening model*,[26] and a *supported employment model*.[27] The most efficacious of these models appears to be the supported employment model. This model utilizes extensive "job coaching" for the individual returning to work. A job coach is assigned to provide early guidance for the worker in the employment setting. Over time, the job coach fades cues and assistance level, allowing the individual to take on greater responsibility for job performance.

SERVICE DELIVERY

Vocational rehabilitation services have been traditionally delivered as a distinctly different and separate process apart from the medical rehabilitation of patients served. In fact, in many instances, vocational rehabilitation is not allowed to occur until the patient has reached some type of maximum medical improvement or medically permanent and stationary status. In the case of the traumatically brain-injured patient, however, vocational rehabilitation has come to be viewed as an integral part of the planning for medical rehabilitation.

Outcome, in general, is heavily dependent upon the extent to which resolution of deficits arising from injury can be achieved, which is, in part, dependent upon the experience and nature of personnel and technological advances available to a given client in his recovery. The vocational end product will, therefore, be equally dependent upon the nature of services delivered prior to vocational rehabilitation service delivery and upon the nature of the injury sustained.

It is very important that the vocational rehabilitation counselor have a working knowledge of at least some of the prerequisite skills which should be addressed by the medical rehabilitation of the TBI patient. The counselor should take the opportunity to address these issues openly with the medical rehabilitation team in order to ensure that the vocational rehabilitation goals are recognized and integrated within the overall rehabilitation plan. These matters will be discussed more fully in later sections of this chapter.

In treating the traumatically brain-injured client, we can employ an approach common to all vocational rehabilitation as put forth by Rubin and Roessler:[1]

Good vocational adjustment by individuals with disabilities is the final objective of the vocational rehabilitation process. To achieve good vocational adjustment, several objectives must be reached:

1. The client should receive all information necessary to understand the role and function of the rehabilitation agency and its service providers.
2. The client should be properly informed of the purpose and expected outcomes of all services in which he or she is asked to participate.
3. A sound vocational counseling relationship must be developed early and maintained throughout the rehabilitation process.
4. All information necessary for the development of an accurate diagnosis should be acquired.
5. A comprehensive diagnostic process should precede the development of a rehabilitation plan.
6. The counselor and client should jointly develop an appropriate rehabilitation plan.
7. Each service called for by the rehabilitation plan should be thoroughly rendered and closely monitored.
8. Each case should be efficiently terminated.

From these objectives, it is clear that the participant in the vocational rehabilitation process is expected to play an active role in the process. However, the traumatically brain injured client has specific needs due to cognitive, behavioral, physical, social, psychological, and emotional factors that will definitively influence any vocational rehabilitation planning. Zuger and Boehme[28] relate several commonly encountered areas of difficulty in aligning perceptions between the TBI client and the VRC. They cite the idea that many persons with TBI believe that their level of functioning will return to preinjury levels and few anticipate significant problems in returning to work. This may occur as a result of a protective denial process, a simple lack of awareness of deficits, or a neurologically based inability to appreciate deficits. Zuger and Boehme indicate that frequently the person with TBI will be unwilling to shift vocational expectations and may be resistant to VRC recommendations or suggestions.

Thus, Rubin and Roessler's[1] model should be expanded to include:

1. Prevocational counseling utilizing a team approach.
2. Early vocational rehabilitation counselor interaction with the client.
3. Vocational testing and/or work evaluation.
4. Vocational rehabilitation planning.
5. Vocational rehabilitation outcome determination.
6. Follow-up.

Prevocational Counseling and Preparation

Life History

One purpose of prevocational counseling is to provide a forum in which information can be gathered concerning the client's relevant life history. This information includes a review of academic, social, familial, medical, and vocational information. This information should be brought together in a cohesive fashion to enable the vocational rehabilitation counselor a broad perspective of the client. Once obtained, life history information is combined with information about current medical status and/or anticipated limitations arising from cognitive, behavioral, physical, social, psychological, or emotional factors.

Self-Worth

It is particularly important that the individual's self-concept and self-worth be evaluated, both as they existed prior to injury and as they exist at the time of commencement of vocational rehabilitation services.

Marinelli and Dell Orto[29] state, "The impact of physical impairment on an individual's self-concept, body image, and social interactions is well documented.[30-34] Self-concept may be affected whether disability is totally or permanently disabling or moderate in effect...the impact of physical impairment on self-concept is also related to the premorbid personality of the client. Therefore, in the case of adventitious disability, it is helpful for the counselor to know something about the client's previous personality. Unless clients, their families, or the referring agency can provide an adequate psychosocial history, the counselor may not be aware of the self-concept the client had before the trauma. If the client had a history of poor self-concept and accompanying feelings of inadequacy, the trauma-accident may intensify those feelings. Similarly, an angry young man who, through his own impulsiveness, suffered a spinal cord injury in an auto accident may manifest exaggerated hostility."

Melamed, Groswasser, and Stern[35] reviewed relations between acceptance of disability, involvement in vocational activities, and subjective rehabilitation status (SRS) in 78 TBI patients one to two years following discharge from rehabilitation. The *subjective rehabilitation status* was defined as the individual's gratification of basic needs, physical well-being, emotional security, and family, social, economic, and vocational needs. These authors reported the highest SRS to be found among patients who were employed in the open labor market. Lower SRS was found in patients employed under protected conditions; they also reported their work to be different than their expectations. Unemployed patients who lived active lives reported higher SRS than unemployed patients living passive lives. Both of these, however, showed lower SRS than employed patients. The authors attributed work involvement and SRS to the degree of acceptance of disability.

Vocational rehabilitation is often viewed as the final stage in the rehabilitation process for the traumatically brain-injured patient. It is, however, instead, a culmination of the efforts of many medical and allied health professionals' efforts combined with those of the traumatically brain-injured individual. Consequently, it becomes extremely important that the vocational rehabilitation professional be familiar with the aforementioned parameters of an individual. It is in this way that the individual is both understood and treated as a whole.

Deficit Identification and Resolution

Initiation of vocational rehabilitation should be undertaken as a continuation of the overall rehabilitation process, rather than to await the resolution of all medical problems. These can include ongoing cognitive, behavioral, physical, psychological, social, and/or emotional problems. One of the most frequent mistakes of practice is initiation of vocational rehabilitation services without adequate attention to problems in these areas. That is not to say that a person with deficits in one or more of these areas is not a suitable vocational rehabilitation candidate but, rather, certain of these deficits, either in isolation or in combination with other deficits, may be such that failure in the vocational rehabilitation process is all but certain.

To that end, the vocational rehabilitation counselor must develop a keen awareness of the potential client's status in the medical rehabilitation process. The professional must be able to discern, either from other allied health professionals or from his or her own judgment, whether observed deficits will be adequately resolved by the time vocational rehabilitation is the primary focus of treatment. Likewise, the professional must be able to determine whether observed deficits, without further attention, will interfere with or cause the failure of the vocational rehabilitation plan.

Deficits which are not expected to be resolved must be considered for their impact on the vocational rehabilitation plan. Some physical deficits, for example, may be dealt with by physical alteration of the work site or by provision of additional equipment in the work site to compensate accordingly. Cognitive deficits may require a restructuring of work responsibilities, perhaps with inclusion of fail-safe procedures to monitor task completion or reassignment of selected responsibilities to other personnel.

Patients with significant psychological and/or emotional disturbances cannot reasonably be expected to be successful in a vocational rehabilitation process. At the same time, there are some patients for whom the vocational rehabilitation process serves an important role in their psychological and emotional recovery. The vocational rehabilitation counselor, then, must have access to his peers in other disciplines so as to secure information regarding the individual's psychosocial status and the intended treatment in this arena and the expected resolution of same.

Prevocational Testing

In the prevocational counseling phase of interaction with the traumatically brain-injured client, the vocational rehabilitation professional may determine that prevocational testing would assist in focusing allied health treatment to activities more specifically geared to return to work. The provision of said information can be helpful, not only to the therapists working with the patient but, also, in adjustment to disability discussions.

Care should be taken, however, to avoid an overreliance on standardized testing data. Burns et al.[11] reported that 38% of VRC's surveyed relied "moderately" and "very heavily" on standardized testing. This can be problematic in that many persons with TBI may actually have some measure of preserved functioning relative to previously learned job tasks. TBI generally affects old and new information processing differentially. New information is frequently problematic in terms of assimilation for the brain-injured individual. Often, it is new learning that is necessary in novel job placements and, therefore, most challenged.

Vocational Rehabilitation Prerequisites

As has been stated, one of the most unfortunate, yet common, mistakes in vocational rehabilitation of the traumatically brain-injured individual has to do with premature return to work. All too often, brain-injured individuals are readied for vocational return without adequate attention being paid to resolution of deficits in the physical, cognitive, emotional, psychological, communicative, or social realms. This appears to occur due to a lack of understanding of the importance of resolution of deficits in these realms combined with a seeming naïveté concerning the complexities of vocational participation.

The vocational rehabilitation counselor is in a critical position to provide feedback about whether deficits in all realms have been adequately dealt with so as to allow for successful involvement in vocational rehabilitation. Early participation by the vocational rehabilitation counselor can provide insight for other allied health professionals for suitable goal setting as outlined above and can also help to ensure a common understanding of the point of readiness for vocational rehabilitation. In the sections that follow, we will examine specific areas of deficit as listed above in more detail.

Physical Deficits

In many cases, work evaluators will not work with a client who has not been medically released by previously involved physicians. From a physical standpoint, it is generally best if the client is medically stable and, if possible, permanent and stationary ("maximal medical improvement" is used in some jurisdictions). However, with the head-injured individual, it is not unusual for there to have been a vast array of physicians for a variety of reasons, and medical stability may not be completely attained by the time it becomes advisable for vocational rehabilitation service to be initiated.

Vocational rehabilitation with such a client can be taken in steps according to the status of medical releases. Vocational testing can be undertaken for the client who would benefit from progression in the vocational rehabilitation process even if some medical issues remain unresolved. Vocational testing could include interest testing, paper-and-pencil aptitude testing, and physical evaluation of unaffected areas of the client's body. It may be assumed, for example, that a client with a back injury as well as a head injury will likely require sedentary types of positions. In this way, the process moves forward, allowing the client to be continually motivated toward vocational goals. Progression in this fashion also allows for significant time savings until the point at which the vocational rehabilitation process can become more focused. There can be clear therapeutic benefit from participation in these activities as well.

The vocational rehabilitation counselor should pay particular attention to mobility, balance and coordination, ambulation, vision, visual perceptual issues, and overall strength and endurance, both from a muscular as well as cardiorespiratory perspective. Very close attention should also be paid to vestibular function, as these deficits are often overlooked. The reader is referred to Chapters 6 and 13 in this volume for in-depth review of these subjects.

It should be remembered that maximal physical restoration will broaden vocational opportunities available to the injured individual. To that end, the vocational rehabilitation counselor should be in early communication with physical and occupational therapists as well as the treating physiatrist to encourage goal setting which approaches maximal physical restoration vs. "functional" physical restoration. Many therapists differentiate functional skills from normal skills as they qualify a patient's skills. The term *functional* implies a minimalistic capability and may not adequately consider the rigorous demands of the vocational setting.

Psychological Deficits

Motivation and attitude are two major factors which most frequently affect a client's entry into the vocational rehabilitation process. Unresolved issues relative to adjustment to disability can work together with problems in motivation and attitude as significant barriers to vocational rehabilitation success. Difficulties in these arenas call for intensive counseling efforts to assist in resolution of these problems.

Behavioral observation of the client involved in therapeutic programs can assist in determining client readiness for vocational rehabilitation. If resistance is seen in the medical rehabilitation process, it may be reasonable to expect resistance in the vocational rehabilitation arena as well. It is important that these matters be carefully reviewed and considered as they will likely impact the success of vocational rehabilitation.

It should be noted, however, that, occasionally, it is necessary to continue to address motivation and adjustment to disability during vocational rehabilitation. The importance of awareness and acceptance of deficits has been identified by Ezrachi et al.[19] A careful appraisal of the client's status in this area should be undertaken. In fact, it is useful, sometimes, to use the vocational rehabilitation process as a tool in the adjustment to disability process. Since the most common reasons for job separation include interpersonal relationship and substance abuse problems, the VRC would be well advised to ensure that vigorous investigation into these areas has been undertaken prior to vocational rehabilitation programming. Treatment of these problems will be crucial to the individual's long-term vocational success.

The client's feelings of anxiety, stress, fear, or apprehension regarding return to competitive gainful employment should be considered. It is important that the vocational rehabilitation counselor maintain contact with the psychologist or counselor involved in the rehabilitation process to obtain a first-hand understanding of any potential problems in these areas. Second, it may be advisable for conjoint interaction between the vocational rehabilitation counselor and the psychologist to strategize methods to address such problems. Review of personality testing which may have been conducted by a treating counselor or psychologist can provide tremendous insight into variables which may influence the manner in which vocational rehabilitation should be pursued. The results of the MMPI, Taylor-Johnson Temperament Analysis, and the FIRO-B can be quite useful when properly interpreted and integrated into the vocational rehabilitation process.

It should not be assumed that a return to work is always in the client's best interest. While most therapists would agree that vocational involvement represents ongoing therapeutic exercise from cognitive, physical, communicative, social, and psychological perspectives, the client may view vocational return from a more pragmatic perspective. Simply stated, whether the client will benefit financially from returning to work should be determined. This single point can have a major impact on the success of vocational rehabilitation programming and the advisability of undertaking same.

There can be many reasons that a client does not desire a return to work. These can include loss of income from an undisclosed disability insurance policy, loss of income from social security, or return to lesser stability in income as in cases of seasonal workers who are injured on the job. Secondary gain is, occasionally, a problem in progression of a traumatically brain-injured individual through the rehabilitation process. Issues which contribute to secondary gain can be quite varied. A lack of desire to work in order to maintain dependency, a desire to maintain immigration status for the injured individual or family which may have been allowed into the country during the rehabilitation process, or more complicated emotional problems can arise. In cases such as these, it is important to be in a position where the individual's ability to perform activities of daily living (ADL's) and/or job functions can be contrasted to willingness to do the same. Here again, it is important to have close contact with allied health professionals in order to gain adequate understanding of these matters.

Cognitive Deficits

Cognitive deficits associated with an individual's traumatic brain injury will vary according to the severity of the injury and location of lesions. The client's abilities and limitations need to be explored and acknowledged with vocational rehabilitation geared toward the functional abilities of the client. Cognition must be carefully measured in order to guide the client in the right direction for future employment. The quality of the cognitive rehabilitation effort preceding vocational rehabilitation will directly impact the viability of any vocational rehabilitation plan. Great care must be taken to ensure that appropriate cognitive rehabilitation efforts were undertaken to secure commensurate success in vocational rehabilitation.

It is not unusual for a traumatically brain-injured person to have major cognitive problems which interfere with returning to work. These deficits can take many forms, i.e., deficits in attention, memory, judgment, or problem-solving capabilities. Cognition can be best viewed as a hierarchical process, such that one skill builds upon another and, when all skills are present, the person is able to attend, organize information, remember, problem-solve, and reason.

The vocational rehabilitation counselor should look for information regarding specific cognitive deficits in attention, perceptual feature identification, categorization, cognitive shift, problem solving, reasoning, and cognitive distance. The patient must be able to maintain a focus of attention (vigilance) and shift focus of attention at will in the presence of multisensory stimuli (cognitive shift). Shifting of attention should be done with a minimal loss of accuracy and with a minimum amount of time. The individual must be able to deal with all perceptual information available and apply this information discriminately to categorical processes. Abilities in the areas of attention, perceptual feature identification, or categorization bear directly upon skills for problem solving and reasoning.

Bjerke[36] discusses evaluation of memory function in 190 patients with TBI. Interestingly, patients with mild head injuries were observed to report greater difficulty with memory function as compared to patients with more severe head injuries. Neuropsychological test results did not correspond well with the levels of reported difficulty for either patients of mild head injury nor for those of more severe injury. Thus, the vocational counselor may be faced with seemingly conflicting information which will require consideration and resolution within the scope of the overall vocational process.

Melamed et al.[37] explored the relationship between attention capacity limitations and abilities to perform work activities. *Capacity limitation* was identified as difficulties in dual task performance requiring simultaneous attention and response to two sources of stimulation. The authors showed that individuals with poor performance in capacity limitation were less likely to return to work. Thus, the need for adequate resolution of basic cognitive processes is underscored. The impact of these deficits on job performance and retention can be considerable.

Since cognitive function is of paramount importance to vocational rehabilitation, the reader is referred to Chapter 12 in this volume for a comprehensive review of cognitive skills and remediation.

Communication Deficits

Effective communication in the vocational setting is critical to vocational success. The client should be able to communicate at a minimal level in order to be classified as vocationally feasible, and more complex positions will, without doubt, require more advanced communication skills. Assembly-type work, for example, may require lesser communication skills. Communication abilities should be consistent with required skills, no matter what the position.

Specifically, the vocational rehabilitation counselor should obtain information regarding auditory comprehension capabilities, skills in auditory figure-ground, and expressive language skills which are both verbal and written. The client's speech intelligibility (how well speech can be understood by a listener) should be adequate to the work position. Disorders which compromise intelligibility can lead to faulty or reduced communication at the work site. It is hard to imagine a work site where such communication problems would be welcomed.

Voice or fluency disorders may also negatively impact a person's ability to communicate adequately in a work setting. Some voice disorders (e.g., when a person's ability to manipulate vocal intensity is impaired) may cause co-workers or supervisors to misunderstand the client's communicative intent. A loudly spoken utterance could be construed as impatient or angry, whereas a soft utterance could communicate shyness or a lack of confidence.

Similarly, the client who is dysfluent may fail to communicate when necessary, due to embarrassment or difficulty being understood, or co-workers may avoid the individual for the same reasons.

The client must be able to understand what is said to him, both in quiet and background noise situations. The client must be able to understand directions which may be provided, either orally or in writing, and must be able to retain the information. Auditory and visual processing skills are often disrupted by competing stimuli. The potential for disruption may not be apparent from casual observation or even from more in-depth vocational testing. Unfortunately, without appropriate observation during simulated work circumstances, subtle difficulties in attention and cognitive shift can go undetected. Lastly, the client's graphic skills must be considered. The client must be able to both receive and give information in a written format in many work positions. This entails not only the ability to code and decode information but also entails some fine motor skills for writing.

Social Deficits

The vocational setting offers a wealth of opportunity for social interaction. As a consequence, social skills, or deficits therein, become quite apparent in the vocational environment. The client's ability to interact with co-workers and supervisors must be carefully measured and analyzed as to its anticipated impact on the vocational rehabilitation placement. A higher level of socially appropriate skills will enhance the number of vocational choices available to the individual.

Several aspects of socially appropriate behaviors which should be considered are listed below:

1. The client must be able to respect personal space of co-workers.
2. Clients are much more successful in vocational settings when they can spontaneously exchange social pleasantries.
3. Inappropriate language in the workplace can be problematic, depending upon the site. (In some work sites, however, rough language may be more the norm.)
4. The individual must be able to interface with members of the opposite sex in a way which respects social mores and maintains appropriate social distance.
5. The individual should be able to recognize his place in the organization and any limitations or expectations commensurate with that place, e.g., it may not be appropriate for a clerk in a medical office to refer to the physician on a first name basis or for an employee to blow up at a supervisor.
6. The client should be able to use manners well, without over- or underutilization of politeness.
7. An individual who continues to be emotionally labile may have difficulties fitting into some work settings.
8. Clients with impulse control disorders have substantial difficulties in most work settings and may require the longest periods of job coach utilization or supported employment.

Timing

As the prerequisites for vocational rehabilitation are considered, the timing of vocational rehabilitation services in relation to the client's progression through medical and therapeutic rehabilitation must be coordinated. If progress in all areas is not considered carefully, vocational rehabilitation services can begin too early, leading to undesirable results.

One of the best indicators for initiation of vocational rehabilitation services is stabilization of progress in the various rehabilitation disciplines. In circumstances where the client is making minimal gains in the medical rehabilitation model, the vocational rehabilitation counselor's involvement may enhance the ability to progress further. In contrast, if medical or therapeutic rehabilitation has not been adequate, or is incomplete, and the client has not obtained necessary prerequisite skills for vocational rehabilitation involvement, the client may fail in vocational rehabilitation, thereby adding substantial difficulty to future rehabilitation programming.

The impact of vocational failure on the individual's psychological and emotional status cannot be overstated. Likewise, success in the vocational rehabilitation arena can be expected to have a substantially positive impact on the client's overall status. It is critical that the client's psychological well-being be carefully considered as the medical rehabilitation process moves to a vocational one.

Vocational Counseling

Conveyance of Roles and Responsibilities

The initial client contact should begin with a clear setting of expectations outlining what the counselor can and cannot provide. Likewise, it is the vocational rehabilitation specialist's responsibility to convey expectations concerning the client's participation in the vocational rehabilitation process.

Explanation of Benefits

Information regarding all vocational rehabilitation benefits for which the client is eligible should be provided in a concrete and detailed way. It may be necessary, from time to time, to review this information in a concrete fashion which will allow for suitable repetition of the information and better retention by the client.

It may also be helpful for the counselor to review the services rendered to the client with significant others. Many clients begin the vocational rehabilitation process having had second-hand experience with vocational rehabilitation via a friend or family member. Services which were delivered to those individuals may be different due to many circumstances: differing state laws governing those cases, differing insurance benefits applicable to those cases, or different disabilities which might have required different processes. It is most helpful to discuss these matters openly and in advance of any rehabilitation planning, in order to alleviate any misunderstandings and align expectations.

Estimation of Vocational Goals

It is critical that the counselor obtain information about the client's vocational goals and contrast those goals to what the client's actual benefits provide for. It is often effective for the vocational rehabilitation counselor to have the client paraphrase or repeat the benefits for which he or she is eligible. In this way, the counselor can gauge the client's understanding of the process and the benefit that will be provided.

The counselor will gain valuable information from discussion of the client's vocational goals. The person with traumatic brain injury is often at a loss for an accurate understanding of the impact of the traumatic brain injury on his/her vocational future. More often than not, the client will not be able to estimate his/her vocational rehabilitation potential. Any over- or underestimation will provide good therapeutic fodder for prevocational counseling interaction. Plaum and Speight[38] discuss motivation for achievement in connection with rehabilitation measures. They found that vocational therapists' ratings and *Konstanzer Erfolgs-Misserfolg Batterie* (Constanci success-failure battery) (KEMB) findings showed that less severely disabled patients tended to hold unrealistically high objectives, while more severely disabled patients tended to strongly orientate their motivation on the specific deficits associated with the organic brain damage, thus arriving at possibly more reality-adjusted objectives. Persons who have sustained TBI anticipate few, if any, problems in returning to work.[28] They frequently underestimate the difficulties they will encounter compared to rehabilitation professionals.[39] It is at this stage that the vocational rehabilitation professional may desire ongoing interaction with a psychologist, psychiatrist, or a counselor who may be involved with the client.

Dependency

Prevocational guidance allows a counselor to develop rapport with the client and, in the establishment of that rapport, to evaluate dependency issues. Dependency is often fostered through the medical model of recovery, and the counselor must address dependency issues appropriately. Egocentricity and self-centeredness may develop due to the fact that all attention has been focused on the client through the weeks or months of medical recovery. The counselor must assist the client in realizing that the real world and society are very different from the sheltered environment from which he or she is emerging. The client must come to realize that his roles and responsibilities will change once the vocational rehabilitation phase gets under way. It is not, "What can therapy do for me with hard work?" but rather, "What can I do for an employer with hard work?". This transition can occur smoothly if the client is well prepared both prior to and after vocational rehabilitation has begun.

Job Analysis and Description

As the counseling process proceeds, a job description and work history should be obtained from the client. This vital information is important in determining the client's understanding of his preinjury job. This information, together with the work history, can be invaluable to treaters assisting in the medical rehabilitation process for goal definition.

It should be understood that it is not unusual for the client's job description to vary from the job description and work history obtained from the previous employer. A key indicator of the client's level of functioning is often how easily a reasonably complete job description and work history can be obtained by the counselor. This information is then compared with information obtained from other appropriate sources. Discrepancies in descriptions should be discussed and resolved with the client.

Once the job analysis has been reviewed by both the client and the employer, the client's current or anticipated abilities can be matched to the job analysis. The vocational counselor's goal is to utilize all information provided to attempt to determine whether the job analysis remains suitable for the injured worker. Obviously, a comparison of the patient's current or anticipated functional skills to those defined by the job analysis will provide all rehabilitation personnel with important information regarding goal setting and directions of therapeutic intervention.

Vocational Testing/Work Evaluation

When a client is ready for vocational rehabilitation services, work experience following the original injury is usually minimal or nonexistent. It is, therefore, advantageous for vocational testing and work evaluation to be incorporated into the vocational rehabilitation plan. These services allow for the client and the vocational rehabilitation counselor to obtain a realistic understanding of the client's potential for future vocational directions. With information gleaned from a work evaluation, the vocational rehabilitation counselor can assess a client's readiness to work, either part-time or full-time. The work evaluation may also point to the need for a work adjustment/work hardening program, which will be discussed further. It should be recognized that the information realized from work evaluation can be as valuable as any obtained from standardized testing. Information should be taken from both sources in order to prognosticate most accurately about a person's ability to return to work. It should also be remembered that even this information may not accurately reflect a person's abilities in previously learned tasks.

Vocational testing may include 1) interest testing, 2) aptitude testing, 3) standardized work samples, and 4) work samples designed to measure specific abilities. The reader is referred to the Appendix for a detailed review of numerous assessment tools utilized in vocational testing.

Work evaluation may include 1) standardized work samples designed to measure specific skills in question, 2) actual work samples taken from a previous position that will need to be completed in that position (i.e., assembling wheelbarrows, barbecues, etc.), 3) evaluation at the previous or similar type of employment setting, 4) evaluation via a set of work tasks which will be undertaken in a new occupation, or 5) a combination of the above. Work evaluation also allows assessment of the client's basic worker characteristics, including work quality and quantity. Work evaluation which samples previously performed work tasks are likely to be most prognostically accurate of ability to return to a former position.

Work adjustment involves utilizing information collected from vocational testing and work evaluation to develop or improve basic worker characteristics or specific work skills via a short-term work placement as a prelude to return to the real work force. During this phase, a job coach may be required to assist in accomplishment of these goals. The use of job coaches has been well documented in terms of its usefulness.

A job coach is an individual who works with the client in close proximity, training and assisting the client to become productive in the chosen work environment. The job coach usually accompanies the client, on a short-term basis, to any new-found temporary or permanent employment opportunity and is later transitioned out of the workplace following achievement of stability in the workplace.

Kreutzer et al.[40] describe a supportive approach to employment using job coordinators or job coaches and utilizing a number of compensatory strategies within the process.

West et al.[41] described three case studies illustrating types of intervention, including job placement, job site and off-site training, advocacy, and compensatory strategies, and ongoing assessment of maintenance of social and productive gains in order to assist with job retention. They suggested intensive and long-term intervention and support in order to achieve effective return to employment.

Wehman et al.[42] reported return to work of persons with traumatic brain injury and a supported employment approach. They looked at individuals with a mean latency of seven years and a mean period of unconsciousness of 53 days. Thirty-six percent of the referred clients had achieved competitive postinjury employment compared with 91% of the same group who were competitively employed before injury. Job retention was 71% with most jobs in warehouse, clerical, and service-related occupations following treatment. A mean of 291 hours of job coaching was required to place and maintain all clients in supported employment. Haffey and Abrams[43] reported a mean of 85 hours per client of job coach time.

Nisbet and Hagner[44] point out that there are a few potential pitfalls to utilization of a job coach. They cite difficulty fading the job coach from the workplace, undue attention to and potential stigmatization of the supported employee, the fact that the presence of the job coach may be obtrusive and alter the manner in which other employees behave, and the cost-effectiveness of long-term job coach support. Nisbet and Hagner suggest several "natural" work site support options which can be used to transition away from job coach support and into so-called natural supports. These options consist of using co-workers to create a mentor, training consultant, job-sharing, or attendant option, as appropriate.

Work hardening placement allows physical, cognitive, social, and psychological and emotional abilities to be developed in a specific job position. Work hardening programs are utilized to assist the client in building strength and endurance as well as stabilizing specific vocational skills. These programs can sometimes be designed and overseen by occupational therapists under the supervision of a physician in circumstances where there is no vocational rehabilitation benefit available for reimbursement.

The work hardening experience provides an opportunity for the client to make mistakes and learn from feedback in a real-world setting. The work setting can be thought of as "disposable" in that the goal of a work hardening program is to conduct "vocational therapy" in order to perfect skills in a number of areas so the client can move on to a more permanent position. The vocational rehabilitation specialist must keep open communication so as to assist the employer in providing a nurturing environment which will allow the client to develop improved productivity in the work placement.

The client has an opportunity to adjust and accommodate while relearning old job skills as well as new ones. This process may require several months to complete, and it is important that the majority of behavioral deficits be resolved in this setting before returning the client to his former position or to a new job. Some authors have reported set-up of work hardening opportunities within hospital settings.[43,45] The work hardening experiences available in these settings are fairly diverse and provide easy access for monitoring of performance.

The work hardening process should be monitored frequently and may require adjustments, both in terms of the placement and in accompanying therapeutic treatments. Frequently, information obtained from the work hardening setting can be provided to therapists working with the individual in order to better focus therapeutic activities toward vocational requirements.

Avocational placements, or volunteer positions, may also provide this type of intervention. The client can be assisted in developing positive worker characteristics and skills in avocational settings. Avocational settings can be established in a community setting by most vocational rehabilitation counselors through community contacts.

Work in parks and recreation areas are particularly useful, for example. These settings offer varied environments from museum settings to gardening. Volunteer positions are available, and the need to have a work evaluator or job coach present is not usually a problem. Avocational placements can sometimes provide experience and opportunities for learning, allowing the individual to become employable at a later date.

Vocational Rehabilitation Planning

Perhaps the most crucial aspect of the vocational rehabilitation process involves development of the overall vocational rehabilitation plan. The planning which is undertaken must be realistic and can only be well actualized following development of a written rehabilitation plan. Vocational rehabilitation plans differ in cost, time, and effectiveness in returning the brain-injured individual to work. Ideally, the counselor presents a plan to the individual which considers not only his interests, but his emotional, cognitive, psychological, and physical abilities and limitations. The plan is developed in concert with the individual and considers the labor market of the individual's intended discharge community as well as job availability within that labor market.

In the development of the plan, consideration must be given to potential problematic areas. These include, but are not limited to: 1) actual vs. stated motivation for the client's return to work, 2) the client's cognitive abilities, 3) the client's emotional profile, 4) physical deficits and limitations, 5) family support and interactions, 6) financial gain/need, 7) litigation, 8) self-esteem and self-concept, 9) work ethic, 10) work history, 11) preinjury work characteristics, 12) current and preinjury personality factors, 13) adjustment to disability, 14) transferable skills, 15) age, 16) the general employment index in the intended discharge geographical area, 17) employer prejudices regarding head injury and/or other disabilities, 18) general medical stability, 19) the presence or absence of a seizure disorder or other neurologic deficits, and 20) potential areas of conflict arising from various secondary gain issues.

Vocational rehabilitation plans for the brain-injured client can take a number of forms. It is occasionally possible to evolve from one plan to another since the vocational rehabilitation process is a dynamic one. The following vocational rehabilitation outcomes are listed in order of preference, in descending order, as plans which have been successfully utilized for brain-injured individuals.

1. Return to work: This is reemployment of the client by the same employer in the same job and work setting. A return to work plan may initially incorporate part-time hours, slowly building to full-time employment as the client becomes capable of handling all job responsibilities.
2. Modified work: This is reemployment of the client by the same employer in the same job, but with changes or modifications to the work process or station to assist the client to work within various physical or cognitive restrictions.
3. Alternative work: This is reemployment with the same employer in a similar or different job that is within the client's medical limitations. This can also be an attempt by the client to

utilize transferable skills with the same employer in a different job which the client has the ability to perform in a satisfactory manner.

4. Direct placement: This is employment with a new employer, either in a new job or preinjury job description that utilizes the employee's remaining transferable skills. This can range from utilizing skills obtained from hobbies, preinjury occupation, or past formalized training or education.

5. On-the-job training: This is employment with a new employer willing to provide adequate training to an employee in a new job. Often, some of the financial responsibility is shared with the employer during the course of on-the-job training and, frequently, the client continues to receive insurance or employer benefits throughout the on-the-job training experience.

6. Formalized schooling or training: This involves vocational schooling or academic instruction in a classroom setting with internships, where appropriate, directed at employment in new occupations.

7. Self-employment: This type of plan is designed to establish an independent business which is a self-sustaining enterprise. The bulk of responsibility lies with the client in establishing and maintaining success of the business entity.

Our experience would suggest that brain-injured individuals generally experience more success in the following five types of plans: 1) return to work, 2) modified job, 3) alternative work, 4) direct placement, and 5) on-the-job training (with a job coach). This mirrors the success of vocational rehabilitation plans, in general, as reported by the California Workers' Compensation Institute.[46]

Formalized schooling and self-employment are generally less successful due to the fact that, with the head-injured population, cognitive deficits frequently limit the individual's ability to benefit from such plans. New learning must take place in either of these plans, and problem-solving skills are heavily utilized. Again, this correlates well with the general population of disabled individuals for whom vocational rehabilitation plans are developed. Formalized schooling plans have less success in returning an individual to work than nonschooling plans.[47]

As a vocational rehabilitation plan is developed, it is important that all parties involved with a particular individual be consulted and agreement reached as to the vocational direction of choice. The vocational rehabilitation counselor will need to continue close monitoring of the individual throughout execution of the plan. Due to the nature of deficits seen following head injury, a lack of structure or direct intervention by the vocational rehabilitation counselor can cause a rehabilitation plan to fail. Continued contact with all concerned parties throughout execution of a plan allows for early recognition of problems and referral to various medical and therapeutic resources for resolution of problems before they become permanent road-blocks to success. The vocational rehabilitation counselor must anticipate problems and needs throughout the design and implementation of the rehabilitation plan and communicate these to the other professionals involved in the case.

Any rehabilitation plan should be phased to closure. The vocational counselor can expect various difficulties in the employment setting(s) prior to closure. It is not unusual for problem solving or restructuring of the plan to be required as the client progresses in the working environment(s). The vocational rehabilitation counselor's role is to assist in problem identification and problem solving.

Roles and Responsibilities

The vocational rehabilitation counselor must address the following skills:

1. Developing an effective résumé to account for lost work time due to recovery from the traumatic brain injury.

2. Role-playing activities for answering questions involving observed deficits.

3. Developing appropriate answers for specific questions that are directly related to the occupation the client wants to pursue.
4. Developing structured concrete job searching techniques with regular monitoring by the vocational rehabilitation counselor or job placement specialist.

Employment Monitoring

Once employment has been obtained, the vocational rehabilitation counselor takes on the additional responsibility of monitoring the client's performance. The majority of plan problems occur at this juncture, due to a lack of familiarity by the counselor with the necessity of closely monitoring clients with brain injuries in relation to their actual work load and employment setting.

Sale et al.[20] review reasons for separation from supported employment. They noted that reasons include the following: 1) interpersonal relationship problems, 2) issues related to the employment setting, 3) mental health problems, 4) criminal activity, 5) poor attendance, 6) low motivation, and 7) transportation problems. These authors noted that an unsuccessful placement was usually associated with a series of events leading to the separation decision rather than a single isolated event. The majority of separations occurred in the first six months of employment, suggesting a need for closest oversight during this period. Of course, even with fairly aggressive and comprehensive programming, job separations cannot be avoided altogether. In fact, Ben-Yishay et al.[45] reported a general decline in employment over a three-year period following such rehabilitative programming. At discharge, 64% of clients achieved competitive levels of employment, with 30% achieving noncompetitive levels of employment. At one year postdischarge, the figures were 63% and 28%, respectively; at two years, the figures were 59% and 25%, respectively; and at three years, they were 50% and 22%, respectively.

VOCATIONAL REHABILITATION OUTCOME DETERMINATION

It is important to review the timing and reasons for cessation of vocational rehabilitation. The counselor must determine if the client will be able to be successful in pursuit of the vocational rehabilitation plan. Where the expectation for success exists, the client should be taken through the plan wherever resources permit. Should the counselor determine that the client cannot be successful through vocational rehabilitation, nonfeasibility must be stated and services terminated.

There are circumstances where, even in the presence of adequate medical, rehabilitative, and vocational services, clients may not be able to benefit from vocational rehabilitation and may be deemed *vocationally nonfeasible.*

The reason(s) for nonfeasibility should be clearly reported, and it should be recalled that a determination of nonfeasibility does not necessarily preclude later reinitiation of vocational rehabilitation efforts. Nonfeasibility may occur for a variety of reasons, including medical restrictions, obtained employment, moving out of the area, substance abuse, failure to follow through with responsibilities as outlined in the vocational rehabilitation plan, or a simple declination of vocational rehabilitation services. The counselor may determine that a suspension of services is in order, or may decide that termination of services is necessary. These decisions should always be made in consideration of the overall rehabilitation picture and following consultation with other professionals involved in the case.

In cases of vocational nonfeasibility for clients with disabilities other than brain injury, vocational rehabilitation benefits typically stop and clients must fend for themselves through other private or social agencies. Application of these policies to the brain-injured individual, however, may represent a dire error and may result in regression in one or more areas of achievement.

Idle time for the brain-injured individual can be problematic, as the individual may not know how, or have the opportunity, to fill nonstructured time productively. Authors have noted that clients may become involved in crime, alcohol, drugs, negative relationships, medical deterioration, and may move to institutionalization or reinstitutionalization, seemingly related to idle time.[20,21] If a client is deemed nonfeasible for competitive or sheltered work settings, continued vocational rehabilitation efforts should be considered, not for the purpose of achieving traditional vocational rehabilitation goals, but for maintaining goals already achieved through the medical rehabilitation process.

The counselor can assist in locating part- or full-time volunteer settings, possibly utilizing a job coach, thereby requiring minimal monitoring by the employer. Volunteer placements can enhance the quality of life for the individual and assist in building self-esteem/self-concept. It may also assist in maintaining the individual at a particular level of functioning, avoiding return to medical treatment.

Continuing vocational rehabilitation benefits, in this manner, can certainly be cost-effective, since the individual will be able to more readily mainstream into society. The vocational rehabilitation counselor and case manager can develop a fairly dependable system through which they can monitor an individual effectively by collection of information provided by an employer or co-workers in the volunteer setting.

Both vocational and avocational involvement maximize demands placed upon an individual. Usually, the environment will demand all that an individual has to offer by way of physical, communicative, cognitive, social, and psychological/emotional skills. In fact, in many circumstances, the vocational/avocational setting can be expected to further these skill sets. As meaningful participation in the community occurs, the likelihood of regression is necessarily diminished.

Lastly, vocational/avocational participation allows for return to a more normalized rhythm of living. The concept of rhythm of living refers to the usual progression from a home environment to an alternative environment for participation in activities which occupy much of the day. These activities may be preschool and school activities for young individuals, or vocational activities for older individuals. These rhythms are established from a very early age and are integral to "normal" life.

Expectations for behavior change with each setting and the medical and vocational rehabilitation programs need to prepare the individual to be able to respond to these changing expectations. As postacute rehabilitation programs developed in the late 1970's and early 1980's, several models of care were devised. Some of these models called for the removal of the TBI patient to remote or rural settings, ostensibly to relieve the individual of the stresses of daily urban life and to allow the treating facility greater flexibility of treatment without the close and sometimes critical scrutiny of the community. More information has come to the fore, however, regarding environmental (ecological) validity and the impact of the treatment environment on generalization. Wehman et al.[27] point to the importance of "real work" settings in vocational rehabilitation. Golden et al.[48] advocate for both community reintegration and vocational rehabilitation services to be provided in "real" community and employment settings.

FOLLOW-UP

The provision of follow-up services is dependent upon three variables: 1) funding; 2) commitment by the rehabilitation professional; and 3) acceptance by the client. Provision for follow-up services may be required in the vocational rehabilitation or workers' compensation laws of a particular state. While 60–90 days of follow-up is common, persons with traumatic brain injury may require longer periods of observation.[45]

In establishing objectives for follow-up, the counselor should consult with other health professionals involved in the case, any financially responsible party, and the client. Close attention should be paid to what will be accomplished by the follow-up and whether the client will truly benefit from it.

The purpose of follow-up should be designed to ultimately enhance the quality of the individual's lifestyle. It should provide an opportunity for recommendations for further medical or other care. Follow-up should provide a review of new or different job responsibilities or placements to ensure compatibility with both the original vocational rehabilitation plan and the client's current capabilities. Congruence with skills and ability to perform job tasks safely should be primary concerns.

The counselor should be interested in whether the client has done or is doing anything which will compromise further health or successful completion of the plan. This may include motor vehicle or other accidents, hospitalization, substance use or abuse, failure to continue various medical or therapeutic treatments as recommended, and so on. A check with the local department of motor vehicles may show problems with traffic citations, substance abuse, or accidents.

Overall, the counselor conducting follow-up is interested in how the employee is doing on the job. The employer-employee relationship should be investigated together with work quality and quantity. Tardiness and absenteeism should be reviewed. The client's security in the position should be considered.

Follow-up services allow for problems to be discovered early on in the vocational rehabilitation process. Early discovery may allow for intervention to occur, thereby reducing the likelihood of job termination. Fine-tuning and modification of job duties and responsibilities can be performed both proactively and reactively, improving the placement for the client and the employer.

SUMMARY

Although vocational rehabilitation for the traumatically brain-injured individual represents a formidable task, success is possible through a multilevel, *aggressive* process. Considerable effort on the part of the vocational rehabilitation specialist is required, in terms of his own counseling skills as well as his directive/managerial prowess in utilizing the skills of allied health professionals. Indeed, when all members of the rehabilitation team are brought to the point of seeing themselves as part and parcel to the vocational rehabilitation process, the likelihood of a successful outcome is enhanced tremendously.

REFERENCES

1. Rubin, S. E. and Roessler, R. T., *Foundations of the Vocational Rehabilitation Process*, 3rd Edition, Pro-Ed, Austin, TX, 1987.
2. Dikmen, S., Machamer, J., and Temkin, N., Psychosocial outcome in patients with moderate to severe head injury: 2-year follow-up, *Brain Injury*, 7, 113, 1993.
3. Brooks, N., Psychosocial assessment after traumatic brain injury, *Scand. J. Rehabil. Med. Suppl.*, 26, 126, 1992.
4. Jacobs, H. E., The Los Angeles head injury survey: Procedures and preliminary findings, *Arch. Phys. Med. Rehabil.*, 69, 425, 1988.
5. Rao, N., Rosenthal, M., Cronin-Stubbs, D., Lambert, R., Barnes, P., and Swanson, B., Return to work after rehabilitation following traumatic brain injury, *Brain Injury*, 4, 49, 1990.
6. McMordie, W. R., Barker, S. L., and Paolo, T. M., Return to work (RTW) after head injury, *Brain Injury*, 4, 57, 1990.
7. Gonser, A., Prognose, Langzeitfolgen und berufliche Reintegration 2–4 Jahre nach schwerem Schadel-Hirn-Trauma [Prognosis, long-term sequelae and occupational reintegration 2–4 years after severe craniocerebral trauma], *Nervenarzt*, 63, 426, 1992.
8. Englander, J., Hall, K., Stimpson, T., and Chaffin, S., Mild traumatic brain injury in an insured population: Subjective complaints and return to employment, *Brain Injury*, 6, 161, 1992.
9. Johnson, R., Employment after severe head injury: Do the Manpower Services Commission schemes help? *Injury*, 20, 5, 1989.

10. Hallauer, D. S., Prosser, R. A., and Swift, K. F., Neuropsychological evaluation in the vocational rehabilitation of brain injured clients, *J. Appl. Rehabil. Counseling*, 20, 3, 1989.

11. Burns, P. G., Kay, T., and Pieper, B., A Survey of the Vocational Service System as It Relates to Head Injury Survivors and Their Vocational Needs, Grant No. 0001229, New York State Head Injury Association, 1986.

12. Michaels, C. A. and Risucci, D. A., Employer and counselor perceptions of workplace accommodations for persons with traumatic brain injury, *J. Appl. Rehabil. Counseling*, 24, 38, 1993.

13. Oddy, M., Coughlan, T., Tyerman, A., and Jenkins, D., Social adjustment after closed head injury: A further follow-up seven years after injury, *J. Neurol. Neurosurg. Psychiatry*, 48, 564, 1985.

14. Vogenthaler, D. R., Smith, K. R., Jr., and Goldfader, P., Head injury, an empirical study: Describing long-term productivity and independent living outcome, *Brain Injury*, 3, 355, 1989.

15. van Zomeren, A. H. and van den Burg, W., Residual complaints of patients two years after severe head injury, *J. Neurol. Neurosurg. Psychiatry*, 48, 21, 1985.

16. Rao, N. and Kilgore, K. M., Predicting return to work in traumatic brain injury using assessment scales, *Arch. Phys. Med. Rehabil.*, 73, 911, 1992.

17. Wehman, P., Kregel, J., Sherron, P., Nguyen, S., Kreutzer, J., Fry, R., and Zasler, N., Critical factors associated with the successful supported employment placement of patients with severe traumatic brain injury, *Brain Injury*, 7, 31, 1993.

18. Ruff, R. M., Marshall, L. F., Crouch, J., Klauber, M. R., Levin, H. S., Barth, J., Kreutzer, J., Blunt, B. A., Foulkes, M. A., Eisenberg, H. M., Jane, J. A., and Marmarou, A., Predictors of outcome following severe head trauma: Follow-up data from the Traumatic Coma Data Bank, *Brain Injury*, 7, 101, 1993.

19. Ezrachi, O., Ben-Yishay, Y., Kay, T., Diller, L., and Rattok, J., Predicting employment in traumatic brain injury following neuropsychological rehabilitation, *J. Head Trauma Rehabil.*, 6, 71, 1991.

20. Sale, P., West., M., Sherron, P., and Wehman, P. H., Exploratory analysis of job separation from supported employment for persons with traumatic brain injury, *J. Head Trauma Rehabil.*, 6, 1, 1991.

21. Kreutzer, J. S., Marwitz, J. H., and Wehman, P. H., Substance abuse assessment and treatment in vocational rehabilitation for persons with brain injury, *J. Head Trauma Rehabil.*, 6, 12, 1991.

22. Pampus, I., Rehabilitation Hirnverletzter. Ein erfolgreich abgewickelter Gesamtplan an einem Beispiel aufgezeight [Rehabilitation of brain-injured patients — demonstrated with the help of a successfully performed individual rehabilitation plan (author's transl)], *Rehabilitation (Stuttg)*, 18, 51, 1979.

23. Hackspacher, J., Dern, W., and Jeschke, H. A., Interdisziplinare Zusammenarbeit in der Rehabilitation — Problemlosungen nach schwerem Schadelhirntrauma [Interdisciplinary cooperation in rehabilitation — problem solving following severe craniocerebral injury], *Rehabilitation (Stuttg)*, 30, 75, 1991.

24. Jellinek, H. M. and Harvey, R. F., Vocational/educational services in a medical rehabilitation facility: Outcomes on spinal cord and brain-injured patients, *Arch. Phys. Med. Rehabil.*, 63, 87, 1982.

25. Prigatano, G. P., Fordyce, D. J., Zeiner, H. K., Roueche, R., Peppig, M., and Wood, B., Neuropsychological rehabilitation after closed head injury in young adults, *J. Neurol. Neurosurg. Psychiatry*, 47, 505, 1984.

26. Thompsen, I. V., Late outcome of very severe blunt head trauma: 10–15 year second follow-up, *J. Neurol. Neurosurg. Psychiatry*, 47, 260, 1984.

27. Wehman, P., Kreutzer, J., Stonnington, H. H., Wood, W., Sherron, P., Diambra, J., Fry, R., and Groah, C., Supported employment for persons with traumatic brain injury: A preliminary report, *J. Head Trauma Rehabil.*, 3, 82, 1988.

28. Zuger, R. R. and Boehme, M., Vocational rehabilitation counseling of traumatic brain injury: Factors contributing to stress, *J. Rehabil.*, April/May/June, 28, 1993.

29. Marinelli, R. P. and Dell Orto, A. E., *The Psychological and Social Impact of Physical Disability*, 2nd Edition, Springer Publishing Co., New York, 1984.

30. Hamburg, D. A., Coping behaviors in life-threatening circumstances, *Psychother. Psychosom.*, 23, 13, 1974.

31. Kolb, C. L. and Woldt, A. L., The rehabilitative potential of a Gestalt approach to counseling severely impaired clients, in *Rehabilitation Counseling with Persons Who Are Severely Disabled*, McDowell, W. A., Meadows, S. A., Crabtree, R., and Sakata, R., Eds., Marshall University Press, Huntington, WV, 1976.

32. Linkowski, M. A. and Dunn, M. A., Self-concept and acceptance of disability, *Rehabil. Counseling Bull.*, 18, 28, 1974.

33. Litman, T. J., The influence of self-concept and life orientation factors in rehabilitation of the orthopedically disabled, *J. Health Hum. Behav.*, 3, 249, 1962.

34. Wright, B. A., *Physical Disability — A Psychological Approach*, Harper & Row, New York, 1960.

35. Melamed, S., Groswasser, Z., and Stern, M. J., Acceptance of disability, work involvement and subjective rehabilitation status of traumatic brain-injured (TBI) patients, *Brain Injury*, 6, 233, 1992.

36. Bjerke, L. G., Hukommelsesfunksjon etter hodeskader [Memory function after head injuries], *Tidsskr. Nor. Laegeforen.*, 109, 684, 1989.

37. Melamed, S., Stern, M., Rahmani, L., Groswasser, Z., and Najenson, T., Attention capacity limitation, psychiatric parameters and their impact on work involvement following brain injury, *Scand. J. Rehabil. Med. Suppl.*, 12, 21, 1985.

38. Plaum, E. and Speight, I., Zur Erfassung der Leistungsmotivation im Zusammenhang mit Rehabilitationsmassnahmen [Assessment of motivation for achievement in connection with rehabilitation measures], *Rehabilitation (Stuttg)*, 27, 140, 1988.

39. Prigatano, G. P. and Fordyce, D. J., Cognitive dysfunction and psychosocial adjustment after brain injury, in *Neuropsychological Rehabilitation after Brain Injury*, Prigatano, G. P., Fordyce, D. J., Zeiner, H. K., Roueche, J. R., Pepping, M., and Wood, B. C., Eds.,, The Johns Hopkins University Press, Baltimore, 1986.

40. Kreutzer, J. S., Wehman, P., Morton, M. V., and Stonnington, H. H., Supported employment and compensatory strategies for enhancing vocational outcome following traumatic brain injury, *Int. Disabil. Stud.*, 13, 162, 1991.

41. West, M., Fry, R., Pastor, J., Moore, G., Killam, S., Wehman, P., and Stonnington, H. H., Helping post-acute traumatically brain injured clients return to work: Three case studies, *Int. J. Rehabil. Res.*, 13, 291, 1990.

42. Wehman, P. H., Kreutzer, J. S., West, M. D., Sherron, P. D., Zasler, N. D., Groah, C. H., Stonnington, H. H., Burns, C. T., and Sale, P. R., Return to work for persons with traumatic brain injury: A supported employment approach, *Arch. Phys. Med. Rehabil.*, 71, 1047, 1990.

43. Haffey, W. J. and Abrams, D. L., Employment outcomes for participants in a brain injury work reentry program: Preliminary findings, *J. Head Trauma Rehabil.*, 6, 24, 1991.

44. Nisbet, J. and Hagner, D., Natural supports in the workplace: A re-examination of supported employment, *J. Assoc. Persons Severe Handicaps*, 13, 260, 1988.

45. Ben-Yishay, Y., Silver, S. M., Piasetsky, E., and Rattok, J., Relationship between employability and vocational outcome after intensive holistic cognitive rehabilitation, *J. Head Trauma Rehabil.*, 2, 35, 1987.

46. California Workers' Compensation Institute, *Vocational Rehabilitation: The California Experience — 1975–1989*, California Worker's Compensation Institute, San Francisco, 1991.

47. Drury, D., Vencill, M., and Scott, J., *Rehabilitation and the California Injured Worker: Findings from Case File Reviews*, A report to the Rehabilitation Presidents' Council of California, Berkeley Planning Associates, Berkeley, CA, 1988.

48. Golden, T. P., Smith, S. A., and Golden, J. H., A review of current strategies and trends for the enhancement of vocational outcomes following brain injury, *J. Rehabil.*, October/November/December, 55–60, 1993.

49. Brandon, T. L., Button, W. L., Rastatter, C. J., and Ross, D. R., *Manual for Valpar Component Work Sample 1: Small Tools (Mechanical)*, Valpar Corporation, Tucson, AZ, 1974[a].

50. Brandon, T. L., Button, W. L., Rastatter, C. J., and Ross, D. R., *Manual for Valpar Component Work Sample 2: Size Discrimination*, Valpar Corporation, Tucson, AZ, 1974[b].

51. Brandon, T. L., Button, W. L., Rastatter, C. J., and Ross, D. R., *Manual for Valpar Component Work Sample 3: Numeric Sorting*, Valpar Corporation, Tucson, AZ, 1974[c].

52. Brandon, T. L., Button, W. L., Rastatter, C. J., and Ross, D. R., *Manual for Valpar Component Work Sample 4: Upper Extremity Range of Motion*, Valpar Corporation, Tucson, AZ, 1974[d].

53. Brandon, T. L., Button, W. L., Rastatter, C. J., and Ross, D. R., *Manual for Valpar Component Work Sample 5: Clerical Comprehension and Aptitude*, Valpar Corporation, Tucson, AZ, 1974[e].

54. Brandon, T. L., Button, W. L., Rastatter, C. J., and Ross, D. R., *Manual for Valpar Component Work Sample 6: Independent Problem Solving*, Valpar Corporation, Tucson, AZ, 1974[f].

55. Brandon, T. L., Button, W. L., Rastatter, C. J., and Ross, D. R., *Manual for Valpar Component Work Sample 7: Multi-Level Sorting*, Valpar Corporation, Tucson, AZ, 1974[g].

56. Brandon, T. L., Button, W. L., Rastatter, C. J., and Ross, D. R., *Manual for Valpar Component Work Sample 8: Simulated Assembly*, Valpar Corporation, Tucson, AZ, 1974[h].

57. Brandon, T. L., Button, W. L., Rastatter, C. J., and Ross, D. R., *Manual for Valpar Component Work Sample 9: Whole Body Range of Motion*, Valpar Corporation, Tucson, AZ, 1974[i].

58. Brandon, T. L., Button, W. L., Rastatter, C. J., and Ross, D. R., *Manual for Valpar Component Work Sample 10: Tri-Level Measurement*, Valpar Corporation, Tucson, AZ, 1974[j].

59. Brandon, T. L., Button, W. L., Rastatter, C. J., and Ross, D. R., *Manual for Valpar Component Work Sample 11: Eye-Hand-Foot Coordination*, Valpar Corporation, Tucson, AZ, 1974[k].

60. Brandon, T. L., Button, W. L., Rastatter, C. J., and Ross, D. R., *Manual for Valpar Component Work Sample 12: Soldering and Inspection (Electronic)*, Valpar Corporation, Tucson, AZ, 1975.

61. Jastak, J. F. and Jastak, S., *Wide Range Interest Opinion Test (WRIOT)*, Jastak Associates, Inc., Wilmington, DE, 1979.

62. Knapp, R. R. and Knapp, L., *COPS (California Occupational Preference System) Interest Inventory*, EdITS, San Diego, 1982.

63. Langmuir, C. R., *Oral Directions Test*, The Psychological Corp., New York, 1974.

64. *Vocational Evaluation System (VES): Administration Manual*, 4th Edition, The Singer Company Career Systems, Rochester, NY, 1982.

65. Bennett, G. K., Seashore, H. G., and Wesman, A. G., *Differential Aptitude Tests (DAT): Administrator's Manual*, Harcourt, Brace, Jovanovich, New York, 1982.

66. Knapp, L. and Knapp, R. R., *CAPS (Career Ability Placement Survey) Technical Manual*, EdITS, San Diego, 1984.

67. Duckworth, J. C. and Anderson, W. P., *MMPI Interpretation Manual for Counselors and Clinicians*, Accelerated Development, Inc., Muncie, IN, 1986.

68. Nash, L., Ed., *Taylor-Johnson Temperament Analysis Manual*, Western Psychological Services, Los Angeles, 1980.

69. Beck, A. T., Ward, C. H., Mendelson, M., Mock, J., and Erbaugh, J., An inventory for measuring depression, *Arch. Gen. Psychiatry*, 4, 561, 1961.

70. Schutz, W. C., *COPE: A FIRO Awareness Scale*, Consulting Psychologists Press, Inc., Palo Alto, CA, 1962.

71. Gluck, G. A., *Psychometric Properties of the FIRO-B: A Guide to Research*, Consulting Psychologists Press, Inc., Palo Alto, CA, 1983.

72. Jastak, S. and Wilkinson, G. S., *The Wide Range Achievement Test — Revised*, Western Psychological Services, Los Angeles, 1984.

73. Connolly, A. J., Nachtman, W., and Pritchett, E., *KeyMath Diagnostic Test*, American Guidance Service, Circle Pines, MN, 1976.

APPENDIX: VOCATIONAL REHABILITATION ASSESSMENT TOOLS

Valpar Component Work Sample 1: Small Tools

The Valpar Component Work Sample 1 (VCWS-1)[49] measures a person's ability to understand and work with various small hand tools such as pliers, screwdrivers, and wrenches. Also, VCWS-1 evaluates the frustration tolerances, the perseverance, and physical abilities of the evaluee. This test also allows observation of the client's ability to perform long, repetitive tasks; the client's manual dexterity; and the client's experience working with the various small tools in use. In the open labor market, the work activities which relate to the work component are characterized by emphasis on actual manual skills in relation to application of tools to related materials.

Valpar Component Work Sample 2: Size Discrimination

The Valpar Component Work Sample 2 (VCWS-2)[50] evaluates a person's ability to visually discriminate sizes using nuts and bolts on a board with various screws attached. This test allows observation of the evaluee's eye/hand coordination and bilateral dexterity since the bolts and nuts are manipulated physically. Jobs related to the VCWS-2 include performing work using gauges, calipers, and other tools. Examining and measuring for purposes of grading and sorting and working within prescribed tolerances and standards are evaluated.

Valpar Component Work Sample 3: Numerical Sorting

The Valpar Component Work Sample 3 (VCWS-3)[51] evaluates the ability of a person to sort, categorize objects, and file by a numerical code. This work sample relates to vocations which involve activities such as examining, sorting, grading, keeping records and receipts, recording and transmitting verbal or coded information, posting numerical data, posting verbal data, and other similar activities.

Valpar Component Work Sample 4: Upper Extremity Range of Motion

The Valpar Component Work Sample 4 (VCWS-4)[52] was developed to be a nonmedical or nonoccupational therapy measurement of the range of motion and work tolerances of the client in relation to the upper body. This test evaluates the client's use of upper arms, shoulders, forearms, wrists, elbows, hands, fingers, and thumbs. This work sample is particularly helpful in providing insight into the client's fatigue level, finger dexterity, and tactile sense abilities. This work sample measures abilities that are needed in jobs calling for handling, reaching, fingering, feeling, and visual orientation. The mechanics of the work sample allow the evaluator to view the various muscle groups in action relative to the fingers and wrists as well as other parts of the body. Coordination and perceptual skills are also evaluated in a practical manner by observation.

Valpar Component Work Sample 5: Clerical Comprehension and Aptitude

The Valpar Component Work Sample 5 (VCWS-5)[53] measures the client's ability to perform a variety of clerical tasks and the client's ability to learn new tasks. This test measures clerical ability and aptitude in a variety of areas including alphabetical filing, telephone answering, bookkeeping, and typing.

Valpar Component Work Sample 6: Independent Problem Solving

The Valpar Component Work Sample 6 (VCWS-6)[54] evaluates the client's ability to perform work tasks that require visual comparison of colored shapes. The major focus of this test includes decision-making and instruction-following abilities. Samples of these types of work activities include verifying computations, record keeping, and checking items for accuracy and consistency.

Valpar Component Work Sample 7: Multilevel Sorting

The Valpar Component Work Sample 7 (VCWS-7)[55] evaluates a person's ability to make decisions while participating in work tasks requiring physical manipulation and visual discrimination. This work sample allows the evaluator to observe the client's orientation, organization, and approach in regard to color, task, letter and number discrimination skills, decision processing and ability at a very simple level, together with physical manipulation skills.

Valpar Component Work Sample 8: Simulated Assembly

The Valpar Component Work Sample 8 (VCWS-8)[56] evaluates the person's ability to perform work at an assembly-line task requiring repetitive physical manipulations and measures a person's use of the upper extremities. This test measures the client's ability to perform jobs which are assembly-line in nature in which material moves toward and away from workers on the assembly line. This work task is also used to determine standing and sitting tolerances for evaluees entering or returning to the labor force.

Valpar Component Work Sample 9: Whole Body Range of Motion

The Valpar Component Work Sample 9 (VCWS-9)[57] is a measure of agility in various gross body movements of the trunk, arms, hands, legs, and fingers, as they relate to the physical capacities of various work tasks. This test sample tends to be very tiring. This test closely relates to the client's actual functional ability in performing job tasks such as kneeling, stooping, crouching, reaching, handling, feeling, fingering, and seeing found in various jobs.

Valpar Component Work Sample 10: Tri-level Measurement

The Valpar Component Work Sample 10 (VCWS-10)[58] evaluates a person's ability to perform very simple to very precise inspection and measurement tasks. Various job activities related to this work component include working with hands, tools, or standards, following set techniques and procedures, and exercising judgment and decision-making skills.

Valpar Component Work Sample 11: Eye-Hand-Foot Coordination

The Valpar Component Work Sample 11 (VCWS-11)[59] evaluates a person's ability to use his eyes, hands, and feet simultaneously in an organized and coordinated manner. The evaluator has an opportunity to observe the client's concentration, reaction time, planning, and learning as they relate to the work sample. Various jobs which are related to this work sample include starting and stopping, as well as observing the function of, machines, perceiving relations between moving objects, and planning the order of successive operations.

Valpar Component Work Sample 12: Soldering and Inspection (Electronic)

The Valpar Component Work Sample 12 (VCWS-12)[60] evaluates a person's ability to acquire and apply basic skills necessary to perform soldering tasks varying in levels of difficulty. Valpar-12 is designed to provide information regarding the client's eye-hand coordination, dexterity, ability to measure accurately, ability to follow instructions, visual acuity, frustration tolerance, attentiveness, and judgment. Jobs related to this work activity include processing or repairing materials, fabricating, and examining and measuring for the purpose of grading and sorting.

The Wide Range Interest Opinion Test (WRIOT)

The WRIOT[61] was designed to consider many areas and levels of activities as they may relate to various occupations. The test includes a range of unskilled labor through technical operations to professional and managerial positions. The test is not limited to its ability to measure specific occupations but provides insight into personality and motivational concerns as well. Categories of the WRIOT include art, literature, music, drama, sales, management, office work, personal service, protective services, social service, social science, biological science, physical science, numbers, mechanics, machine operation, outdoor, athletics, sedentariness, risk, ambition, chosen skill level, sex stereotype, agreement, negative bias, and positive bias.

The California Occupational Preference System (COPS) Interest Inventory

The COPS[62] is designed to assist individuals in career decision and future vocational direction. The COPS is a systematically developed measurement test providing information on occupational clusters which may be used as entry to most occupational information systems. The job categories evaluated by the COPS system include science, professional; science, skilled; technology, professional; technology, skilled; consumer economics; outdoor; business, professional; business, skilled; clerical; communication; arts, professional; arts, skilled; service, professional; service, skilled.

Oral Directions Test (ODT)

The ODT[63] assesses the client's ability to follow directions presented by verbal directions. This test is particularly useful for individuals with limited education and written skills, since the skills required to complete the items on this test range from basic literacy to above the junior high school level. The test is designed so that increase in difficulty occurs in progression. This test also provides information about the client's skills in taking and understanding oral directions.

Singer Vocational Evaluation System (VES): Small Engine Repair

The Singer VES[64] engine service work sample evaluates the client's ability to perform on job tasks that are common in many jobs related to the engine service field. The evaluation check points include 1) disassembling the engine, 2) making specified engine checks, 3) changing the oil, 4) adjusting the points, 5) selecting and gapping a new spark plug, 6) assembling the engine, and 7) cleaning the work area.

Other information is gathered through observation of the client's learning ability, attentiveness to taped instructions, and utilization of a filmstrip. The work sample allows the evaluator to observe the client in a real work situation involving complicated cognitive processing.

The Differential Aptitude Tests (DAT) Mechanical Reasoning Test

The DAT Mechanical Reasoning Test[65] is useful in making decisions as to the client's ability in occupations that require knowledge in the principles of commonly encountered physical forces. Occupations that require somewhat higher skill levels include mechanics, carpenters, maintenance persons, assemblers and assembly-line workers, and other physical manipulation occupations.

The Differential Aptitude Tests (DAT) Verbal Reasoning Test

The DAT Verbal Reasoning Test[65] measures the client's ability to understand concepts stated in words. The test is focused on the evaluation of the client's ability to think constructively, to find commonalities among apparently different thoughts and concepts, and to manipulate concepts on an abstract level. The verbal test is useful in predicting the ability to be successful in fields that require understanding of complex verbal relations and concepts.

The Differential Aptitude Tests (DAT) Spatial Relations Test

The DAT Spatial Relations Test[65] measures the client's ability to deal with concrete materials through visualization. This test is useful in determining how a client will perform in jobs that require one to imagine how an object would look if made from a given pattern or how a specified object would look if rotated in a given direction. These abilities are needed in such fields as dress designing, drafting, architecture, art, dye making, and decorating.

The Differential Aptitude Tests (DAT) Numerical Ability Test

The DAT Numerical Ability Test[65] is designed to test an individual's understanding of numerical concepts and facility in handling numerical relationships. The numerical ability test is important for such occupations as mathematics, physics, chemistry, engineering, and other occupations in which quantitative thinking is essential. Other occupations utilizing numerical ability information are jobs such as laboratory assistant, bookkeeper, statistician, and shipping clerk, and skilled positions such as carpenter and tool maker.

The Differential Aptitude Tests (DAT) Language Usage/Spelling Test

The DAT Language Usage/Spelling Test[65] is intended to measure the client's ability to detect errors in grammar, punctuation, and capitalization. The items on the test reflect skills in formal and informal writing in various types of occupations. The test is highly predictive of success in a variety of educational or formalized training situations.

The Differential Aptitude Tests (DAT) Clerical

The DAT Clerical[65] measures the ability to work under time constraints in the areas of filing, coding, keypunching, stockroom work, and similar occupations. The major factor of this test is clerical speed and accuracy rather than specific ability.

The Differential Aptitude Tests (DAT) Abstract Reasoning Test

The DAT Abstract Reasoning Test[65] is designed to provide a nonverbal measurement of the client's reasoning ability.

The Career Ability Placement Survey (CAPS) Mechanical Reasoning Test

The CAPS Mechanical Reasoning Test[66] was designed to measure the client's ability to understand basic, frequently-encountered mechanical principles and laws of physics. This test is useful for gaining information for clients interested in employment in the technical fields including construction, engineering, and all mechanical careers as well as many scientific pursuits.

The Career Ability Placement Survey (CAPS) Spatial Relations Test

The CAPS Spatial Relations Test[66] assesses how well a person can mentally picture and position objects in space in relation to given information. Vocational fields which specifically utilize this skill are careers in engineering, arts, technical and scientific fields, and designing and fabrication of materials.

The Career Ability Placement Survey (CAPS) Verbal Reasoning Test

The CAPS Verbal Reasoning Test[66] is designed to measure the ability to reason logically, given statements, facts, and possible conclusions which may be drawn from the given information. The ability to reason accurately when dealing with verbal relations is an important consideration in vocational trade schools as well as other types of formal education.

The Career Ability Placement Survey (CAPS) Numerical Ability Test

The CAPS Numerical Ability Test[66] measures the client's ability to reason with numbers at the level required in basic dealings and manipulations with quantitative materials. This ability is useful to varying degrees in occupations within the scientific, technical, business, and clerical fields.

The Career Ability Placement Survey (CAPS) Language Usage Test

The CAPS Language usage Test[66] measures the clients ability to utilize the English language from a written and oral communication standpoint. This skill is necessary in many jobs where written and oral communication play an important role such as vocations in the areas of clerical, business, instruction, and most other white-collar and professional occupations.

The Career Ability Placement Survey (CAPS) Word Knowledge Test

The CAPS Word Knowledge Test[66] measures the client's ability to understand the precise meaning of words. This test measures the client's ability to use words in oral and written communication. This aptitude is specifically useful in not only the communication field but also in science, engineering, business, clerical, and most white-collar professions in the service area.

The Career Ability Placement Survey (CAPS) Perceptual Speed and Accuracy Test

The CAPS Perceptual Speed and Accuracy Test[66] measures the client's ability to accurately perceive small details within combinations of numbers, symbols, and letters. This aptitude test is specifically important in determining the client's ability in filing, coding, and data entry work, and all similar occupations which demand a great deal of precision as well as speed.

The Career Ability Placement Survey (CAPS) Manual Speed/Dexterity Test

The CAPS Manual Speed/Dexterity Test[66] is a motor coordination test to determine how well a client can make rapid and accurate movements with his/her hands. This ability is needed in precision and manual work in a technical or arts field as well as in most skilled trades within various occupations.

The Minnesota Multiphasic Personality Inventory (MMPI)

The MMPI[67] was developed as a complex psychological instrument designed to assist in diagnosis of mentally disordered patients into different categories of neurosis and psychosis. It has developed, however, over time, to be used in various settings, including employment agencies, university counseling centers, mental health clinics, schools, and industry. Most important, the MMPI has been expanded to include a person's behavior, thought patterns, attitudes, and strengths, which is extremely useful in assisting any vocational evaluation process.

The Taylor-Johnson Temperament Analysis Test

The Taylor-Johnson Temperament Analysis test[68] was designed to serve as a quick and convenient method of measuring a number of important, comparatively independent personality tendencies or behavioral variables which influence not only vocational adjustment but also personal, social, marital, parental, family, and scholastic traits. One interesting aspect of the Taylor-Johnson Temperament Analysis test is that it has the ability to identify emotionally troubled individuals before the emotional problem becomes acute. The test was not designed to measure serious abnormalities or disturbances but does provide information about adjustment problems which may require immediate improvement.

Another interesting factor of the Taylor-Johnson Temperament Analysis test is that the test allows comparisons in which one person records his or her impression of another person. The Taylor-Johnson Temperament Analysis criss-cross testing is not only valuable for diagnostic purposes and understanding an individual but also helps the individuals involved in the testing to better understand themselves or one another.

The Beck Depression Scale

The Beck Depression Scale[69] measures the client's emotional profile in relation to depression and current adjustment to life difficulties.

The COPE

The COPE[70] is a test designed to evaluate the client's use of defense mechanisms. The COPE attempts to identify normal coping situations which clients may use under stress or duress. Categories include denial, isolation, projection, regression, or turning against self. The COPE is very useful in determining how a client will react to an employment situation dealing with co-workers or supervisors.

The Fundamental Interpersonal Relations Orientation-Behavior (FIRO-B)

The FIRO-B[71] measures three fundamental dimensions of interpersonal relationships: inclusion, control, and affection. *Inclusion* scores assess the degree to which a person associates with others and how a person associates. The *affection* score reflects the degree to which a client becomes emotionally involved with others surrounding him. The *control* score measures the extent to which a client assumes responsibility, makes decisions, or dominates others around him. This test allows comparison of "expressed" vs. "desired" levels of inclusion, control, and affection.

The Wide Range Achievement Test (WRAT)

The WRAT[72] assesses three areas of academic ability. These include spelling, arithmetic, and reading decoding ability. Scores are provided in grade equivalencies.

The KeyMath Test

The KeyMath Test[73] assesses mathematical ability, particularly computational skills and math application skills.

15

Case Management of Brain Injury: An Overview

Jan Wood

CONTENTS

INTRODUCTION

Persons with traumatic brain injury (TBI) present with some of the most challenging constellations of deficits related to injury of any diagnostic group. Injury to the central nervous system impacts the individual so pervasively that most systems are either directly impaired or indirectly impaired because of their interdependence with other impaired systems. As we think more pragmatically and less physiologically, we can see a direct translation of physical systems impairments and the havoc these impairments wreak on the more functional systems of family, work, socialization, etc. Of course, all systems relate to one another and, as such, treatment of a specific system will necessarily impact other systems as well. The rehabilitation of a person with TBI requires a wide variety of professional services and tremendous coordination of effort in order to be appropriately comprehensive.

Since the late 1970's and early 1980's, advances in the field of trauma care and neurosurgery have allowed victims of traumatic brain injuries to survive the initial insult and live longer than ever before. As a result, the needs of people with traumatic brain injury are constantly changing, and the demands placed upon family members and caregivers to locate appropriate resources and treatment continue for the remainder of that individual's life. The availability of resources and treatment is ever-changing and, thus, there has been a growing demand to have one person coordinate these services within the scope of that individual's funding resources.

Funding sources can be public, such as Medicare/Medicaid; private, as in accident and health or workers' compensation; or simply personal funding provided by the individual or family members. In the past, coordination of complicated resources and treatment fell to social workers, nurses, claims adjustors, family members, and caregivers. Today, the case coordinator role is given the title of *case manager*.[1]

CASE MANAGEMENT: ROLES AND RESPONSIBILITIES

Case management is not new to the world of catastrophic disability. The concept surfaced after World War II when people with spinal cord injury began to survive and live productive lives due to advances in medical/rehabilitative care and treatment. There developed a need for intervention on the part of an injured individual for coordination of necessary medical services. The first proponent of this innovative concept, seeing case management as a means of controlling costs while providing the most appropriate services allowable under policies, was the insurance industry.

The field continued to grow and develop until, in 1991, the Case Management Society of America and the Independent Case Management Association along with other national associations developed the first standardized definitions and policies regarding case management. The definitions of *case management*[1] are as follows:

Case Management is a collaborative process that promotes quality care and cost effective outcomes which enhance the physical, psychosocial, and vocational health of individuals. It includes assessing, planning, implementing, coordinating, and evaluating health related service options.

Case management is primarily a process directed at coordinating resources and creating flexible, cost-effective options for catastrophically or chronically ill or injured individuals on a case-by-case basis to facilitate quality, individualized treatment goals. The case manager should facilitate communication and coordination between all members of the health care team involving the patient and family in the decision-making process in order to minimize fragmentation of the health care delivery system. The case manager educates the patient and all members of the health care delivery team about case management, community resources, insurance benefits, cost factors, and issues in all related topics so that informed decisions may be made. The case manager is the link between the individual, the providers, payers, and the community. The case manager should encourage appropriate use of medical facilities and services, improve quality of care, and maintain cost effectiveness on a case-by-case basis. The case manager is an advocate for the patient, as well as the payer, to facilitate a win/win situation for the patient, the health care team, and the payer.

The process of case management should include the following basic elements:

1. Identification of high-risk/high-cost cases
2. Assessment of the patient, the patient's needs, and the treatment goals
3. Development of a treatment plan, in conjunction with the health care team and attending physician, which is responsive to the needs and the goals of the patient
4. Implementation of needed services in a cost-effective and organized manner
5. Ongoing evaluation of the treatment plan in relationship to the desired patient outcome
6. Evaluation of case management interventions to promote quality services and evaluate the effectiveness of case management relative to the desired and/or optimal outcomes

With these definitions in mind, the case manager should positively impact the lives of people with brain injuries, enhancing medical care and the quality of life available to these individuals. Case managers are truly advocates and, if a survivor of brain injury were likened to a wheel, the case manager would be at the hub.

As the hub of this important process, the case manager should have basic knowledge of the following key areas: funding sources, treatment resources, social welfare benefits, vocational rehabilitation services, medicine, and, most important, acceptance of disability and social issues. The case manager should operate with a knowing eye, utilizing current knowledge of available medical and therapeutic technologies, be able to provide authorizations for needed equipment and services to current caregivers, write comprehensive, cohesive reports, and conduct themselves well on the telephone. They need to be able to oversee the dollars and the "sense" of all that is necessary to relieve the effects of the brain injury.

There are two general types of case management services. These are *internal* and *external*. Internal case managers are directly employed by companies who utilize case management services such as insurance companies, hospitals/facilities, and health maintenance organizations, whereas external case managers are contracted to represent an insurance company or a hospital or an attorney. Internal and external case managers differ in their individual roles and how they work throughout the case management process. They do hold in common the combined roles of coordinators and educators/facilitators.

Those case managers who are internal case managers follow procedures that are governed by their employer. Case management services are quality controlled and cost driven, and the case managers are interested in achieving positive outcomes and client independence. Many times they have direct authority to be the decision maker. Other times, they report directly to an in-house supervisor, an adjuster, a claims manager, or a utilization review coordinator.

Within a hospital-based/facility-based internal case management program, the case manager coordinates all the services that are available through that particular facility based on the client needs. In addition, they may become involved in discharge planning. It is possible that an in-house hospital/facility case manager could work directly with an insurance internal or external case manager. This can be an ideal situation in the continuum of care with maximum outcome.

External case managers are contracted for case management services for a specific disability or to do an evaluation and make recommendations for medical treatment and services. The scope of the case management services are dependent upon the agreed contract. If hired by an attorney, the case manager may be asked only to do an evaluation and make recommendations regarding lifetime care and the continuation of rehabilitation. In other situations, an insurance company may contract with the case manager to provide the full range of case management coordination and services. In this instance, the case manager does not have the authority to be the decision maker but would report to someone within the company with their recommendations, and the case manager would receive the authority to provide the recommended services.

Whether a case manager is an internal case manager or an external case manager, it remains the common goal to facilitate maximum independence through the provision of rehabilitation treatment, services, and education. In working with a client with a brain injury, the case manager identifies needs, facilitates communication, recommends appropriate treatment plans, develops and coordinates services, monitors and assesses ongoing progress, and monitors cost of the case.[2] In order to achieve these objectives, it is imperative that the case manager have early involvement in the case. Ideally, the case manager should be in contact with the trauma facility, the physician, and the injured individual within the first 24 to 48 hours following injury. He/she needs to establish early personal contact with the family. This will allow early coordination of claims and rehabilitation issues and development of an early understanding of the individual with the brain injury, the family, and interaction between the two.[2]

The case manager needs to obtain a preinjury history regarding the primary language, educational achievement, and work history of the injured individual. The existence of substance abuse problems should be determined. The family situation should be assessed to determine whether there are small children, teenagers, elderly adults, or extended family issues to be considered. The case manager should also be aware of any family members that have substance abuse problems. The primary spokesperson for the family must be identified. This may be the spouse, a parent, a sibling, or even a friend. There needs to be a discussion of benefits which focuses on what services are available to the injured individual and the family in the way of monetary, medical, and rehabilitative support.

The case manager should make the family aware of medical and rehabilitative facilities, their relative assets and liabilities, and which programs are appropriate for their family member. Transfers should be facilitated, as quickly as possible, to an appropriate medical or rehabilitation center.[3]

Discussion should be held with the patient, if possible, the family, and the carrier regarding all medical and rehabilitation issues. After meeting with the patient, the family, the carrier, the physicians, and the treating staff, outcome goals should be established and discharge planning should be discussed. Ideally, these goals should be agreed upon prior to the commencement of treatment and all parties should be in agreement including the patient, where possible, the carrier, the family, the treating staff and physicians, the case manager, and the attorney.

At the same time, identification of potential sources of conflict must be made. These may include the influence of secondary gain motivators, such as supplemental income, third-party litigation, immigration status, or issues pertaining to family adjustment.

Careful monitoring of the treatment process should be ongoing to track progress toward, and achievement of, treatment goals. This is time-intensive and may require daily contact with the injured individual, the family, and the facility; however, the case manager should never lose sight of the goal of independence and should be aware of the time to reduce involvement and allow independence. Communication is an integral part of this process and, as such, the case manager needs to be able to address the concerns of the patient, the family, the carrier, and the treatment team accurately, diplomatically, and comfortably.

The case manager may become the primary source of resource information for the family. Education should begin early so that the family can gain experience in making educated decisions with regard to continued care and treatment options available to their loved one. Many case managers find that another benefit to educating families as to the intricacies of traumatic brain injury is that families can better assist in observing quality of care.

Lastly, there needs to be careful consideration and integration of vocational rehabilitation possibilities early on in the treatment process to maintain an expectation of return to work and continuation of the work ethic.[4] Information on vocational rehabilitation is presented in Chapter 14 of this volume.

FUNDING SOURCES AND BENEFITS

The case manager must operate within the limitations of the funding sources that are available to the survivor of brain injury.[5] Typically, there are four main funding sources: *public funding, accident and health insurance, workers' compensation,* and *third-party litigation.*

Public Funding

Public funding may consist of Medicare,[6] Medicaid, MediCal, Department of Vocational Rehabilitation, State Victims of Violent Crimes funds, school district funds, or governmental health insurance funds such as those used in the national health care programs of Canada, England, Australia, and many European countries. The case manager needs to be able to quickly identify what can be authorized under these programs since there are varying limitations as to what equipment, services, and other benefits can be provided.

It is always useful to understand the motivations which drive decisions made by personnel of different funding sources regarding authorization, or withholding of same, for treatment. Generally, sources such as state or federally funded ones are less motivated to provide rehabilitation services. Usually, they are mostly interested in whether a service is allowed under existing guidelines as well as whether the provider of those services is registered with, or authorized by, the funding organization. Unfortunately, there is often less interest in the patient's need for services or in whether prescribed services will enhance the quality of life for the patient, reduce the cost of care, or provide long-term reduction in cost of care by reducing level of dependence.

On the other hand, some governmental funding sources may be more interested in what services are required and less with what they will cost. This is the case, particularly, for those patients covered by governmental insurance plans outside the United States. Some governmental plans are beginning to use case management services, however, in an effort to gain a better understanding of resource availability and exercise some control over resource utilization.

The case manager attempting to utilize public funding sources will need to be persistent in pursuit of such funding. It is sometimes useful to encourage families to call upon elected officials to enlist their support in securing funding. Bureaucratic systems require a great deal of time and effort to obtain funding. In some cases, it is helpful to be aware of public law which may mandate provision of services (e.g., Public Law 94-142 pertaining to school district funding) or to be aware of precedent cases which may have been funded for similar services (e.g., Veterans' Administration funding).

Accident and Health Insurance

Most policies have limits as to the amount of money that can be spent over the lifetime of an individual or have time limitations on certain services where, for example, only 60 or 90 days of rehabilitation will be authorized. The more severe limitations are typically seen with HMO plans. There is usually more flexibility available under non-HMO accident and health policies. In any situation, the case manager must determine the most appropriate treatment plan within the scope of the available benefits. It is important that contact be made as quickly as possible, particularly in the situation where there are time limitations involved in benefit availability.[7]

In some instances, it becomes necessary to provide services other than those specifically allowed under the insurance contract to facilitate the best treatment for the patient with brain injury. Successful arguments can frequently be made regarding the advisability of extension of contract coverage for services or facilities which are not usually covered. These arguments are often successful when presented in terms of the cost savings to be realized on an immediate basis by utilization of the alternative or noncovered services or facilities.[2,8] An example of this would be the use of skilled nursing facility patient days to fund participation in a postacute rehabilitation facility.

The case manager should be aware that arrangements such as these are not usually made at the claims level. Many companies utilize internal case managers in order to assist in such determinations and maintain oversight on catastrophic cases for the carrier. Thus, the external or independent case manager may need to request that the carrier's case manager become involved in any decision regarding provision of extracontractual services. The external case manager then acts as a liaison between the accident and health insurer and the injured to facilitate appropriate services.

Once again, the motivation of the carrier will come into play in the decision-making process for provision of services. Generally speaking, the driving force tends to be one of short-term cost containment. This arises from the fact that, often, the accident and health contract has specific time limitations applicable to benefit provision. This varies, however, with whether the injured individual was the employee covered by the policy or a family member of same.

When the injured person is also the employee, contract coverage may be terminated at one year after the last premium is paid by the employer. Of course, COBRA (Consolidated Omnibus Budget Reconciliation Act) protection may extend the coverage period; however, these are expensive and, therefore, prohibitive for many persons, especially when household income drops by the amount of the injured person's paycheck. When the individual with brain injury is a family member of the employee, however, contract coverage will continue unless the employee changes employment or the employer changes accident and health companies. In the circumstance of an injured dependent, the carrier may take a somewhat longer term view of the case with short-term cost containment becoming less crucial.

In any event, the case manager should be prepared to discuss how a recommended treatment plan will provide either more service for the same amount of money, thereby requiring less treatment time overall, or how the treatment plan will provide the same treatment for less money. The case manager should not choose or recommend a facility on the basis of cost but, rather, communicate the benefits of a chosen facility within the framework of this perspective to a potentially reluctant carrier.[9]

Workers' Compensation

Those individuals that have been injured while on the job come under the umbrella of workers' compensation, with a limited number of exceptions (Jones Act for seamen and railroad workers). Workers' compensation is a "no-fault" system which allows for all medical treatment that is reasonable and necessary to cure and relieve the effects of the injury. In cases where the individual is seriously injured, medical treatment may be required over the remainder of that individual's life.

Currently, major issues in the workers' compensation arena focus on medical cost containment, controls over escalating medical costs, the appropriateness of treatment, and determination of whether treatment will improve functional independence. The case manager must have knowledge of these issues in order to select the most appropriate treatment plan and goals for the industrially injured.[10,11] The case manager should also be attuned to differences in workers' compensation benefits and their administration since these benefits vary from state to state.

As is sometimes seen with accident and health coverage, workers' compensation carriers may utilize an internal case management staff. This staff may be separate from, or part of, the claims staff. In any event, it may be necessary for the external case manager to coordinate with a carrier's internal case management staff.

The workers' compensation carrier is generally motivated to reduce the long-term costs associated with care for a catastrophically injured worker by provision of the best medical and rehabilitative services early on in the recovery process. The carrier is usually less interested in short-term cost savings which might be available by choice of less expensive treatment facilities. The workers' compensation carrier is motivated to have a broad and long-term perspective on how cost and quality of care interact on both a short- and long-term basis. The case manager must be in a position to demonstrate how this will be accomplished by any medical or rehabilitative venue which is to be proposed.

Third-Party Litigation

Case management for litigation cases can be quite different from other types of case management. The litigious process often requires that positions concerning both immediate and long-term care needs be taken. As the litigation process can be simplistically viewed as one of negotiation, the parties to this process may adopt views and positions which are seemingly extreme as they move through a process which will culminate in a settlement or judgment with which all parties must live.

The parties to the defense often have a goal of minimizing the financial impact of any case. Some approach the process by expert evaluation and testimony. Others combine evaluation and testimony with attempts to direct the care and rehabilitation of the injured individual. The case manager may be in a position to provide expert testimony and/or case management services pertaining to required treatment or care.

The parties for the plaintiff often have the goal of securing required treatment for the individual. They also attempt to address long-term needs of the individual to ensure that these matters are provided for as best as possible from a financial perspective. The case manager may be used to secure appropriate care and/or treatment for the individual. They may also be asked to participate in expert testimony or life-care planning. It is not within the scope of this chapter to address life-care planning in detail, and the case manager desiring to conduct this type of work should carefully prepare for same.

Since litigation cases may not always have intact funding sources for securing care and treatment, the case manager may need to solicit services for the injured individual on a lien basis. Care should be taken to carefully disclose the nature of the case to the provider, allowing the potential provider of service to discuss the legal issues with the individual's attorney. The merits of the actual legal case may impact the willingness of the treating facility to accept the case on a lien basis. The case manager should be aware that, in cases where less than ideal judgments or settlements are reached, the case manager and/or providers may be approached, after the fact, to discount bills substantially. Thus, these cases carry some financial risks not typical to other types of funding.

The case manager must be vigilant regarding the fact that some cases may have third-party litigation pending though the primary payer source is workers' compensation or accident and health insurance. The presence of pending third-party litigation has been observed, in some cases, to negatively impact the overall direction of ongoing rehabilitation efforts.

In cases where there is no other funding source available, the case manager may be able to utilize public funding sources, either singly or in combination, in order to secure care and/or treatment for the injured individual. Care should be taken to advise all parties that the care and/or treatment is being provided on the basis of what can be paid for, as opposed to what is ideal for the individual, to avoid undesirable liability issues later on.

CONTINUUM OF CARE

With the explosion in growth and development of new brain injury/head trauma programs, the traditional modes of fragmented medical and rehabilitation treatment are no longer appropriate to meet the complex needs of this population.[12] The ideal system flows from onset of the injury/disease and is designed to achieve the maximum recovery and lowest long-term costs. This may include early acute management, treatment in an acute rehabilitation center, and treatment in a postacute rehabilitation center. These may be followed by outpatient or home and community rehabilitation programming and may continue with long-term care, thereby illustrating the continued need for case management services. As a person with a head injury enters this system, his needs tend to evolve with each step in the recovery process. Education of both the injured individual and the family should be ongoing throughout the continuum of care.

The continuum of care begins with admission to the emergency room or trauma center. After possible surgical intervention, the individual may be transferred to the intensive care unit or general medical unit, remaining in an acute hospital setting. Depending upon the severity of the injury, the individual may be transferred to an acute rehabilitation center or begin to receive structured rehabilitative therapies while in the intensive care unit or acute setting. Should the individual remain in a comatose or persistent vegetative state, a coma stimulation program may be initiated in an attempt to improve arousal and level of awareness.

Postacute rehabilitation services, covering both transitional living facilities and community reentry programs, were developed in the late 1970's in direct response to the less-than-desirable discharge options available then following acute rehabilitation. In the majority, these are community-based residential programs and serve to facilitate reentry or reintegration into society at the highest functional level possible for a given individual. As such, they are often an appropriate interim step between the acute rehabilitation hospital and return to home. When necessary, the individual may continue on to a day treatment or outpatient program where ongoing rehabilitation and vocational issues can be further addressed. Behavioral rehabilitation programs exist for those individuals who exhibit severe behavioral problems during recovery that are difficult to control.[13]

When home is not a suitable discharge option, a supervised living program may be considered as a logical next step. These are usually group living situations which often use resources within the community for day activities. In addition, specialized long-term care facilities exist for those individuals who require skilled nursing or constant monitoring, or who, for other reasons including behavior, are not able to return to the homes and communities from which they came.[11,14]

FACILITY ASSESSMENT

The case manager, as can be seen, must certainly have up-to-date information regarding resources that can be utilized for a given individual's continuum of care. This places a great deal of responsibility on the case manager to develop a thorough understanding of available resources. The question which must be carefully and critically posed, then, concerns what to look for in a head injury rehabilitation program.[3,8,9,15] The following outlines a number of areas to which the effective case manager needs to give further attention:

I. Facility experience
   A. How long has the facility been open?
   B. Is it specialized in brain injury?
   C. Does it handle behavioral problems?
   D. What do they consider to be their specialty, i.e., community reentry, vocational rehabilitation, return to work?
II. Personnel qualifications
   A. What are the personnel qualifications?
      1. Does the program employ all professional staff?
   B. Does the program employ or contract with:
      1. A physical therapy staff?
      2. An occupational therapy staff?
      3. A speech-language pathology staff?
      4. An educational therapy staff?
      5. A community staff?
      6. A neuropsychology staff?
      7. A clinical psychology staff?
      8. A vocational rehabilitation counseling staff?
      9. A nursing staff?
      10. A recreational therapy staff?
      11. A social services staff?
   C. Do the above-mentioned staff have professional licensure?
      1. If so, are these licenses available for review?
   D. Is each professional assigned to one facility 100% of the time or do they move around?
   E. Does the licensed professional provide more than half the treatments for his/her discipline or is an assistant used?
   F. Does the program have a medical director?
   G. Does the program regularly obtain medical consultations for patients' health issues?
   H. Does the program regularly obtain medical consultations for patients' program issues?

    I. Does the program have a core of senior staff with more than two to three years of treatment experience?

    J. Has the core of senior staff been employed by this program for longer than two years?

III. Peer review

    A. Is the opinion of the professional community outside the program favorable?

    B. Does the program seek input for programming purposes from the case manager involved?

    C. Is the staff able to answer questions concisely, in layperson's terms, and in a manner which makes sense?

    D. Is senior and treating staff readily available for consultations or to answer questions?

IV. Services provided

    A. Is the program setting consistent with the patient's preinjury lifestyle and/or the anticipated discharge setting?

    B. Is therapy performed in a setting separate from the living environment?

    C. Is the program residential?

        1. If so, is therapy also performed in the residential setting?

    D. Is therapy regularly conducted in community settings?

    E. Is the majority of therapy conducted on a one-on-one, therapist-to-client basis?

    F. Has the facility been operational for at least two years?

    G. Is the program able to prepare the patient for the intended discharge setting?

    H. Are the programs custom-tailored to meet the individual patient's needs?

 V. Patient evaluation criteria

    A. Was the evaluation performed by other than marketing staff?

    B. Did the evaluation include a thorough review of cost, medical records, and medical/rehabilitative care and treatment?

    C. Did the evaluation include a detailed projection of treatment costs?

        1. If not, is this available?

    D. Did the evaluation include an estimate of discharge living status, i.e., independent, nursing home, parent's home, etc.?

    E. Did the evaluation provide a length of time the required program will take to accomplish the goals stated in the evaluation?

    F. Did the evaluation include objective, quantifiable goals for treatment to be evaluated against?

    G. Did the evaluation provide you with more information than you had before the evaluation?

VI. Communication and documentation

    A. What are the reporting requirements of the facility?

    B. Are the reports clear, concise, and easy to read?

    C. Are appropriate goals set?

    D. What is the treater's approach to education of the injured individual and family?

VII. Price structure

    A. Is fee-for-service billing available as a billing option?

    B. Is the program billing easily audited?

    C. Does the program provide complete reports with billing?

    D. Are detailed reports available from all professional staff?

    E. Does the program participate in discounting practices?

    F. Does the program charge for evaluation services?

    G. Does the program charge only a per diem rate?

        1. If there is a per diem rate, how many hours of therapy services are available within the per diem?

WORKING WITH THE TBI PATIENT

Many case managers work not only with catastrophic cases but also with other disabilities which would not be considered catastrophic injuries. Traumatic brain injury, spinal cord injury, and burn patients are generally considered to be catastrophically injured individuals. The traumatically brain-injured patient differs from any other patient in that the involvement of a case manager has the potential for lasting the longest period of time.

The majority of traumatically brain-injured individuals will have long-lasting demonstrable deficits. The process of recovery and rehabilitation is a long-term one. The need for environmental structure and environmental modification cannot be overstated with this population. Of course, the rehabilitation process seeks to reduce the dependence upon environmental modification and structure. However, it is fair to say that various levels of severity of injury, together with varying personalities, will culminate in equally variable needs for environmental modification and structure.

Perhaps one of the most striking differences in case management of the traumatically brain-injured patient has to do with the pervasiveness of deficits. There seems to be no other disability in which functional realms are so diversely impacted. Traumatic brain injury can result in cognitive, emotional, psychological, physical, communicative, social, educational, recreational, perceptual, visual, intellectual, and vocational impairments. The injury frequently brings about changes in family structure.[12]

It is important to realize that, as the case manager interacts with the individual and his/her family, the very nature of observed changes in personality for the injured individual and for roles and responsibilities within the family mandates an interaction with the individual and his family on a highly personal and private level. It is far too easy to misinterpret these changes and to be caught up in them. It is also easy to personalize behaviors of either the injured individual or his family. It is of paramount importance that the case manager be able to be of support to the injured individual and his family, yet, at the same time, maintain a professional distance that will allow maintenance of objectivity in the long term.

The psychological and emotional impact of case management of the traumatically brain-injured patient on the case manager can be considerable. As such, the case manager must frequently evaluate level of personal involvement contrasted to personal detachment in order to efficaciously maintain professional objectivity.

The case manager should ensure that treaters have a full understanding of preinjury dynamics involved in personality, family, social, academic, vocational, and medical matters. There is perhaps no stronger influence on outcome than preinjury characteristics in these areas. There is frequent assumption made about skill sets in one or more of these areas by allied health professionals. Likewise, there is frequent projection of personal morals, values, and cultural norms by allied health professionals to their patients. The case manager should be ever vigilant for these occurrences and should attempt to ensure that the medical and rehabilitative care is directed to the morals, values, and cultural norms of the injured individual and his family. Counseling can be invaluable in the pursuit of a good balance therein.

The case manager needs to be aware of the role of iatrogenesis in the management of the traumatically brain-injured patient. *Iatrogenesis* refers to treatment-induced conditions and, as such, can arise not only from surgical intervention but from pharmacological intervention as well. The case manager should scrutinize all pharmacological and surgical interventions and consider those together with other life events which may be occurring concomitantly in the injured individual's life. It is not uncommon to find that iatrogenic conditions (e.g., medication side effects) are treated inappropriately. Medication side effects may very well be treated by additional medications rather than by titration of medication dosage.

The case manager should realize that there is perhaps no other disability category in which intensity of treatment and dollars expended, especially early on, equate with dollar savings and better outcomes in the long term.[8,16] The case manager should understand that the traumatically brain-injured patient is quite capable of learning, in the vast majority of cases. As a consequence, therapy should be conducted in a fashion which facilitates learning and has, as its basis, the idea that the brain-injured patient can, in fact, learn.

SUMMARY

The case manager carries on a delicate balancing of meeting the needs of the TBI patient and meeting the needs of all other parties involved. It is not uncommon for financial or legal parties, in particular as referral sources, to wield significant pressures for the case manager to utilize specific approaches to the rehabilitation process. The case manager must carefully evaluate the influence of all motivators on decisions of a case. The primary rule of thumb to be followed is that, if the injured individual will gain substantial benefit from a particular treatment, all other parties will benefit. The temptation may be present to lean in the direction of a plaintiff or defense attorney, for example, or in the direction of a parent or spouse. However, the case manager must be able to maintain a neutral high ground which focuses on the needs of the injured individual first, considering the needs and desires of others secondarily.

The goal of the case manager in the brain injury case is to positively impact the individual's life in order to minimize long-term changes in living and occupational status and to improve independence and minimize disability level. All goals should support each other and must be congruent with each other.

The case manager is an integral part of the rehabilitation process and, as such, has a responsibility to enhance the overall process. Good, thorough rehabilitation is a winning scenario for society, the funding source, the family, the case manager, and, most important, the person with traumatic brain injury.

REFERENCES

1. Definition of case management, *The Case Reporter*, 1, 1991, December.
2. Gambosh, M. F., Who's in charge? *Continuing Care*, 28, 1991, July.
3. Durgin, C., Rath, B., and Dales, E., The cost of caring, *Continuing Care*, 28, 1991, November.
4. Meeks, K., Balfour, J., Merritt, R., and Seifker, J. M., Guidelines for supervision of medical case management, *NARPPS J. News*, 6, 251, 1991.
5. Batavia, A. I., Book reviews: The payment of medical rehabilitation services: Current mechanisms and potential models, *J. Rehabil. Adm.*, 14, 90, 1990.
6. France, R. G. and Goodrich, D. F., The medicare prospective payment system: Implications for rehabilitation managers, *J. Rehabil. Adm.*, 12, 33, 1988.
7. Kowlsen, T., The balancing act, *Continuing Care*, 18, 1991, July.
8. Ashley, M. J., Krych, D. K., and Lehr, R. P., Cost/benefit analysis for post-acute rehabilitation of the traumatically brain-injured patient, *J. Insurance Med.*, 22, 156, 1990.
9. McNeill, B. E., A case manager's guide to provider evaluation, *Case Manage. Advisor*, Special Report, 1990.
10. McIntyre, K. J., Marriott medical management: Nurses help cut work comp medical bills, *The Case Manager*, 32, 1991, July-September.
11. Goka, R. S., Case management: A rehabilitation physician's perspective, *J. Insurance Med.*, 23, 1, 1991.
12. Adams, H. R., The silent epidemic — Brain injury, *Calif. Workers' Compensation*, 11, 1992, February.
13. Goldstein, J. K., Neurobehavioral rehabilitation, *Continuing Care*, 11, 1992, March.
14. Winn, J. and Sierra, R., Case management: Cooperation among disciplines, *J. Insurance Med.*, 23, 258, 1991.
15. Arakaki, A. and Goka, R. S., Centers of excellence: Choosing the appropriate rehabilitation center, *J. Insurance Med.*, 23, 66, 1991.
16. Ashley, M. J., Persel, C. S., and Krych, D. K., Changes in reimbursement climate: Relationship among outcome, cost, and payer type in the post-acute rehabilitation environment, *J. Head Trauma Rehabil.*, 8, 1993.
17. Case management: a building block for health care reform, *CMSA*, April, 1993.
18. Case management — a resource that is working...quality care and cost containment, *Natl. Assoc. Advancement Case Manage.*, May, 1993.

INDEX

A